MW00837050

SpringerWienNewYork

Marc Sindou
Editor

Practical Handbook of Neurosurgery

From Leading Neurosurgeons

Volume 1

Cranial Approaches, Vascular, Traumas, Cerebrospinal Fluid, Infections

SpringerWienNewYork

Prof. Dr. Marc Sindou
Department of Neurosurgery, Hôpital Neurologique P. Wertheimer, University of Lyon, Lyon, France

SpringerWienNewYork is part of
Springer Science+Business Media
springer.at

Cover Illustrations: Stefan Kindel
Typesetting: Thomson Press (India) Ltd., Chennai, India
Printing: Strauss GmbH, 69509 Mörlenbach, Germany

Printed on acid-free and chlorine-free bleached paper
SPIN: 12186914

With 184 (partly coloured) Figures

Library of Congress Control Number: 2009927205

ISBN 978-3-211-84819-7 (3 Volumes) SpringerWienNewYork

PREFACE

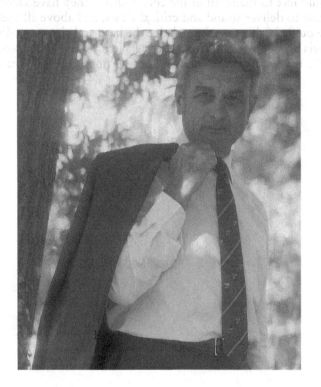

"*Practical Handbook of Neurosurgery*" invites readers to take part in a journey through the vast field of neurosurgery, in the company of internationally renowned experts. At a time when the discipline is experiencing a (detrimental) tendency to segment into various subfields and scatter in the process, it can be worthwhile to collect a number of practical lessons gleaned from experienced and leading neurosurgeons.

The book also aims to present numerous important figures in the neurosurgical community, with a brief overview of the vitae and main contributions for each. We must confess that we were sad that some of the most active members were unable to participate, likely due to time constraints. We are however fortunate that the majority were able to take part. As such, though not exhaustive, the book does represent an anthology of contemporary neurosurgeons.

At the very beginning of the project, our intention was to make a "pocketbook". But month after month it became obvious that the work would be much more expansive; ultimately we produced three volumes. Nevertheless we hope that all the three volumes together will remain easily accessible and a daily companion. The pocket has to be more like a travel bag!

We would like to thank all of the contributors; they have sacrificed their valuable time to deliver sound and critical views, and above all useful guidelines. We would also like to acknowledge the hard and rigorous edition work of Mrs. Silvia Schilgerius at Springer-Verlag Vienna. Finally, we would like to wish you the reader an exciting journey, one we hope you will both enjoy and learn from.

CONTENTS

Volume 1: Cranial Approaches, Vascular, Traumas, Cerebrospinal Fluid, Infections

CRANIAL APPROACHES

MICRONEUROSURGERY: PRINCIPLES, APPLICATIONS, AND TRAINING

M. G. YAŞARGIL

THE IMPACT OF MICROTECHNIQUES ON THE DEVELOPMENT OF NEUROSURGERY

To fully discern and accept the significance of microneurosurgery a clear interpretation and grasp of its components is essential (see Table 1).

The history surrounding the evolution of the operating microscope, microvascular surgical techniques, rediscovery of the cisternal, vascular and parenchymal compartments of the CNS, as well as documentation of the surgical outcome and clinical results in the treatment of saccular aneurysms, various types of cranio-spinal lesions: AVMs, cavernomas, extrinsic and instrinsic tumors, occlusive cerebrovascular diseases, intractrable temporal seizures and spinal disc-herniation, have been presented in numerous publications within the past 50 years [15, 19, 22, 26, 44, 46, 53, 65, 69, 78, 107, 116, 118]. A brief summary of these processes and developments follows.

HISTORY OF MICROSCOPES AND OPERATING MICROSCOPES

The history of microscopes has been presented in many previous publications (34, 74, 99, 119, 149). Ernst Abbe, physicist, mathematician and astronomer at the Friedrich Schiller University Jena, Germany, was able to perfect the development of the microscope while working with his friends, Carl Zeiss, founder of the company of the same name, and Otto Schott, a chemist and founder of the famous glass company of the same name, which produced high quality glass for lenses. During the 1870s, while experimenting with water emission objective lenses, Abbe devised the equation of "angular aperture". This accomplishment brought Zeiss to the forefront of microscope technology. By the 1880s, using oil immersion objective lenses, a numerical aperture of 11.4 was finally reached, allowing light microscopes to resolve two points only 0.2 μm apart. With the exception of some very unusual immersion fluids or ultraviolet light, the above remains the limit today [1]. The electron microscope (1932) and scanning tunneling technology (1981) finally revealed the nanometric dimensions of intra- and intercellular structures.

Keywords: microneurosurgery, surgical techniques

Table 1. Microsurgical axioms summarizing personal experience

1. Microneurosurgery encompasses a cogent, cohensive concept comprising noninvasive approaches along the natural pathways of the cisternal systems, to reach the lesions of the central nervous system and to completely and skillfully eliminate them, the goal being to achieve, a "pure lesionectomy".
2. Microneurosurgery requires intensive, long-term training of one to two years (or preferably, longer) in the cadaver- and/or animal-laboratory, mastering the details of specific surgical neuroanatomy, acquiring proficiency using bipolar coagulation and the high-speed drill, learning the microtechniques of dissection and repair of extra- and intracranial vessels and nerves, as well as dura, arachnoidea, and pia, and practicing the art of surgical approaches and techniques, the ultimate goal being to optimize the reciprocal balance between the "mental eye", vestibulo-visual system, and manual dexterity of the surgeon.
3. Microtechniques present a significant and unequivocal advance in neurosurgery.
4. Microneurosurgery is superior to all other contending specialties in neurotherapy. It offers to patients a proven and more effective therapy, and shields them from academic discussion.

Table 2. Development of optical instruments for surgery from a personal view

Magnifying loupe		Operating microscope	
1823	Binocular opera glass	1921	Brinel-Leitz Monocular
1876	Saemisch	1921	Nylen-Person Monocular
c. 1880	E. Abbe/Zeiss	1922	Holmgren-Zeiss/Jena Binocular
1886	Westien and Schulze	1925	Hinselmann-Zeiss/Jena Binocular, colposcope
1886	Westien and von Zehender	1938	Tullio-Zeiss/Jena Binocular, floorstand
1899	Axenfeld	1953	OPMI 1 Binocular, floorstand
1910	Telescopic binocular loupe/Zeiss		Littman (Zeiss/Oberkochen): (later ceiling mounted changeable magnification) stereoscopic vision in sharp focus through narrow surgical corridors; coaxial light; beam-splitter: observer tube, cameras
1911	von Hess		
1913	von Rohr and Stock		
1948	Riechert		
1951	Guiot	1960	Littmann (Zeiss/Oberkochen) Binocular diploscope
1965	Drake	1972	Heller-Schattmaier-Yaşargil Binocular, floorstand (Contraves): counterbalanced stand; floating movements; mouth switch to release the brake system; electrical eyepiece warmer
		1992	Hensler-Yaşargil (modified Zeiss Contraves floorstand stand attached to an OPMI F1, Zeiss microscope optic)

Good illumination, stereoscopic vision, magnification changer, and good mobility of the stand are valuable requisites of an operating microscope for the neurosurgeon. Various types of magnifying spectacles were introduced by otologists, ophthalmologists and neurosurgeons (see Table 2) [67, 70]. All these spectacles permit free movement of the head but they fail to provide stereoscopic vision in the depths of a narrow neurosurgical approach. Furthermore, adequate illumination in the depths of a neurosurgical field is lacking.

A monocular monoscope was applied to surgery in 1921 by otologist Carl Olof Nylen in Stockholm, Sweden. Together with his teacher Holmgren he envisioned and pioneered micro oto-surgery and published the developmental process in his 1954 paper [59]. The monocular microscope had to be fixed to the patients' head. In 1922, Gunnar Holmgren used a binocular microscope, attached to the operating table. Another pioneer of otologic surgery, George Shambaugh Jr. was the first to use the microscope routinely for the one stage Lempert fenestration operation, beginning as early as 1939 [81].

L.H. Wullstein, another pioneer of otosclerosis surgery, arranged the construction of an easily movable microscope consisting of a 10× Leitz magnifier mounted on the stand swivelarm of a dental engine. Using this particular microscope, Wullstein carried out more than 1000 operations from 1949 to 1953. Perritt [63], Harms [28], Barraquer [8] pioneered microtechniques for operations on the eye [8, 28, 63, 104].

Under the guidance of H.L. Littmann, Zeiss engineers finally succeeded to construct a versatile binocular operating microscope, OPMI-1, which was introduced in 1953 [48]. This achievement was welcomed by otologists, ophthalmologists, vascular, plastic, reconstructive surgeons and neurosurgeons.

1. FLOATING OPERATING MICROSCOPE [116]

After extensive research, a completely balanced floating microscope with adjustable counterweights mounted on the microscope stand was developed at the Department of Neurosurgery, University Hospital Zurich, Switzerland with the assistance of Contraves Company. This ingenious and sophisticated system allows the operating microscope to be easily and quickly brought into any desired position during neurosurgical procedures. The addition of a mouth switch permits horizontal and vertical movements, thus the surgeon can move the microscope around the operating field, and remains well in focus then continues the flow of the procedure. The prime aim of the neurosurgeon is to concentrate on dissection and elimination of the lesion and not to battle with the microscope (Fig. 1).

2. ACCESSORIES TO THE MICROSCOPE [54, 116]

For assisting and education purposes co-observation equipment, such as a binocular tube and closed circuit television, can be attached to a beam splitter

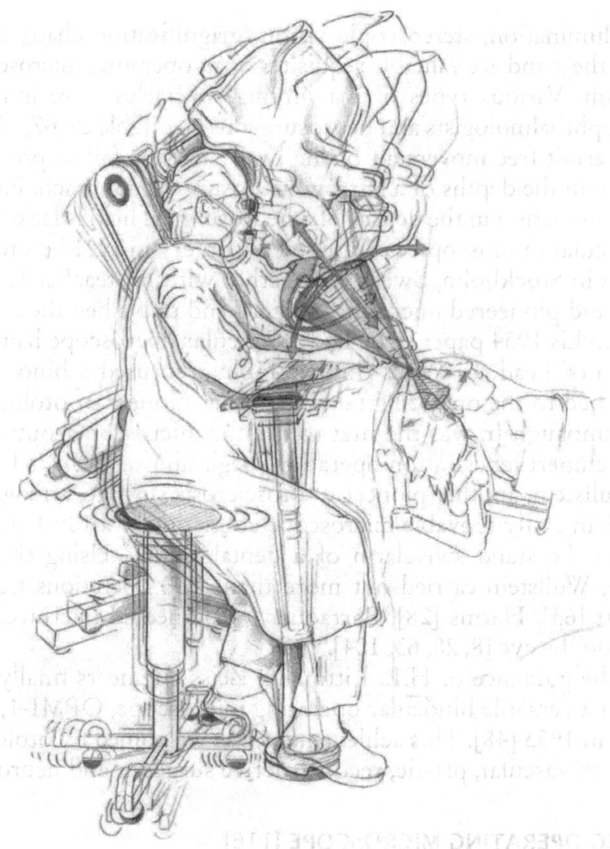

Fig. 1. Artist's impression of the combined range of mobility between the hydraulic chair, arm rest, and microscope, with mouth switch, for the seated surgeon. These can all be adjusted in unison. Taken from [88]; illustration by P. Roth

between microscope body and binocular tube. An operation can be recorded and still camera photographs taken for documentation. Recordings and photographs are instructive supplements for teaching purposes. Prior to a re-operation (for recurrent tumor for instance), it is of great value to have the opportunity to study the previous recorded surgical procedure.

3. APPLICATION OF MICROTECHNIQUES TO CLINICAL NEUROSURGERY

W. House was a pioneer of microtechniques in his exploration of the internal auditory canal and removal of acoustic neurinomas (1961). His success stimulated and challenged neurosurgeons [29, 30]. Kurze and Doyle [45], Jacobson et al. [32], Kurze [44], Rand and Kurze [66], Lougheed and Tom [50], Pool and Colton [64], Jannetta and Rand [35], all reported on the application of the microscope in neurosurgery. The operating microscope proved to be of particular value for operations on avascular or poorly vascularized organs such as the middle ear, and on the cornea and the lens of the eye. However, the availability of the microscope for surgery on the brain, a complex and highly vascular organ, provided the means and the stimulus to develop new approaches and atraumatic techniques to ensure preservation of normal vital structures and vessels.

The cerebral vascular procedure of thrombectomy for an occluded MCA has been performed without an operating microscope by Driesen, Scheibert, Schillito, Welch, Chou (see [115]), and the procedure of bypass graft of a saphenous vein between the extra- and intracranial carotid arteries has been performed by Woringer and Kunlin [103]. Technically, all procedures were successfully accomplished, but surgical outcomes were not satisfactory.

In 1960, Jacobson and Suarez, using an OPMI operating microscope (Zeiss), achieved convincing progress in suturing of the common carotid artery in mongrel dogs, with good surgical results [31]. Six years later in the same laboratory at the University of Vermont, Burlington, microvascular techniques were developed that could be applied to brain arteries embedded within their cisternal-arachnoidal network [20]. The first successful anastomosis between the superficial temporal artery and anterior temporal cortical artery was performed on a mongrel dog on March 30, 1966. During the ensuing 7 months, 34 bypass procedures on dogs were successful and remained patent [20]. These new and evolving surgical techniques led to the design of appropriate instrumentation, and especially of microsuture material. Bipolar coagulation technology allowed coagulation of fine caliber vessels, and therefore precise hemostasis was assured. Surgical tactics, the planning of a procedure, the concepts of operating were influenced by all these developments, and evolved accordingly.

MICROSURGICAL INSTRUMENTS [112, 116 VOL. IV B, 119]

1. BIPOLAR COAGULATION-TECHNOLOGY

In 1940, Greenwood introduced the use of two point coagulation to neurosurgery [23]. This concept was later perfected by Malis and is known as bipolar coagulation, which causes no current spread or radiation of heat to surrounding tissue [55]. Bipolar coagulation is crucial to accomplishing successful neurosurgery, and has been instrumental in promoting new concepts. Without bipolar coagulation the microsurgical approaches, tactics and concepts we currently apply, would be impossible [20, 114, 115, 118]. Less familiar are the bipolar coagulation ball electrodes, also developed by Malis. These can be used effectively to shrink vascular lesions such as hemangioblastomas, meningiomas, and cavernomas by very gently stroking the surface of these tumors with the ball, at a bipolar setting appropriate to the size, vascularization and location of the lesion [25–60]. Cold water irrigation during and following coagulation is recommended [53, 55].

The size, shape, weight, balance and spring of the bipolar coagulation forceps are important features of their design. Bayonet shaped bipolar forceps are available in many different lengths from 2 cm to 13.5 cm working length (2 cm and 3.5 cm for surface work, and longer forceps as dissection progresses deeper). A bayonet shape avoids the surgeon's hand blocking the field of vision. A moderate degree of spring aids in tissue dissection with the forceps. All forceps are insulated to prevent short circuit of current into tissue that may come into contact with the shaft of the forceps. The tips of bipolar forceps are available in various widths, 0.4 mm, 0.7 mm, 1 mm, and 1.3 mm. When applying coagulation, the vessel should not be tightly squeezed between the tips. When coagulating a larger diameter vessel, using brief bursts of current, along a short length of the vessel at a power of 15–25 Malis units is recommended. This usually prevents the tips from "sticking". Bipolar forceps are in constant use for dissection, and coagulation, therefore it is advisable to prepare

Table 3. Instrument innovations in microneurosurgery

Counter balanced operating microscope stand can be attached to a binocular microscope, diploscope, triploscope, 2-D or 3-D videoscope monitor
Bipolar coagulation
Electrically powered perforator and craniotome and drill bits
Double-pronged spring hook for scalp and muscle flap
Flexible dura dissector
Self-retaining brain protection with malleable spatula
Ultrasound suction apparatus
Ultrasound detector
Brain and nerve stimulator, and monitoring
Microinstruments

- Spring loaded bayonet bipolar coagulation forceps in seven different lengths (20–135 mm working length) and four different tip sizes (0.4–1.3 mm)
- Ring tipped tumor or aneurysm grasping forceps with and without teeth
- Bayonet-shaped scissors in four different lengths (50–135 mm working length) with straight and curved blunt tips
- Biopsy rongeurs in two different lengths and six different jaw sizes
- Micro-Rongeur with malleable shaft
- Tumor-grasping forks in four different tip sizes and forked forceps
- Suction tips: four lengths (50–150 mm) and five diameters (1.5–4.5 mm)
- Regulator for suction pressure
- Dissectors: 20 various shapes and sizes
- Clips: 180 aneurysm clips, various shapes and sizes, hemoclips, temporary clips, microclips
- Microsuture
- Mobile tip mirror (5.0–7.0 mm), endoscopes

High quality cotton pledgets
Hydraulic surgeon's stool
Hydraulic arm support
Hydraulic instrument table for scrub nurse
Neuronavigation (not used by the author)

a whole series for each surgery. Forceps can then be cleaned frequently, and the tips cooled in a solution, which helps to prevent their "sticking".

Basic microneurosurgical instruments are summarized in Table 3.

2. SUCTION SYSTEM

A suction pump with a pressure-regulating mechanism can be adjusted according to the intraoperative situation, for instance high for tumor suction and for hemorrhage, low when opening the sylvian fissure, and when dissecting vessels and aneurysms and nerves. A round, smooth, atraumatic surface of the suction tip prevents injury to the brain and vasculature. Suction tubes are available in various lengths and diameters, which can be interchanged depending on the depth of the surgical field, the nature of the dissection and consistency of the tissue and the fluids to be eliminated. Equally important, the suction tube functions as a retractor at low pressure, drawing tissue, tumor, a vessel, or a nerve to one side during dissection. On many occasions this dispenses with the need to apply the self retaining brain retractor. Coordinated with the bipolar forceps, the suction tube can act as a blunt dissector [116].

For the debulking or enucleation of tumors the suction apparatus is very effective for soft tumors. Tough, hard tumors can be excised with a knife, scissors, or bipolar cutting loop. The ultrasonic aspirator (CUSA) system supplies continuous irrigation and suction to aspirate emulsified tissue 1–2 mm from the tip, and is most efficient for all types of tumors.

Frequent irrigation of the operative field with fluid at 37°C minimizes tissue adhesion to instruments, removes blood and tissue debris, and maintains a clear operative field. Irrigation delivery systems have been developed, to attach to the various instruments (suction tube, bipolar forceps). A presoaked sponge affords a form of continuous irrigation.

3. PROTECTIVE RETRACTION DEVICES [116, VOL. IV B]

Ideally, retraction devices should not compress the brain, but provide a shield of protection. As discussed previously, the suction tube can be used to retract tissue: the area of the suction tube is narrow and the period of retraction is brief, due to the fact that dissection is continuously moving around the lesion, therefore the risk of damage to normal tissue is reduced. A cotton ball saturated with fluid constitutes a simple, non-injurious retractor, positioned, for instance, between tumor capsule and normal tissue. During dissection of the Sylvian fissure, interhemispheric fissure, cerebral sulci, cerebellopontine cistern for example, moistened cotton balls are placed, one at each end of the fissure, sulcus, etc., in increasing sizes, as dissection progresses, maintaining a delicate retraction. Sponges with strings attached have many applications: (1) protection of normal, exposed tissue, (2) retraction, (3) absorb fluids (CSF or blood), (4) fluid can be gently aspirated without damage to tissue beneath the sponge (when opening the dura, a sponge can be placed over the brain and suction applied to absorb CSF), (5) when profuse bleeding occurs, the same method of sponge beneath suction tube can be applied, (6) dissection (a sponge held in the bipolar forceps, and using stroking motions, tumor is coaxed from a vessel wall), (7) once the tumor has been debulked, 2 or 3 sponges are placed inside the tumor sac to give it substance, during dissection of the sac from surrounding tissue. The sac is thus easier to grasp and manipulate, (8) a sponge can be positioned to temporarily displace tumor or normal tissue a little, during dissection, (9) to press and spread bone wax over bony hemorrhage, (10) placed over hemostatic agent (surgical, gelfoam) to firm the position.

4. VESSEL AND ANEURYSM CLIPS [116, VOL. I]

Temporary vascular clips differ from permanent aneurysm clips. They have a lower closing pressure to prevent damage to the vessel wall and endothelial lining. Temporary clips are golden in color to distinguish them from permanent clips, as they should not be implanted to permanently occlude an aneurysm or vessel. A selection of temporary clips with their appliers are available on the field, at every surgical procedure in preparation for any unanticipated hemorrhage that may occur. Should the wall of a small arterial vessel be injured, 2 small golden clips can be applied, one distal and one proximal to the injury. The previous oozing of blood can be cleaned by suction placed over a sponge for protection of the vessel. The injured wall is then clearly visible, can be closed by bipolar coagulation at Malis setting 15 or 20, and the clips removed. If the injury is on the posterior surface, the vessel can be rotated to reveal the hole by placing a flat sponge over the vessel and using the suction tube at low pressure to rotate.

Aneurysm clips are available in many sizes and in a variety of curved and angled shapes, to accommodate the diverse anatomic configurations and sometimes uncommon situations presented in patients. Unnecessary, repetitive opening of the aneurysm clips' blades is to be avoided as this reduces the

Table 4. Microneurosurgical concepts

1. Rediscovery of cisternal anatomy, which allows exploration of all the lesions of the CNS through subarachnoid pathways: "cisternal navigation"
2. Recognition of the compartmental anatomy of the CNS and the related predilection sites of the lesions (neoplastic, vascular, infectious, toxic, degenerative,c ongenital)
3. Complete elimination of the lesion: "pure lesionectomy"
4. Meticulous hemostasis (bipolar coagulation technology)
5. Exploration without rigid brain retraction but applying protective dynamic retraction
6. Reconstruction and repair of central and peripheral nerves
7. Reconstruction and repair of extra- and intracranial arteries and veins, pia and arachnoidea
8. Creation of specific transosseous windows to the skull

closing pressure. The technique of stepwise obliteration of an aneurysm is described in detail in ref. 116, vol. I (see Table 6).

5. NEURO-NAVIGATION

With the emergence of high-quality intraoperative imaging using computed tomography and/or magnetic resonance imaging, the first integrated microscope navigation systems were developed which can be used effectively in cases of skull base tumors. The concept of microscope-based neuronavigation consists of superimposing the localization and extension of a lesion on to the microscope field of view through contours. The integration of preoperative functional data from magnetoencephalography and functional MRI, resulting in so-called "functional neuronavigation" can lead the way towards future improvements in the field of microneurosurgery. Other advances of note such as the use of tumor fluorescence, using 5-aminolevulinic acid or autofluorescence, show promising results [88]. Brain shift and spatial resolution of the implemented techniques should not be underestimated, and therefore applying this technology may give a false sense of surgical security and confidence. Personally I prefer to use the ultrasound detector to check for residual tumor.

The most relevant and reliable method for evaluating the location of a lesion and devising a surgical strategy, remains the thoroughly trained, multidimensional "mental eye" of the surgeon, which has acquired proficiency related to laboratory training and clinical knowledge and experience, combined with the accomplished evaluation of visualization technology. This is currently the most reliable guide and qualified method to determine a diagnosis and define a concept of treatment and design a surgical strategy.

6. MICRONEUROSURGICAL CONCEPTS

To master the techniques of microneurosurgery, it is necessary to become familiar with the detailed surgical and radiological anatomy of the cisternal, vascular and parenchymal systems, the course and variation of arteries and veins, and the distinct architecture of gyral segments and connective fibers in neopallial, archi-, paleopallial, and central areas of white matter, lentiform nucleus and brain stem [96, 97, 116, 120]. Altogether there are at least 50 compartments in each cerebral hemisphere, 8 compartments in each of the cerebellar hemispheres and 9 compartments of spinal cord, which provide natural pathways to approach the lesions, to achieve accurate exploration and dissection of adjacent vasculature, and to preserve the hemodynamics and homeostasis of the brain.

7. CISTERNAL ANATOMY REVIVED

Key and Retzius [38], by injecting the subarachnoid space with blue dye, were able to demonstrate the cisternal anatomy of the brain, and confirmed that the cisterns intercommunicate and are compartmentalized. They showed the relationship of the cerebral vessels to the arachnoid and to the numerous trabeculae which suspend these vessels from the walls of the cisterns. Their findings remain valid today, although appreciation of the importance of cisternal anatomy for neurosurgery had to await the introduction of the operating microscope. Performing procedures under the operating microscope has contributed to progress in understanding anatomy, and has defined the importance of precise dissection of the subarachnoid cisterns in the exposure of cerebral aneurysms, arteriovenous malformations, and extrinsic and intrinsic tumors.

The traditional definition of the subarachnoid space as consisting of a freely communicating channel for the flow of CSF is an inadequate explanation, and fails to correspond to the findings at operation under the microscope. The arachnoid partitions the subarachnoid space into relatively discrete chambers, possibly retarding and directing the flow of CSF. These barriers to CSF are seen in numerous locations, providing a rationale for naming them as individual subarachnoid cisterns (Figs. 2 and 3). Microneurosurgical procedures presented us with the opportunity to revise our knowledge of compartmentalization of the subarachnoid cisterns, because we are able to view them

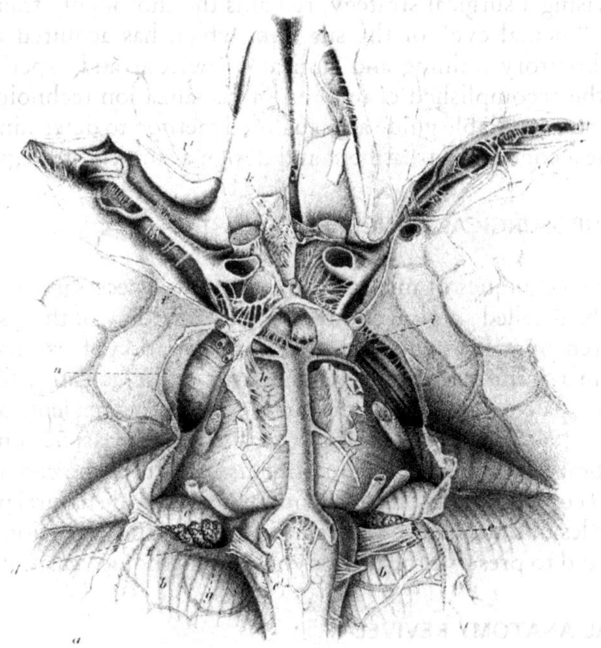

Fig. 2. Original figure from Ref. [38], showing a dissection of the basal cisternal compartments (olfactory, chiasmatic, Sylvian, carotid, interpeduncular, crural, prepontine, cerebellopontine, and anterior spinal cisterns)

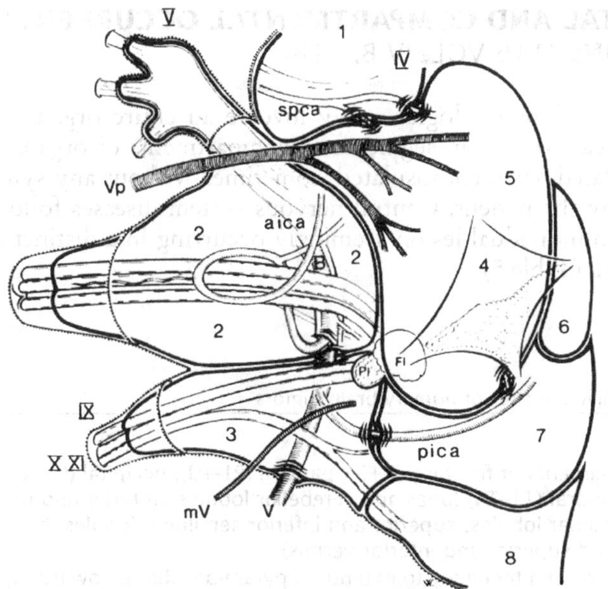

Fig. 3. Artist's impression of the left-sided infratentorial cisterns with the structures they encase (*1* junction between cisterna ambiens and quadrigemina, *2* cerebellopontine cistern, *3* lateral cerebellomedullary cistern, *4* 4th ventricle, *5* superior cerebellar cistern, *6* superior vermian cistern, *7* cisterna magna, and *8* cervical subarachnoid space). Taken from [88]; illustration by P. Roth

in their natural physiological state, fully distended with CSF. Knowledge of the cisternal anatomy allows precise exploration of intra- and extra-axial intracranial lesions along the "cisternal pathways". The lesion can be circumferentially dissected, observing cisternal anatomy, and the parent arteries and main draining veins can be secured, thereby achieving control of cerebral hemodynamics.

In chapter 1 of "Microneurosurgery, volume I" cisternal anatomy and compartmentalization is reviewed in detail [60, 116]. A concept of the subarachnoid space is presented that attempts to describe the actual observations at operation as accurately as possible. In current neurosurgical nomenclature, these terms are commonly used, and continue to be relevant when describing dissection and exposure of intracranial and arachnoidal lesions and their accompanying cranial nerves and vasculature. The predilection sites of vascular, neoplastic, malformative, and degenerative lesions in these compartments can be defined precisely. Further advances in radiological imaging, and developmental and functional anatomy will give more detailed insight into the cisternal anatomy and physiology of arachnoid fibers and trabeculae [124].

SEGMENTAL AND COMPARTMENTAL OCCURRENCE OF LESIONS [116 VOL. IV B, 118]

Diseases of various etiologies rarely involve an entire organ or the entire body. A disease occurs in segments or compartments of organs, sometimes entirely isolated, even encapsulated, sometimes without any symptoms and unnoticed by the patient. Central nervous system diseases follow a regular pattern, each individual lesion seemingly occurring in a distinct segment or compartment (Table 5).

Table 5. Predilection sites of primary brain tumors

1. Neopallial
   a. Gyral segments of frontal (F1–F3), parietal (P1–P3), occipital (O1–O3), and temporal (T1–T4) lobes and cerebellar lobules (anterior and posterior quadrangular lobules, superior and inferior semilunar lobules, biventral lobule, tonsil, and superior and inferior vermis)
   b. Gliomas have a tendency to extend, in pyramidal shape, toward the ventricle
   c. Gliomas of neopallial, archi- and paleopallial, intraventricular, white matter, basal ganglia and central nuclei remain in their compartments; however, in high grade gliomas after radiotherapy and incomplete surgical removal, they may disseminate
2. Archi- and paleopallial (limbic, paralimbic)
   a. Mesiobasal temporal (temporal pole, amygdala-hippo- and parahippocampus)
   b. Insular (anterior, posterior, entire)
   c. Cingulate gyrus (anterior, middle, posterior)
   d. Posterior frontoorbital gyri and septal region
   e. Combined a–d
3. Midline
   a. Only caudate head (rare), never body or tail of caudate nucleus
   b. Lentiform nucleus (extremely rare)
   c. Corpus callosum (anterior, middle, posterior part)
   d. Pre- and retrolentiform region of the white matter
   e. Diencephalon (hypothalamus infero-anterior or supero-posterior; thalamus anterior or posterior [pulvinar]); only malignant gliomas in late phase transgress the borderline between hypothalamus and thalamus
   f. Mesencephalon (dorsal, ventral, lateral, central)
   g. Pons-medulla oblongata (dorsal, ventral, central)
4. Intraventricular
   a. Lateral ventricles (anterior horn, cella media, or atrium)
   b. Third ventricle
   c. Aquaduct
   d. Fourth ventricle
5. Cervical, thoracic, and lumbar spinal cord (dorsal, lateral, central)

The occurrence of extrinsic cranio-spinal tumors (meningiomas, neurinomas, craniopharyngiomas, adenomas, chordomas, chondrosarcomas and epidermoids) in specific cisternal compartments had already been clearly understood by the founding generation of neurosurgeons. The predilection sites of brain lesions such as AVMs, cavernomas, and the various types of intrinsic tumors can now be demonstrated with modern neurovisualization technology, coordinating three planar or three dimensional studies with all modalities. Despite these advances, the topographic description of intrinsic lesions of the brain continues to be the traditional terminology related to the "lobar" concept. This is by no means wrong, but imparts insufficient data and fails to define comprehensively the accurate location of a lesion in a particular parenchymal compartment(s) of the CNS. Intrinsic lesions occur in compartments of the neopallial, archi-pallial and paleo-pallial (limbic-paralimbic) systems, in the basal ganglia, in compartments of the white matter of the dien-, and mesen-, metencephalon, in the cerebellum, spinal cord and in the 4 compartments of the ventricular system [116 IV B, 120, 121, 122].

The generally accepted concept that gliomas grow in an infiltrative manner is not a convincing hypothesis. Glial tumors compress and displace but do not infiltrate into or follow connective fibers, and they do not transgress connective fibers until a very late phase of grade IV tumors. This segmental/compartmental concept has been reinforced by recent studies with diffusion tensor imaging and 3 planar MRI. Gliomas within neopallial, archi- and paleopallial, white matter, basal ganglion, diencephalon, brainstem and intraventricular compartments usually exhibit a sharp borderline to neighboring compartments. Nevertheless, as the limbic system encircles the brainstem and the telencephalon, topographically the appearance of limbic gliomas on MRI can be fairly confusing, because they may simulate a multi-lobar tumor, particularly in cases in which the gliomas involve the mesiotemporal, posterior frontoorbital, septal and insular compartments of the limbic system all at once. This segmental and compartmental occurrence of diseases, with different vascularization patterns of each compartment, creates for the surgeon and radiation-therapist the opportunity to offer a favorable form of therapy and pursue an efficient treatment regime to a successful and beneficial conclusion. Recurrence of low-grade gliomas always occurs in the same location even after decades. In approximately 95% of high-grade gliomas recurrence occurs in the same place; in 1–2%, dissemination is observed, and in about 2–3%, the recurrence is multicentric.

1. CRANIOTOMIES

Each craniotomy requires thorough studies of the architecture of the bone in the intended surgical region (CT) and the course and variation of arteries and veins and venous sinuses (CTA, MRA, MRV). The optimal size of craniotomy is chosen to improve the operating field of vision, minimize brain retraction, and provide multiple surgical angles for dissection. Various approaches have been devised and described [3–5, 9, 16, 25, 27, 33, 36, 37, 62, 71, 72, 78, 80, 89, 94, 116, 120–122]. Sustained application of endeavors resulted in mastering of combined approaches, for instance, transsphenoidal-transSylvian, transSylvian-transcallosal, and supracerebellar-transtentorial explorations in one session. The use of the power drill is indispensable for precise achievement of these approaches. Perfection of drilling-skills and learning the complex anatomy of the skull base and the arachnoid space in the laboratory is strongly recommended.

2. THE CAVERNOUS SINUS

The final hurdle in skull base surgery has finally been surmounted. Due to the vital structures passing through, the internal carotid artery, the cranial nerve of oculomotion, and the trigeminal nerve, the cavernous sinus has long been approached with the appropriate respect, and was not entered surgically because continued oozing of venous blood obstructed the surgical view. In the 1980s Vinko Dolenc was the first to enter the cavernous sinus for the purpose of treating internal carotid artery aneurysms and carotid cavernous fistulas, controlling venous bleeding with Surgicel and compression [17, 18]. His technique has been refined (in part with the advent of fibrin glue) and, for those who have trained long and extensively, the cavernous sinus is on the verge of being tamed [40]. The combined pterional pretemporal transcavernous approach achieves a wide exposure and is currently employed to treat saccular aneurysms in the cavernous sinus and at the level of the upper third of the basilar artery, including the basilar tip [41–43]. The treatment of cavernous tumors (meningiomas, chordomas) has become possible and total resection is possible, in cases without severe adhesions.

3. CISTERNAL APPROACHES

Due to the limited space of this chapter a detailed presentation of the cisternal approaches cannot be given. The exploration and elimination of the various intracranial and intraspinal, extrinsic and intrinsic lesions has been described in extenso in former publications [108, 111, 116 vol. I, III B, IV B, 111, 120, 122].

4. CEREBROVASCULAR MICROSURGERY

Alexis Carrel pioneered the basic vascular surgical techniques in the animal laboratory (1902–1940) [10, 75]. In 1953 Michael E. DeBakey began routine clinical application of vascular surgery. Concomitant advances in the diagnosis of arterial disease with improved angiography, followed by Duplex ultrasonography, CTA, MRA, and the availability of anticoagulants, contributed to improvements [49]. The application of extracranial vascular surgical techniques to intracranial arteries necessitated the recognition of the distinct relationship of the cerebral vasculature to the cisterns and the necessity of maintaining a constantly bloodless surgical field. This became possible with the combined application of the operating microscope, bipolar coagulation, microinstruments and microsutures, later complemented by ultrasound flowmetry and fluoroscopy. Microneurosurgical techniques ultimately permitted preservation of arteries and veins down to 0.5 mm in size by meticulous dissection, repair and reconstruction within the cisternal-arachnoidal system. Exploration and elimination of saccular aneurysms, AVMs, cavernomas, hemangioblastomas also became possible [9, 18, 24, 43, 52, 92, 93].

Surgical concepts, techniques, tactics and results have been published in six volumes of "Microneurosurgery" [116]. In Table 6, surgical concepts are summarized.

Although impressive improvement of endovascular techniques has been documented, current neurosurgery needs to develop confidence and dexterity

Table 6. Microsurgery of intracranial saccular aneurysms, AVMs and cavernomas

Aneurysms (see Microneurosurgery, vols. I and II)

Transcisternal exploration of the proximal and distal segments of the parent artery(ies)

Recognition of the geometry and wall-condition of the aneurysms

Control of hemodynamics in parent arteries using proximal and distal temporary clips (maximum 3 minutes)

Taming, shaping, shrinkage, deflation and neck creation of dysmorphic saccular aneurysms using bipolar coagulation techniques, temporary and pilot clips (see Figure 208A-B in Microneurosurgery, vol. I, pp 253-254)

Complete elimination of aneurysm, particularly the inferiorly bulging parts and, if necessary, graft/bypass in case of large or giant aneurysms.

Arteriovenous malformations (see Microneurosurgery, vol. IIIA, B)

Perilesional helical exploration, identification and elimination of the feeding arteries

Temporary microclips of the small periventricular perforating arteries, bipolar coagulation

Consideration of specific hemodynamics in a given case related to the venous drainage, particularly the condition of the straight sinus (stenosis or occlusion)

Creation of new venous drainage

Cavernomas

The introduction of MRI technology markedly facilitated the diagnosis of cavernomas in CNS. Symptomatic cavernomas causing hemorrhages or seizures or neurologic and mental deficits should always be operated. Applying microtechniques they can be precisely explored and removed, saving adjacent venous anomalies (see Microneurosurgery, vols. IIIB and IVB).

in cerebrovascular microsurgery and advance techniques, because ultimately, surgical therapy provides the most definitive solution to cerebrovascular lesions.

5. REVASCULARIZATION OF THE BRAIN

Reconstructive surgery of extracranial brain arteries has become, in the second half of the 20th century, a routine procedure involving vascular surgeons, neurosurgeons and interventional radiologists who aimed to create new ideas to attain the best and most effective treatment.

Extra-intracranial bypass and intracranial bypass procedures have been well established since 1967, and are an integral part of neurosurgery in the treatment of giant aneurysms, skull base tumors and reconstruction of the venous sinuses [6, 11, 12, 21, 24, 61, 68, 73, 77, 79, 84, 86, 91, 92, 102, 115]. In cerebrovascular occlusive disease, indications for EC–IC bypass requires careful evaluation and assessment [7]. However, a certain group of patients with compromized hemodynamics due to an insufficient collateral system, can be relieved from their burden of cerebrovascular ischemic events by this procedure.

The advent of quantitative MRI angiography as well as SPECT and PET promises to be of great value in determining those patients who may benefit [12, 96]. The excimer laser-assisted non-occlusive anastomosis (ELANA) technique is proving to be a successful alternative surgical technique to the classical procedure of suturing the vessels [95].

6. EPILEPSY SURGERY

Anterior transSylvian selective amygdalohippocampectomy, introduced in 1973, is performed in patients with medically intractable mesiotemporal seizures, as indicated by an epileptologist [100, 113, 117]. This alternative to standard temporal lobectomy provides outstanding outcomes for seizure control. Microneurosurgical dissection achieves atraumatic opening of the anterior Sylvian fissure and the amygdalohippocampectomy can be accomplished without injuring the surrounding cerebrovascular system and neopallial and related white matter [88].

7. SPINE SURGERY

Microsurgical techniques are applied to spinal surgery for disc disease, as well as for extrinsic and intrinsic extra- and intramedullary tumors, AVMs, cavernomas, and hemangioblastomas. Quadrilaminectomy has proven a practical and suitable method to approach and completely remove these lesions [39, 51, 52, 57, 105, 108–111]. Hemilamintomy and microdiscectomy for lumbar disc surgery have advantages over open surgery as no spinal fixation is necessary

[2, 101, 106]. The spinal arachnoid cisternal space is also compartmentalized. A fenestrated arachnoidal septum exists between the dorsal median sulcus of the spinal cord and dura from C2 through Th10–11 and divides the dorsal spinal cistern into two compartments [57]. Meticulous manipulation to preserve the arachnoid aids in identifying the dorsal median sulcus. Precise closure of the pia, arachnoidea, and dura hinders dural-pial adhesions.

8. TRAUMA

Having vivid memories of personal experiences treating the open wounds of cranio-spinal injuries (1967–1970), the application of microtechniques seemed, initially, to be superfluous to others and was therefore opposed. Soon, however, after observing the effectiveness of meticulous exploration and removal of debris and hematomas, repair of vessels, precise hemostasis and exact closure of wounds, microtechniques became accepted.

9. CADAVER AND ANIMAL LABORATORY TRAINING

Theoretical learning methods are provided in abundance, whereas the technical, surgical aspects in the field of neurosurgery seem to be underappreciated.

Practical learning in well-equipped microneurosurgical laboratories provides a means to broaden knowledge of anatomy and acquire dexterity in microsurgical techniques, such as the appropriate use of the operating microscope, microsurgical instruments, drilling and dissection skills. Furthermore, microsurgical training will further enhance the capabilities of the "mental eye" of the surgeon.

DISCUSSION

The components of microneurosurgical concepts can be defined as follows: availability of appropriate tools, instruments, and equipment, thorough training in a laboratory dedicated to microneurosurgery to acquire broader neuroanatomical perspectives, and to adapt to the operating microscope while perfecting microsurgical techniques and improving skills with tools, instruments, and equipment; finally, establishing teamwork and interactive dialog with neuroradiologists, neuroanesthesiologists, neuropathologists and neurosurgical nurses in the OR, ICU and ward to promote optimal care of patients.

Considering these challenging developments, young colleagues are encouraged and advised of the absolute necessity, to spend at least one year in a laboratory setting, training in surgical neuroanatomy and microsurgical technique. The employment of advanced robotic technology in neurosurgery will require us to be far more accurate and knowledgable in neuroanatomy and neurophysiology and will demand confidence and precision in surgical maneuvers, methods and manipulations [87]. Aboud et al. [3] introduced an innovative lifelike model emulating the normal human anatomy and dynamic vascular filling found in real surgery. This model gives us the unique opportunity to develop and practice a wide range of skills, for example opening the Sylvian fissure, suturing microanastomoses, dissecting and clipping artificial aneurysms, and practicing neurosurgical approaches in general.

The most effective surgery is always that administered by the trained "mental eye" and hands of a surgeon. I am convinced the coming generation will participate with zeal, in advancing, developing and improving the field of neurosurgery, and in creating innovative ideas and initiating sound concepts for the benefit of our patients.

Ongoing laboratory experience throughout a neurosurgeon's career is critical for the microsurgeon to learn new techniques and procedures and to refresh and refine a knowledge of anatomy. Hands-on laboratory dissection courses and individualized cadaver dissection opportunities are excellent means for fine tuning seldom-used techniques [3, 114, 123].

FUTURE

In the information era, for the modern neurosurgeon, it is of importance to understand and master the interpretation of the many radiological imaging techniques, to implement neuronavigation in surgery and teaching, and to assist in developing even more advanced microscopes (such as with oscillating objectives to improve depth perception), microsurgical instruments, and 3D-television cameras with fluctuating objectives. In the field of neuroradiological imaging, diffusion tensor imaging and white matter tractography, although in their preliminary clinical phase, seem very promising techniques [47, 76, 83, 98]. They open exciting new possibilities for exploring features of the central nervous system anatomy that are invisible in vivo. These techniques have already expanded our current neuroanatomical knowledge, for example, the anatomic connectivity of cortical and subcortical structures, the somatotopical anatomic connectivity of cortical and subcortical structures, and the somatotopical organization of white matter tracts such as the pyramidal tract and medial lemniscus system [14, 58]. There is a parallel revival of interest in the anatomy and dissection of white matter tracts [76, 98, 121]. More recent studies have shown the relationship between intra-axial lesions, (gliomas, arteriovenous malformations, and cavernomas) to the adjacent white matter tracts. Preoperative neurosurgical planning and postoperative assessment of lesionectomy are defined according to the relationship of fiber systems to the lesion and whether they are impaired, displaced or intact [13, 83]. Optimally, intraoperative navigation with real-time information from ultrasound (parenchymography), MRI and CT, as well as tractography would be ideal to direct the process of dissection and serve as a pilot, guiding the procedure to accomplish a pure lesionectomy. Five categories of tract alteration in relation to a lesion have been described by Lazar et al., namely: normal, deviated, interrupted, infiltrated, or degenerated [47]. Interestingly, they also showed that after lesion resection, the white matter tracts appeared more similar to normal anatomy, compared to the contralateral side. Tract alteration had disappeared which correlated with improvement or preservation of motor function, when lesions were associated with the pyramidal tract. Their findings corroborate well with the concept that "glial tumors grow initially from a focus of abnormal cells in the white matter, in specific architectonic areas that are phylogenetically more recently evolved" [116]. As stated previously, these tumors, in the early and intermediate phase of their existence, as they grow, remain primarily restricted to their sectors of origin and split the surrounding white matter fibers. It is important to remember that the white matter consists not only of myelinated and unmyelinated fibers, but also of migrating stem cells, microglia, a specialized capillary and arachnoidal system, CSF channels, and a cellular and fluidal immune system.

CONCLUSIONS

The fundamental concepts of microneurosurgery are based on control of cerebral vasculature and hemodynamics, which includes exploration of main cerebral vasculature, also sulcal arteries and the arteries and veins surrounding cerebral lesions. As summarized in Table 1, successful fulfillment of these concepts is dependent on: (1) a clear understanding and recognition of the compartmental anatomy of the cisternal and parenchymal (neo-, paleo-, and archipalleal) and ventricular systems, (2) knowledge of the compartmental and segmental occurrence of gliomas and cerebral vascular lesions such as AVMs and cavernomas, (3) being well acquainted with instruments, bipolar coagulation, suction (regulation and CUSA), pledgets and sponges, (4) skilled reconstruction of arteries and veins using microsurgical techniques.

Acknowledgements

I wish to convey my sincere thanks and appreciation to Ruben Dammers, MD for his dedicated and enthusiastic assistance and to Dianne C. H. Yaşargil, RN for reviewing the text.

References

[1] Abbe E (1886) The new microscope. S Ber Jena Ges Med 2: 107-108

[2] Abernathey CD, Yaşargil MG (1990) Technique of microsurgery. In: Williams RW, McCulloch JA, Young PH (eds) Principles and techniques in spine surgery. Aspen Publishers Inc., Rockville, pp 271

[3] Aboud E, Al-Mefty O, Yaşargil MG (2002) New laboratory model for neurosurgical training that simulates live surgery. J Neurosurg 97: 1367-1372

[4] Al-Mefty O, Ayoubi S, Smith RR (1991) The petrosal approach: indications, technique, and results. Acta Neurochir Suppl (Wien) 53: 166-170

[5] Apuzzo ML, Heifetz MD, Weiss MH, et al. (1977) Neurosurgical endoscopy using side-viewing telescope. J Neurosurg 46: 398-400

[6] Ausman JI, Moore J, Chou SN (1976) Spontaneous cerebral revascularization in a patient with STA-MCA anastomosis. J Neurosurg 44: 84-87

[7] Barnett HJ, Peerless SJ (1985) Failure of extracranial-intracranial arterial bypass to reduce the risk of ischemic stroke. Results of an international randomized trial. The EC/IC Bypass Study Group. N Engl J Med 313: 1191-1200

[8] Barraquer JI (1956) The microscope in ocular surgery. Am J Ophthalmol 42: 916-918

[9] Bertalanffy H, Seeger W (1991) The dorsolateral, suboccipital, trancondylar approach to the lower clivus and anterior portion of craniocervical junction. Neurosurgery 29: 815-821

[10] Carrel A, Guthrie CC (1906) Uniterminal and biterminal venous transplantations. Surg Gynecol Obstet 2: 266

[11] Charbel FT, Meglio G, Amin-Hanjani S (2005) Superficial temporal artery – MCA bypass. Neurosurgery 56(Suppl 1): 186-190

[12] Chater N, Spetzler R, Tonnemacher K, Wilson CB (1976) Microvascular bypass surgery. Part 1: Anatomical studies. J Neurosurg 44: 712-714

[13] Chen X, Weigel D, Ganslandt O, Buchfelder M, Nimsky C (2007) Diffusion tensor imaging and white matter tractography in patients with brainstem lesions. Acta Neurochir 149: 1117-1131

[14] Concha L, Gross DW, Beaulieu C (2005) Diffusion tensor tractography of the limbic system. Am J Neuroradiol 26: 2267-2274

[15] Conforti P, Tomasello T, Albanese V (1984) Cerebral revascularization. Nuova Librario, Padua, Picifi

[16] Derome PJ (1985) Surgical management of tumors invading the skull base. Can J Neurol Sci 12: 345-347

[17] Dolenc V (1983) Direct microsurgical repair of intracavernous vascular lesions. J Neurosurg 58: 824-831

[18] Dolenc VV, Skrap M, Sustersic J, Skrbec M, Morina A (1987) A transcavernous-transsellar approach to the basilar tip aneurysms. Br J Neurosurg 1: 251-259

[19] Donaghy RM (1996) History of microneurosurgery. In: Wilkins RH, Rengachary SS (eds) Neurosurgery, 2nd edn, vol I. McGraw-Hill, New York, pp 37-42

[20] Donaghy RMP, Yaşargil MG (eds) (1967) Micro-vascular surgery: Report of first conference, October 6-7, 1966, Mary Fletcher Hospital, Burlington, Vermont. Georg Thieme, Stuttgart

[21] Ferguson GG, Drake CG, Peerless SS (1977) Extracranial-intracranial arterial bypass in the treatment of giant intracranial aneurysm. Stroke 8: 11

[22] Flamm ES (1997) History of neurovascular surgery. In: Greenblatt SH (ed) History of neurosurgery. AANS, Park Ridge, pp 259-288

[23] Greenwood J Jr (1940) Two point coagulation. A new principle and instrument for applying coagulation current in neurosurgery. Am J Surg 50: 267-270

[24] Hakuba A (ed) (1996) Surgery of the intracranial venous system. Springer, Tokyo

[25] Hakuba A, Liu S, Nishimura S (1986) The orbitozygomatic infratemporal approach: a new surgical technique. Surg Neurol 26: 271-276

[26] Handa H (ed) (1973) Microneurosurgery. Gaku Shoin Ltd., Tokyo

[27] Hardy J (1969) Transsphenoidal microsurgery of the normal and pathological pituitary. Clin Neurosurg 16: 185-216

[28] Harms H (1953) Augenoperationen unter dem binocularen Mikroskop. Ber Dtsch Ophthalmol Ges 58: 119-122

[29] House HP, House WF (1964) Historical review and problem of acoustic neuroma. Arch Otolaryngol 80: 599-604

[30] House WF (1961) Surgical exposure of the internal auditory canal. Laryngoscope 71: 1363-1385

[31] Jacobson JH II, Suarez EI (1960) Microsurgery in anastomosis of small vessels. Surg Forum 11: 243-245

[32] Jacobson JH II, Wallman LJ, Schumacher GA, Flanagan M, Suarez EL, Donaghy RM (1962) Microsurgery as an aid to middle cerebral artery endarterectomy. J Neurosurg 19: 108-115

[33] Jannetta PJ (1967) Arterial compression of the trigeminal nerve at the pons in patients with trigeminal neuralgia. J Neurosurg 26(Suppl): 159-162

[34] Jannetta PJ (1968) The surgical binocular microscope in neurological surgery. Am Surg 34: 31

[35] Jannetta PJ, Rand RW (1966) Trigeminal neuralgia. Microsurgical technique. Bull Los Angeles Neurol Soc 31: 93-99

[36] Kawase T, Toya S, Shiobara R, Mine T (1985) Transpetrosal approach for aneurysms of the lower basilar artery. J Neurosurg 63: 857-861

[37] Kelly PJ, Alker GJ Jr, Goerss S (1982) Computer-assisted stereotactic microsurgery for the treatment of intracranial neoplasms. Neurosurgery 10: 324-331

[38] Key A, Retzius G (1875–1876) Studien in der Anatomie des Nervensystems und des Bindesgewebes, vols I & II. Norstad, Stockholm

[39] Klekamp J, Samii M (2007) Surgery of spinal tumors. Springer, Berlin

[40] Krayenbuhl N, Hafez A, Hernesniemi JA, Krisht AF (2007) Taming the cavernous sinus: technique of hemostasis using fibrin glue. Neurosurgery 61: E52; discussion E52

[41] Krisht AF, Kadri PAS (2003) Microsurgical anatomy of the cavernous sinus. Tech Neurosurg 8: 199-203

[42] Krisht AF (2005) Transcavernous approach to diseases of the anterior upper third of the posterior fossa. Neurosurg Focus 19(2): E2

[43] Krisht AF, Krayenbuhl N, Sercl D, Bikmaz K, Kadri PA (2007) Results of microsurgical clipping of 50 high complexity basilar apex aneurysms. Neurosurgery 60: 242-250; discussion 250-242

[44] Kurze T (1964) Microtechniques in neurological surgery. Clin Neurosurg 11: 128-137

[45] Kurze T, Doyle JB (1962) Extradural intracranial (middle fossa) approach to the internal auditory canal. J Neurosurg 19: 1033-1037

[46] Lang WH, Muchel F (1981) Zeiss microscopes for microsurgery. Springer, Berlin, Heidelberg, New York

[47] Lazar M, Alexander AL, Thottakara PJ, Badie B, Field AS (2006) White matter reorganization after surgical resection of brain tumors and vascular malformations. Am J Neuroradiol 27: 1258-1271

[48] Littmann H (1954) Ein neues Operations-Mikroskop. Klin Monatsbl Augenheilkd Augenärztl Fortbild 124: 473-476

[49] Loftus CM, Kresowif TF (2000) Carotid artery surgery. Thieme, New York, Stuttgart

[50] Lougheed WM, Tom M (1961) A method of introducing blood into the subarachnoid space in the region of the circle of Willis in dogs. Can J Surg 4: 329-337

[51] Malis LI (1978) Intramedullay spinal cord tumors. Clin Neurosurg 25: 512-539

[52] Malis LI (1979) Microsurgery for spinal cord arteriorvenous malformation. Clin Neurosurg 26: 543-555

[53] Malis LI (1979) Instrumentation and techniques in microsurgery. Clin Neurosurg 26: 626-636

[54] Malis LI (1981) Neurosurgical photography through the microscope. Clin Neurosurg 28: 233-245

[55] Malis LI (1996) Electrosurgery. Technical note. J Neurosurg 85: 970-975

[56] Malpighi M (1661) Duae epistole de pulmonibus. Florence

[57] Nauta HJ, Dolan E, Yaşargil MG (1983) Microsurgical anatomy of spinal subarachnoid space. Surg Neurol 19: 431-437

[58] Nucifora PG, Verma R, Lee SK, Melhem ER (2007) Diffusion-tensor MR imaging and tractography: exploring brain microstructure and connectivity. Radiology 245: 367-384

[59] Nylen CO (1954) The microscope in aural surgery, its first use and later development. Acta Otolaryngol 116(Suppl): 226-240

[60] Ono M, Kubik S, Abernaty CD (1990) Atlas of the cerebral sulci. Thieme, Stuttgart

[61] Peerless SJ (1976) Techniques of cerebral revascularization. Clin Neurosurg 23: 258-269

[62] Perneczky A, Tschabitscher N, Resch KDM (1993) Endoscopic anatomy for neurosurgery. Thieme, Stuttgart

[63] Perritt RA (1958) Micro-ophthalmic surgery. XVIII. Belgica, Concil Ophthal

[64] Pool JL, Colton RP (1966) The dissecting microscope for intracranial vascular surgery. J Neurosurg 25: 315-318

[65] Rand RW (1969) Micro-neurosurgery. CV Mosby, St. Louis

[66] Rand RW, Kurze T (1965) Micro-neurosurgical resection of acoustic tumors by a transmeatal posterior fossa approach. Bull Los Angel Neuro Soc 30: 17-20

[67] Riechert T (1948) Die Operationen an der WS und am Rückenmark. In: Bier A, Braun H, Kümmel H (eds) Chirurgische Operationslehre, vol 2. JA Barth, Leipzig, p 753

[68] Reichman OH (1971) Experimental lingual-basilar arterial microanastomosis. J Neurosurg 34: 500-505

[69] Rhoton AL Jr (1979) Microsurgical anatomy of the posterior fossa cranial nerves. Clin Neurosurg 26L: 398-462

[70] Rohr M, Stock W (1913) Über eine achromatische Brillenlupe schwacher Vergrößerung. Klin Monatsbl Augenheilkd 51: 206-210

[71] Samii M, Ammirati M, Walter GF (1992) Surgery of skull base meningiomas. Springer, Berlin

[72] Samii M, Mathies C (1997) Management of 1000 vestibular schwannomas (acoustic neuromas): Hearing function in 1000 tumor resections. Neurosurgery 40: 248-262

[73] Samson DS, Boones L (1998) Extra-intracranial arterial bypass; past performance and current concepts. Neurosurgery 3: 79-86

[74] Schierbeek A (1959) Measuring the invisible world. The life and works of Antoni van Leeuwenhoek FRS. With a biographical chapter by Maria Rooseboom. Abelard-Schuman, New York

[75] Schlich T (2007) Nobel Prizes for surgeons: In recognition of the surgical healing strategy. Int J Surg 5: 129-133

[76] Schmahmann JD, Pandya DN (2007) Cerebral white matter – historical evolution of facts and notions concerning the organization of the fiber pathways of the brain. J Hist Neurosci 16: 237-267

[77] Schmiedek P, Gratzl O, Spetzler R, Steinhoff H, Enzenbach R, Brendel W, Marguth F (1976) Selection of patients for extra-intracranial arterial bypass surgery based on rCBF measurements. J Neurosurg 44: 303-312

[78] Seeger W (1978) Atlas of topographical anatomy of the brain and surrounding structures. Springer, Wien

[79] Sekhar LN, Bucur SD, Bank WO, Wright DC (1999) Venous and arterial bypass grafts for difficult tumors, aneurysms, and occlusive vascular lesions: evolution of surgical treatment and improved graft results. Neurosurgery 44: 1207-1223; discussion 1223-1204

[80] Sekhar LN, de Oliveira E (1999) Cranial neurosurgery. Thieme, Stuttgart

[81] Shambaugh GE (1939) Surgery for otosclerosis. Indications, techniques and results. Fortschr Hals-Nas-Ohrenheilkd 8: 367-428

[82] Shillito J (1967) Intracranial arteriotomy in three children and three adults. In: Donaghy RMP, Yaşargil MG (eds) Micro-vascular surgery. Georg Thieme, Stuttgart, pp 138-142

[83] Smits M, Vernooij MW, Wielopolski PA, Vincent AJ, Houston GC, van der Lugt A (2007) Incorporating functional MR imaging into diffusion tensor tractography in the preoperative assessment of the corticospinal tract in patients with brain tumors. Am J Neuroradiol 28: 1354-1361

[84] Spetzler RF, Carter LP, Selman WR, Martin NA (1985) Cerebral revascularization for stroke. Thieme-Stratton, New York Stuttgart

[85] Spetzler RF, Chater N (1976) Occipital artery-middle cerebral anastomosis for cerebral artery occlusive disease. Surg Neurol 2: 235-238

[86] Spetzler RF, Chater NL (1980) Microvascular bypass surgery. Part 2: Physiological studies. J Neurosurg 53: 22-70

[87] Spicer MA, van Velsen M, Caffrey JP, Apuzzo ML (2004) Virtual reality neurosurgery: a simulator blueprint. Neurosurgery 54: 783-797; discussion 797-788

[88] Stummer W, Pichlmeier U, Meinel T, Wiestler OD, Zanella F, Reulen HJ (2006) Fluorescence-guided surgery with 5-aminolevulinic acid for resection of malignant glioma: a randomised controlled multicentre phase III trial. Lancet Oncol 7: 392-401

[89] Sugita K (1985) Microneurosurgical atlas. Thieme, Stuttgart

[90] Sundt TM Jr (1979) Neurovascular microsurgery. World J Surg 3: 53-65, 127

[91] Sundt TM Jr, Fode NC, Jack CR Jr (1988) The past, present, and future to extracranial bypass surgery. Clin Neurosurg 34: 134-153

[92] Sundt TM Jr, Piepgras DG (1979) Surgical approach to giant intracranial aneurysms. Operative experience with 80 cases. J Neurosurg 51: 731-742

[93] Sundt TM Jr, Piepgras DG, Stevens LN (1991) Surgery for supratentorial arterivenous malformations. Clin Neurosurg 37: 49-115

[94] Tew JR, van Loveren HR (1994) Atlas of operative microneurosurgery. WB Saunders, Philadelphia

[95] Tulleken CA, Verdaasdonk RM, Berendsen W, Mali WP (1993) Use of the excimer laser in high-flow bypass surgery of the brain. J Neurosurg 78: 477-480

[96] Türe U, Yaşargil MG, Krisht AF (1996) The arteries of the corpus callosum: a microsurgical anatomic study. Neurosurgery 39: 1075-1084; discussion 1084-1075

[97] Türe U, Yaşargil MG, Al-Mefty O, Yaşargil DCH (2000) Arteries of the insula. J Neurosurg 92: 676-687

[98] Türe U, Yaşargil MG, Friedman AH, Al-Mefty O (2000) Fiber dissection technique: lateral aspect of the brain. Neurosurgery 47: 417-426; discussion 426-427

[99] Turner GLE (1972) The study of the history of the microscope. Proc R Microsc Soc 7(2): 121-149

[100] Wieser HG, Yaşargil MG (1982) Selective amygdalohippocampectomy as a surgical treatment of mesiobasal limbic epilepsy. Surg Neurol 17: 445-457

[101] Williams RW (1978) Microlumbar discectomy. A conservative surgical approach to the virgin herniated disc. Spine 3: 175-182

[102] Wolfe SQ, Tummala RP, Morcos JJ (2005) Cerebral revascularization in skull base tumors. Skull Base 15: 71-82

[103] Woringer E, Kunlin J (1963) Anastomose entre le carotide primitive et la carotide intra-craniennet ou la sylvienne par greffon selon la technique da la suture suspendue. Neurochirurgie 9: 181-188

[104] Wullstein H (1953) Technik und bisherige Ergebnisse de Tympanoplastik 87: 308

[105] Yaşargil MG (1969) Surgery of vascular malformations of the spinal cord with the microsurgical technique. Clin Neurosurg 18: 257-265

[106] Yaşargil MG (1977) Microsurgical operation for herniated lumbar disc. In: Advances in Neurosurgery, vol 4. Springer, Berlin, pp 81

[107] Yaşargil MG (1985) History of microneurosurgery. In: Spetzler RF, Carter LP, et al. (eds) Cerebral revascularization. Thieme, Stuttgart, pp 28-33

[108] Yaşargil MG, Antic J, Laciga R, de Preux J, Fideler RW, Boone SC (1976) The microsurgical removal of intramedullary spinal hemangioblastomas. Report of twelve cases and a review of the literature. Surg Neurol 1976: 141-148

[109] Yaşargil MG, Perneczky A (1976) Operative Behandlung der intramedullaren spinalen Tumoren. In: Schiefer W, Wieck HH (eds) Spinale raumfordernde Prozesse. Verlag Peri Med, Erlangen, pp 299-312

[110] Yaşargil MG, Symon L, Teddy P (1984) Arteriovenous malformations of the spinal cord. Adv Tech Stand Neurosurg 11: 61-102

[111] Yaşargil MG, Tranmer BI, Adamson TE, Roth P (1991) Unilateral partial hemilaminectomy for the removal of extra- and intramedullary tumors and AVMs. Adv Tech Stand Neurosurg 18: 113-132

[112] Yaşargil MG, Vise WM, Bader DC (1977) Technical adjuncts in neurosurgery. Surg Neurol 8: 331-336

[113] Yaşargil MG, Wieser HG, Valavanis A, von Ammon K, Roth P (1993) Surgery and results of selective amygdala-hippocampectomy in one hundred patients with nonlesional limbic epilepsy. Neurosurg Clin N Am 4: 243-261

[114] Yaşargil MG (2005) From the microsurgical laboratory to the operating theatre. Acta Neurochir (Wien) 147: 465-468

[115] Yaşargil MG, Donaghy RMP, Fisch UP, Hardy J, Malis LI, Peerless SJ, Zingg M, Borer WJ, Littmann H, Voellmy HR (1969) Microsurgery applied to neurosurgery. Georg Thieme, Stuttgart

[116] Yaşargil MG (1984–1996) Microneurosurgery in 6 volumes. Georg Thieme, Stuttgart

[117] Yaşargil MG, Teddy PS, Roth P (1985) Selective amygdalo-hippocampectomy. Operative anatomy and surgical technique. Adv Tech Stand Neurosurg 12: 93-123

[118] Yaşargil MG (1999) A legacy of microneurosurgery: memoirs, lessons, and axioms. Neurosurgery 45: 1025-1092

[119] Yaşargil MG (2000) The history of optical instruments and microneurosurgery. In: Barrow DL, Kondziolka D, Laws ER, Traynelis VC (eds) Fifty years of neurosurgery. Lippincott, Williams & Wilkins, Philadelphia, pp 105-142

[120] Yaşargil MG, Krisht AF, Türe U, Al-Mefty O, Yaşargil DCH (2002) Microsurgery of insular gliomas, Part I: Surgical anatomy of the Sylvian cistern. Contemp Neurosurg 24: 1-8

[121] Yaşargil MG, Türe U, Yaşargil DCH (2004) Impact of temporal lobe surgery. J Neurosurg 101: 725-738

[122] Yaşargil MG, Türe U, Yaşargil DCH (2005) Surgical anatomy of supratentorial midline lesions. Neurosurg Focus 18(6): E1

[123] Yonekawa Y, et al. (1999) Laboratory training in microsurgical technique and microvascular anastomosis. Oper Tech Neurosurg 2: 149-158

[124] Zhang M, An PC (2000) Liliequist's membrane is a fold of the arachnoid mater: study using sheet plastination and scanning electron microscopy. Neurosurgery 47: 902-908; discussion 908-909

[125] Zollner F (1949) Mikroskopstativ fuer Operation. Laryngol Rhinol Otol 28L209

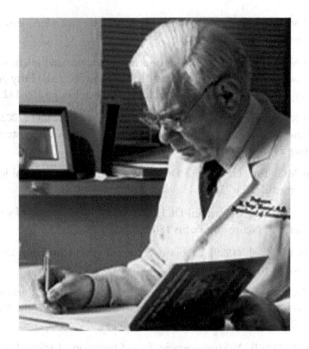

Mahmut Gazi Yaşargil

In 1994, Professor Yaşargil accepted an appointment as professor of neurosurgery at the University of Arkansas for Medical Sciences in Little Rock, where he is still active in microneurosurgical practice, research, and teaching. Professor M. Gazi Yaşargil was born on July 6, 1925, in Lice, Turkey. In 1953, he began his neurosurgical residency at the University of Zürich, under Professor Hugo Krayenbühl. From 1965 to 1967 he was a research-fellow in microvascular surgery at the University of Vermont, Burlington, under Professor R.M. Peardon Donaghy, where he learned microsurgical techniques, which were then applied to the cerebral arteries in the animal laboratory. After returning to Zürich, he performed the first cerebral vascular bypass surgery using the surgical microscope on October 30, 1967. Since then, he shaped microneurosurgery with innovative instrumentation, such as the floating microscope, microsurgical instruments, and ergonomic aneurysm clips and appliers. The emergence of microneurosurgery and the consequences hereof for his patients have been summarized in his 6-volume monograph.

Contact: M. Gazi Yaşargil, Department of Neurosurgery, University of Arkansas for Medical Sciences, 4301 W. Markham Street #507, 72205 Little Rock, AR, USA
E-mail: williamsronaldaa@uams.edu

ENDOSCOPY: PRINCIPLES AND TECHNIQUES

E. DE DIVITIIS

INTRODUCTION

Neurosurgery, compared to other medical and surgical specialties, is a relatively recent one. Indeed, it is considered as one of the most rapidly evolving and flourishing. During the second half of the last century and the past few years, this field has made a well noticed advance in evolving ideas and surgical tools in the attempt to attain the lowest rates of morbidity and mortality in a safe, feasible, limited, yet practical way. Among those tools has been the endoscope. It first emerged as a diagnostic tool, shifted with time to become a surgical one, passed through an era of struggle to survive among other practical tools, and lastly has strongly re-emerged and gained popularity as the sole visualizing tool in more neurosurgical approaches.

Aiming to clarify the evolving role of the endoscope in neurosurgery, the historical background of neuroendoscopy, its past and recent applications in the field of brain surgery, the milestones of its technological advancements will be reviewed.

Minimal invasiveness is a surgical approach modality designed to minimize trauma, maximize outcomes and enable patients to quickly return to their normal life.

The goal for using endoscopes for surgery is to reduce the tissue trauma when compared with traditional "open surgery". In addition, the use of side-viewing capability and better lighting produces much better viewing inside the operative field than traditional surgery. However, minimally invasive endoscopic surgery is certainly not a minor surgery. As a matter of fact, despite several advantages for the patient, such as reduced blood loss, shorter hospital stay, decreased postoperative pain and quicker return to normal activities, some complications must be taken into account. The procedure is not completely risk-free and can produce complications ranging from infection to death. Risks and complications include the following: bleeding, infection, blood vessel injury, CSF leak. Some disadvantages for the surgeon also exist: difficult handling of the instruments, restricted maneuverability, difficult eye–hand coordination, learning curve. Despite these problems, it is certainly

Keywords: neuro-endoscopy, approaches, techniques, skull base

true that the advent of the endoscope has produced ripples of enthusiasm and progress in the field of modern neurosurgery.

HISTORICAL BACKGROUND

The development of endoscopic neurosurgical applications can be traced back to the XIXth century and continues in the present awaiting the next coming revolution that will change the view to this era to be an intermediate one, while shifting to the really new era from the prospective of that revolution. As a matter of fact, Philipp Bozzini is considered the spiritual father of the endoscope [10]. He invented the first simple model, the "Lichtleiter", an eye piece and a mirror reflecting a candle light, which he demonstrated in the year 1806. Limited illumination and visualization together with painful application, yet it is always considered a breakthrough. More than 70 years later, around 1877, Max Nitze revolutionized the field [15], using an optical system consisting of a train of lenses and a glowing platinum wire as a source of illumination [14]. He has been also the first to consider the documentation ability of the endoscope via photography and the first to apply cutting loops during endoscopic procedures, changing the view from diagnosis to intervention [15]. It has not been until the year 1910 for the endoscope to be applied in a neurosurgical procedure by Lespinasse [12], who operated upon two hydrocephalic infants applying a cystoscope for endoscopic choroid plexectomy [18]. Yet, Dandy is considered the father of neuroendoscopy. Concerning endoscopic third ventriculostomy, Mixter has been the first to report such a procedure in 1923 [18]. In 1935, Scarff performed the procedure with novel instruments: he used an endoscope with irrigation system, advanceable cauterization and ventriculostomy tips. Ventricular endoscopy started to gain land among few neurosurgeons who started to realize its benefits, considering the available facilities at that time.

It seems that the field of endoscopy and particularly that of neuroendoscopy entered then a stage of hibernation for more than two decades for many reasons, among them: inadequate illumination, poor image quality, advent of ventricular CSF shunting, last but not least, the birth of microneurosurgery in the early sixties of the last century offering more practical solutions for the endoscopic drawbacks, together with feasibility of approaching brain and skull base lesions through different novel trajectories.

Hopkins and Storz are credited for the renaissance of endoscopy [5]. Many technical advances lead to their innovative endoscope, "a Hopkins rod lens system with an external light source transmitted through incoherent glass fibers attached to the telescope", that has been shown for the first time in 1967. It is worth clarifying that Hopkins invented his rod lens system in 1959. Compared to the previous train of lenses system of Nitze, this system offered greater light transmission, a wider view, better image quality, and a smaller diameter for the system [5]. Two years earlier to Hopkins's invention,

Hirschowitz, in 1957, developed the fiberscope. Karl Storz inspired these two main ideas. We have come finally to the modern form of the endoscope that has been applied since then with little if any new advances.

Technical advances in image capturing and processing also took part in the field of endoscopy. Among them are the CCDs (charge-coupled devices), which have been incorporated in the endoscopic systems, resulting in improved image quality and decrease in size.

The modern era of neuroendoscopy can be identified with the role of T. Fukushima, who in 1973 reported the use of a ventriculofiberscope as a new technique for endoscopic diagnosis and operation [11]. He was followed in 1974 by Olinger and Ohlhaber, who used an eighteen-gauge microscopic-telescopic needle endoscope. Yet, it has not been until 1977, when Apuzzo et al. started to apply the concept of adjunctive endoscopy during the conventional microneurosurgical procedures. They reported the use of a side-viewing endoscope to control the angles hidden from the prospect of a microsurgical approach [1]. Again, due to the inferior image quality of the endoscopes compared to that of the surgical microscopes, this technique was not very popular. In the neurosurgical historic perspective, Apuzzo et al. [1] are credited for the concept of adjunctive endoscopy. During the eighties, neurosurgeons started to explore the extra capabilities of ventriculoscopy, both in diagnosis and interventions.

ENDOSCOPES

The endoscope offers three main advantages: (i) improvement of the illumination because of a light source that brings the light in the surgical field; (ii) better definition of the anatomical details because of the use of high-definition lenses and the closer view of the scope that allows an augmented definition of the details at the tumor–tissue interface; (iii) marked increase of the angles of visualization with the use of angled lenses, allowing to see in areas otherwise hidden to the microsurgical vision and giving a different perception of the anatomy. Thus, the endoscope can increase the precision of the surgery and permit the surgeon to differentiate different tissues, so that a selective removal of the lesion can be achieved. However, one of the current limitations of the modern endoscopes is that they provide a bidimensional image. The lack of stereoscopy can be overcome with training, though, with the multiangled vision, with the fine understanding of all the lights and shadows of the image, with fixing the multiple landmarks during the operation and, in one word, with the knowledge of the surgical anatomy that the endoscope has pushed again.

Currently, different types of endoscopes exist and are classified either as fiber-optic endoscopes (fiberscopes) or rod lens endoscopes. The endoscopes specifically designed for neuroendoscopy can be classified into four types: (i) rigid fiberscopes, (ii) rigid rod lens endoscopes, (iii) flexible fiberscopes,

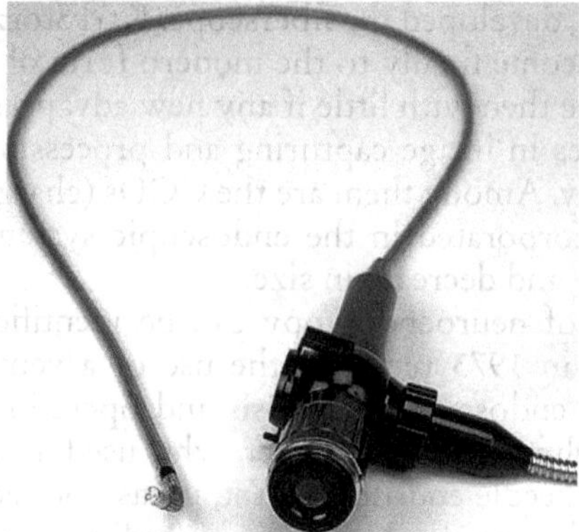

Fig. 1. Example of flexible endoscope

(iv) steerable fiberscopes. These different endoscopes have different diameters, lengths, optical quality, number and diameter of working channels, all of which vary with size. The choice between them should be made on the basis of the surgical indication and personal preference of the surgeon.

1. FLEXIBLE (STEERABLE) ENDOSCOPES

The properties of optic fibers permit the steerable fiberscopes to orient the tip up and downwards (Fig. 1) [4]. The angle of bending varies in the different models. Modifying the orientation of the optical fibers, the surgeon can orientate the instruments to reach all of the structures to visualize. This system makes looking and working around corners. The rigid part of the scope is attached to a mechanical or pneumatic holder. The diameter of the scope is usually between 2.3 and 4.6 mm, depending upon the number of optic fibers. The number of operative channels varies from one to three; the best device is the three-channel endoscope (one working channel for introduction of instruments and two independent channels for irrigation and aspiration). The diameter of the working channel is usually approximately 1.0 mm, allowing the introduction of 3-French (1 mm) different flexible miniaturized instruments, such as scissors, grasping and biopsy forceps, monopolar electrodes and Fogarty balloon. A dedicated peel-away sheath is essential to introduce the endoscope to reach the target.

2. RIGID ROD LENS SCOPES

Rod lens endoscopes consist of three main parts: a mechanical shaft, glass fiber bundles for light illumination, and optics (objective, eyepiece, relay system).

The angle of view of rod lens endoscopes ranges from 0° to 120°, according to the objective, but objectives with an angle greater than 30°–45° are not

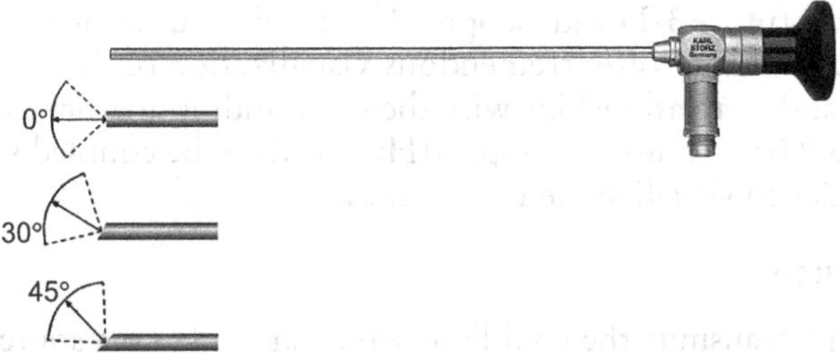

Fig. 2. Example of rigid rod-lens endoscope, zero-degree and angled lenses

very useful in neuroendoscopy. The 0° scope provides a frontal view of the surgical field and minimizes the risk of disorientation [17] and is generally used during the majority of the operation. The angled objectives offer additional advantages, allowing to look around the corners.

The rod lens rigid endoscope is commonly used through a sheath, connected to a cleaning-irrigation system which permits cleaning and defogging of the distal lens, thus avoiding repeated entrances and exits from the surgical field. Preferably, the scopes used are without any working channel (diagnostic endoscopes) and the other instruments are inserted sliding alongside the sheath and using the latter as a guide for the correct direction. The diameter of rod lens endoscope varies between 1.9 and 10 mm, but for endoneurosurgery usually endoscopes with a diameter of 2.7–4 mm are used. It is not advisable to use smaller endoscopes because the smaller the diameter of the lens, the less light it can transport. It has been estimated that for each 10% of increase of diameter there is a 46% percent increase in light transmitted, but endoscopes larger than 2.7 mm can be too bulky and requiring larger approaches.

3. ENDOSCOPIC INSTRUMENTATION

3.1 Video camera and monitor

In order to properly maneuver the instruments under fine control, the endoscope is connected to a dedicated video camera and the endoscopic images are projected onto a monitor placed in front of the surgeon. Additional monitors can be placed in varying locations in the operating room, as well as outside in the hallways or adjacent rooms, to permit other members of the team to watch the surgery.

Several types of endoscopic video cameras are available, the most common of which utilize a 3-CCD sensor which provides a better color separation, more brilliant colors and a sharper image with higher contrast than the 1-CCD cameras, which process all three fundamental colors in one chip. Most modern endoscopic cameras are analog.

A further improvement of the resolution of both the video cameras and the monitors is represented by the high-definition (HD) technology, which is ready for the future 3-D endoscopes. The continuous improvements in endoscopic image quality offer tremendous visualization of the operative field, of the lesion and its relationships with the surrounding anatomical structures. A full HD 16:9 flat monitor (1080p, 60 Hz) needs to be coupled with the HD camera in order to visualize the HD images.

3.2 Light source

The endoscope transmits the cold light which arises from a source inside the surgical field through a connecting cable made of glass fibers. Currently, in endoscopic surgery xenon light sources are used. They have spectral characteristics similar to those of the sunlight, with a color temperature of approximately 6000 K, which is "whiter" than the classic halogen light (3400 K). The power of the unit is commonly 300 W. The flexible connecting cable is made of a bundle of glass fibers that brings the light to the endoscope, virtually without dispersion of visible light [14]. Furthermore, the heat (composed by infrared light) is poorly transmitted by the glass fibers, thus reducing the risk of burning the tissues.

3.3 Surgical instruments

For the endoscopic approach, the instruments need to be inserted along the same axis as the endoscope and need to maintain the same position with respect to the endoscope for their entire length. For this reason they need to be straight and not bayoneted. This is mainly due to two peculiarities of the endoscopic approach: (i) the visibility of only that which is beyond the distal lens of the scope and (ii) the panoramic and multiangled view afforded by the endoscope. With regard to the first point, while the microscope produces magnification from a distant lens, and light is transmitted from the lamp of the microscope to the surgical field, so that the surgeon can follow the entrance of the instruments from the outside, the vision provided by the endoscope is maintained completely inside the surgical field. The instruments are inserted blind in the surgical field with the concomitant risk to injure the anatomical structures until the tip of the instrument becomes visible once it has passed beyond the distal lens, unless the endoscope is removed and inserted every time a different instrument is used.

Since the introduction of the endoscopic approaches, new instruments have been designed that meet the following criteria [2, 3, 14]:

- move easily and safely in a limited surgical corridor;
- be well-balanced and ergonomic for safe handling, while avoiding any conflict between the surgeon's hands, the endoscope and other instruments that may be present in the same corridor;
- allow the surgeon to work in every visible zone of the surgical field provided by the endoscope.

3.4 Bleeding control

One of the most difficult and common problems of endoscopic surgery is the control of bleeding.

Monopolar coagulation is usually easy to obtain. However, bipolar coagulation is preferable, either alone or in association with hemostatic agents. Consequently, different dedicated bipolar forceps have been designed, with various diameters and lengths, which have proven to be quite effective in bleeding control.

Recently, the radiofrequency technology for either monopolar and bipolar coagulation has been introduced. Radiofrequency instruments have two main advantages over the electric ones: the spatial energy dispersion with radiofrequency is minimal, with concomitant minimal risk of injury to the surrounding anatomical structures; radiofrequency bipolar forceps do not need to be used with irrigation or to be cleaned every time.

3.5 Video documentation

Documentation and storage of intraoperative images and movie clips is of increasing importance for education and documentation. Although video recording is not mandatory, having the possibility to document either still images or video clips of the surgical procedure is quite important for a series of reasons. It is possible to review the operation and, if any mistakes are made, learn and know how to avoid them in future; to obtain pictures for publication or produce video clips to teach residents, course attendees, etc.; to store the material in an electronic library; to use the material for legal purposes.

3.6 Other instruments

Modern neurosurgery, no matter if with microsurgical and/or endoscopic technique, uses special instruments and devices that are quite helpful even if not absolutely needed [4].

Image-guided neuronavigation systems are very useful for intraoperative identification of the anatomic structures involved in the procedure. This is specially true in case of distorted anatomy due to a particular growth pattern of the lesion which causes the classic landmarks being not easily identifiable. In such cases, neuronavigation can help to maintain the surgeon's orientation.

Prior to performing sharp dissections or incisions and whenever the surgeon thinks it is appropriate (especially while working very close to vascular structures), it is of utmost importance to use the microDoppler probe to insonate the major arteries. The use of this device, frequently used in endoscopic skull base surgery, should be recommended every time a sharp dissection is made, to minimize the risk of injury to major arteries.

3.7 Preoperative planning

Preoperative radiological investigations are the same as for the microsurgical approaches. They include magnetic resonance imaging (MRI), computed tomography (CT), angiography, etc. These exams provide the neurosurgeon information about the peculiar anatomical conditions concerning the tumor itself and the bone and anatomical structures involved in the approach.

Such studies are important for the planning of the approach and the removal strategy and to be used with the image-guided surgery systems (namely, the neuronavigator).

ENDOSCOPIC TECHNIQUES AND INDICATIONS

Neuroendoscopy can be used to treat a variety of pathologies [3, 4]. The more frequent indications are obstructive hydrocephalus, intra-paraventricular lesions, intraneural cysts, multiloculated hydrocephalus marsupialization, colloid cysts, pituitary adenomas and skull base approach.

In most of the neurosurgical cases treated with neuroendoscopic technique, a single drill hole is need for the approach. The hole site and the path that the neuroendoscope follows through the cerebral parenchyma to reach the target vary in relation to the type of surgery and the location of the lesion. The preoperative magnetic resonance multiplanar images permit to set the exact position of the drill hole and the more convenient path.

1. ENDOSCOPIC THIRD VENTRICULOSTOMY

Endoscopic third ventriculostomy is the most used procedure in neuroendoscopy [3, 4, 13]. By this technique, a communication between the anterior part of the third ventricle and the interpeduncular cistern is accomplished. Generally, the procedure is performed under general anesthesia; the endoscope is entered through a burr hole placed in front of the coronal suture, 2 cm away from the midline. The foramen of Monro is identified with its anatomical landmarks (choroid plexus, fornix, venous corner) (Fig. 3). Once the third ventricle is entered, through the foramen of Monro, the anatomical landmarks of the floor are recognizable: mammillary bodies, infundibular recess and the tuber cinereum (Fig. 4). The floor is perforated between the infundibular recess in front and the mammillary bodies behind. Then, the perforation is dilated by a Fogarty catheter. The interpeduncular cistern is entered with the endoscope to ascertain the existence of a good communication and the tip of the basilar artery comes under vision (Fig. 5). In case of some bleeding, bipolar coagulation, irrigation and balloon dilatation can be used.

This technique is the method of choice in treating occlusive hydrocephalus due do stenosis of the aqueduct (Fig. 6). A prerequisite of a successful endoscopic third ventriculostomy is the patency of the distal liquoral pathways.

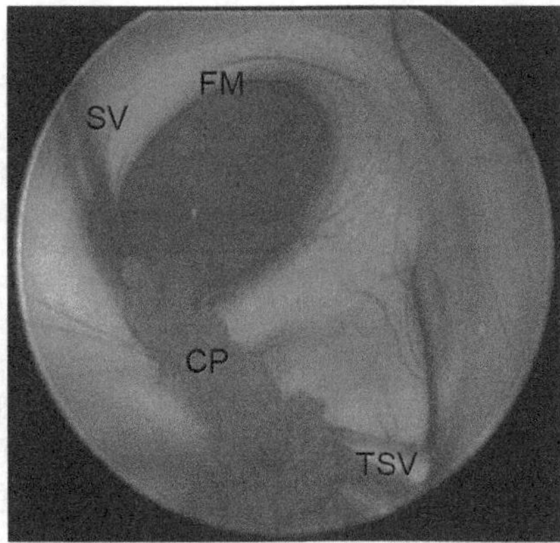

Fig. 3. Endoscopic view of the right foramen of Monro. The choroid plexus and the venous corner (septal vein and thalamo-striate vein) are recognizable. *FM* Foramen of Monro; *CP* choroid plexus; *SV* septal vein; *TSV* thalamo-striate vein

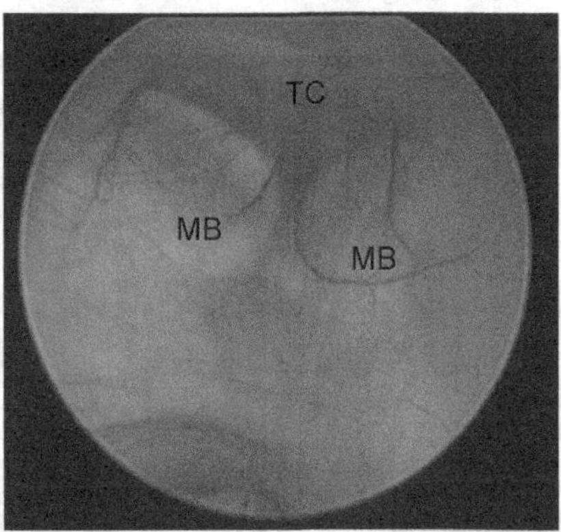

Fig. 4. Endoscopic view of floor of the third ventricle seen as soon as the foramen of Monro is entered. The landmarks formed by the mammillary bodies (*MB*) and the tuber cinereum (*TC*) are recognizable

2. COLLOID CYSTS

The choice of endoscopy as treatment modality depends on the adequacy of the surgeon experience and skill and the adequacy of the endoscopic equipment. The surgical technique is briefly reported [3, 4, 9]. The endoscope is inserted in the lateral ventricle of the non-dominant hemisphere through a burr hole in front of the coronal suture. The colloid cyst is usually identified filling the foramen of Monro (Fig. 7); the cyst wall is coagulated, punctured and opened as widely as possible in order to aspirate the colloid material. The capsule of the cyst is elevated from the fornix, coagulated and removed.

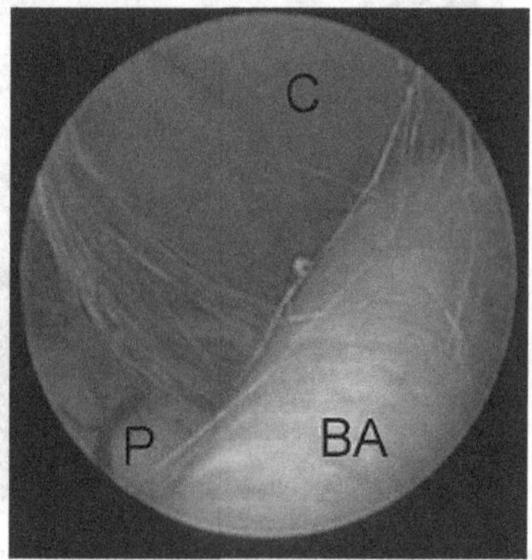

Fig. 5. Endoscopic view of the interpeduncular cistern after the endoscopic third ventriculostomy has been performed. The basilar artery (*BA*) and the anterior surface of the pons (*P*), together with the clivus (*C*) are recognizable

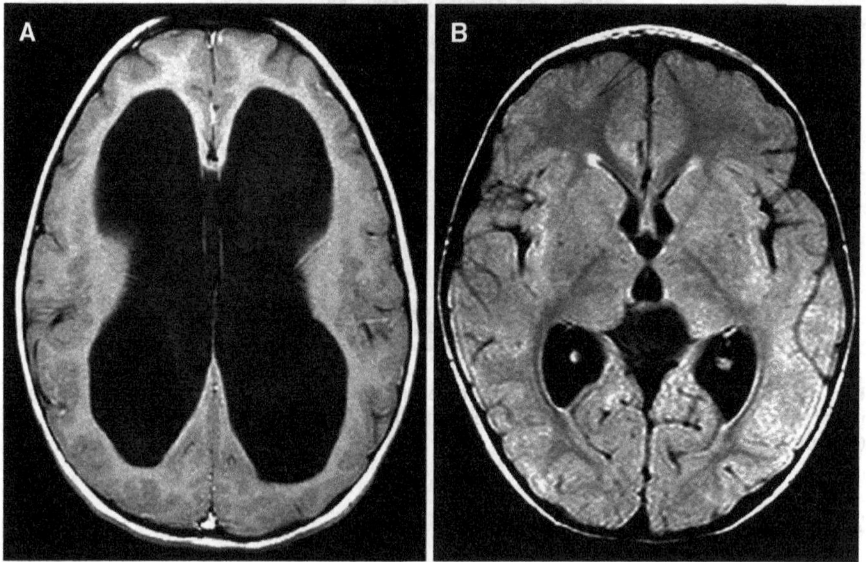

Fig. 6. Pre-operative (**A**) and post-operative (**B**) axial MRI of a case of a supratentorial hydrocephalus treated by endoscopic third ventriculostomy

In case it is strictly adherent to the surrounding vital structures, the remnant must be left in place to avoid complications.

The treatment is successful in 60–90% of cases treated by endoscopy (Fig. 8). The unsuccessful cases can be retreated by neuroendoscopy or by a transcranial approach.

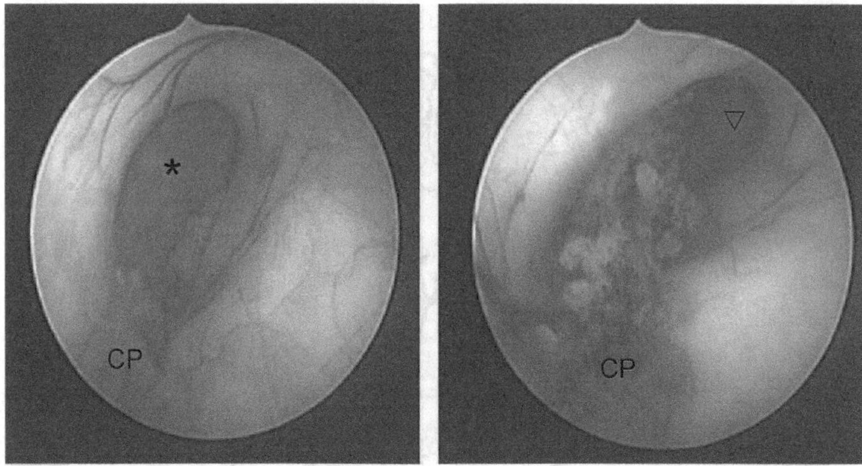

Fig. 7. A Endoscopic view of a colloid cyst of the third ventricle protruding through the foramen of Monro. **B** The same case after the cyst emptying and capsule resection. *Asterisk*: cyst capsule; *arrowhead*: third ventricle seen through the foramen of Monro after the removal of the cyst

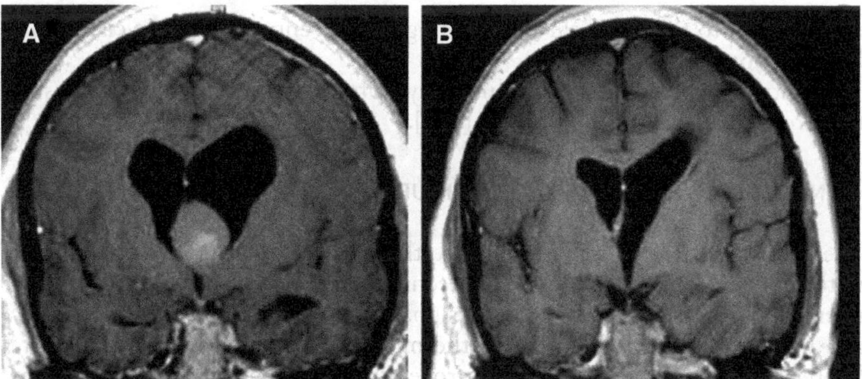

Fig. 8. Pre-operative (**A**) and post-operative (**B**) axial MRI of a case of a colloid cyst of the III ventricle

3. ARACHNOID CYSTS

Endoscopy is one of the multiple surgical strategies in the management of symptomatic arachnoid cysts. It aims for neuroendoscopic reduction of the cyst by establishing a communication between the cyst and the CSF pathway (Fig. 9). To avoid the closure of the stomy following the procedure, a large opening and the removal of fragments of the cyst wall as widely as possible are absolutely required. In order to improve the results, particularly when the cyst is associated with hydrocephalus, an association between fenestration

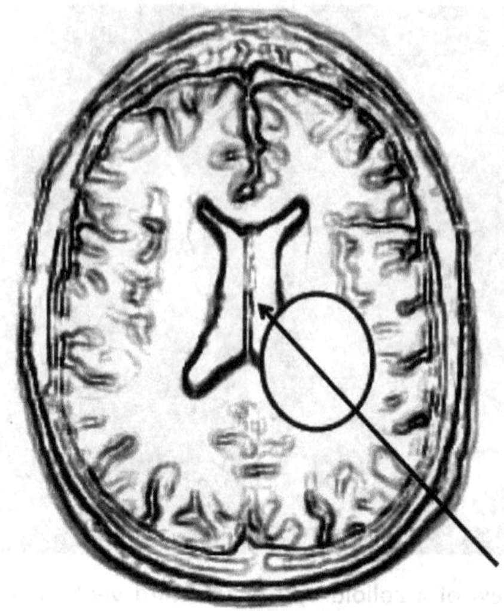

Fig. 9. Schematic drawing of the technique of fenestration of a paraventricular arachnoidc yst

of the cyst into the ventricle and opening of the ventricle into the cistern has been proposed.

Control of the cyst size and clinical symptoms are usually obtained, using this procedure, in 71–81% of cases [3, 4].

4. ENDOSCOPIC ENDONASAL TECHNIQUE

The endoscopic endonasal approach to the sellar region is a recent evolution of the conventional transsphenoidal technique performed with the operating microscope. This method can be designated as "pure" pituitary endoscopy and not only as a complement to the microscopic intervention – the term "pure" being applied to a surgical procedure in which the endoscope is the only optical device being used.

The endoscopic endonasal transsphenoidal approach to the sella is performed via an anterior sphenoidotomy, through the enlargement of the natural sphenoid ostium, with a rigid diagnostic endoscope, and without the use of a transsphenoidal retractor. Three main steps make up this surgical procedure: nasal, sphenoidal and sellar [7].

During the nasal step the endoscope (18 cm in length, 4 mm in diameter) is inserted in the chosen nostril up to the middle turbinate. The endoscope is then advanced inside the nasal cavity up to the choana and along its roof, in the sphenoethmoid recess, until the natural sphenoid ostium is reached.

The sphenoid step starts with the coagulation of the sphenoethmoid recess and the detachment of the nasal septum from the sphenoid prow using a

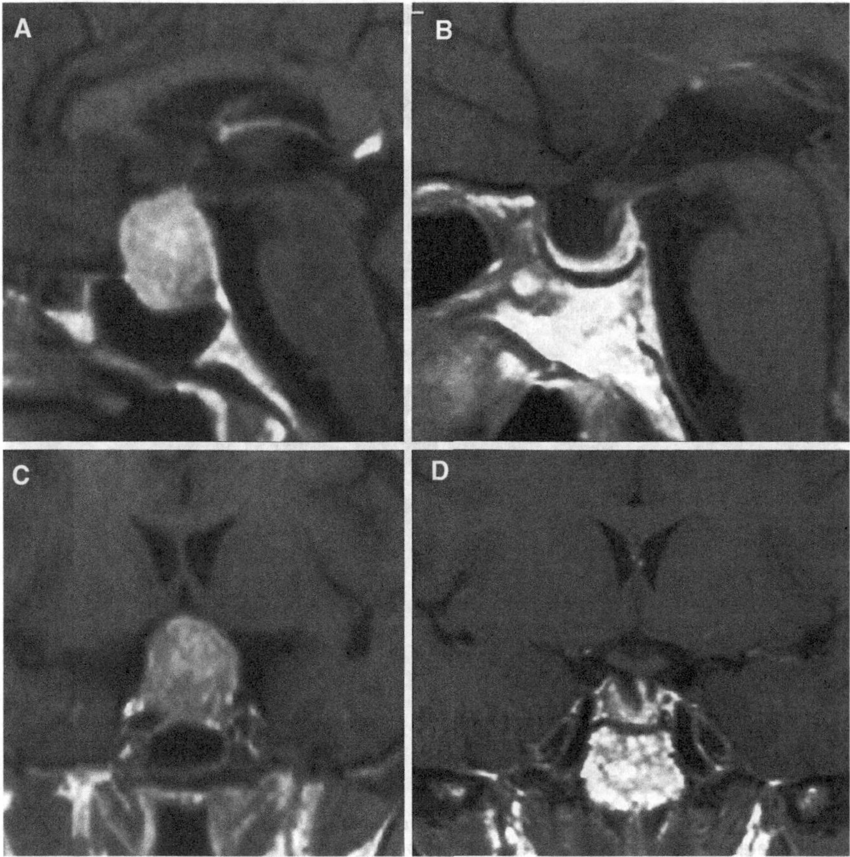

Fig. 10. Pre-operative (**A**, **C**) and post-operative (**B**, **D**) contrast-enhanced sellar MRI of a case of intra-suprasellar pituitary macroadenoma

microdrill. Once the anterior wall of the sphenoid sinus is exposed on both sides, it is removed all around with different bone punches.

During the sellar step, the endoscope can be held by a second surgeon in order to free both the surgeon's hands. Alternatively a longer scope (30 cm in length, 4 mm in diameter) can be used and fixed to an autostatic holder. The sellar floor is opened and the dura incised with a telescopic blade. The sellar lesion is then removed with different curettes depending on the size and position of the pituitary tumor (Fig. 10). After lesion removal the sellar floor is repaired, when necessary, with different autologous or heterologous or synthetic materials, according to the common guidelines.

The main advantages of the endoscopic procedure arise from the absence of the nasal speculum and from the use of the endoscope that discloses its bet-

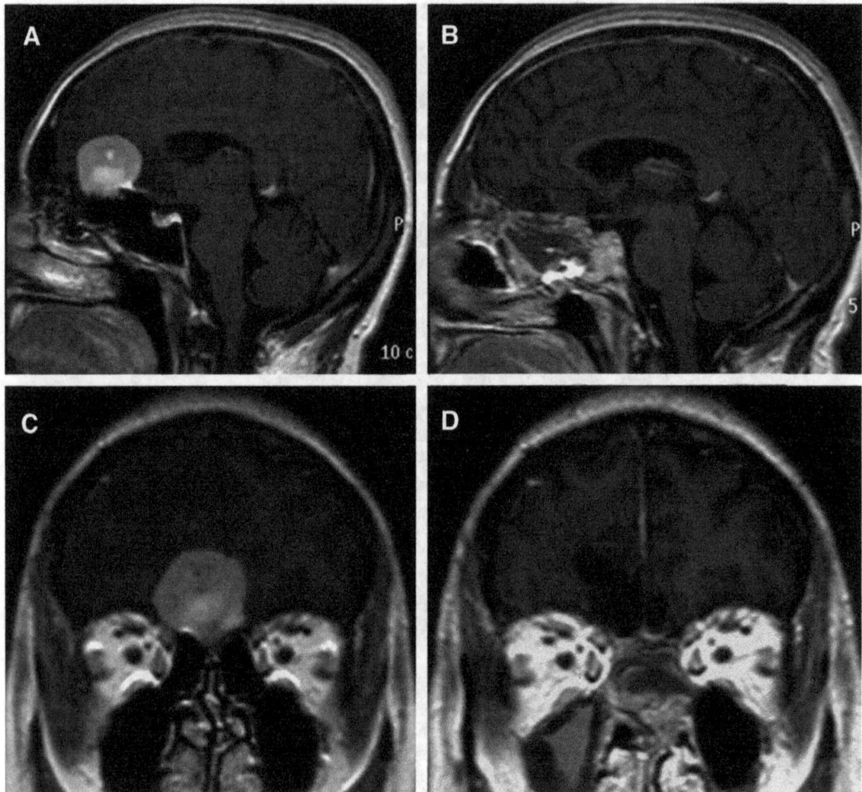

Fig. 11. Pre-operative (**A, C**) and post-operative (**B, D**) contrast-enhanced sellar MRI of a case of suprasellar (tuberculum sellae) meningioma

ter properties, permitting a wider vision of the surgical field, with a close-up "look" inside the anatomy. The whole procedure is less traumatic. No post-operative nasal packing is necessary thus improving significantly the patient's compliance [6].

With this standard transsphenoidal approach, however, it is difficult to provide complete visualization of the extrasellar lesions. To overcome this limitation, modifications of the approach have been developed for the removal of such lesions. The so-called extended transsphenoidal approach is a modification of the standard one, allowing for additional bone resection of cranial base to reach several areas from the "crista galli" to the craniocervical junction. This approach has become an alternative to transcranial surgery for several skull base tumors, such as suprasellar meningiomas (Fig. 11), craniopharyngiomas, clival chordomas, etc. [8].

ADVANTAGES AND RESTRICTIONS

The endoscope in neurosurgery is increasingly used as a minimally invasive treatment of a wide spectrum of intracranial pathologies [3, 4]. That reflects the current tendency of modern neurosurgery to aim towards minimalism, allowing for a less invasive treatment of neurosurgical pathologies. Endoscopic procedures encourage excellent compliance on the part of the patients, particularly those already operated on by a transcranial approach, who can compare the two experiences and appreciate the reduced postoperative discomfort. Often, through a single burr hole it is possible to manage several lesions through anatomical cavities. In such a way, obstructive hydrocephalus, intracranial cysts and some small intraventricular tumors can be easily removed. Concerning the use of the endoscope in transsphenoidal surgery, the wider vision offered by this device, not only of the sellar cavity but of the whole sellar and parasellar areas (clivus, planum, sphenoidale) and also around the sphenoid sinus (pterygo-maxillary fossa and cervico-medullary junction) caused an enlargement of the indications and of the extension of this approach, thus demanding new and more effective and sophisticated instruments to safer manage new situations [8].

Beside the many advantages provided by the use of the endoscope in neurosurgery, there are several limitations which should be not underestimated: (i) there is a steep learning curve before becoming confident with the peculiar neuroendoscopic anatomy; (ii) the initially reduced ability makes operative times longer (several hours during the first attempts); (iii) the endoscope provides bidimensional, flat images that are inferior to the three-dimensional images provided by the microscope; (iv) the endoscope offers vision on the video-monitor without the sense of deepness that can be gained with the surgeon's experience, executing in-and-out movements; (v) dedicated instruments, such as microforceps, microscissors, mono- and bipolar coagulation, ad hoc designed are absolutely essential; (vi) the bleeding control, either venous and arterial, may be difficult to obtain.

HOW TO AVOID COMPLICATIONS

Reducing the complication rate to 0% is a goal that is most of the times quite difficult to obtain. More realistic are the efforts towards minimizing the complications, specially the major ones, to an acceptable rate. In order to accomplish such task, several tips can be used and several tricks can be avoided.

1. The first important recommendation is to dedicate time and efforts to perform anatomical dissections and attend hands-on workshops to become confident with the surgical anatomy, fix the landmarks, learn how to handle the instruments and the endoscope, etc.

2. Play video games. In fact, it has been demonstrated that playing video games improves the eye–hand coordination, which is basic in endoscopic surgery.
3. Learn from the others' experience and try to avoid the complications already described.
4. Avoid quick movements in proximity to the surgical target.
5. The correct function of each component must be always checked before surgery.
6. Two complete sets of each endoscopic component should be available for each operation.
7. Work bimanually during the crucial steps of the endonasal procedure.

CONCLUSIONS

It is certainly true that the advent of endoscopy has produced ripples of enthusiasm and progress similar to those seen when a sizable stone is thrown into a relatively quiescent pound [6]. It is imperative that young neurosurgeons and residents become familiar and comfortable with the endoscopic techniques and hopefully they can contribute to the evolution and development of these surgical methods which are currently on their way. Despite the many advantages which have been clearly outlined previously, the endoscope has also many features that are currently suboptimal because of the cumbersome nature of the endoscopes themselves and of the lack of intelligently designed appropriately miniaturized instruments to complete the use of this wonderful viewing tool.

References

[1] Apuzzo ML, Heifetz MD, Weiss MH, Kurze T (1977) Neurosurgical endoscopy using the side-viewing telescope. J Neurosurg 46: 398-400

[2] Cappabianca P, Alfieri A, Thermes S, Buonamassa S, de Divitiis E (1999) Instruments for endoscopic endonasal transsphenoidal surgery. Neurosurgery 45: 392-395; discussion 395-396

[3] Cappabianca P, Cinalli G, Gangemi M, et al. (2008) Application of neuroendoscopy to intraventricular lesions. Neurosurgery 62(Suppl 2): SHC575-SHC598

[4] Cinalli G, Cappabianca P, de Falco R, Spennato P, Cianciulli E, Cavallo LM, Esposito F, Ruggiero C, Maggi G, de Divitiis E (2005) Current state and future development of intracranial neuroendoscopic surgery. Expert Rev Med Devices 2: 351-373

[5] Cockett WS, Cockett AT (1998) The Hopkins rod-lens system and the Storz cold light illumination system. Urology 51: 1-2

[6] de Divitiis E (2006) Endoscopic transsphenoidal surgery: stone-in-the-pond effect. Neurosurgery 59: 512-520

[7] de Divitiis E, Cappabianca P, Cavallo LM (2003) Endoscopic endonasal transsphenoidal approach to the sellar region. In: de Divitiis E, Cappabianca P (eds) Endoscopic endonasal transsphenoidal surgery. Springer, Wien New York, pp 91-130

[8] de Divitiis E, Cavallo LM, Cappabianca P, Esposito F (2007) Extended endoscopic endonasal transsphenoidal approach for the removal of suprasellar tumors: Part 2. Neurosurgery 60: 46-58; discussion 58-49

[9] Decq P, Le Guerinel C, Brugieres P, Djindjian M, Silva D, Keravel Y, Melon E, Nguyen JP (1998) Endoscopic management of colloid cysts. Neurosurgery 42: 1288-1294; discussion 1294-1286

[10] Engel RM (2003) Philipp Bozzini – the father of endoscopy. J Endourol 17: 859-862

[11] Fukushima T, Ishijima B, Hirakawa K, Nakamura N, Sano K (1973) Ventriculofiberscope: a new technique for endoscopic diagnosis and operation. Technical note. J Neurosurg 38: 251-256

[12] Grant JA (1996) Victor Darwin Lespinasse: a biographical sketch. Neurosurgery 39: 1232-1233

[13] Hellwig D, Grotenhuis JA, Tirakotai W, Riegel T, Schulte DM, Bauer BL, Bertalanffy H (2005) Endoscopic third ventriculostomy for obstructive hydrocephalus. Neurosurg Rev 28: 1-34; discussion 35-38

[14] Leonhard M, Cappabianca P, de Divitiis E (2003) The endoscope, endoscopic equipment and instrumentation. In: de Divitiis E, Cappabianca P (eds) Endoscopic endonasal transsphenoidal surgery. Springer, Wien New York, pp 9-19

[15] Mouton WG, Bessell JR, Maddern GJ (1998) Looking back to the advent of modern endoscopy: 150th birthday of Maximilian Nitze. World J Surg 22: 1256-1258

[16] Powell MP, Torrens MJ, Thomson JL, Horgan JG (1983) Isodense colloid cysts of the third ventricle: a diagnostic and therapeutic problem resolved by ventriculoscopy. Neurosurgery 13: 234-237

[17] Siomin V, Constantini S (2004) Basic principles and equipment in neuroendoscopy. Neurosurg Clin N Am 15: 19-31

[18] Walker ML (2001) History of ventriculostomy. Neurosurg Clin N Am 12: 101-110, viii

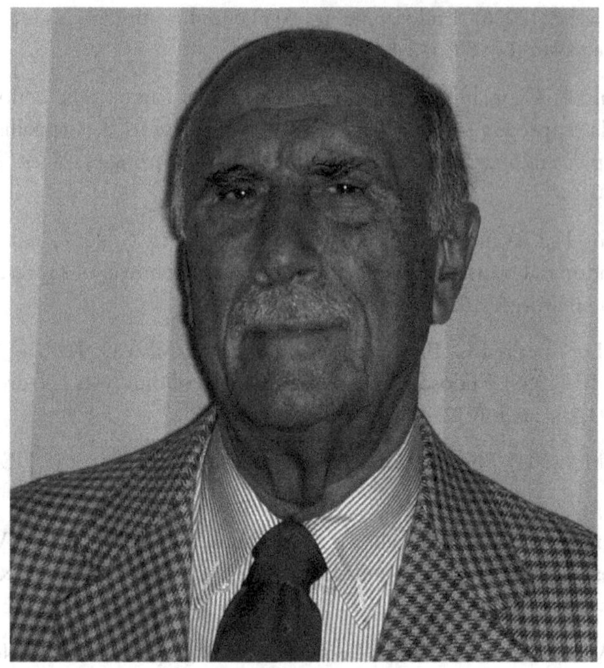

Enrico de Divitiis

Enrico de Divitiis is Professor and Chairman of Neurosurgery at the Università degli Studi di Napoli Federico II of Naples. He is chairman of the Italian Board of Neurosurgery Professors.

He is former president of the Italian Society of Neurosurgery (SINch) and member of many international scientific societies (American Association of Neurological Surgeons – AANS, Congress of Neurological Surgeons – CNS, Sociètè de Neurochirurgie de Langue Française – SNLF, European Society for Stereoctactic and Functional Neurosurgery – ESSFN). He is member of the editorial board of Neurosurgery, member of the advisory board of Operative Neurosurgery and of Journal of Neurosurgical Sciences and president of Italian College of University Neurosurgery Professors. He was organizer of twenty national and international congresses. He participated with personal communications in more than 420 national and international congresses, and has been invited speaker more than 200 times. He is author of more than 300 publications of neurosurgical interest, most of them reported in the Index Medicus/Current Contents/ Journal of Citation Reports, and of 18 books or book chapters.

Contact: Enrico de Divitiis, Department of Neurological Sciences, Division of Neurosurgery, Università degli Studi di Napoli Federico II, Via Sergio Pansini 5, 80131 Napoli, Italy
E-mail: dediviti@unina.it

IMAGE-GUIDED RADIOSURGERY USING THE GAMMA KNIFE

L. D. LUNSFORD

INTRODUCTION

Image guided brain surgery became a reality in the mid-1970s after the introduction of the first methods to obtain axial imaging using computed tomography (CT) [9]. The recognition of cranial disease much earlier in its clinical course prompted the need for concomitant minimally invasive technologies to both diagnose and to treat the newly recognized brain tumors and vascular malformations. Subsequently, the development of magnetic resonance imaging (MRI) spurred further interest in accurate, safe, and effective guided brain surgery. Stereotactic radiosurgery (SRS) was the brain child of the pioneering brain surgeons, Lars Leksell and Erik-Olof Backlund at the Karolinska Institute [4, 5]. Stereotactic guiding devices were adapted to newly evolving imaging techniques, ranging from encephalography to angiography, CT, and MRI. These new techniques prompted further evaluation of stereotactic radiosurgery, a field envisioned by Leksell in 1951. His concept that ionizing radiation could be cross fired to destroy or inactivate deep brain targets without a surgical opening proved to be an enormous step forward in minimally invasive surgery. Under the watchful eye of Leksell, Gamma knife technologies gradually expanded in their role and their usage exploded across the field of neurosurgery [1–3, 6–13].

Our efforts at the University of Pittsburgh began in 1987 with the introduction of the first 201 source Cobalt-60 Gamma knife, which was the fifth unit manufactured worldwide [7]. Since that time, more than 9000 patients have undergone Gamma knife radiosurgery at the University of Pittsburgh Medical Center. Our efforts first began with usage of the original U unit. Since 1987 we have introduced each successive generation of the Gamma knife, starting with the B unit, the robotic assisted C unit, the 4C unit which advanced software capabilities, and the next generation and fully robotic Perfexion® Gamma knife (Fig. 1). Continuing incorporation of new imaging techniques, advanced long-term outcome studies, and multi-disciplinary care have facilitated the incorporation of Gamma knife radiosurgery into its application to more than 10% of patients undergoing neurosurgical cranial procedures at our center. Radiosurgery has refined the role of more invasive surgical tech-

Keywords: radiosurgery, Gamma knife, image guided radiosurgery

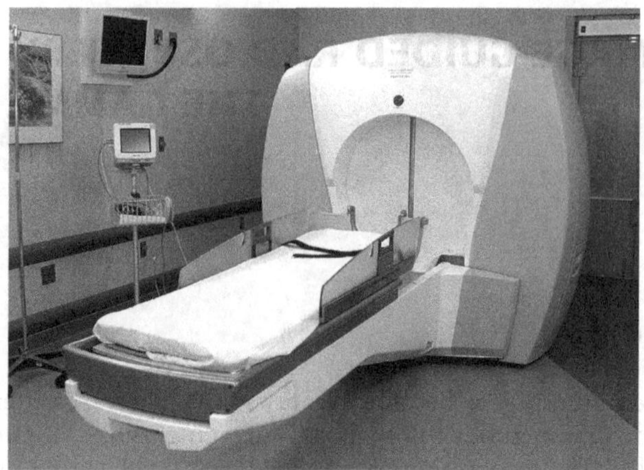

Fig. 1. The Leksell Perfexion Gamma Knife

niques and promoted better patient outcomes. When microsurgical brain surgery is incomplete because of the location or nature of the tumor, subsequent radiosurgery facilitates the ultimate goal: reduced morbidity, better clinical outcomes associated with long-term prevention of tumor growth, obliteration of vascular malformations, or non-invasive lesion creation in patients with movement disorders, chronic pain, or epilepsy.

RATIONALE

Stereotactic radiosurgery represents the penultimate model of image-guided and minimally invasive brain surgery. Using stereotactic guiding devices coupled with high resolution CT, MRI, positron emission tomography (PET) or magnetic source imaging, we can target critical brain structures. Decision making related to the role of radiosurgery has expanded during the more than 20 years of experience since its potential was first tested. Long-term outcome studies have confirmed the benefits of radiosurgery as a primary therapeutic option for many primary brain tumors, especially those of the skull base, and brain metastases, as well as various functional neurosurgery indications such as trigeminal neuralgia, essential tremor, obsessive compulsive disorders, and mesial temporal lobe epilepsy. SRS has a major role in the adjuvant treatment of subtotally removed tumors of the skull base, selected glial neoplasms, and residual or recurrent pituitary tumors. For surgeons involved in the use of SRS, a different goal of patient management was needed: tumor control as opposed to tumor elimination *plus* patients with a stable or improved neurological examination.

Extensive studies at our center and many others have confirmed the role of Gamma knife radiosurgery in the management of many benign skull base tu-

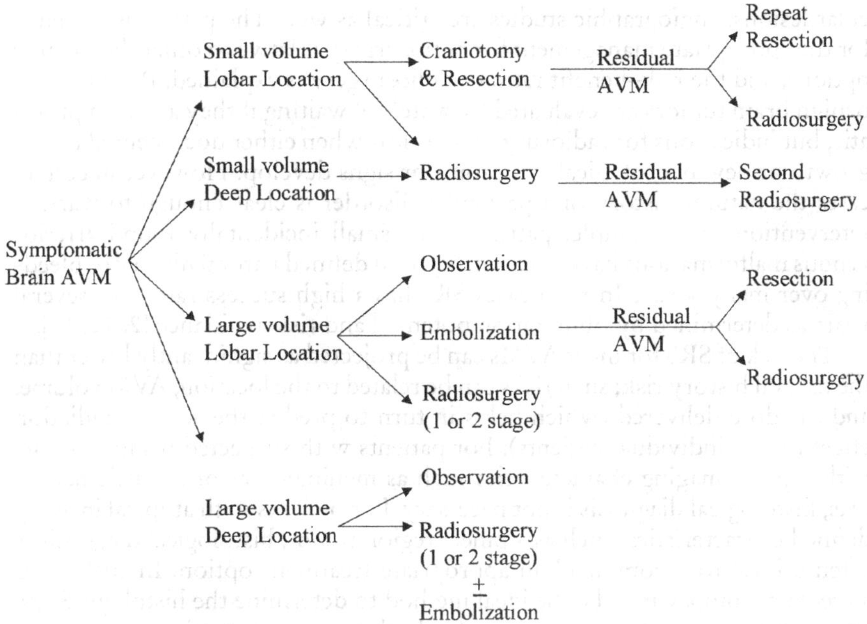

Fig. 2. A decision tree for selection of management options for patients with arteriovenous malformations. Similar decision tree analyses that can be used for skull base tumors, brain metastasis, and trigeminal neuralgia are available via the internet on the National Guidelines Clearinghouse

mors such as acoustic and other non acoustic neuromas, meningiomas, and pituitary tumors. Its use in the primary cost effective care of patients with metastatic cancer to brain is now well established [1, 13]. SRS is successful in the care of the majority of patients with brain metastases that are not associated with extensive mass effect at the time of clinical recognition. Finally, emerging indications for radiosurgery include management of epilepsy, a resurgence of interest in medically refractory behavioral disorders, and even in the potential treatment of patients with obesity. All discussions related to the role of radiosurgery are based on an analysis of the risks or benefits of observation, alternative surgical techniques, the potential role of fractionated radiation therapy and chemotherapy (for malignant tumors) in comparison to what defined benefits of SRS are feasible. A typical decision making analysis is shown in Fig. 2 relative to the management of arteriovenous malformations.

1. THE TECHNIQUE OF GAMMA KNIFE STEREOTACTIC RADIOSURGERY

Patients are evaluated during clinical consultation, at which time we review all pertinent imaging studies. Such studies generally include high resolution MRI for tumors or in preparation for functional procedures. For patients with vascular lesions, angiographic studies are critical as well. The patient is screened for the appropriate management for radiosurgery relative to other therapeutic options, and the risk–benefit ratio of radiosurgery is explained. Patients with benign brain tumors are evaluated by watchful waiting if they are asymptomatic, but indications for radiosurgery are clear when either documented tumor growth or new neurological symptoms or signs develop. However in certain cases the natural history of a particular disorder is clear enough to warrant intervention. For example, patients with small incidentally found arteriovenous malformations have a reasonably well defined natural history of bleeding over many years. In such cases SRS has a high success rate over several years as determined by obliteration potential and risk avoidance [2, 10, 11].

The risk of SRS for most AVMs can be projected as significantly lower than the natural history risk; such risks can be related to the location, AVM volume, and the dose delivered (which helps in turn to predict the adverse radiation effect risk in individual patients). For patients with suspected benign tumors with typical imaging characteristics such as meningiomas or acoustic neuromas, histological diagnosis is not necessary. For patients with atypical imaging defined characteristics, such as a pineal region tumor, histological diagnosis is often critical to recommend an appropriate treatment option. In such cases stereotactic biopsy may be the ideal method to determine the histology. Since we use the same stereotactic system for both open stereotactic surgery as we do in radiosurgical cases, in selected cases a patient may undergo diagnosis and treatment in the same sitting. This requires excellent neuropathological expertise to confirm the clinical suspicion during the procedure itself.

Radiosurgery has primary indications in the management of arteriovenous malformations unsuitable for microsurgical intervention, a primary management role in the care of skull base tumors such as acoustic neuromas and meningiomas, an adjuvant role in the management of most patients with pituitary tumors, and a primary role in the management of metastatic cancer to the brain. Additional adjuvant roles include boost radiosurgery in patients who have malignant glial neoplasms that have progressed despite prior management.

DECISION-MAKING

Indications and results are briefly summarized below.

1. ARTERIOVENOUS MALFORMATIONS

At our center, 1300 patients with vascular malformations of the brain have undergone radiosurgery in a 21 year interval. In properly selected patients, the goal of obliteration can be achieved in between 70–95% of patients, depending on the volume and the dose that can be delivered safely. Radiosurgery is especially valuable for deep-seated AVMs for which there is no other microsurgical option. At the present time, embolization strategies as part of the spectrum of options for arteriovenous malformations facilitates flow reduction but not volume reduction. Because of this, its role in preparation for conventional stereotactic radiosurgery has remained controversial. In the future, embolization strategies that facilitate the radiobiological response of subsequent radiosurgery may be more beneficial. For dural vascular malformations, radiosurgery followed immediately by embolization of the fistulous connections is a better staged strategy that provides both short term (early embolization benefit) and long-term response (as the radiosurgical obliterative response develops). SRS needs to precede the embolization so that the entire target can be visualized.

At our center we preferentially place the stereotactic frame, target the dural AVM using MRI and angiography, perform SRS, and immediately return the patient to the interventional suite with a femoral sheath in place to complete the embolization procedure.

Cavernous malformations that have bled twice and are located in deep seated brain locations respond to radiosurgery with a slow reduction in their subsequent bleeding rate, within a latency interval generally of approximately two years. Our studies have confirmed that once a patient has bled twice from a cavernous malformation, the annual rate of a third or additional bleeds may be as high as 33% per year. After two years, the annual bleed risk diminishes to less than 1% per year. Developmental venous anomalies, which are often seen adjacent to cavernous malformations are never treated by SRS. Occlusion of these aberrant venous drainage channels runs the risk of venous infarction.

2. SKULL BASE TUMORS

More than 1300 acoustic neuromas have undergone radiosurgery at our center. Over the course of the last 20 years, radiosurgery has become a primary management strategy for small to medium sized acoustic neuromas, achieving facial nerve preservation rates in virtually all patients, a 50–70% chance of preservation of hearing levels, and a rapid return to pre-radiosurgical employment and lifestyle. The long-term tumor control rate is 98% in patients who undergo radiosurgery with doses of 12–13 Gy at the tumor margin [12]. Highly conformal and selective radiosurgery is possible using the Gamma knife which allows this procedure to be done in a single session with precise intracranial guidance and stereotactic head frame fixation (Fig. 3).

Skull base meningiomas similarly can be treated, and have responded well. In a series of more than 1000 meningiomas treated over the last 21 years long-term tumor growth control rates are achieved in more than 95% of patients with low grade meningiomas [3]. Radiosurgery is an adjuvant management strategy for patients with more aggressive Grade II or malignant Grade III men-

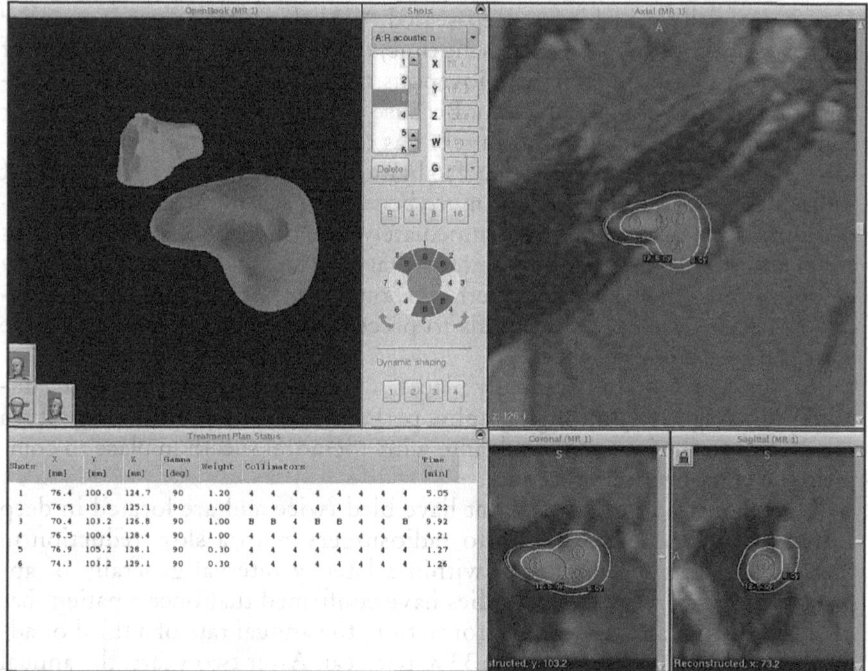

Fig. 3. Dose plan for an acoustic neuroma

ingiomas, but such tumors require multimodality management. Outcomes may require multiple surgical procedures, SRS, and fractionated radiation therapy.

Pituitary adenomas are generally managed first by transsphenoidal resection. However, for tumors that are recurrent or residual after surgery, or located primarily de novo in the cavernous sinus, Gamma knife radiosurgery may be a primary option. It is very effective in preventing tumor growth control, but higher doses are necessary to achieve endocrine relapse for patients who have endocrine active tumors such as growth hormone or ACTH secreting tumors. With current highly conformal and selective dose planning techniques, pituitary radiosurgery is possible immediately adjacent to the optic chiasm – as long as the dose to the optic apparatus is kept below 8–10 Gy in a single procedure. SRS also has a very important role in the management of other lower skull base tumors, especially tumors involving the jugular bulb, the trigeminal nerve, and as an adjuvant management in the treatment of aggressive chondrosarcomas or chordomas of the skull base.

3. METASTATIC CANCER

In 2500 patients who have undergone radiosurgery for metastatic cancer, we have found that long-term tumor growth control rate can be achieved in most patients without the need for invasive brain surgery. Depending on the tumor primary, long-term tumor control rates are achieved between 67 and 95% of patients [1]. Most patients now die of systemic disease rather than intracranial progression, a major shift in the paradigm of management of metastatic cancer affecting the brain. SRS has additional major benefits in comparison to other conventional therapies. As a single day procedure, during which multiple brain metastases can be treated, it does not delay the concomitant use of chemotherapy or radiation techniques that are needed to improve control of the systemic cancer.

We have not detected major differences in survivals in patients with one to four brain metastases. Long-term survivals have been confirmed in breast, lung, renal, and melanoma metastatic disease, especially when control of systemic disease is obtained. For patients with non small cell lung cancer with a solitary brain metastasis, median survivals often exceed two years. We cannot confirm that additional fractionated external beam radiation therapy improves survival, because repeat SRS is used for salvage management if new brain disease develops. For patients with long-term survival potential, elimination of the late cognitive disorders after whole brain radiation therapy is highly desirable.

Surgical removal is necessary for patients with large metastatic tumors who have symptomatic mass effect at the time of presentation. Tumor bed radiosurgery can be used to treat the peritumoral cavity in order to reduce the risk of delayed local recurrence as well as to avoid the long-term risks of whole brain radiation therapy. The new Perfexion model Gamma knife is an ideal tool for the treatment of multiple brain metastases scattered in widely different areas of the brain.

4. GLIAL NEOPLASMS

At our center more than 700 patients have been treated for brain gliomas ranging from Grade I to Grade IV. SRS can be considered as a primary management strategy for residual or recurrent primarily solid pilocytic astrocytomas. It is especially valuable for patients without cystic changes and achieves local control in more than 85% of patients. SRS is an alternative option for the management of small volume, sharply bordered Grade II tumors (astrocytomas and oligodendrogliomas). Such tumors are defined with high definition MRI using both contrast enhanced T1 and T2 studies. SRS is considered as an adjuvant strategy to provide boost radiation in patients with malignant gliomas, generally those patients who have failed conventional management with surgery, radiation and chemotherapy.

5. FUNCTIONAL NEUROSURGERY

Gamma knife SRS, which facilitates application of small volume, very precise lesions within the brain, has been used effectively in more than 800 patients with trigeminal neuralgia at our center. Long-term results indicate that 70–90% of patients achieve pain control. Results are best for patients who have failed medical management for typical trigeminal neuralgia, but who have not failed a prior surgical procedure. The typical dose is 80 Gy using a 4 mm collimator to focus the beams at the root entry zone of the trigeminal nerve as defined by volumetric MRI, including 1 mm T2 volume slices to define the nerve. In selected cases CT imaging is used to define the nerve if the patient cannot have an MRI because of prior surgery or other medical issues such as a prior pacemaker placement. The latency until pain relief is between a few days and several months, during which time medicines are slowly tapered as pain control is achieved. SRS can be repeated for patients who develop a relapse. Trigeminal radiosurgery is most often used for patients with typical trigeminal neuralgia who are elderly or have medical co-morbidities that make them poor candidates for microvascular decompression. We prefer SRS to percutaneous pain management strategies as an initial treatment for appropriate patients because it has a high success rate and a low risk of delayed trigeminal sensory loss (less than 10% of patients develop changes in facial sensation).

Since its first development of radiosurgery in 1967, the Gamma knife has been used to create selective deep seated brain lesions for advanced movement disorders, especially essential tremor. Typically a radiosurgical dose of 120–140 Gy is delivered to the ventrolateral nucleus of the thalamus as identified by high resolution MRI. As a closed skull procedure physiological confirmation of the anatomically defined target is not possible. If bilateral symptoms are noted, we typically wait at least one year before proceeding with a contralateral thalamic lesion. Since the procedure does not require reversal of anticoagulants or antiplatelet agents, GK SRS is especially valuable for patients not eligible for deep brain stimulator implantation. The interval for full lesion development is typically 3–6 months.

Leksell originally proposed development of the Gamma knife in order to create 4–6 mm lesions in the anterior internal capsule in patients with advanced medically refractory behavioral disorders such as severe anxiety neuroses and obsessive-compulsive disorders. New investigative techniques are under evaluation for the possible role of radiosurgery for temporal lobe epilepsy and for chronic obesity (ventrolateral hypothalamotomy). At present both animal models and patient experience indicate that radiosurgery for medial temporal lobe epilepsy achieves comparable Engel class I results to microsurgical hippocampectomy, with a latency of about one year until the full effect occurs.

SURGICAL TECHNIQUE

The patient is brought into the hospital as an outpatient and given mild intravenous conscious sedation using Medazaolam and Fentanyl. Under

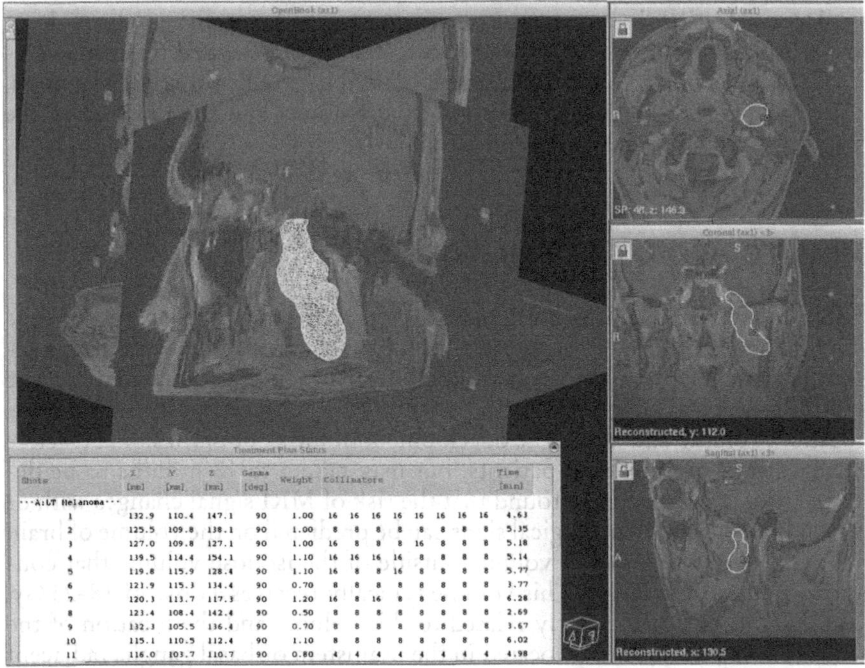

Fig. 4. Patient with metastatic melanoma tracking via the trigeminal nerve from the maxillary sinus region to the cavernous sinus. This patient had already failed local radiation and immune therapy

local anesthesia (a mixture of marcaine and xylocaine), the Leksell Model G stereotactic head frame is attached to the head using titanium pins. Appropriate frame shifting is based on the location of the target. Frame shifting is less important using the new Perfexion Gamma Knife which facilitates treatment of patients with lesions scattered throughout the brain or even in the inferior skull base and paranasal sinuses. We currently use both the Leksell 4-C and Leksell Gamma Knife Perfexion Units, which maximizes the precision and appropriate robotic positioning. Patients subsequently undergo high resolution imaging, most commonly MRI or CT for patients ineligible to have an MRI scan. Lower skull base lesions have generally both MRI and CT imaging performed (Fig. 4). Image fusion is used frequently for enhanced recognition of selective targets. Using the new Perfexion unit, extracranial disease can be treated effectively. Dose planning is performed using high speed workstations, and final treatment decisions are made by an experienced medical team including neurological surgery, radiation oncology and medical physics. Extracranial disease may also require consultation with appropriate colleagues in otolargyngology or head and neck surgery.

Dose selection is based on extensive experience published throughout the world's literature. The maximal dose, marginal dose, and isodose selected to cover the margin are based and modified by the histological diagnosis, the expected radiobiological response, the volume, and the location of the target.

HOW TO AVOID COMPLICATIONS

After undergoing Gamma knife radiosurgery, patients are discharged on the day of the procedure. Other than mild headache after stereotactic frame removal, patients are able to resume their regular activities immediately. The risk of long-term adverse radiation effects (ARE) are related to lesion type, location, volume and dose. The development of intra- or perilesional reactive changes vary in individual patients, but may take 3 to 18 months to be detected. For AVMs we have found that the risk of MRI signal changes with or without associated neurological signs can be predicted on the volume of brain receiving 12 Gy or more, a volume outside of the isodose volume that conforms to the AVM target. This volume typically receives a dose of 18–23 Gy. The risk of ARE are directly related to this volume and the location of the AVM. As expected, AVMs located in the brainstem or basal ganglia (adjacent to the internal capsule) are more likely to have either temporary or permanent new neurological symptoms. Prior exposure to radiation may also increase the chance of subsequent ARE after radiosurgery. It is also estimated that 4% of the normal population may have special sensitivity to radiation, and are therefore more likely to suffer ARE. Typical imaging sequences performed on most patients include scans at six months, one year, two years and four years for assessment of response. Both tumor growth control is assessed as well as the risk of developing peritumoral reactive changes. Such changes may have minimal contrast enhancement but prolonged T2 signal changes compatible with edema formation. Such patients are treated with a brief course of corticosteroids.

Long-term risks of radiation necrosis are detected by serial imaging. To date, no additional imaging technologies including PET or SPECT has been particularly useful in sorting out tumor response versus radiation injury. For patients who have long-term effects suggestive of radiation injury after a corticosteroid trial of approximately two weeks, we try to switch patients to a combination of oral vitamin E and Trental. This is continued for approximately three months. Long-term risks published in our experience suggests that the risk of adverse radiation effects range from 3–10%. We have found that certain indications have a higher risk of ARE. For example, cavernous malformations have a higher risk of ARE at doses that do not have such risks when an AVM is treated. We suspect that chronic iron deposition in the gliotic brain surrounding the cavernous malformation may serve as a radiation sensitizer. When a dose reduction was instituted for cavernous malformations, the ARE risk declined substantially.

The ability to minimize risks can best be enhanced by highly conformal and highly selective treatment plans and selection of the appropriate dose, modified by the volume and the radiobiological response. Fortunately, multiple outcome studies have now confirmed the necessary doses that are required to achieve the overall radiobiological goal. Over the course of 20 years, a gradual dose de-escalation strategy has significantly reduced complications. It is likely that further dose de-escalation will have an adverse effect in terms of long-term tumor growth control, and therefore it is likely that in the future, to enhance tumor response for more aggressive tumors, a gradual dose escalation study will be necessary.

CONCLUSIONS

Stereotactic Gamma knife radiosurgery based on a discussion of comprehensive selection options and precise high resolution intraoperative management, is a critical component of modern neurosurgery. It is estimated that 10% of all neurosurgery, and as much as 15–20% of all intracranial brain surgery can be most safely and best performed using stereotactic radiosurgical techniques. The Gamma knife represents a technology which has been applied in more than 500,000 patients worldwide, with more than 400 outcome studies presented from our center alone over the last 20 years. Proper patient selection, review of appropriate treatment options, and a risk–benefit analysis are critical in the selection of any neurosurgical procedure. Radiosurgery using the Gamma knife represents an important technology that is now firmly established in the field of contemporary brain surgery.

References

[1] Bhatnagar AK, Flickinger JC, Kondziolka D, Lunsford LD (2006) Stereotactic radiosurgery for four or more intracranial metastases. Int J Radiat Oncol Biol Phys 64: 898-903

[2] Flickinger JC, Kondziolka D, Lunsford LD, Pollock BE, Yamamoto M, Gorman DA, et al. (1999) A multi-institutional analysis of complication outcomes after arteriovenous malformation radiosurgery. Int J Radiat Oncol Biol Phys 44: 67-74

[3] Kondziolka D, Mathieu D, Lunsford LD, Martin JJ, Madhok R, Niranjan A, et al. (2008) Radiosurgery as definitive management of intracranial meningiomas. Neurosurgery 62: 53-58; discussion 58-60

[4] Lunsford LD (1996) Lars Leksell. Notes at the side of a raconteur. Stereotact Funct Neurosurg 67: 153-168

[5] Lunsford LD (1993) Stereotactic radiosurgery: at the threshold or at the crossroads? Neurosurgery 32: 799-804

[6] Lunsford LD, Flickinger J, Coffey RJ (1990) Stereotactic Gamma knife radiosurgery. Initial North American experience in 207 patients. Arch Neurol 47: 169-175

[7] Lunsford LD, Flickinger J, Lindner G, Maitz A (1989) Stereotactic radiosurgery of the brain using the first United States 201 cobalt-60 source Gamma knife. Neurosurgery 24: 151-159

[8] Lunsford LD, Kondziolka D, Bissonette DJ, Maitz AH, Flickinger JC (1992) Stereotactic radiosurgery of brain vascular malformations. Neurosurg Clin N Am 3: 79-98

[9] Lunsford LD, Martinez AJ (1984) Stereotactic exploration of the brain in the era of computed tomography. Surg Neurol 22: 222-230

[10] Pollock BE, Flickinger JC, Lunsford LD, Bissonette DJ, Kondziolka D (1996) Factors that predict the bleeding risk of cerebral arteriovenous malformations. Stroke 27: 1-6

[11] Pollock BE, Flickinger JC, Lunsford LD, Bissonette DJ, Kondziolka D (1996) Hemorrhage risk after stereotactic radiosurgery of cerebral arteriovenous malformations. Neurosurgery 38: 652-659; discussion 659-661

[12] Pollock BE, Lunsford LD, Kondziolka D, Flickinger JC, Bissonette DJ, Kelsey SF, et al. (1995) Outcome analysis of acoustic neuroma management: a comparison of microsurgery and stereotactic radiosurgery. Neurosurgery 36: 215-224; discussion 224-219

[13] Rutigliano MJ, Lunsford LD, Kondziolka D, Strauss MJ, Khanna V, Green M (1995) The cost effectiveness of stereotactic radiosurgery versus surgical resection in the treatment of solitary metastatic brain tumors. Neurosurgery 37: 445-453; discussion 453-445

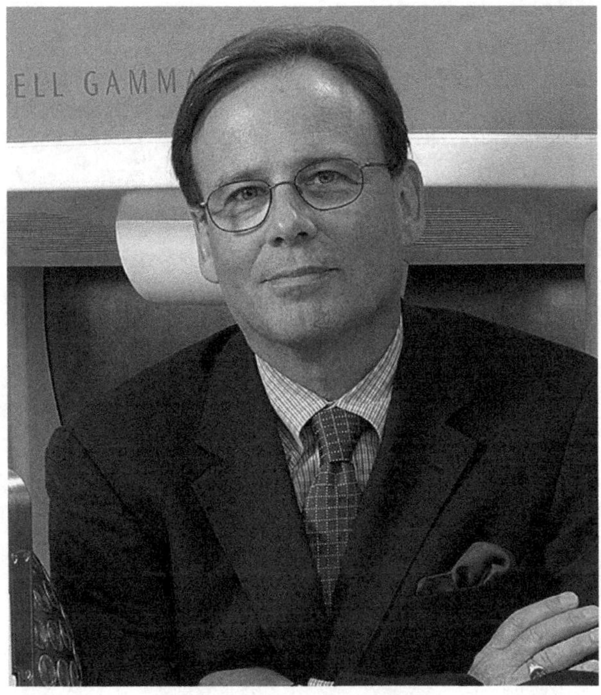

L. Dade Lunsford

L. Dade Lunsford, MD, FACS, is Lars Leksell Professor of Neurological Surgery, Distinguished Professor University of Pittsburgh, Director of the Center for Image Guided Neurosurgery, and Director of the Neurosurgery Residency Program at the University of Pennsylvania at Pittsburgh. He completed medical school at Columbia University College of Physicians and Surgeons, residency training in neurosurgery at the University of Pittsburgh, and fellowship training in stereotactic technologies and radiosurgery at the Karolinska Institute. Dr. Lunsford's primary interests are related to image-guided surgery, innovation in brain tumor management, stereotactic radiosurgery, and patient long-term outcome studies related to the use of modern minimally invasive technologies. His basic science and clinical studies have helped to substantiate the role of radiosurgery and other minimally invasive techniques in the armamentarium of modern neurosurgery.

Contact: L. Dade Lunsford, University of Pittsburgh Medical Center, Presbyterian B400, 200 Lothrop Street, Pittsburgh, PA 15213, USA
E-mail: lunsfordld@upmc.edu

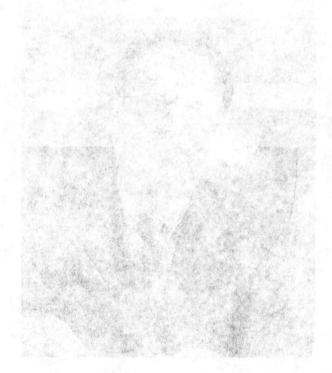

HOW TO PERFORM SURGERY FOR INTRACRANIAL (CONVEXITY) MENINGIOMAS

P. M. BLACK

INTRODUCTION

Convexity meningiomas are important tumors historically and in contemporary neurosurgery. Felix Plater provided their first recognizable description in 1614 and the first successful surgical removal was by Pecchioli in Siena in 1847 [10]. It was Cushing in 1922 who decided to group many previous meningeal tumors under the general name "meningioma". In the 1920s, Cushing also established techniques for their removal that became the standard for these tumors. Walter Dandy, Leo Davidoff, Colin McCarty, Lindsay Simon, Jacques Philippon, Giovanni Broggi, Charles Wilson, Ossama Al-Mefty, Robert Ojemann, and many others are among the surgeons who have carried forward the understanding of their optimum care in the twentieth century [1]. In the last decade, improved imaging, navigation, and concepts of minimally invasive surgery have begun to create a quiet revolution in the management of these tumors [2].

RATIONALE

1. *Goal of management*. The goal of management is to relieve brain compression without damaging cortical veins or compressed cortex and to prevent recurrence of tumor.

2. *Location and anatomy*. Convexity meningiomas originate in the meninges of the cerebral hemispheres; they constituted 51% of the author's series of 807 meningiomas [1]. It is historically believed that they arise from arachnoid cap cells. The arachnoid layer is often intact, making their removal from eloquent cortex possible without deficit; however, for large meningiomas or for atypical and anaplastic meningiomas, there may be significant disruption of the arachnoid and adherence or invasion to the brain tissue. These tumors may often be very large before they are detected. They produce symptoms by compression of the brain under them – if above motor cortex, contralateral weakness; for vision, visual field loss; for frontal or temporal speech areas, aphasia. They also may cause seizures.

Keywords: intracranial tumors, meningiomas, convexity meningiomas, microsurgery

DECISION-MAKING

1. DIAGNOSIS

The diagnosis of a convexity meningioma is usually made by CT or MRI scanning. Contrast material is necessary to see the tumor appropriately – without contrast, it may be almost invisible as its signal characteristics are very similar to those of the brain. Meningiomas are dural-based lesions with well-circumscribed margins that indent the brain but do not invade it. They are very characteristic but may occasionally be mimicked by a dural-based metastasis or even inflammation such as sarcoidosis. They may cause significant hyperostosis of overlying bone, a feature that confirms meningioma as the diagnosis (Fig. 1). Other imaging modalities do not contribute significantly to the routine diagnosis. If there is an important differential with metastasis, however, PET scanning with somatostatin receptors can establish the diagnosis definitively.

2. INDICATIONS FOR SURGERY

The major therapeutic options for convexity meningiomas are to observe or remove them. Unlike some skull base meningiomas, radiation including radiosurgery is not usually considered an option in the primary care of these tumors. An exception may be in an elderly patient with severe medical problems contraindicating surgery. Many convexity meningiomas, especially in patients over the age of 65, can simply be observed. There is about a 35% chance that they will grow over a five-year period [13]. Our general approach is to observe many convexity meningiomas as the first treatment; however,

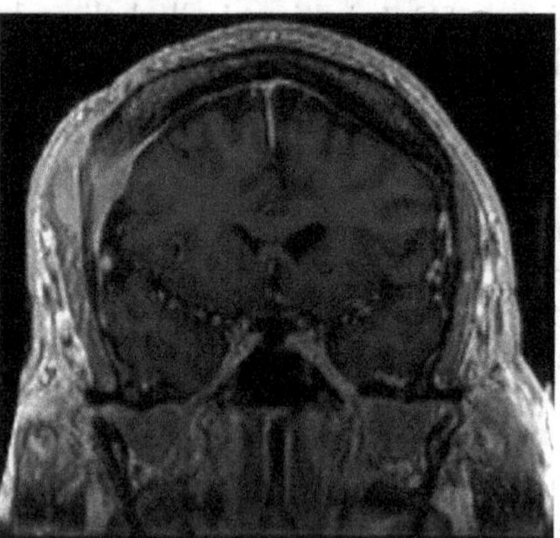

Fig. 1. Convexity meningioma which has also eroded through bone

there are certain conditions which indicate that surgery should be done as the initial step.

Indications for surgery at our center are as follows:

1. Symptoms attributable to tumor compression
2. Demonstrated growth with sequential scans
3. Size over 4 cm diameter
4. Apparent invasion of brain
5. Significant peritumoral edema
6. Patient preference
7. Need for diagnosis

Our decision-making algorithm is as follows:

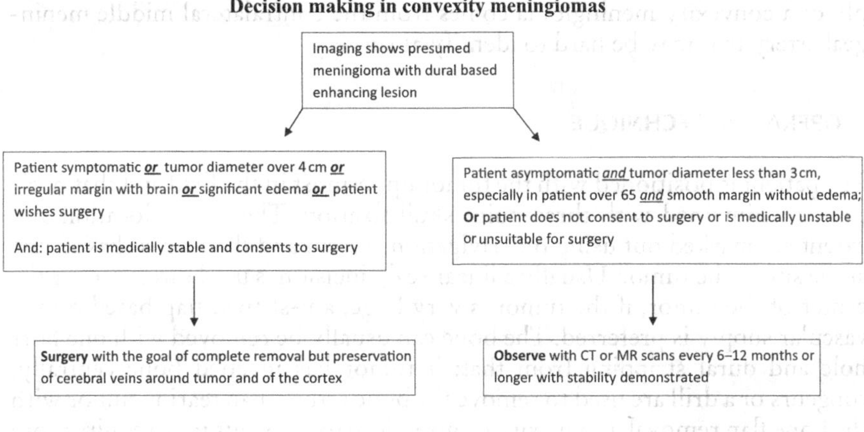

Decision making in convexity meningiomas
Imaging shows presumed meningioma with dural based enhancing lesion
Patient symptomatic or tumor diameter over 4 cm or irregular margin with brain or significant edema or patient wishes surgery
And: patient is medically stable and consents to surgery
Patient asymptomatic and tumor diameter less than 3 cm, especially in patient over 65 and smooth margin without edema;
Or patient does not consent to surgery or is medically unstable or unsuitable for surgery
Surgery with the goal of complete removal but preservation of cerebral veins around tumor and of the cortex
Observe with CT or MR scans every 6–12 months or longer with stability demonstrated

3. PREOPERATIVELY, THERE ARE SEVERAL TESTS THAT SHOULD BE DONE AND QUESTIONS THAT SHOULD BE ANSWERED

1. Do I have the imaging I need? Can I see the veins around the tumor on the MRI? Is the MRI an appropriate scan for navigation? (We have found that a navigation system is extremely helpful for minimally invasive resection of these lesions including bone flap planning and identification of veins.)
2. Should embolization be carried out preoperatively? (In general, we embolize only very large or apparently very vascular tumors, fewer than 5% of our convexity meningiomas.)
3. Is the patient medically stable and are the patient's blood tests including coagulation studies acceptable?
4. Has appropriate surgical consent been obtained?

SURGERY

1. PREPARATION

Most of our convexity meningiomas are now done with the help of a navigation system that assures accurate localization of the tumor. Preoperatively, it is important to assure the proper scan sequences are done and they have been loaded into the system satisfactorily.

For the removal, an ultrasonic aspirator is usually helpful and loop cautery may be useful. For very vascular tumors, the contact YAG laser can help resect with hemostasis. The operating microscope is helpful for relation to the brain.

In our experience, embolization has only been needed in tumors over 5 cm that appear hypervascular on preoperative MR. Sometimes the vascular supply of a convexity meningioma comes from the contralateral middle meningeal artery that may be hard to identify at surgery.

2. OPERATIVE TECHNIQUE

The patient is positioned with the tumor uppermost in the field and that position is maintained with three-point skull fixation. The tumor location and extent are marked out using the navigation system and the hair is shaved just at the site of the tumor. Usually a linear scalp incision is used directly over the center of the tumor; if the tumor is very large, a u-shaped flap based on the vascular supply is preferred. The bone can usually be removed with one burr hole and dural stripping from that; if tumor has invaded bone centrally, rongeurs or a drill are used to remove the bone rather than tearing tumor with the bone flap removal. Convexity tumors close to the sinus may require more careful stripping of dura from bone.

We take care not to open the dura initially much beyond the tumor margin to prevent venous congestion and infarction. It is extremely important to watch for cortical veins as the dura is opened; a cottonoid patty placed over the brain surface as the dura is opened is a useful technique. The dura is the origin of the tumor, so it is removed with the lesion. After the tumor is removed, it may be possible to get a wider excision margin, and we aim for a 1 cm margin if possible, taking all the dural tail seen on preoperative imaging.

Before removing a large tumor from the brain surface, it is important to internally core out the tumor with a loop cautery or cavitron; this allows internal decompression and gradual dissection from even eloquent cortex rather than trying to mobilize a large mass. Great care should be taken to avoid veins surrounding the tumor and to be as gentle as possible with the brain surface. Lifting up on the tumor as you dissect it from brain is potentially dangerous because deep white matter tends to come with it.

For dural closure, we replace the dura with pericranium or Alloderm (LifeCell, Branchburg, NJ), making a watertight closure. We avoid cadaver or bovine tissue because of the potential problem of slow viral infection.

We replace the bone flap with a plating system to hold it in place. If it is extensively involved with tumor, we will use a methylmethacrylate cranioplasty; if there is partial involvement, we will drill out the area that is hyperostotic. Postoperatively the patient is cared for in the neurosurgical ICU for an average of one night before returning to the ward. The average length of hospital stay is 3 days.

3. LONG-TERM RESULTS

Most convexity meningiomas can be completely removed; occasionally because of their proximity to the sagittal sinus or to cerebral veins they cannot be resected completely. We achieved a Simpson Grade I removal in more than 95% of convexity meningiomas, a finding similar to others [3, 4, 6, 11].

Recurrence. Several studies have evaluated the effect of tumor removal on recurrence – the most comprehensive is that of Jaaskelainen et al., who found a recurrence rate of 3% at 5 years for benign tumors completely removed, 9% at 10 years and 21% at 25 years [3].

Since most convexity tumors can have a Simpson Grade I removal, they provide an important test of the role of histological grade in recurrence. We noted that 88.3% of our convexity tumors were grade 1, 9.8% grade 2, and 1.8% grade 3. If the benign tumors in our series were separated into those that were completely benign and those that had some atypical features, the recurrence rate for the benign group was zero, whereas the "borderline atypical" group had a 5-year recurrence rate of 33%, which is in the same range as the atypical tumors. Grade 3 tumors had a recurrence rate of 78% at five years. Thus for convexity tumors the biology of the tumor is the most important criterion for recurrence [9].

Several authors have reviewed histological features that predict recurrence; chief among them is the MIB-1 or other proliferative index [5, 7, 12].

Adjunctive therapy. Radiation may be a useful adjunctive therapy for grade 2 and 3 meningiomas of the convexity. Our approach is to irradiate all grade 3 meningiomas after the first operation but for other histological grades to select cases on an individual basis depending on the decision of our tumor board.

In our series, 3 of 16 patients with grade 2 meningiomas (18%) received adjuvant radiation following initial surgery. These tumors did not recur within the time period of our study, whereas 4 patients who did not receive initial adjuvant radiation after the initial operation later required radiation for recurrent tumors.

There is controversy about postoperative radiation therapy. Modha and Gutin suggest that all grade 3 tumors, and grade 2 tumors subtotally excised, with brain invasion or with an MIB-1 index of ≥4.2% should be treated with fractionated radiotherapy [8].

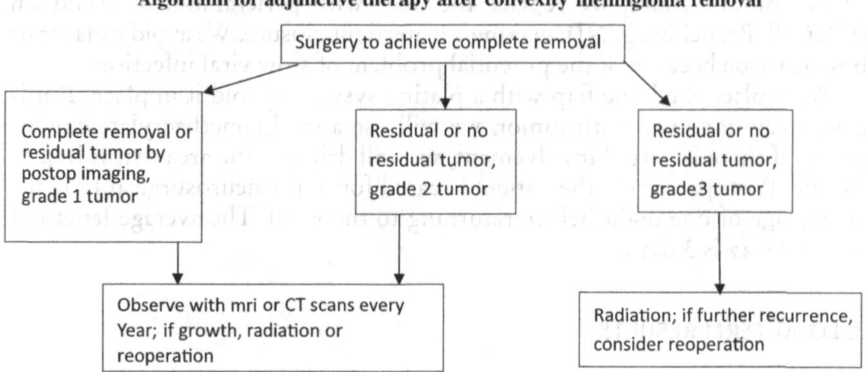
Algorithm for adjunctive therapy after convexity meningioma removal
Surgery to achieve complete removal
Complete removal or residual tumor by postop imaging, grade 1 tumor
Residual or no residual tumor, grade 2 tumor
Residual or no residual tumor, grade3 tumor
Observe with mri or CT scans every Year; if growth, radiation or reoperation
Radiation; if further recurrence, consider reoperation

4. COMPLICATIONS

In our series, there was no surgical mortality. The overall surgical morbidity was 5.2%: Complications included new neurological deficit in 1.7% of patients, a 0.6% incidence of postoperative hematoma and an infection rate of 2.9%. There were two cardiac complications, which occurred in the 65 years or older group. There was no significant difference in morbidity between patients under and over age 65.

These are similar to other reports. Yanno et al. reported a 4.4% morbidity rate in patients under age 70 and 9.4% in patients over age 70 [13].

HOW TO AVOID COMPLICATIONS

An important initial step in avoiding complications is to be sure the tumor is localized correctly and that cardiac and other conditions have been carefully evaluated preoperatively. During the surgery itself, there are two major potential problems to avoid: injury to cerebral veins and injury to the cortex and white matter as the tumor is removed. Although we did not have venous infarction in our series, it can be a devastating problem that gives new neurological deficit and problematic seizures. The veins must be preserved, if necessary by sharp dissection from the tumor; and if there is very dense adherence, a small amount of tumor can be left on them. When dissecting the tumor off the cortex and white matter, it is important to avoid coagulating vessels that may supply adjacent cortex and not to pull up on the white matter.

CONCLUSIONS

Convexity meningiomas are among the most satisfying tumors a neurosurgeon can treat. The major issue is often when to remove them, but there is a tendency to have earlier surgery as our surgery becomes less invasive using navigation techniques. Moreover, early surgery removes the worry that tumor may grow or change, and has an acceptable morbidity of 5.5%. The tumor grade is particularly important in the long-term outcome of patients.

References

[1] Al-Mefty O (1995) Meningiomas. WB Saunders, Philadelphia

[2] Black P, Morokoff A, Zauberman J (2008) Surgery for extra-axial tumors of the cerebral convexity and midline. Neurosurgery 63: 427-433; discussion

[3] Jaaskelainen J, Haltia M, Servo A (1986) Atypical and anaplastic meningiomas: radiology, surgery, radiotherapy, and outcome. Surg Neurol 25: 233-242

[4] Kamitani H, Masuzawa H, Kanazawa I, Kubo T (2001) Recurrence of convexity meningiomas: tumor cells in the arachnoid membrane. Surg Neurol 56: 228-235

[5] Kim YJ, Ketter R, Henn W, Zang KD, Steudel WI, Feiden W (2006) Histopathologic indicators of recurrence in meningiomas: correlation with clinical and genetic parameters. Virchows Arch 449: 529-538

[6] Kinjo T, Al-Mefty O, Kanaan I (1993) Grade zero removal of supratentorial convexity meningiomas. Neurosurgery 33: 394-399; discussion 399

[7] Maiuri F, De Caro MB, Esposito F, Cappabianca P, Strazzullo V, Pettinato G, de Divitiis E (2007) Recurrences of meningiomas: predictive value of pathological features and hormonal and growth factors. Neurooncology 82: 63-68

[8] Modha A, Gutin PH (2005) Diagnosis and treatment of atypical and anaplastic meningiomas: a review. Neurosurgery 57: 538-550; discussion 538-550

[9] Morokoff AP, Zauberman J, Black PM (2008) Surgery for convexity meningiomas. Neurosurgery 63: 427-433

[10] Patil DG, Laws ER Jr, Meningioma. history of the tumor and its management. In: Pamir N, Black P, Fahlbusch R (eds) Meningiomas: a comprehensive text. Elsevier, Philadelphia (in press)

[11] Simpson D (1957) The recurrence of intracranial meningiomas after surgical treatment. J Neurol Neurosurg Psychiatry 20: 22-39

[12] Yamasaki F, Yoshioka H, Hama S, Sugiyama K, Arita K, Kurisu K (2000) Recurrence of meningiomas. Cancer 89: 1102-1110

[13] Yano S, Kuratsu J (2006) Indications for surgery in patients with asymptomatic meningiomas based on an extensive experience. J Neurosurg 105: 538-543

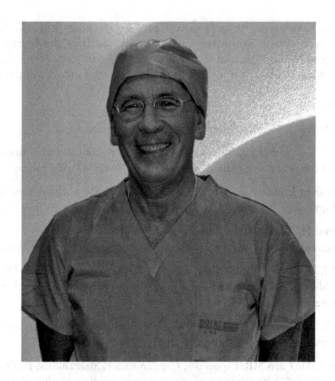

Peter M. Black

Peter Black is Franc D. Ingraham Professor of Neurosurgery at Harvard Medical School, Founding Chair of the Departments of Neurosurgery at Brigham and Women's Hospital, and Chair emeritus of the Department of Neurosurgery at Children's Hospital. He has had a long interest in meningiomas, working with Mr. Steven Haley to create the Meningioma Project. He is Chair of the Editorial Board of Neurosurgery and sits on numerous foundations and editorial boards. He has received many awards including the Charles Wilson award, Rofeh award, the Pioneer award of the Children's Brain Tumor Foundation, and the distinguished service award from the Section on Tumors. Dr. Black directs a molecular biology laboratory that investigates growth and invasion in meningiomas. His bibliography includes 13 books and five hundred papers. He is president-elect of the World Federation of Neurosurgical Societies. He has mentored over a hundred trainees and is very proud of the productivity of his former trainees, many holding prominent academic positions.

Contact: Peter M. Black, Department of Neurosurgery, Brigham & Women's Hospital, 75 Francis St, Boston, MA 02115, USA
E-mail: pblack@partners.org

THE "DANGEROUS" INTRACRANIAL VEINS

M. SINDOU

INTRODUCTION

No doubt that number of so-called unpredictable post-operative complications are likely to be related to iatrogenic venous damages. They manifest as locally developed edema, regional or diffuse brain swelling, some being fatal because of uncontrollable intracranial hypertension, and/or hemorrhagic infarcts, sometimes devastating and erroneously attributed to default in hemostasis. Ignoring the venous structures during surgery would lead to such disastrous consequences.

The main "dangerous" veins are classically the major dural sinuses, the deep cerebral veins and some of the dominant superficial veins like the vein of Labbé. A complete and detailed pre-operative setting including venous angio-MR, and if necessary digital substraction angiography with late venous phases, helps to determine optimal surgical strategy. A sustained effort during surgery to always respect and sometimes reconstruct the venous system is an obligation for the surgeon.

RATIONALE

Good knowledge on the surgical anatomy and physiology of the intracranial venous system is of prime importance [3, 5, 9–11, 14].

1. THE DURAL SINUSES (Fig. 1)

The major dural sinuses – foremost the superior sagittal sinus (SSS) – carry a considerable amount of blood. The anterior third of SSS receives the prefrontal afferent veins; its posterior radiological landmark is the coronal suture. It is generally admitted that its sacrifice is well tolerated. Actually mental disorders, personality changes, loss of recent memory with a general slowing of thought processes and activity, or even akinetic mutism, may occur if sacrificed or if frontal veins are compromised. The midthird receives the numerous and voluminous cortical veins of the central group. Interruption of this portion entails high risks of bilateral hemiplegia and akinesia. The posterior third, as well as the torcular Herophili, which receives the straight sinus, drains a considerable amount of blood. Interruption would inevitably provoke potentially fatal intracranial hypertension.

Keywords: intracranial veins, major dural sinuses, brain, anatomy, vascular

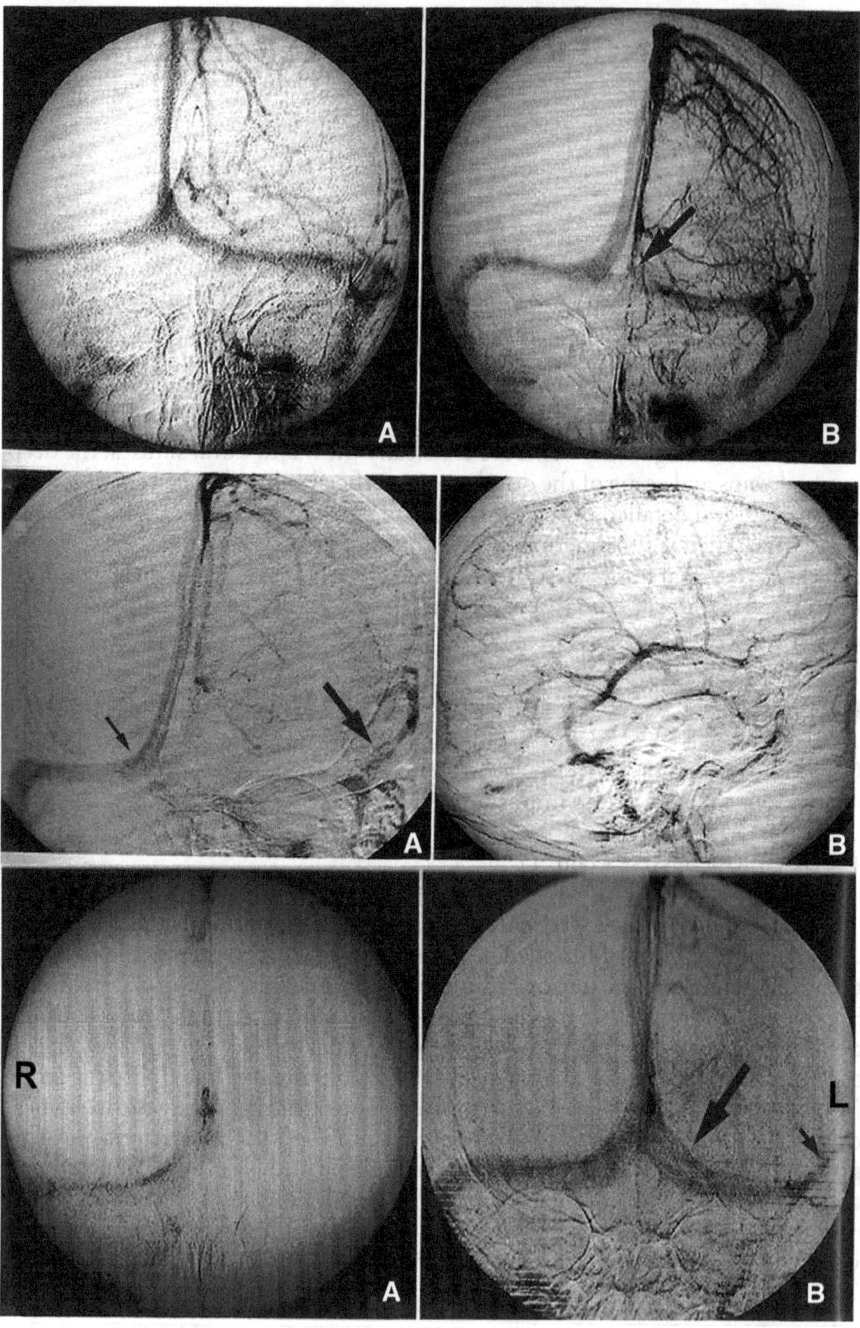
A
B
A
B
R
A
L
B

The lateral sinuses (LS) ensure a symetric drainage in only 20% of the cases; in the extreme one LS may drain the SSS in totality, most often the right one, and the other the straight sinus.

The transverse sinus (TS) may be atretic on one side, the sigmoid sinus segment draining the inferior cerebral veins (i.e. the Labbé system).

The sigmoid sinus (SS) drains the posterior fossa. It receives the superior and the inferior petrosal sinuses and also unconstant veins coming from the lateral aspect of pons and medulla. It has frequent anastomoses with the cutaneous venous network through the mastoid emissary vein. When the sigmoid segment of the lateral sinus is atretic, the transverse sinus with its affluents drains toward the opposite side.

All these anatomical configurations have surgical implications and must be taken into account before considering interrupting a sinus (Fig. 2).

2. THE SUPERFICIAL CEREBRAL VEINS

Any of the superficial cerebral veins of a certain calibre has presumably a functional role. However, as shown by experience, some of them are more "dangerous" to sacrifice than others. The superficial veins belong to three "systems": the midline afferents to the SSS, the inferior cerebral afferents to the TS and the superficial sylvian afferents to the cavernous sinus. These three systems are strongly interconnected, but in very variable ways from one individual to another.

Midline afferent veins enter into the SSS. They are met during interhemispheric approaches. Seventy percent of sagittal venous drainage is evident within the sector four centimeters posterior to the coronal suture; it corresponds to the central group. Sacrifice of the midline central group is risky. The sacrifice of the other midline veins, unless they are of large calibre, does not appear so hazardous. The vein of Trolard, or superior anastomotic vein, links the superficial sylvian system to the SSS. It usually penetrates the SSS in the post-central region.

Inferior cerebral veins are cortical bridging veins that channel into the basal sinuses and/or into the deep venous system. They are met in the skull base approaches. Juxta-basal veins may be sacrificed only if they are small and do not contribute predominantly to the system of Labbé. The vein of Labbé, or inferior anastomotic vein, creates an anastomosis between the superficial sylvian vein and the TS before its junction with the SS. Necessity of the respect

Fig. 1. *Upper row:* **A** Left carotid angiogram, AP projection. The SSS is drained equally by both lateral sinuses (LS). **B** Left carotid angiogram, AP projection. The right LS drains totally the SSS, the left one drains the straight sinus (arrow). *Middle row:* Left carotid angiogram; AP (**A**) and lateral (**B**) projections. The SSS exclusively drains into the right LS (small arrow). The left transverse sinus is atretic; the remaining sigmoid sinus drains the vein of Labbé (large arrow). *Lower row:* **A** Right carotid angiogram, AP projection; **B** left carotid angiogram, AP projection. The sigmoid sinus is absent on left side so that the left transverse sinus (large arrow) and its tributaries, especially vein of Labbé (small arrow), are drained toward the contralateral side

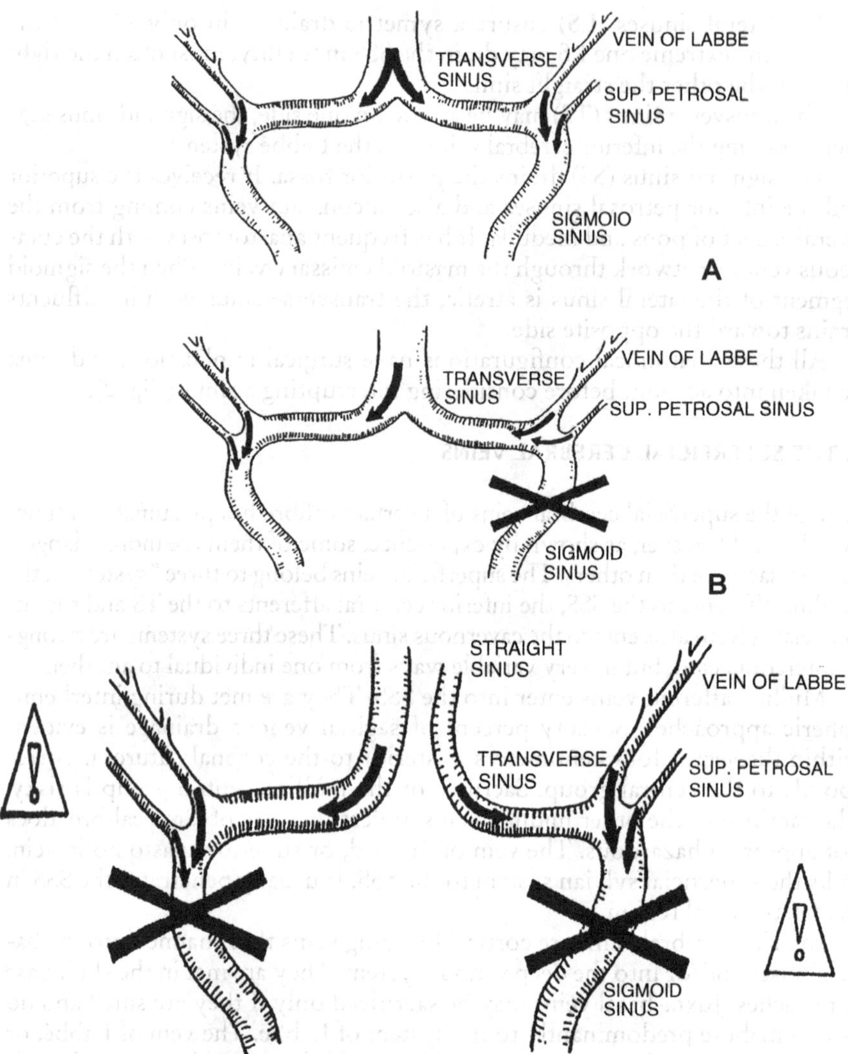

Fig. 2. *Upper and middle rows*: When both lateral sinuses (LS) are well-developed (*upper row*), interruption of one LS (*middle row*) may theoretically be tolerated. *Lower row*: When one LS drains exclusively the SSS and the other one the straight sinus (a frequent configuration), interruption of either one entails high risks for hemispheres, deep cerebral structures and Labbé vein(s)

of vein of Labbé, especially in the dominant hemisphere, is mandatory to avoid posterior hemispheric infarction.

The superficial sylvian vein is formed by anastomosis of the temporosylvian veins; these veins are connected with the midline veins upward and

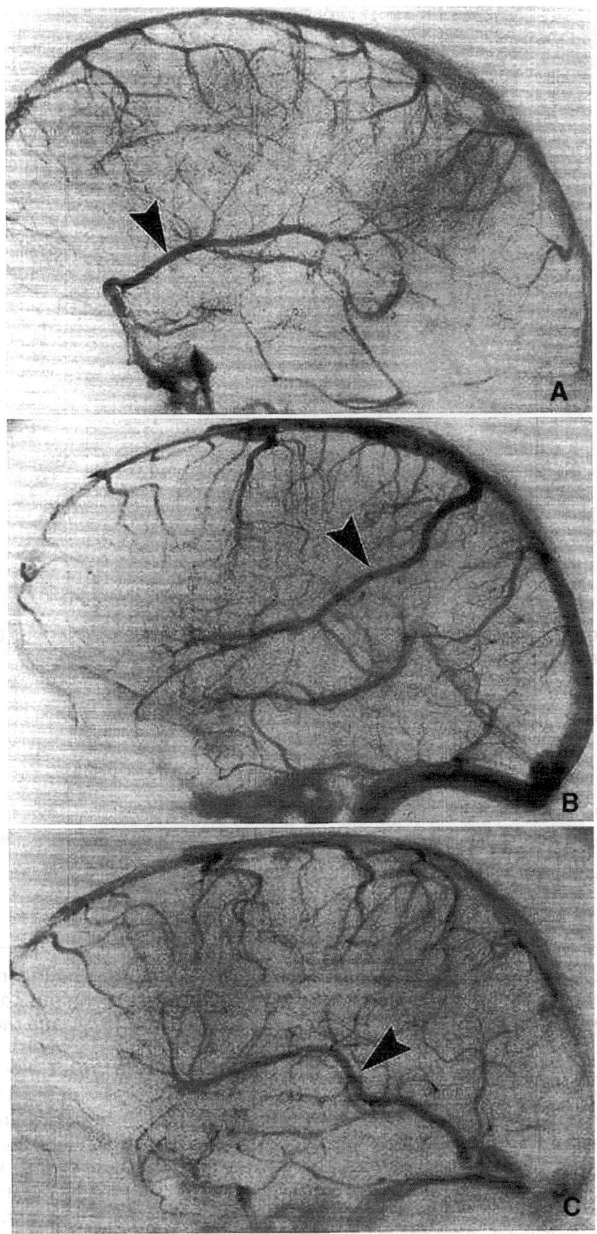

Fig. 3. Variations of superficial venous system. **A** The anterior drainage by the superficial sylvian vein is predominant. **B** The sss is predominant; the post-central vein drains the bigger part of the superficial sylvian vein territory (through Trolard anastomotic vein). **C** The lateral sinus is predominant; it drains almost all the superficial sylvian vein territory (through Labbé vein)

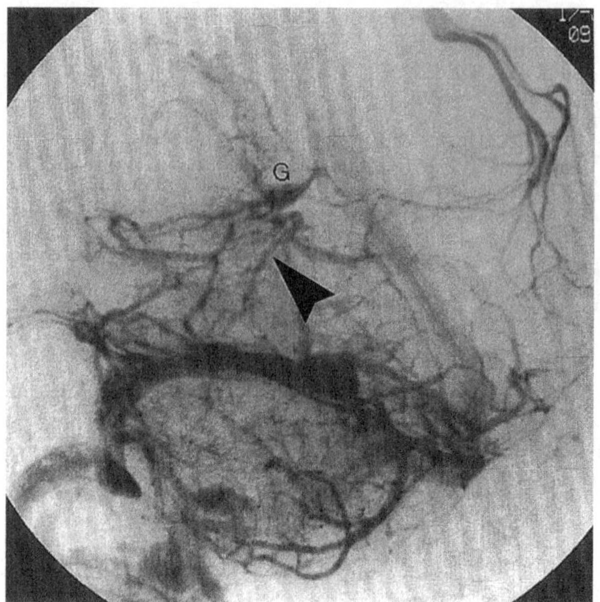

Fig. 4. Posterior fossa venous system by vertebral injection. Vein of Galen (*G*), precentral vermian vein (arrowhead)

the juxtabasal temporal veins downward. It enters predominantly the cavernous sinus, either directly or through the sphenoparietal sinus. Many variations are possible. Sacrificing the superficial sylvian vein is risky when it is of large calibre and poorly anastomosed.

Skull base approaches must be prepared taking into account the anatomical organization of the superficial venous system (see details and literature quotations in references [3, 10, 11]) (Fig. 3, 5, bottom).

Fig. 5. *Top*: Deep cerebral veins and landmark of the interventricular venous confluence. DSA by carotid injection, venous phase, lateral view. The interventricular venous confluence (circle) is formed by confluence of the septal veins (*2*), caudate veins (*3, 4*), and thalamo-striate veins (*5*). Confluence gives rise to the internal cerebral vein (*1*). On lateral view, this confluence has an almost constant situation and corresponds to the interventricular foramen of Monro. This point may contribute a useful anatomical imaging reference. (Confluence of internal cerebral veins and basilar veins [*B*] gives Galen vein [*G*]. *Bottom*: Superficial veins involved in (supratentorial) skull base approaches. Three groups of veins can be distinguished: the middle afferent frontal veins, the inferior cerebral veins (i.e. the Labbé system) and the sylvian veins. These three groups can be delimited by three "triangles". (1) The triangle corresponding to the frontal group of veins (FV) is delimited by the three following landmarks: interventricular venous confluence (circle), bregma (*B*) and the anterior limit of anterior cranial fossa (*A*). (2) The triangle corresponding to the inferior group (*ICV*) is delimited by the interventricular confluence (circle), torcular (*T*) and jugular foramen (*J*). (3) The triangle corresponding to the anterior sylvian group (*ASV*) is delimited by the interventricular confluence (circle), anterior limit of anterior cranial fossa (*A*) and jugular foramen (*J*) landmarks. Skull base approaches must be designed so that the prominent venous drainage(s) be respected

3. THE DEEP VEINS OF THE BRAIN

The deep cerebral veins are the ones which drain toward the deep venous confluent of Galen (Fig. 5, top). The denomination of venous confluent is appropriate since – in addition to the two internal cerebral veins – the Galenic system receives the two basilar veins, and also veins from the corpus callosum, the cerebellum (mainly through the vermian precentral vein) and the occipital cortex. A good knowledge of the deep veins is important for surgery in the lateral ventricles and of course in the third ventricle and pineal region [2].

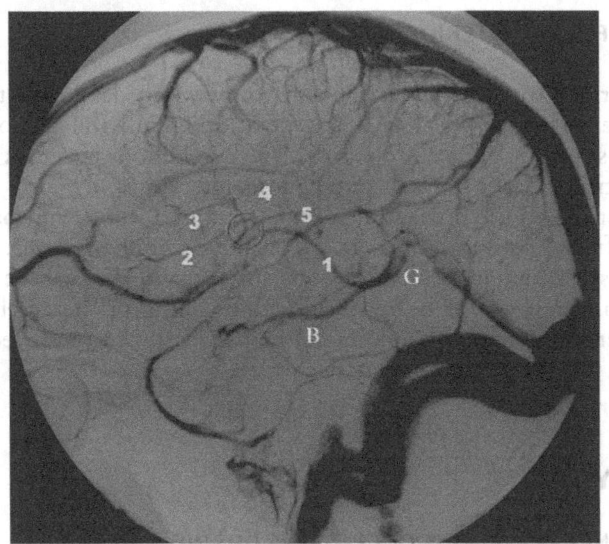

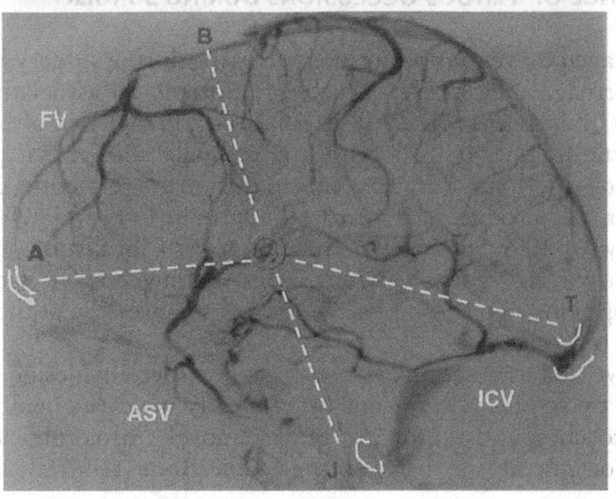

There is a general agreement that the sacrifice of the vein of Galen or of one of its main tributaries should be considered as a high risk, although animal experiments and a few reported clinical observations showed otherwise.

The thalamostriate vein represents an important anatomic landmark when accessing the third ventricle through the lateral ventricle by the interthalamo-trigonal approach. It drains the deep white matter of the hemisphere, the internal capsule and the caudate nucleus. This vein has to be sometimes sacrified in this approach. Consequences vary depending on the authors: from little or none to venous infarction of basal ganglia. Because consequences can be severe, sacrificing the thalamostriate vein is justified only if widening the exposure of the third ventricle is absolutely necessary [4].

4. VEINS OF THE POSTERIOR FOSSA

It is important to consider venous anatomy when dealing with posterior fossa surgery (Fig. 4) [7]. The sitting position entails the risk of air embolism from sinus and/or vein opening. The cerebellum is at risk of swelling and infarction in the eventuality of venous interruption.

The sacrifice of the precentral vermian vein in order to approach the pineal region from posterior, is generally considered not dangerous.

The classical statement that the superior petrosal vein can be interrupted without danger needs to be reconsidered. Swelling of the cerebellar hemisphere after sacrificing a (voluminous) petrosal vein is not unfrequently observed and venous infarction may occur.

SURGERY

1. AVOIDANCE OF VENOUS OCCLUSIONS DURING SURGERY

The role played by venous occlusions occurring during surgery in post-operative hemorrhagic infarcts is undeniable. Important, the association of venous sacrifice to brain retraction entails significantly higher risk of brain damage than retraction alone. It has been experimentally shown that parenchymal retraction of one hour duration, in opposition to retraction combined to venous sacrifice, produces a subcortical infarct in 13% and 60% of animals, respectively [6]. Retraction of the brain provokes a local congestion by compressing the cortical venous network, reduction in venous flow by stretching the bridging veins, and thrombosis of veins if compression of the retractor or a cotonoïd is prolonged.

Excessive brain retraction can be avoided by specially designed approaches obeying two principles: the one of minimally invasive opening: the "keyhole" approaches, and the one of bone removal: "osteotomies" associated with craniotomy at the base of the skull. Bone removal associated to craniotomies for skull base approaches by increasing the field-view angle and the working-cone [1, 12] protect from important retraction and consequently avulsing veins. Extended approaches (as fronto-basal, orbital, zygomatic, orbito-zygomatic, at the level of the roof of the external auditory meatus, transpetrosal or extreme lateral of the foramen magnum) have become classical. Limited opening of the dura mater to the minimum required is most effective to avoid excessive retraction by the self-retractor. In the eventuality of necessary prolonged retraction, releasing the retractor from time to time decreases damaging phenomena. Removing the blade for approximately five minutes every fifteen minutes is considered beneficial.

It may happen that a bridging vein acts as a limitation. To be preserved, the vein has to be dissected free from arachnoid and cortex at a length of 10–20 mm [13]. It also may happen that a big vein inside a fissure or a sulcus performs as an obstacle. Because interruption would entail the risk to provoke "a cascade" of intraluminal coagulation of the neighbouring pial veins it is justified to attempt its preservation. If conservation seems difficult, before deciding sacrifice a gentle temporary clamping for a few minutes with a microforceps or a small temporary clip may be useful to test the absence of consecutive regional congestion.

2. REPAIR

When an important vein has been ruptured, its reconstruction may be considered. For this purpose the silicone tubing technique has been developed. "A silicone tube that is most suitable to the size of the vein origin is selected and inserted into the distal segment of the vein and fixed with a 10-0 monofilament nylon circumferential tie. The other end of the silicone tube is then inserted into the proximal end of the vein and tied [8]."

Frequent is the circumstance in which a wound is made in a vein wall during dissection. Rather than to coagulate the vein, hemostasis can be attempted by simply wrapping the wall with a small piece of Surgicel. If this is not sufficient, obliteration of the wound can be made by a very localized microcoagulation with a sharp bipolar forceps or by placing a single suture with a 10-0 nylon thread. But in all cases, whatever the technique used, quality of hemostasis has to be checked by jugular compression at the neck or with local patency test using two forceps, as classical in microvascular surgery.

When a major dural sinus has been injured or needs to be occluded, its repair is advocated [3, 10, 11].

CONCLUSIONS

Respect of the intracranial venous system results from a constant belief of the importance of preserving veins and a sustained effort to do it during the whole operation.

Surgery on the intracranial venous system requires good neuro-images to work on. Venous angio-MR, as a complement of conventional MRI is mandatory. In supplement, digital substraction angiography with late venous phases can be of prime importance to determine surgical strategy especially in "difficult tumors". For these reasons neurosurgeons must incite neuroimaging colleagues to be full-partners in the neurosurgical management.

References

[1] Alaywan M, Sindou M (1990) Fronto-temporal approach with orbito-zygomatic removal. Surgical anatomy. Acta Neurochir (Wien) 104: 79-83

[2] Apuzzo ML (1977) Surgery of the third ventricle. Williams & Wilkins, Baltimore

[3] Auque J (1996) Le sacrifice veineux en neurochirurgie. Evaluation et gestion du risque. Neurochirurgie 42(Suppl 1): 32-38

[4] Delandsheer JM, Guyot JF, Jomin M, Scherpereel B, Laine E (1978) Accès au troisième ventricule par voie interthalamo-trigonale. Neurochirurgie 24: 419-422

[5] Hakuba A (ed) (1996) Surgery of the intracranial venous system. Embryology, anatomy, pathophysiology, neuroradiology, diagnosis, treatment. First international workshop on surgery of the intracranial venous system at Osaka September 1994. Springer, Tokyo

[6] Kanno T, Kasama A, Shoda M, Yamaguchi C, Kato Y (1989) A pitfall in the interhemispheric translamina terminalis approach for the removal of a craniopharyngioma. Significance of preserving draining veins. Part I. Clinical study. Part II. Experimental study. Surg Neurol 32: 111-115, 116-120.

[7] Matsushima T, Rhoton AL Jr, de Oliveira E, Peace D (1983) Microsurgical anatomy of the veins of the posterior fossa. J Neurosurg 59: 63-105

[8] Sakaki T, Morimoto T, Takemura K, Miyamoto S, Kyoi K, Utsumi S (1987) Reconstruction of cerebral cortical veins using silicone tubing. Technical note. J Neurosurg 66: 471-473

[9] Schmidek HH, Auer LM, Kapp JP (1985) The cerebral venous system. Review. Neurosurgery 17: 663-678

[10] Sindou M, Auque J (2000) The intracranial venous system as a neurosurgeon's perspective. Review. Adv Tech Stand Neurosurg 26: 131-216

[11] Sindou M, Auque J, Jouanneau E (2005) Neurosurgery and the intracranial venous system. Acta Neurochir Suppl 94: 167-175

[12] Sindou M, Emery E, Acevedo G, Ben-David U (2001) Respective indications for orbital rim, zygomatic arch and orbito-zygomatic osteotomies in the surgical

approach to central skull base lesions. Critical, retrospective review in 146 cases. Acta Neurochir (Wien) 143: 967-975

[13] Sugita K, Kobayashi S, Yokoo A (1982) Preservation of large bridgings veins during brain retraction. Technical note. J Neurosurg 57: 856-858

[14] Yaşargil MG (1984) Microneurosurgery. Microsurgical anatomy of the basal cisterns and vessels of the brain, diagnostic and studies, vol 1. Thieme, Stuttgart

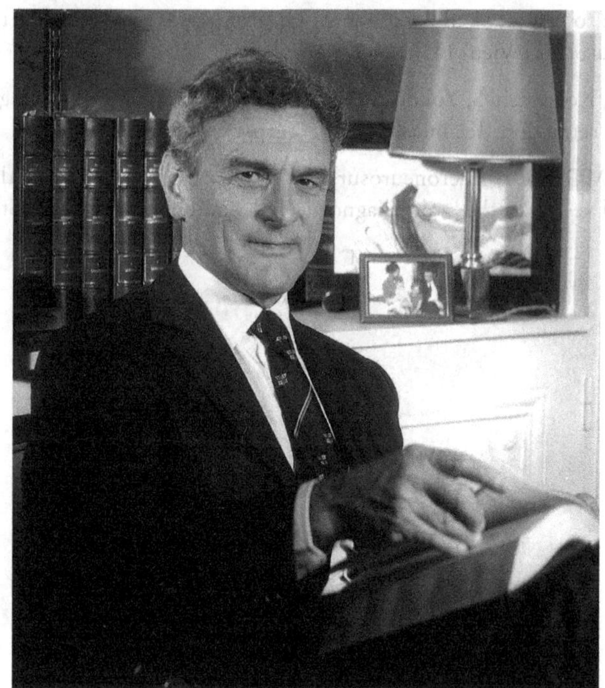

Marc Sindou

Marc Sindou is Professor of Neurosurgery and Chairman of the Department of Neurosurgery at the Hôpital Neurologique P. Wertheimer, Lyon. Born in 1943 in Limoges, he completed in parallel his medical and scientific studies, at the Universities of Limoges, Bordeaux and Paris. Then he applied for residency in neurosurgery in 1969 at the University of Lyon, where a new Institute for Neurosciences had just been created by Pierre Wertheimer, one of the pioneers of French neurosurgery. The institute had 180 beds for neurology and 140 beds for neurosurgery and was served by ten operating rooms, with around 3800 surgical operations per year.

Marc Sindou obtained his M.D. degree in 1972 with the thesis "Anatomical study of spinal dorsal root entry zone. Applications for pain surgery", and same year his Doctorat in Sciences (D.Sc.) with the thesis "Cerebral cortex electrogenesis in humans". After a five-year training in Lyon, he benefited from two fellowships: the first with Professor William Sweet at the Massachusetts General Hospital in Boston, especially for pain surgery, the second with Professor Gazi Yaşargil at Kantonspital in Zurich for training in micro-neurosurgery. He was appointed associate professor in 1982 and became full professor in neurosurgery and chairman of department in 1986.

His research was directed to two different fields. On the basis of his M.D. thesis he developed neurophysiological investigations and surgery in the dorsal root entry zone target for spinal deafferentation pain and focalized spasticity. In the fields of vascular surgery he worked in the laboratory on intracranial venous reconstruction which was then applied to patients harbouring meningiomas.

His main neurosurgical interests, with his large and outstanding team, were (1) functional neurosurgery, including pain, spasticity, epilepsy, trigeminal neuralgia; (2) microsurgery for intracranial aneurysms; (3) skull base meningiomas and meningiomas invading venous sinuses; (4) cranial nerve vascular compression syndromes, and (5) neurophysiology applied to neurosurgery. Surgical personal experience amounts to more than 20000 operations, which gave source to 549 publications.

Marc Sindou has been Founding-member of the International Association for the Study of Pain (IASP) in 1975, President (1998–2001) and Past-president (2001–2005) of the World Society for Stereotactic and Functional Neurosurgery (WSSFN), Vice-President of the European Association of Neurosurgical Societies (EANS) (1999–2003). He is presently President of the Société de Neuro-Chirurgie de Langue Française (SNCLF) (2007–2009). He is member of the editorial boards of a number of prestigious international journals, and has 135 editorials or comments published. He is a teacher in the EANS Training program and was awarded the prestigious "European Lecture" in 2007. He has been honoured by 16 visiting professorships and by 196 invited lectures in 49 different countries.

Main hobbies are: Mountaineering, with a number of summits in the french Alps, but with help of solid guides!, and also playing the piano, preferably when alone! Woody Allen and Umberto Eco are very much appreciated, and (only time to time) Mister Bean. "Resisting-administration" – of course not a hobby – takes part of his daily life.

Last but not least, he is supported by a nice and devoted wife, with whom he has three wonderful children and nine charming but turbulent grand-children.

Above all, Marc Sindou is indebted to all his masters, colleagues, staffs and pupils, from whom he learned so much through professional contacts and personal relationships.

Contact: Marc Sindou, Hôpital Neurologique P. Wertheimer, University of Lyon, 59 Bd Pinel, 69003 Lyon, France
E-mail: marc.sindou@chu-lyon.fr

HOW TO PERFORM SUBFRONTO-ORBITO-NASAL APPROACH FOR ANTERIOR CRANIAL BASE SURGERY

F.-X. ROUX

INTRODUCTION

Subfrontal approaches were first proposed and described by Horsley and Cushing in the early beginning of neurosurgery. These approaches were mostly bifrontal flaps for skull base surgery. First combined craniofacial approaches were described by Dandy [1] in 1941 and by Ray and McLean [6] in 1943 for orbital tumors removal. Principles of transcranial and transfacial surgery were then precised by Smith et al. [8], Ketcham et al. [3] and Derome [2]. Later, enlarged approaches with mobilization of orbital rims and nasal pyramid were proposed. Subfronto-orbito-nasal (SFON) approach was first described in 1978 by Raveh as "anterior extended subcranial approach" for anterior skull base fractures [4, 5]. He extended the indications in 1980 for benign and malignant tumor resection [4, 5]. This approach allows performing a mediofrontonasal monobloc flap including nasal pyramid and orbital rims. We first used it for removal of ethmoidal tumors such as adenocarcinomas but we rapidly discovered the large field of vision given by this approach for anterior cranial fossa, ethmoidal, sphenoidal and maxillary sinuses, internal part of the orbit and clivus as well [7].

RATIONALE

Main goal of this approach is to minimize brain retraction (Fig. 1) during anterior skull base surgery. Other goals are to reach some areas with respect of vasculonervous structures encountered. The SFON flap allows reaching extradural and intradural structures. Extradural structures include anterior skull base, ethmoidal, sphenoidal and even maxillary sinuses with access to clivus, mediosuperior part of orbital contents. Intradural structures include anterobasal part of both frontal lobes with olfactive tracts, jugum with optochiasmatic area, anterior part of the Willis circle and sellar area. Main advantage for intradural access is the minimal frontal lobe retraction. It allows early control of basal vessels such as ethmoidal arteries especially for tumors inserted on the anterior part of the skull. Moreover, this approach is widely modulable and can

Keywords: skull base approaches, fronto-orbital-nasal approach, anterior fossa

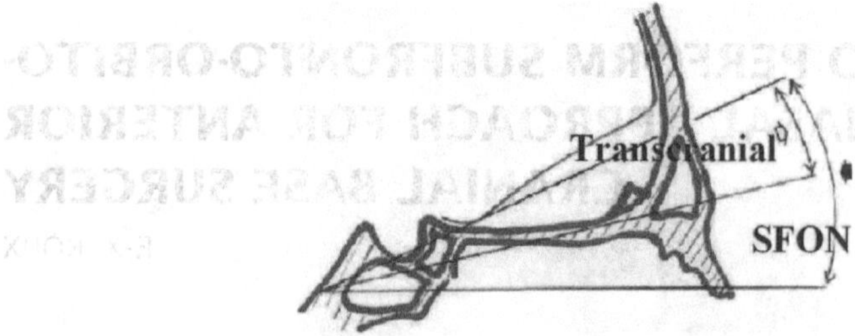

Fig. 1. Compared angles of access for classical subfrontal transcranial and SFON approaches showing minimal retraction and larger view for the latter

be adapted and extended as function of the areas to reach, laterally, upwards or downwards. This highly adaptable approach can be qualified of "swiss-knife" for craniofacial access.

DECISION-MAKING

Basically, the SFON approach allows to reach lesions of the anterior skull-base, of the midline such as sellar, suprasellar or clivus masses, of the superointernal part of the orbit, of sinuses of the face (ethmoidal, sphenoidal, maxillary sinuses) and anterior Willis circle as well. Thus, careful review of preoperative imaging is required to determine precisely if SFON approach is appropriate and to preview the anterioposterior and lateral extension of the approach. Both preoperative CT scan and MRI are mandatory to check bone and cerebral extensions of the lesion to be reached, and study angles between it and the skullbase plane in order to minimize retractions. Frontal sinus extension is not crucial since it is deliberately opened and cranialized. Other important information to check for intradural approach near the sellar area is the prefixed location of the chiasma which may limit dramatically the access to the concerned lesion.

SURGERY

1. POSITIONING

Patient is placed supine, the head fixed in median position and the neck slightly flexed to elevate the head (Fig. 2).

2. INCISION

After minimal shaving, bicoronal skin incision is performed from ear to ear. Care must be taken not to cut the galea which will be dissected and separated

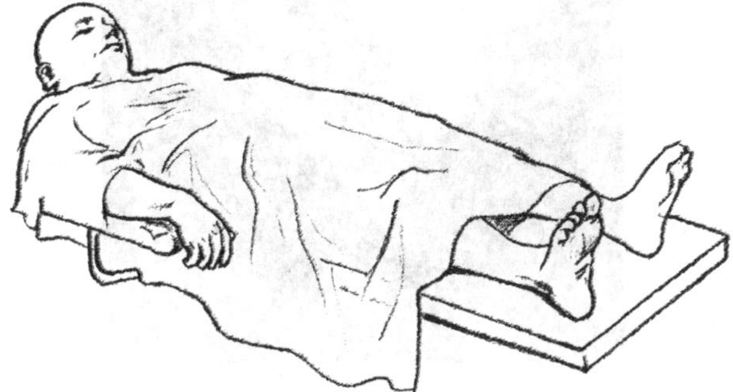

Fig. 2. Operative supine position with the head fixed in median position and the neck flexed slightly to elevate the head (drawing by Marc Harislur)

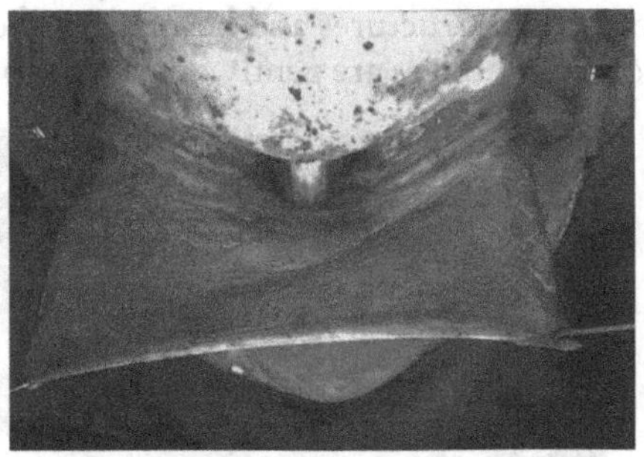

Fig. 3. Pedicled pericranial flap

from the skin starting 3 cm behind the orbital rims, thus sparing both supraorbital nerves.

3. GALEA FLAP

An anterior pediculated galea and pericranial flap is liberated and raised. Its limits are posteriorly the skin incision, and laterally both superior temporal lines. It must be as large as possible, about 8–10 cm laterally and 10–12 cm anteroposteriorly (Fig. 3).

4. SUPRAORBITAL AND PERIORBITAL DISSECTION

Desinsertion of the galea is pursued to the orbital rims and nasal pyramid (Fig. 4). If the bone flap is extended downwards to the lachrymal crests, it may be necessary to cut the lacrymal ducts. To avoid secondary retraction and stenosis of them and consequent post-operative eye watering, lachrymal ducts should be cut obliquely. Then the periorbit is cautiously separated from

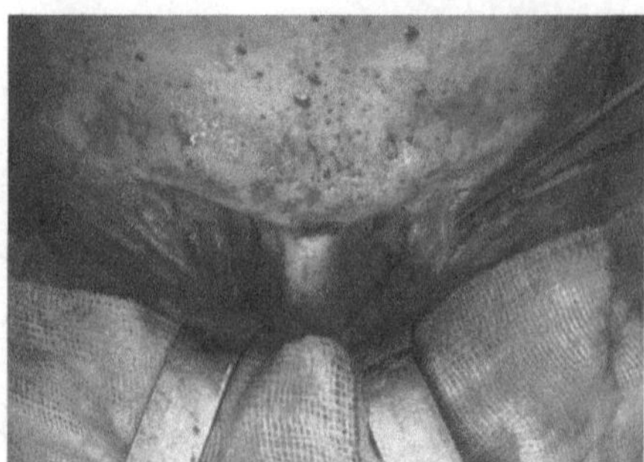

Fig. 4. Desinsertion of nasal pyramid with exposition of orbital rims and supraorbital grooves

the medial wall of the orbit which should not be opened so as avoiding both risks of injury of intraconic structures and herniation of orbital fat in the operative field. Supraorbital pedicles are gently detached from both supraorbital

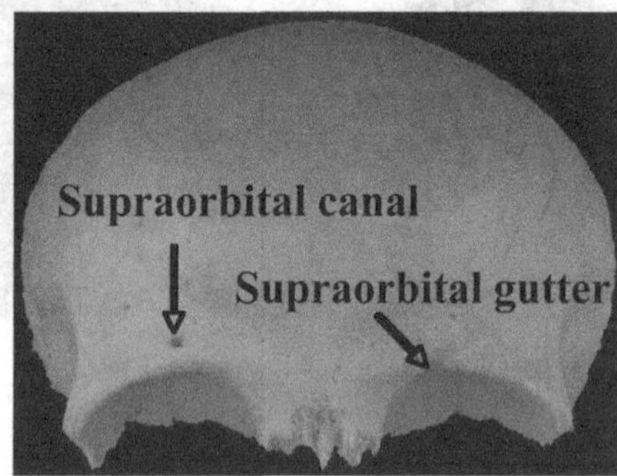

Fig. 5. Frontal bone anatomical piece showing: a supraorbital groove (left) and a closed groove as a supraorbital canal (right)

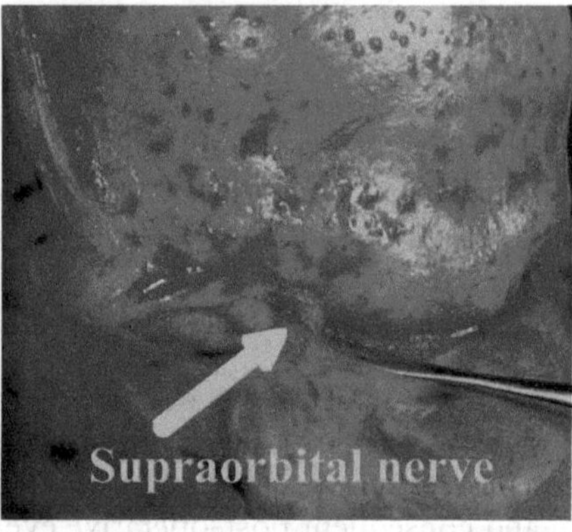

Fig. 6. Desinsertion of supraorbital pedicle within the supraorbital groove

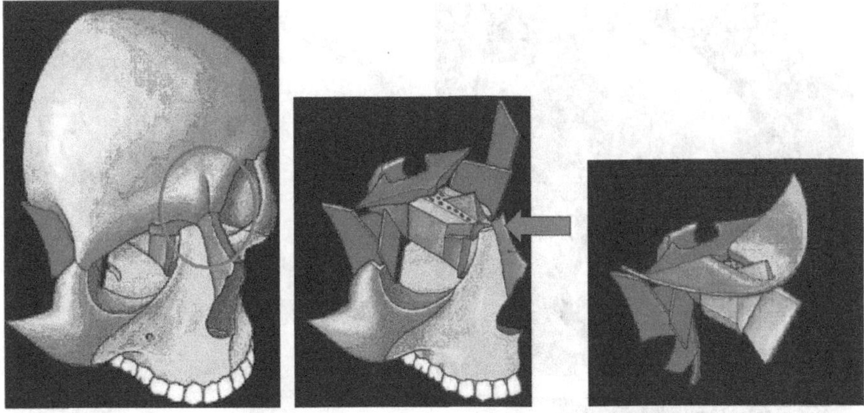

Figs. 7–9. Scheme of craniofacial junction showing the location of the bone flap

grooves (Figs. 5, 6). Sometimes supraorbital gutters appear as canals and will have to be opened with scissors so as to preserve supraorbital nerves.

5. BONE FLAP

Only one burr hole is drilled on the median line facing the superior sagittal sinus in its anterior third. The dura is detached from the bone with a spatula, away in the sagittal sinus, in order to control it and avoid injuring it with the craniotome. The mediofrontal osteotomy is performed so as to raise a monobloc nasofrontal flap (Figs. 7–9). Upper part of the flap is performed with the craniotome starting from the burr hole towards both orbital rims. A flexible retractor is carefully placed in the orbit for retracting the eyeball while cutting, with an oscillant saw, the nasal pyramid and medial and superior walls of the orbits (Figs. 10, 11). Bradycardia may be noted if the eyeball retraction is too important. Then the bone flap is slightly elevated with two periosteal elevators and a vertical osteotomy is performed in front of the crista galli process. At last, the subfronto-orbito-nasal flap is raised in one bloc. Precise location of each lines of cut are shown on Figs. 12–16.

6. FRONTAL SINUS CRANIALIZATION

Frontal sinus is inevitably opened with this flap and it is thus mandatory to cranialize it. All frontal mucosa must be removed and both nasofrontal ducts will be obturated with bone powder, galea and eventually pieces of Surgicel.

7. EXPOSITION OF THE CRIBRIFORM PLATE OF THE ETHMOID

For ethmoidal tumor removal, the superior part of the ethmoid sinuses and the cribriform plates will be exposed. The approach being epidural, conse-

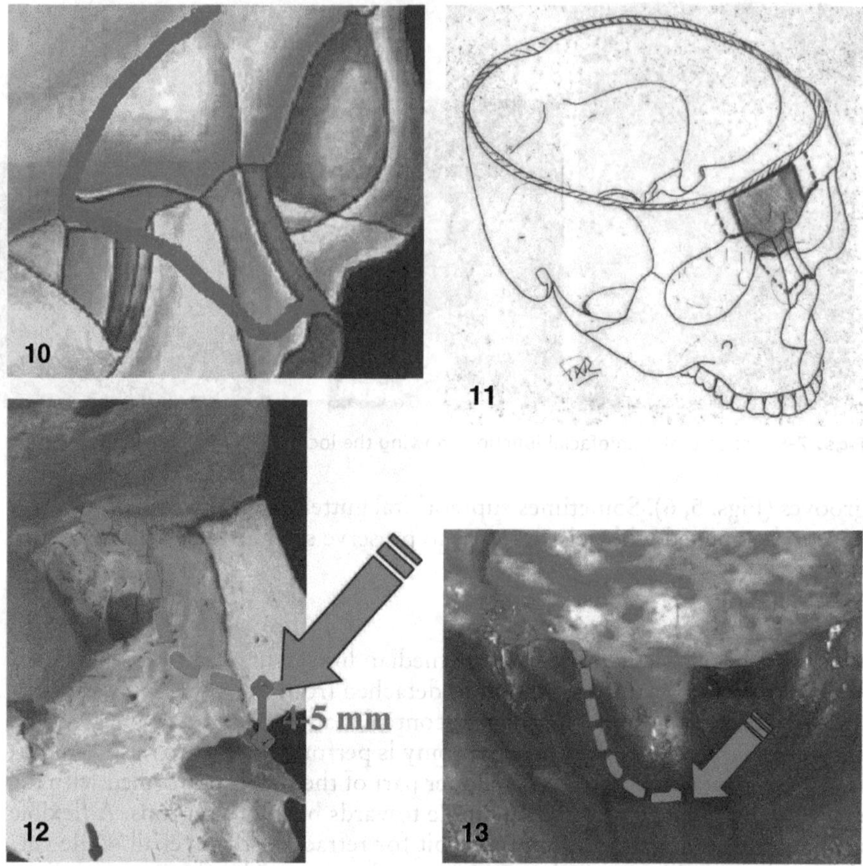

Figs. 10–13. Line of section of the frontal bone (mediofrontal osteotomy) and the nasal pyramid

quently the basifrontal dura will be desinserted from the front to the rear, the posterior limit being the jugum. During this surgical step both olfactive tracts will be coagulated and cut with the bipolar coagulator. This approach allows reaching both ethmoidal and sphenoidal sinuses as well as the maxillar sinuses which have to be controlled in case of wide ethmoidal tumor extending downwards. Opening the posterior part of the sphenoidal sinus allows an approach to the clivus itself, except the upper dead angle of the dorsum sellae.

8. DURA OPENING

The dura opening is performed transversally, entailing cutting the anterior insertion of the superior sagittal sinus (Fig. 17). It can be useful when beginning the procedure to suspend it peripherally on Halsted forceps.

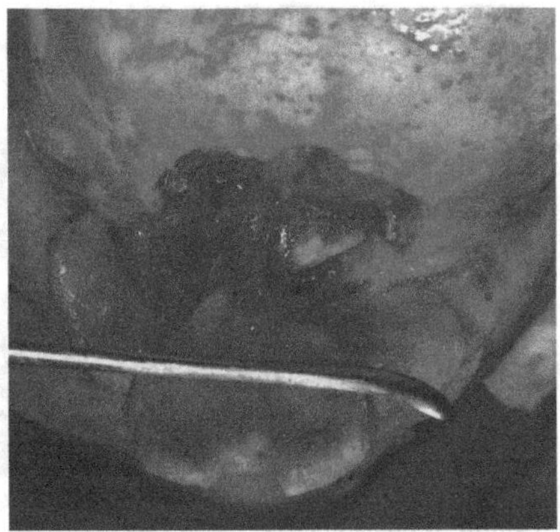

Fig. 14. Detachment of the frontonasal flap after section of the crista galli process

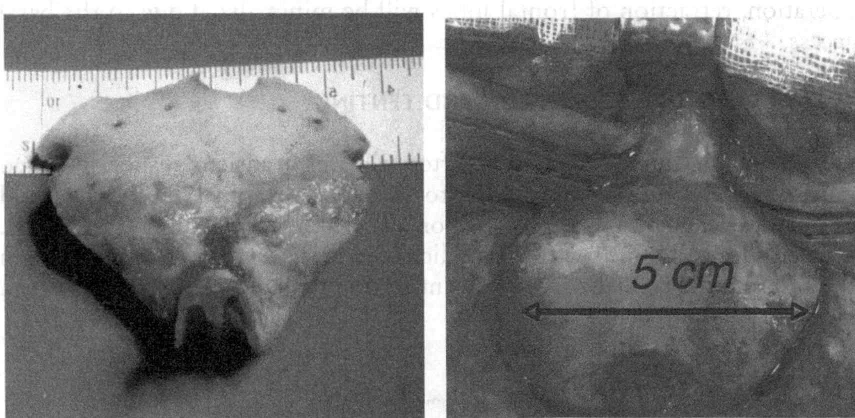

Figs. 15, 16. Frontonasal flap before and after removal

9. DISSECTION OF THE OLFACTORY TRACTS

For an intradural procedure, the dura has not to be detached from the cranial base. It is possible to spare olfactory tracts (at least one in order to preserve as much as possible the olfactory function) by a gentle arachnoidal dissection under smooth retraction of frontal lobes with an autostatic retractor. Biological glue is applied on both tracts to protect them and avoid ischemia or rupture during further dissection and retraction of the frontal lobe. This intradural approach allows exposing all the anterior cranial base, reaching easily the optochiasmatic tracts, the sellar and suprasellar region including the anterior part of the Willis circle. Approach can be lateral in its

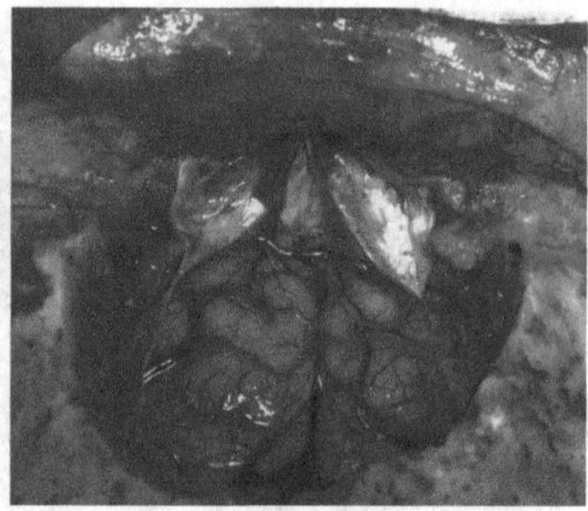

Fig. 17. Dura opening leading to basal access

anterior part and becomes more medial on its posterior part. All along the operation, retraction of frontal lobes will be minimalized due to the basal access.

10. DURA CLOSURE, SUSPENSION AND TENTING

Closure of the dura is performed after releasing transient suspensions and must be totally waterproof in order to avoid cerebrospinal fluid leakage and rhinorrhea. Then peripheral suspension and tenting of the dura is performed. This closure is doubled with the pediculated galea flap which is reclined on the base and the cranialized frontal sinuses and pasted to the dura with fibrin glue and a few stitches.

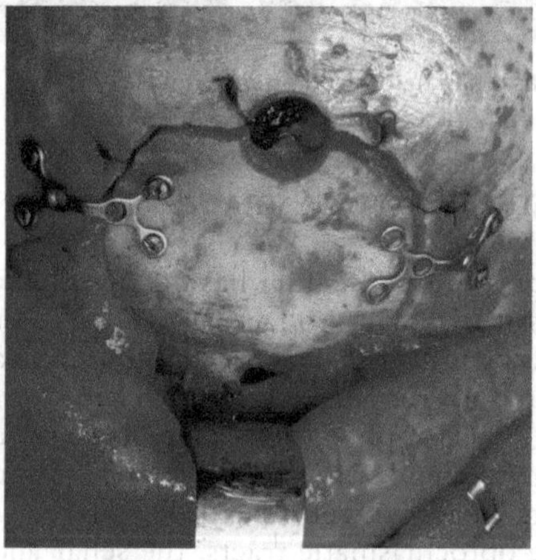

Fig. 18. Fixation of the flap with titanium miniplates (or stitches)

11. BONE FLAP REPOSITIONING

Bone flap is then repositioned and secured with transosseal sutures or titanium miniplates (Fig. 18). We avoid miniplates when the patient is planned for further radiotherapy because of a thinning of the skin with a bad cosmetic result and a higher risk of local infection.

12. SCALP CLOSURE

Scalp is then closed with both subcutaneous and cutaneous sutures with skin clips or stitches.

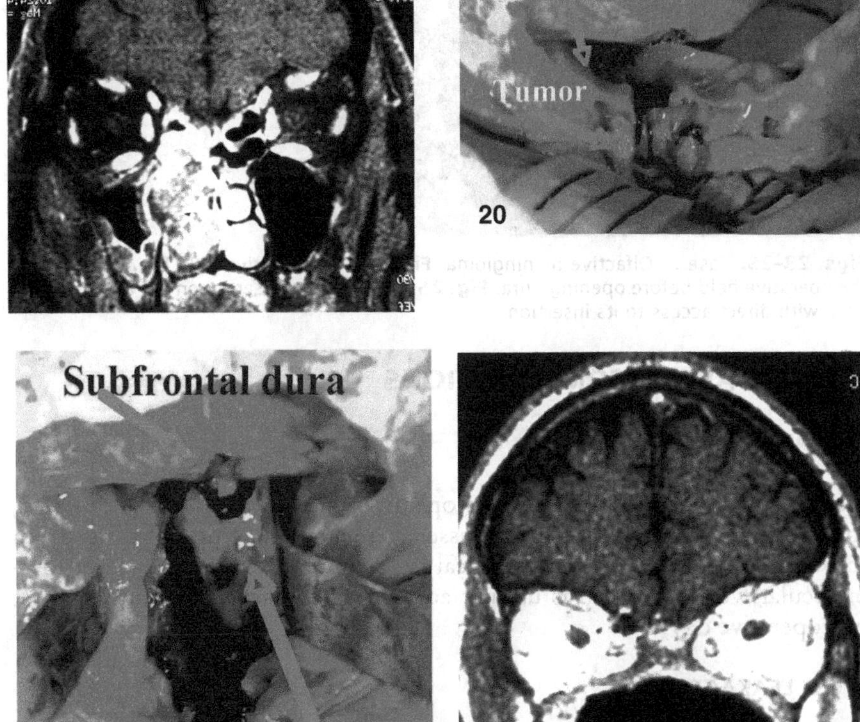

Figs. 19–22. Case 1: Ethmoidal carcinoma. **Fig. 19.** Preoperative MRI showing a T3 tumor invading cribriform plate. **Figs. 20, 21.** SFON approach. **Fig. 22.** Postoperative MRI showing complete removal

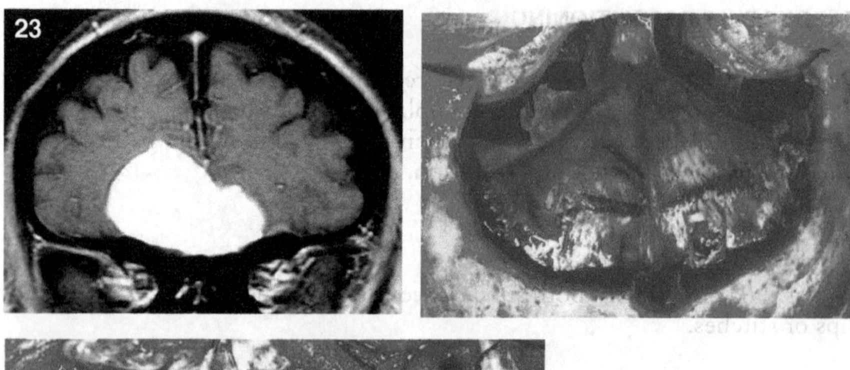

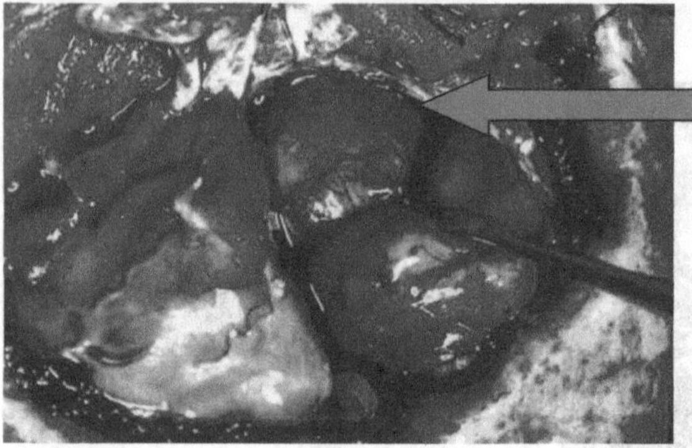

Figs. 23–25. Case 2: Olfactive meningioma. **Fig. 23.** Preoperative MRI. **Fig. 24.** View of the operative field before opening dura. **Fig. 25.** Meningioma inserted on the anterior skull base with direct access to its insertion

HOW TO AVOID COMPLICATIONS

1. GENERAL COMPLICATIONS

General complications such as postoperative hematoma, infection (4.5%), thromboembolism will not be discussed here since they do not differ from those observed in other neurosurgical procedures. Preventive dose of low-molecular-weight heparin is usually administrated early after surgery (first postoperative day).

2. CSF LEAKAGE (3.3%)

One of the most important parts of the procedure to be stressed is a perfect waterproof dural closure. Indeed a possible complication to be avoided is CSF leakage responsible for either rhinorrhea or subcutaneous CSF collection. Therefore a very good and waterproof dural closure is necessary; we use the double galea flap which is reclined onto the cranial base (especially the dura of the base which can be dehiscent) and secured to the dura with fibrin

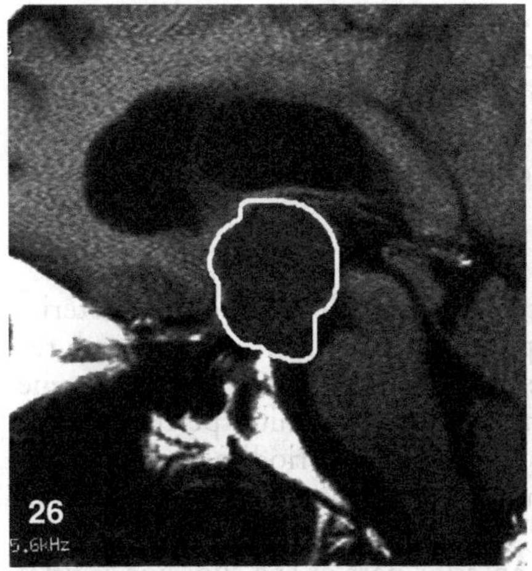

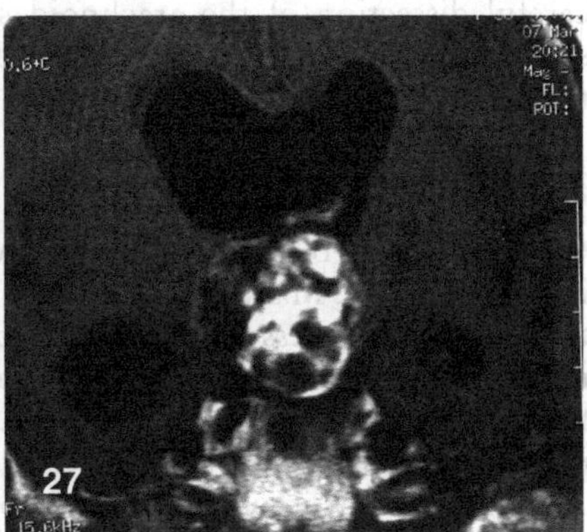

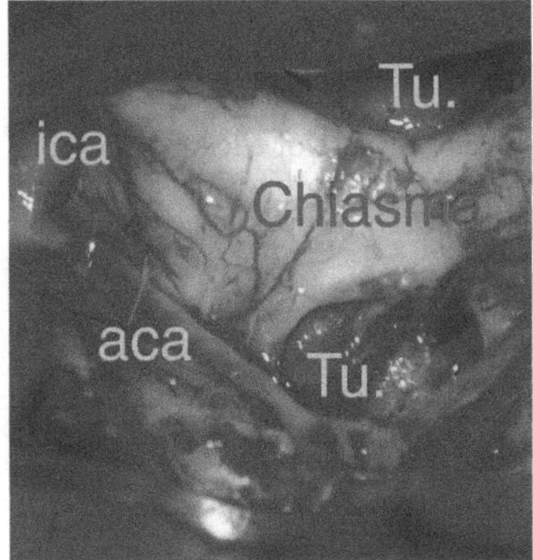

Figs. 26–28. Case 3: Craniopharyngioma. **Figs. 26, 27.** Preoperative MRI. **Fig. 28.** Intradural approach with both vasculonervous structures and tumor (*aca* anterior carotid artery; *ica* internal carotid artery; *Tu* tumor)

glue. In some cases, transient lumbar drainage could be discussed; but we never propose systematically such a drainage considering that the quality of the dural closure should sufficient.

3. NEUROLOGICAL COMPLICATIONS

3.1 Anosmia

Anosmia is unavoidable in ethmoid tumor as well as olfactory meningioma removal since the approach of the cribriform plate requires section of both olfactory tracts. Otherwise, if section of olfactory tracts is not compulsory, anosmia may be avoided when proceeding to intradural approaches with a careful dissection of the arachnoid surrounding the olfactory nerves and strengthening them with fibrin glue. If necessary, sacrifice of one olfactory tract could possibly preserve unilateral olfaction.

3.2 Confusion

Confusion may result from frontal retraction as well as venous or arterial ischemia (3.3%). Main goal of SFON approach is precisely to avoid such retraction. Nevertheless gentle frontal lobe retraction may be mandatory in some instances. CSF drainage in basal cisterns as well as mannitol perfusion may help to decrease this retraction. It must be released periodically during the procedure, and used only if it is really necessary. Great care must be given in avoiding vascular injury or coagulation, especially concerning large anterior frontal veins. If these veins are spared, anterior part of the superior sagittal sinus may be occluded without any consequences.

3.3 Ocular motor palsies, diplopia

Transient oculomotor palsies may often occur because of edema of intraorbital structures. This occurs more likely when the periorbit is opened which should be avoided. Permanent rate of transient postoperative diplopia is about 6.6% in our series.

3.4 Frontal branch of facial nerve injury

Injury of the frontal branch of the facial nerve should never happen. The bicoronal incision must be stopped at least 1 cm above the zygoma process.

3.5 Supraorbital nerve injury

Supraorbital injury may induce hypoesthesia or anesthesia of eyebrow and supraorbital area. It can be avoided by performing a careful subperiosteal dissection of the galea, and releasing the nerves in the supraorbital gutters or canals.

4. WATERING EYES

It can be seen postoperatively (9.9%) if lacrymal ducts are retracted and obstructed. That is why they should be cut obliquely when the approach is extended downwards.

5. MUCOCELE

Late occurrence of a mucocele can be avoided by careful cranialization of the frontal sinus and obstruction of the nasofrontal ducts.

6. ESTHETIC CONSIDERATIONS

Bicoronal scalp incision decreases the risk of an inesthetic visible scar. Frontal median burr hole may sometimes be visible especially after radiotherapy since the skin may become thinner. For same reasons, miniplates used for fixation of the bone flap must be avoided if external radiotherapy is scheduled after surgical procedure.

CONCLUSIONS

SFON approach is a relatively simple approach. It has the advantage of being adjustable depending on the areas and structures to reach. It allows treating a wide field of craniofacial lesions with a limited retraction of cerebral structures. Great care must be taken to perform a perfect and waterproof closure of the dura.

Acknowledgements

I want to thank very much Dr. François Nataf, neurosurgeon in my department, for his great help in the redaction of this paper.

References

[1] Dandy WE (1941) Orbital tumors. Results following the transcranial operative attack. Oskar Piest Publications, New York

[2] Derome P (1972) Les tumeurs sphéno-orbitaires. Possibilités d'exérèse et de réparations chirurgicales. Neurochirurgie 18(Suppl 1): 164

[3] Ketcham AS, Wilkins RH, Van Buren JM (1963) A combined intra-cranial facial approach to the paranasal sinuses. Am J Surg 103: 698-703

[4] Raveh J, Laedrach K, Speiser M, Chen J, Vuillemin T, Seiler R, Ebeling U, Leibinger K (1993) The subcranial approach for fronto-orbital and anterioposterior skull-base tumors. Arch Otolaryngol Head Neck Surg 119: 385-393

[5] Raveh J, Turk J, Ladrach K, Seiler R, Godoy N, Chen J, Paladino J, Virag M, Leibinger K (1995) Extended anterior subcranial approach for skull base tumors: long-term results. J Neurosurg 82: 1002-1010

[6] Ray BS, McLean JM (1943) Combined intracranial and orbital operation for retinoblastoma. Arch Ophthalmol 30: 437-445

[7] Roux FX, Moussa R, Devaux B, Nataf F, Page P, Laccourreye O, Schwaab G, Brasnu D, Lacau Saint-Guily J (1999) Subcranial fronto-orbito-nasal approach for ethmoidal cancers. Surg Neurol 52: 501-510

[8] Smith KR, Klopp CT, Williams JM (1954) Surgical treatment of cancer of the frontal sinus and adjacent areas. Cancer 7: 991-994

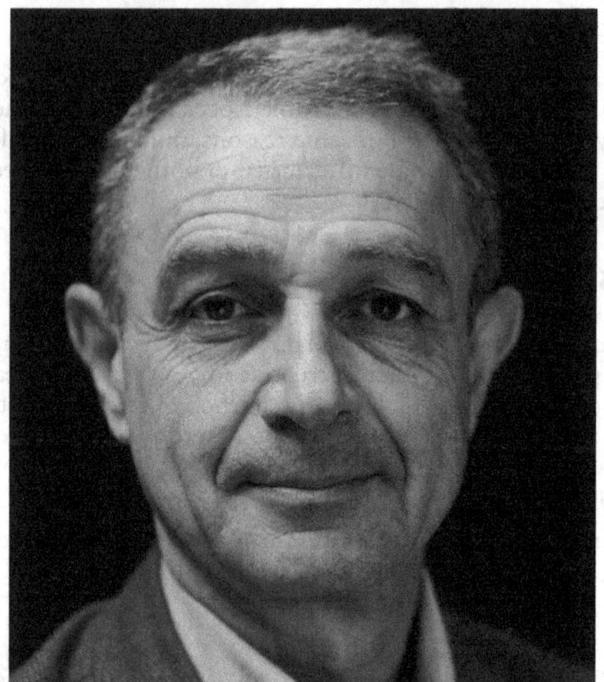

François-Xavier Roux

François-Xavier Roux is Head of the Department of Neurosurgery at Hopital Sainte-Anne, Paris, France.

He was nominated as associate professor in 1985, professor in 1998 and head of department in 2001. He was President of the French Neurosurgical Society from 1998 to 2000. He is well-known for his historical and actual expertise in stereotactic and epileptic surgeries. During the past 25 years, he developed anterior cranial base surgery which is now one of the main activities of the department. His experience concerns particularly ethmoid cancers, olfactory tract meningiomas as well as pituitary and supra sellar tumors. It is in this context that he proposed different techniques and approaches applied to this type of surgery, especially the SFON approach published in 1998, in Surgical Neurology.

He is also very much concerned by cerebral gliomas, particularly oligodendrogliomas, and vascular neurosurgery (aneurysms and AVM's). At last he developed laser neurosurgery since the early 1980s and is the author of 2 books treating this topic.

Contact: François-Xavier Roux, Hôpital Sainte-Anne, 1 rue Cabanis, 75014 Paris, France
E-mail: fx.roux@ch-sainte-anne.fr

HOW TO PERFORM CRANIO-ORBITAL ZYGOMATIC APPROACHES

O. AL-MEFTY

INTRODUCTION

The cranio-orbital zygomatic approach has been in evolution since the frontal approach was first introduced. The addition of both the orbital and zygomatic osteotomies has expanded the limits of neurosurgery to include orbital, craniofacial, and infratemporal pathology. The goal of any skull base approach is to shorten the operative working distance and reduce retraction of the brain while improving exposure. Utilizing the benefits afforded by the cranio-orbital zygomatic approach requires a thorough understanding of the extradural anatomy of the anterior and middle fossae, including the temporal bone, the craniofacial skeleton, and the cavernous sinus.

McArthur and then Frazier were the earliest to incorporate the orbital rim osteotomy with the craniotomy to provide a low frontal approach to the pituitary [11, 17]. Yaşargil in 1969 introduced the pterional approach describing the extradural removal of the sphenoid wing and anterior clinoidal process [23]. Jane et al. resurrected the use of the orbital osteotomy for approaching orbital tumors [15]. Pellerin et al., Hakuba, and Al-Mefty expanded this approach by adding a fronto-orbito-malar osteotomy [6, 13, 20]. Al-Mefty went on to define the cranio-orbital zygomatic approach by combining each of these separate techniques to provide the approach as it is described today [3, 6, 8]. Since then, many authors have described their experiences and modification to this technique [1, 4, 5, 7, 9, 12–14, 18, 20, 21].

RATIONALE

The cranio-orbital zygomatic approach provides the surgeon with a basal exposure of the anterior, middle, and upper ventral middle fossa without retraction of the brain. This approach provides extradural access to the craniofacial skeleton, infratemporal fossa, and paranasal sinuses: frontal, ethmoid, and sphenoid. The internal carotid artery (ICA) can be visualized from its entrance at the skull base through the cavernous sinus extradurally and beyond its bifurcation intradurally as well as the intrapeduncular fossa and the upper

Keywords: cranio-orbital zygomatic approach, skull base surgery, neurosurgical technique, craniotomy

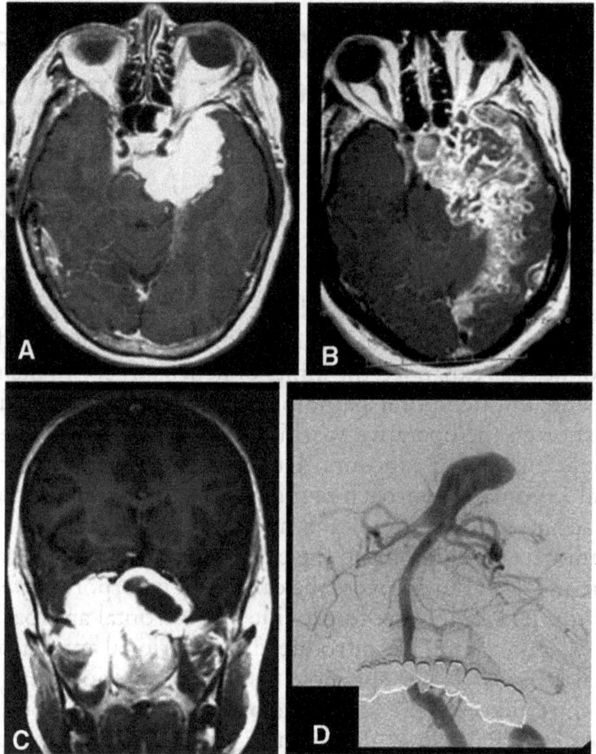

Fig. 1. Example cases that benefit from the utilization of the cranio-orbital zygomatic approach. **A** Sphenocavernous meningioma. **B** Chordoma with extra- and intradural extension with involvement of the cavernous sinus. **C** Juvenile angiofibroma with involvement of the middle fossa and infratemporal fossa. **D** Basilar tip aneurysm

basilar artery complex. Access to the cavernous sinus can be achieved through both intradural and extradural routes. The optic apparatus can be visualized from the optic tracts through the entrance of the optic nerve into the apex of the orbit, as well as provide access to the entire orbit and orbital contents. Additionally, visualization of cranial nerves I through VIII as well as access to the petrous apex is available using this approach. This wide and basal exposure is paramount for the safe treatment for a variety of lesions (Fig. 1) [2, 19, 22].

DECISION-MAKING

Tailored to the nature and extent of lesions in the anterior and middle cranial fossae, variations of cranio-orbital exposures can be used. Each patient should be evaluated individually to determine the most appropriate version [8]. Crucial variables relate to the lesion (pathology, size, and relation to neuro-

Table 1. Tailoring of the cranio-orbital approach

Location of the lesion		Extent of osteotomy
Suprasellar lesions	→	Superior orbital rim
Parasellar lesions, cavernous sinus	→	Superior lateral orbital rim and zygoma
Cavernous sinus, upper clivus	→	Petrous apex
Retropharyngeal, infratemporal	→	Floor of middle fossa
Sphenoid sinus, anterior clivus	→	Frontal sinus, planum sphenoidale

vascular structures) and the patient (age, condition, and anatomy). Detailed radiological studies, including CT scans, MRI, MRA, and MRV are indispensable when selecting the most suitable surgical approach, delineating the tumor relation to surrounding structures and tumor extension. Tailoring of the cranio-orbital approaches is summarized in Table 1.

SURGERY

1. POSITIONING AND PREPARATION

The patient is placed supine. In patients with a small or medium sized tumor, a spinal needle is inserted through a split mattress. Controlled cerebrospinal fluid CSF removal relaxes the brain avoiding brain retraction during the extradural dissection. Approximately 25 ml of CSF is gradually drained with the aid of flow control clamp. The patient's trunk and head are elevated 20°. The head is hyperextended, rotated 20–30° away from the side of the lesion, and tilted slightly. The head is fixed in three point Mayfield head rest. The axis of visualization can be changed by turning the table from side to side. One of the patient's legs is also prepped should a graft of fascia lata, subcutaneous fat, or saphenous vein be needed for reconstruction. Electrodes are inserted for intraoperative monitoring of brain stem auditory evoked responses, and somatosensory evoked potentials, EEG (Fig. 2).

2. SOFT TISSUE DISSECTION

The skin incision is begun 1 cm anterior to the tragus at the level of the zygomatic arch and extended behind the hairline toward the contralateral superior temporal line. Care is taken to cut only through the galea sparing the pericranium. The scalp flap is turned with care to preserve the superficial temporal artery that remains on the temporal muscle. The scalp flap is reflected anteriorly with sharp dissection against the galea, rather than pushing it with a swap, this technique will maintain thick areolar tissue with the pericranium which will be used for reconstruction of the base if needed.

The superficial and deep fasciae of the temporalis muscle are cut 1 cm posterior and parallel to the course of the frontal branches of the facial nerve and

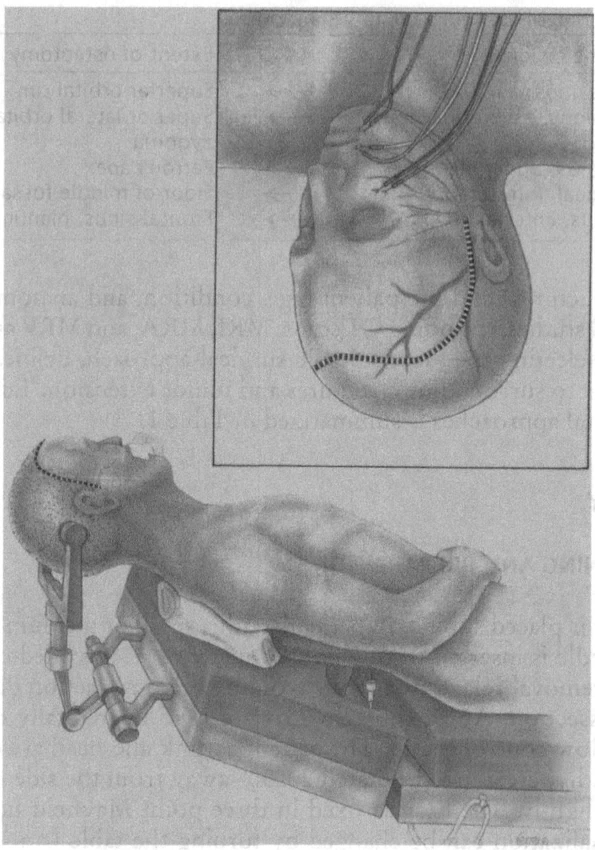

Fig. 2. Position of the patient on the operating table. A lumbar drain has been placed in the lumbar region. The Mayfield headframe is positioned to avoid obstruction to the surgeon. The head is slightly extended and rotation 20° to 30° away from the side of interest. **Inset** The skin incision, represented by the dotted lines, is shown as it relates to the external anatomy, the course of the STA, and the facial nerve, specifically the frontalis branch as it crosses over the zygoma. Needle electrodes have been placed for cranial nerve monitoring

dissected from the muscle fiber, the superficial fascia, fat pad along with the deep fascia are retracted with the skin flap anteriorly (Fig. 3).

3. THE PERICRANIUM

The pericranium is then dissected behind to the skin flap and incised as far posteriorly as needed. The large pericranium flap is reflected forward over the scalp flap. Its intact and vascularized base is dissected free from the roof and the lateral wall of the orbit. This vascularized pericranial flap is crucial for

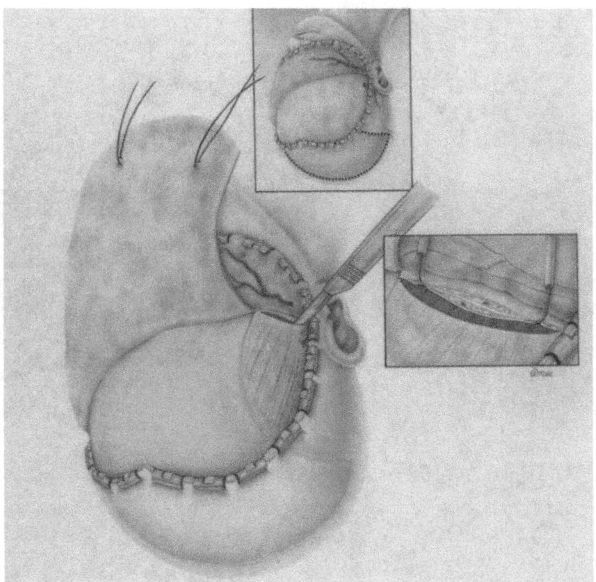

Fig. 3. Top inset The skin flap is dissected sharply from the underlying pericranium and reflected forward. The anterior branch of the STA is transected to avoid retraction injury to the main truck and posterior branch. The dotted lines represent the posterior extent of pericranium dissection. **Main panel** The pericranial flap is reflected forward maintaining a wide anterior base, which preserves its vascular supply. An incision is made through the superficial and deep temporalis fascial layers. **Right inset** The completed subfascial incision showing preservation of the frontalis branch within the fat pad

repairing the floor of the skull base and covering the frontal and ethmoid sinuses at closure to avoid CSF leak. As the intact base of the pericranial flap is dissected free from the orbital rim, the supraorbital nerve is released. If a foramen rather than a notch is present, high speed drill is used to make an osteotomy around this foramen. A collar of bone protects the nerve (Fig. 4).

4. THE ZYGOMA

The temporal fascia is dissected off the zygomatic arch in subperiosteal fashion. The zygomatic arch is incised obliquely at the most anterior and posterior ends. The cuts are made obliquely so that the arch can be anchored during reattachment. The zygoma is then displaced downward with its masseter attachment (Fig. 4).

5. THE TEMPORALIS MUSCLE

The temporalis muscle is incised posterior to the superficial temporal artery course and lifted in subperiostial fashion from the temporal fossa in its en-

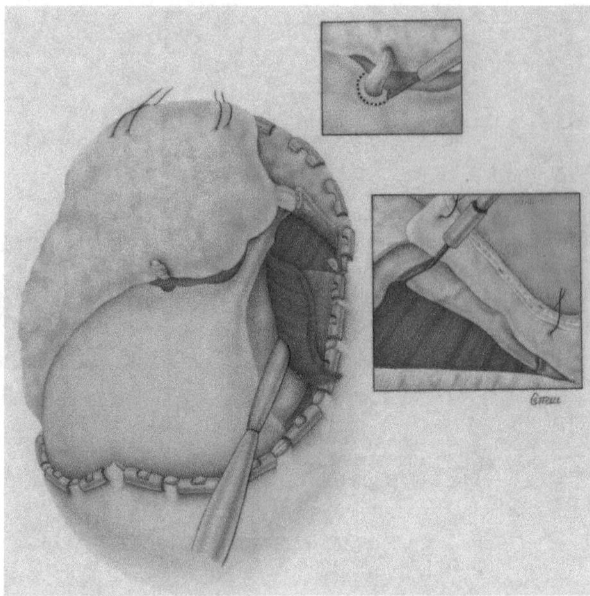

Fig. 4. Top inset When the supraorbital nerve exits a true foramen, an osteotomy is performed to prevent injury to the nerve. **Right inset** A subperiosteal dissection of the lateral orbital rim and zygoma is performed to avoid injury to the frontalis nerve. Oblique cuts are made in the zygoma flush with the malar eminence anterior and at the root of the arch posterior. **Main panel** The temporalis muscle is reflected inferiorly with the zygoma

tirety to preserve the deep temporal arteries and its nerve supply from the third division of the trigeminal nerves (Fig. 4).

6. CRANIOTOMY

A burr hole is placed in the anatomic keyhole located in the depression just behind the suture between the frontal bone and the frontal process of the zygomatic bone. This provides access to the anterior fossa dura and periorbita, separated by the bone of the orbital roof. Burr holes are then placed along the floor of the middle fossa just superior to the root of the zygoma and along the superior temporal line. If necessary a fourth burr hole can be placed posterior to the superior orbital rim and medial to the supraorbital foramen; however, in most instances this hole will enter the frontal sinus. Starting at the burr hole located along the middle fossa floor, the craniotome is directed superiorly and then anteriorly toward the medial aspect of the superior orbital rim. The roof of the orbit will stop the craniotomy. A second cut is made anteriorly along the floor of the middle fossa to the sphenoid wing; the remainder of the cut across the sphenoid wing is made with the Midas Rex B1 attachment. Using a small dissector, the periorbita is dissected from the walls of the orbit. The dissection should begin away from the area of the lacrimal gland as this is typically the thinnest area of the periorbita and therefore prone to laceration. Once the periorbita has been dissected from the bone, a brain spatula should be placed between the periorbita and the bone to protect it from laceration during the orbital osteotomy, carefully avoiding any pressure on the orbital contacts. Using a Midas Rex B1 attachment, a cut is made through the inferior aspect of the lateral orbital rim flush with the malar eminence, then directed superiorly to the keyhole burr hole. A second cut is made through the superior orbital rim medially where the craniotome stopped. Only the thin bone of the orbital roof now attaches the bone flap. Although this can be cracked, we strongly recommend against this practice because the fracture line is inconsistent and may involve the superior orbital fissure or optic canal. Instead, we place a small V-shaped osteotome against the roof of the orbit, visualized in the anatomic keyhole site and direct it to-

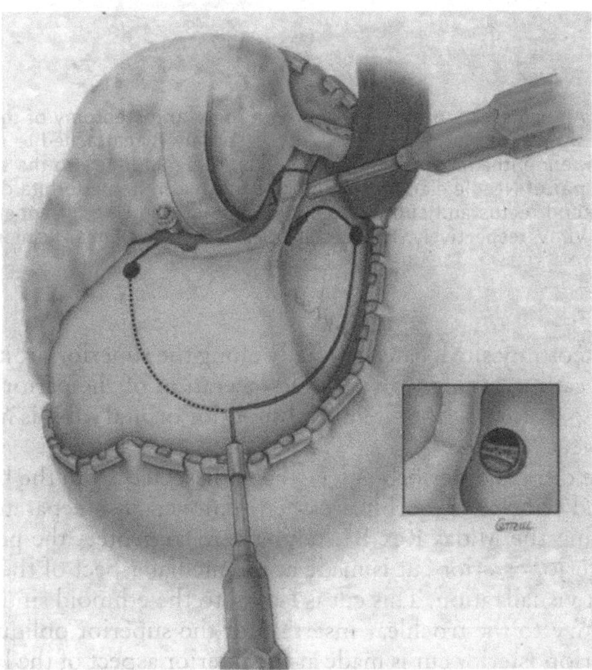

Fig. 5. Right inset A burr hole placed at the anatomic keyhole exposes the anterior fossa dura and the periorbita separated by bone of the orbital roof. **Main panel** Additional burr holes are placed along the floor of the middle fossa, posteriorly along the superior temporal line, and if necessary, medial to the superior orbital rim. The craniotomy is performed by a high-speed drill with a foot attachment. Osteotomies of the super and lateral orbital rims and across the lateral sphenoid wing are made by a high-speed drill without a foot attachment, carefully avoiding laceration to the dura or periorbita. The orbital roof osteotomy is performed using an osteotome placed at the anatomic keyhole

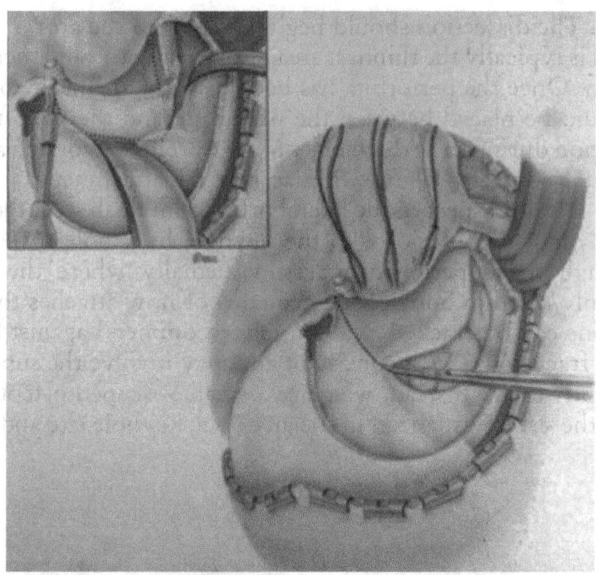

Fig. 6. Inset After dissecting the dura and periorbita, an osteotomy of the superior and lateral orbital walls is performed. The orbital osteotomy is reattached to the craniotomy flap to prevent enophthalmos. Care must be taken to avoid injury to the superior orbital fissure. **Main panel** Needle electrodes are placed through the periorbita directly into the medial and lateral rectus and superior oblique muscles allowing intraoperative monitoring of CNs III, VI, IV, respectively. The dura is opened in a curvilinear fashion and reflected anteriorly

ward the osteotomy site located medially along the superior orbital rim under direct observation, taking care to avoid laceration of the periorbita or dura. The bone flap, including the lateral and superior orbital rims, is now removed as a single piece (Fig. 5).

After the dura and periorbita have been dissected from the bone, the lateral wall and roof of the orbit are then removed in a separate osteotomy (Fig. 6). Using the Midas Rex B1, taking care to protect the periorbita and dura, an anterioposterior cut is made at the medial aspect of the orbital roof under direct visualization. This cut is lateral to the ethmoid sinus taking care to avoid injury to the trochlear insertion of the superior oblique muscle. A second anterioposterior cut is made at the inferior aspect of the lateral orbital wall. These cuts are connected posteriorly, taking care to avoid the superior orbital fissure (SOF). The remaining bone around the SOF, located at the intersection of the lateral wall and roof of the orbit, is removed using a small ronguer or high-speed drill. The optic canal, located at the apex of the orbit, medial to the SOF, is then opened extradurally, and the optic strut is drilled to allow the removal of the anterior clinoid process, exposing the subclinoid portion of the ICA (Fig. 7).

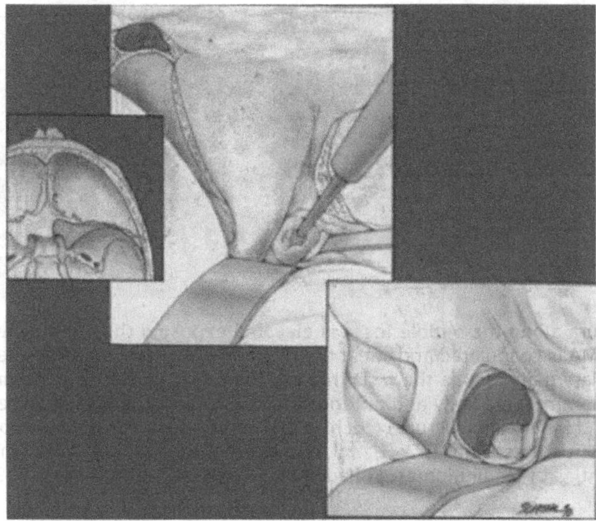

Fig. 7. Main panel The remaining bone of the superior and lateral orbital walls is removed exposing the orbital apex and superior orbital fissure. **Right inset** Drilling of the optic strut allows removal of the anterior clinoid process, exposing the subclinoid portion of the internal carotid artery. **Left inset** Shaded region depicts area of sphenoid bone to be removed extradurally. Reprinted with permission from Al-Mefty O: The cranio-orbital zygomatic approach for intracranial lesions. Contemporary Neurosurgery 14(9): 1-6, 1992

7. EXPOSURE OF THE PETROUS ICA

Starting posteriorly and working anteriorly, the dura along the floor of the middle fossa is elevated. By following the middle meningeal artery, the foramen spinosum is identified and the middle meningeal artery is cut as it exits the foramen. Just medial to the foramen spinosum, the greater and lesser superficial petrosal nerves are identified (GSPN, LSPN) as they exit from the geniculate ganglion through the facial hiatus and run anteriorly in the sphenopetrosal groove. In some case, the bony covering over the geniculate ganglion may be absent. Retraction of the GSPN can cause facial nerve injury and therefore must be avoided. Additionally, we have abandoned and do not recommend transecting the GSPN because it can cause ocular anhydrosis.

Dissection anterior to the foramen spinosum exposes the foramen ovale (V3), foramen rotundum (V2), and superior orbital fissure (III, IV, V-1, and VI). The horizontal portion of the petrous (ICA) lies deep and parallel to the GSPN and posteromedial to the foramen ovale and mandibular branch of the trigeminal nerve. The carotid artery can be unroofed using a diamond drill; however, it is not uncommon for the bony covering of the petrous cartoid to be absent. The Eustachian tube is located lateral to the petrous

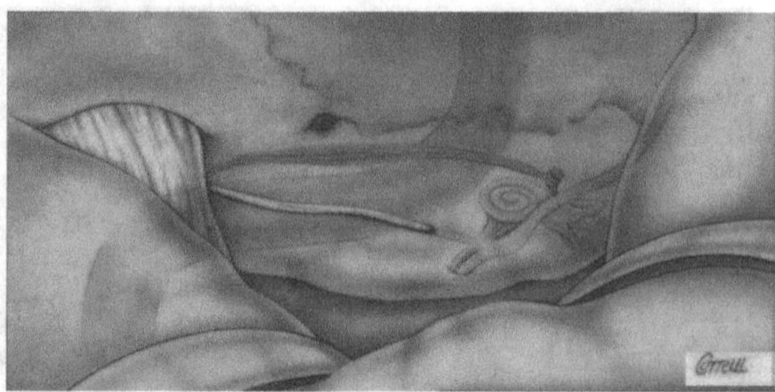

Fig. 8. The dura along the middle fossa is elevated exposing the middle meningeal artery (MMA). The MMA is coagulated and cut at the foramen spinosum exposing the GSPN as it exits the geniculate ganglion via the facial hiatus. The foramen ovale and mandibular branch of CN V are identified medially and anteriorly to the foramen spinosum. The course of the petrous ICA and inner ear structures (cochlea and semicircular canals) are shown in relationship to these structures. Figures 2, 3, 4, 5, 6, 8 are reprinted with permission from Al-Mefty O: Operative Atlas of Meningiomas. Philadelphia, Lippincott-Raven Press, 1998

carotid artery. Exposing the ICA within the petrous bone provides access to the ICA in the event that proximal control and/or a vascular bypass become necessary (Fig. 8).

Sharp dissection of the dural covering over the branches of the trigeminal nerve relaxes the dura for further medial dissection along the middle fossa floor and also exposes the lateral wall of the cavernous sinus. Elevation of the dura further medially and posteriorly along the middle fossa floor allows identification of the arcuate eminence, which is the landmark of the superior semicircular canal (SSC). Unfortunately, the precise position of the SSC can be difficult to appreciate. The SSC lies perpendicular to the petrous bone and about 120° to the course of the GSPN. The internal auditory canal lies at a 45° to 60° with the SSC. Further elevation along the floor will allow identification of the petrous apex. At this point the anterior petrosectomy is performed. The area to be drilled is limited by the trigeminal impression anteriorly, the petrous ICA laterally, the cochlea and facial hiatus posteriorly, and the internal auditory canal inferiorly (allowing access to cranial nerve VII and VII). The cochlea is surrounded by hard compact bone, unlike the bone of the petrous apex, and therefore can be differentiated during drilling of this area. With removal of the petrous apex, the posterior fossa, specifically the petroclival region, is visualized. Removal of the floor of the middle fossa between the foramina ovale and rotundum provides a route of access to the sphenoid sinus. Further removal of the middle fossa floor allows access to the infratemporal fossa through which the posterior wall of the maxillary sinus and nasopharynx can be accessed.

Needle electrodes are placed through the periorbita for intraoperative monitoring of the CNs III, IV, and VI. The dura is opened in a curvilinear fashion and reflected anteriorly.

8. CLOSURE

At the conclusion of the case, the dura must be closed in a watertight fashion using a patch graft as necessary to avoid tension on the brain and to allow tenting to the bone flap to occlude dead space, thereby avoiding epidural fluid collection. In cases where the sphenoid, ethmoid, or maxillary sinuses have been entered, we pack these areas with autologous fat and carefully identify and repair any associated dural openings. Exposure of the frontal sinus is commonly encountered. When exposed, the mucosa is exenterated, the frontal wall is drilled, and the sinus is cranialized by removing the posterior wall. The nasal frontal ducts are occluded with muscle, and the vascularized pericranial flap is placed between the dura and the exposed sinus. We recommend against packing the sinus with foreign material (i.e., bone wax, methylmethacrylate, or hydroxy-apatite) because it can provide a nidus for infection.

The orbital wall ostetomy is reconstructed to the bone flap using craniofacial miniplates. Reconstruction of the orbit reduces long-term enophthalmos. The bone flap is replaced with miniplates, carefully reconstructing the orbital rim to ensure a good cosmetic result. Finally the zygomatic arch is reconstructed using miniplates, and the temporalis muscle is reapproximated.

HOW TO AVOID COMPLICATIONS

Because of the extensive blood supply to the skin flap, necrosis resulting from vascular insufficiency is rare; however, aggressive coagulation of superficial vessels, the application of strong hemostatic clips to the skin edge, or acute folding of the skin flap can interfere with the blood supply and subsequently cause flap complications [7]. The use of thermal coagulation along the temporalis fascia and during the elevation of the temporalis muscle can cause injury to the frontalis branch of the facial nerve and the trigeminal branch to the temporal muscle contributes to the postoperative atrophy of the temporalis muscle [9, 16]. Additionally, we recommend preservation of the STA, not only for its potential use as a vascular bypass, but also for its preserved vascular supply to the temporalis muscle [9]. Postoperative periorbital swelling is common but usually resolves quickly without functional or cosmetic deficits [9, 15].

Entrance into the frontal or other paranasal sinuses is a source of potential complications, including infection, CSF leaks, mucoceles, or pneumocephalus [9, 10]. However, with meticulous dural closure, packing of the exposed sinuses, exenteration of the frontal sinus, and disposal of the instruments from the surgical field after use in the sinus, we have experienced few complications specifically related to these maneuvers [2, 9].

Dissection of the middle fossa floor presents a specific group of complications. We use the operative microscope to aid in this dissection as it provides both improved illumination and better visualization of the structures. As stated earlier preservation and careful dissection of the GSPN are necessary. Additionally, dissection of the branches of the trigeminal nerve can cause postoperative pain, dysesthesia, or masticatory weakness; however, these complications have seldom been encountered in our experience. Careful dissection of the petrous ICA does not need elaboration; however, injury to the Eustachian tube should be avoided because it can cause chronic serous otitis media necessitating the placement of tympanostomy tubes. Finally, bleeding can be encountered during the dissection of the cavernous sinus. It can be brisk but usually is controllable by gently packing the sinus with hemostatic materials.

CONCLUSIONS

The cranio-orbital zygomatic approach is a versatile approach, which can be custom-tailored to the patient's pathology. Its ability to maintain cosmetically appealing results with extensive exposure of the anterior fossa, middle fossa, and petroclival regions with minimal morbidity makes this approach a mainstay in skull base surgery.

References

[1] Alaywan M, Sindou M (1990) Fronto-temporal approach with orbito-zygomatic removal surgical anatomy. Acta Neurochir 104: 79-83

[2] Al-Mefty O (1969) Surgery of the cranial base. Kluwer Academic Publishers, Boston

[3] Al-Mefty O (1987) Supraorbital-pterional approach to skull base lesions. Neurosurgery 21: 474-477

[4] Al-Mefty O, Anand VK (1990) Zygomatic approach to skull-base lesions. J Neurosurg 73: 668-673

[5] Al-Mefty O, Ayoubi S, Schenk MP (1991) Unlocking and entering the cavernous sinus. Perspect Neurol Surg 2: 49-53

[6] Al-Mefty O, Fox JL (1985) Supralateral orbital exposure and reconstruction. Surg Neurol 23: 609-613

[7] Al-Mefty O, Smith RR (1988) Surgery of the tumors invading the cavernous sinus. Surg Neurol 30: 370-381

[8] Al-Mefty O, Smith RR (1990) Tailoring the cranio-orbital approach. Keio J Med 39: 217-224

[9] Al-Mefty O, Smith RR (1993) Combined approaches in the management of brain lesions. In: Apuzzo MLJ (ed) Brain surgery: complication avoidance and management. Churchill Livingstone, New York

[10] Dandy WE (1966) The brain. WF Prior, Hagerstown

[11] Frazier CH (1913) An approach to the hypophysis through the anterior cranial fossa. Ann Surg 57: 145-150

[12] Fujitsu K, Kuwarabara T (1985) Zygomatic approach for lesions in the interpeduncular cistern. J Neurosurg 62: 340-343

[13] Hakuba A, Liu S, Nishimura S (1986) The orbitozygomatic infratemporal approach. A new surgical technique. Surg Neurol 26: 271-276

[14] Hakuba A, Tanaka K, Suziki T, et al. (1989) A combined orbitozygomatic infratemporal epidural and subdural approach for lesions involving the entire cavernous sinus. J Neurosurg 71: 559-704

[15] Jane JA, Park TS, Pobereskin LH, et al. (1982) The supraorbital approach. Technical note. Neurosurgery 11: 537-542

[16] Kadri P, Al-Mefty O (2004) The anatomic basis for surgical preservation of the temporal muscle. J Neurosurg 100: 517-522

[17] McArthur LL (1912) An aseptic surgical access to the pituitary body and its neighborhood. JAMA 58: 2009-2011

[18] Mann WJ, Gilsbach J, Seeger W, et al. (1985) Use of malar bone graft to augment skull base access. Arch Otolaryngol 111: 30-33

[19] Origitano TC, Anderson DE, Tarassoli Y, Reichman OH, Al-Mefty O (1993) Skull base approaches to complex cerebral aneurysms. Surg Neurol 40: 339-346

[20] Pellerin P, Lesoin F, Dhellemmes P, et al. (1984) Usefulness of the orbitofrontomalar approach associated with bone reconstruction for frontotemporosphenoid meningioma. Neurosurgery 15: 715-718

[21] Sekhar LN, Schramm VL Jr, Jones NF (1987) Subtemporal-preauricular infratemporal fossa approach to large lateral and posterior cranial base neoplasms. J Neurosurg 67: 488-499

[22] Smith RR, Al-Mefty O, Middleton T (1989) An orbitocranial approach to complex aneurysms of the anterior circulation. Neurosurgery 24: 385-391

[23] Yaşargil MG (1969) Microsurgery applied to neurosurgery. Georg Thieme, Stuttgart, pp 119-143

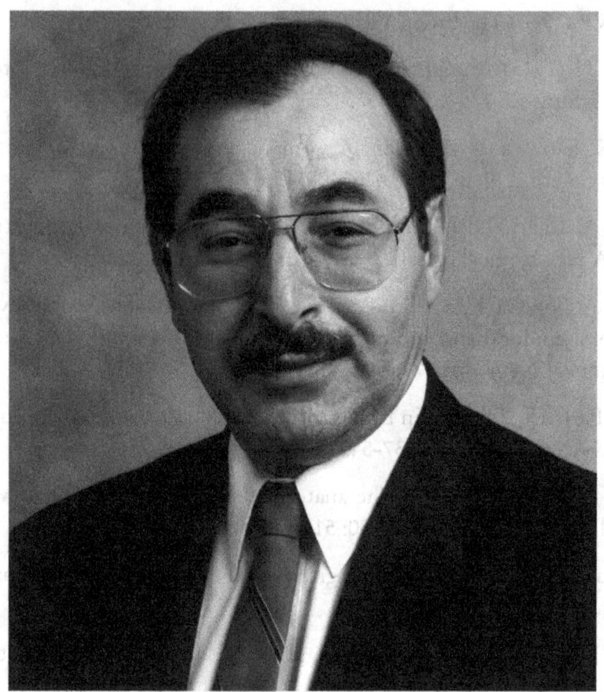

Ossama Al-Mefty

Ossama Al-Mefty is Professor and Chairman of the Department of Neurosurgery at the University of Arkansas for Medical Sciences, a position he has held since 1993. He graduated from Damascus University Medical School in 1972 and underwent neurosurgical residency training at West Virginia Medical Center. It was during his position as a staff neurosurgeon at King Faisal Specialist Hospital in the early 1980s when he developed his abiding interest with skull base surgery. Upon his return to the United States in 1985, he joined the Department of Neurosurgery at the University of Mississippi, where he became professor, and then served as professor of neurosurgery at Loyola University of Chicago prior to his current position as the Robert Watson Endowed Chair in Neurosurgery at the University of Arkansas.

Dr. Al-Mefty is a pioneer in the field of skull base surgery and his expertise is well recognized and highly sought-after throughout the world. He has authored 189 peer-reviewed papers, 74 chapters and 8 books including the seminal textbook Meningiomas. He has given over 700 presentations and has had over 320 invited lectures at meetings and courses around the globe and has been honored with 67 visiting professorships. He is a dedicated teacher and has been faculty and director of well over 50 workshops and hand-on courses. He is on the editorial boards of numerous prestigious journals including Neurosurgery, Contemporary Neurosurgery, Skull Base Surgery, Critical

Reviews in Neurosurgery and Neurosurgical Review. He has received numerous honors including being named the Penfield Lecturer, the first Sugita Memorial Lecturer, the Hakuba Memorial Lecturer, the Dr. Khalifa Bo Rashid Memorial Lecturer, John L. Kemink, M.D. Memorial Lecturer, the First Annual Linda Wolfe Memorial Meningioma Lecturer, Sally Harrington Goldwater Visiting Professors, and the Milam E. Leavens Distinguished Lecturer.

Dr. Al-Mefty is a member of the Society of Neurological Surgeons, the American Association of Neurological Surgeons, the Congress of Neurological Surgeons, and the American College of Surgeons among others. He is President and founding member of the World Academy of Neurological Surgeons, Past President and founding member of the North American Skull Base Society. He is an honorary member of several societies internationally including Skull Base Society of Brazil, Canadian Neuroscience Society, Brazilian Neurosurgical Society, Georgia Neurosurgical Society, Portugal Neurosurgical Society, Turkish Neurosurgical Society, Mexican Society of Neurological Surgery, Japanese Neurosurgical Society, Syrian Society of Neurosciences, and the Chile Neurosurgical Society.

Contact: Ossama Al-Mefty, University of Arkansas for Medical Sciences,
Department of Neurosurgery, 4301 W. Markham, #507 Little Rock, AR 72205, USA
E-mail: keelandamye@uams.edu

HOW TO PERFORM MIDDLE FOSSA/SPHENOID WING APPROACHES

F. UMANSKY

INTRODUCTION

The skull base is a very complex anatomical region with an irregular bony architecture, which is classically divided into anterior, middle, and posterior compartments called fossae. The presence of dural folds, blood vessels, and cranial nerves provides a surgical challenge for even the most experienced neurosurgeon. Several approaches have been described to reach different parts of the middle fossa. These skull base approaches usually require bony drilling for exposure, to control the tumor blood supply, and to minimize brain retraction. Knowledge of anatomy acquired in the laboratory, as well as learning to handle relevant microinstrumentation, including microdrills, is of paramount importance for the young neurosurgeon who is interested in the difficult field of skull base surgery.

In this chapter we will discuss the tumoral pathology of the middle cranial fossa, with an emphasis on intracranial, intradural extra-axial lesions. Special consideration will be given to the most common tumors in this category, sphenoid wing meningiomas. We will discuss surgical approaches, techniques, and complications related to the surgical removal of these challenging lesions.

RATIONALE

1. ANATOMY OF THE MIDDLE FOSSA

The middle cranial fossa is deeper than the anterior fossa, and its lateral parts are larger than its central part. The anterior limit is bounded by the posterior borders of the lesser wings of the sphenoid bone, the anterior clinoid processes (ACP), and the anterior margin of the chiasmatic sulcus. The middle fossa is limited posteriorly by the superior borders of the petrous bones and the dorsum sellae, and laterally by the temporal squamae, the frontal angles of the parietal bones, and the greater wings of the sphenoid (Fig. 1).

The central part of the middle cranial fossa is formed by the body of the sphenoid bone and includes the tuberculum sellae, the sella turcica, middle and posterior clinoid processes, the carotid sulcus, and the dorsum sellae. On

Keywords: skull base approach, middle fossa region, lateral approaches

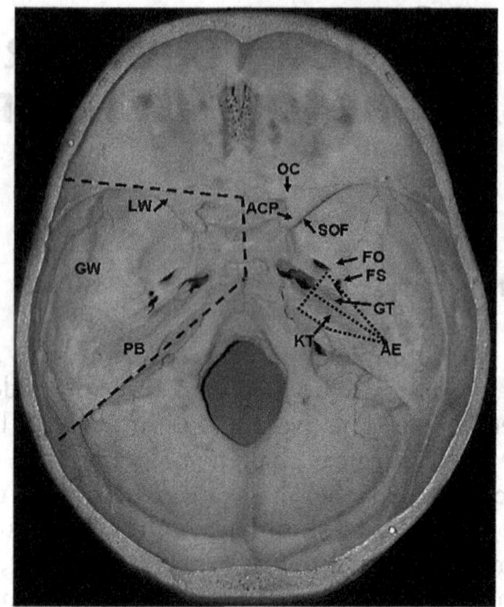

Fig. 1. Endocranial surface of the skull base. The dashed lines on the left side represent the limits of the middle fossa. *ACP* Anterior clinoid process; *AE* arcuate eminence; *FO* foramen ovale; *FS* foramen spinosum; *GT* Glasscock's triangle; *GW* greater wing of the sphenoid bone; *KT* Kawase's triangle; *LW* lesser wing of the sphenoid bone; *OC* optic canal; *PB* petrous bone; *SOF* superior orbital fissure

each side of its central part, the cavernous sinus extends from the medial end of the superior orbital fissure to the apex of the petrous bone.

In the endocranial surface of the middle cranial fossa, there are several bony canals and foramina containing vessels and nerves that are important anatomical landmarks:

1. Optic canal – formed by the anterior and posterior root (optic strut) of the lesser wing. The optic strut separates the optic canal from the superior orbital fissure. The optic nerve (ON) (CN II) and the ophthalmic artery course through the canal.
2. Superior orbital fissure (SOF) – located between the lesser and greater sphenoid wings. The SOF contains the oculomotor (CN III), throclear (CN IV), ophthalmic (CN V, V1), and abducens (CN VI) nerves, as well as a recurrent meningeal artery and the superior and inferior ophthalmic veins.
3. Foramen rotundum – located in the greater wing of the sphenoid, contains the maxillary (CN V, V2) and ovale for the mandibular (CN V, V3) nerves.
4. Foramen spinosum – posterior and lateral to the foramen ovale, contains the middle meningeal artery.
5. Trigeminal impression – located in the petrous apex, contains Meckel's cave and the semilunar ganglion (trigeminal or gasserian ganglion).

6. Upper surface of the petrous bone – presents two grooves for the greater (GSPN) and lesser (LSPN) superficial petrosal nerves. These nerves can be confused with dural strands of the middle fossa floor and are difficult to dissect.
7. Carotid window – the most anterior segment of the intrapetrous carotid artery, covered by a thin bony plate in 75% of our specimens, and by the periosteum only in the remaining 25%.
8. Tensor tympani and eustachian tube – located medial to the foramen spinosum and lateral to the horizontal segment of the petrous carotid.
9. Arcuate eminence – situated posteriorly in the upper surface of the petrous bone, marks the location of the superior semicircular canal.
10. Kawase's triangle (posteromedial middle fossa triangle) [8, 9] – the anterior limit is defined by the lateral border of V3 and the gasserian ganglion. Posteriorly, it is defined by a line parallel, and 13 mm posterior, to the anterior border. The medial limit corresponds to the superior petrosal sinus and the lateral limit is marked by the horizontal segment of the intrapetrous carotid and overlying GSPN.
11. Glasscock's triangle (posterolateral middle fossa triangle) [4] – located lateral to Kawase's triangle, is bounded laterally by a line drawn from the foramen spinosum toward the arcuate eminence, ending at the facial hiatus; medially by the GSPN; and anteriorly by the mandibular division of the trigeminal nerve (V3).

The exocranial surface of the middle fossa includes the infratemporal fossa, the pterygopalatine fossa, and the parapharyngeal and infrapetrosal spaces.

2. CLASSIFICATION OF THE MIDDLE FOSSA TUMORS

Tumors of the middle cranial fossa can be classified in accordance with their anatomical origin from intracranial or extracranial surfaces. By bony erosion, or growth through natural openings/canals, foramina, or fissures of the floor of the middle fossa, tumors can extend from one compartment to another.

2.1 Intracranial tumors

1. Intradural – meningiomas, schwannomas, epidermoids, dermoids
2. Extradural – chordomas, chondrosarcomas, metastases

2.2 Extracranial tumors

1. Infratemporal fossa – juvenile angiofibromas, fibrous dysplasias
2. Pterygopalatine fossa – juvenile angiofibromas
3. Parapharyngeal space – carcinomas

4. Orbital cavity – ON sheath meningiomas, schwannomas, lymphomas, cavernous hemangiomas, ON gliomas, bone lesions (osteomas, dysplasias, aneurysmal bone cysts, metastases, etc.)

3. SPECIAL FEATURES OF MENINGIOMAS, SCHWANNOMAS AND EPIDERMOID/DERMOID CYSTS

3.1 Meningiomas

Meningiomas of the sphenoid wing and middle cranial fossa represent approximately 17–25% of all intracranial meningiomas. This is the third most common site of origin for meningiomas, after the convexity and parasagittal areas.

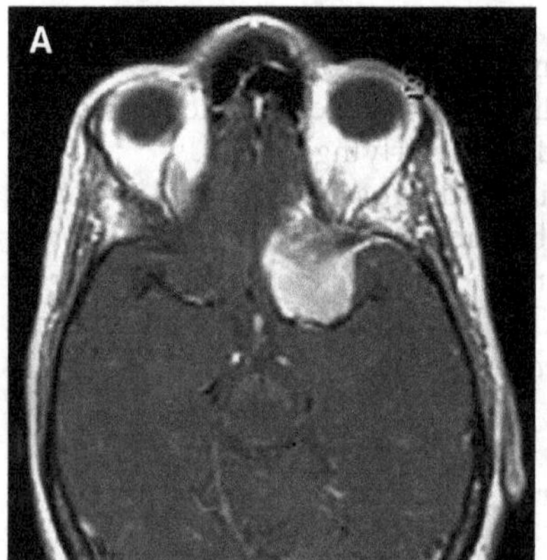

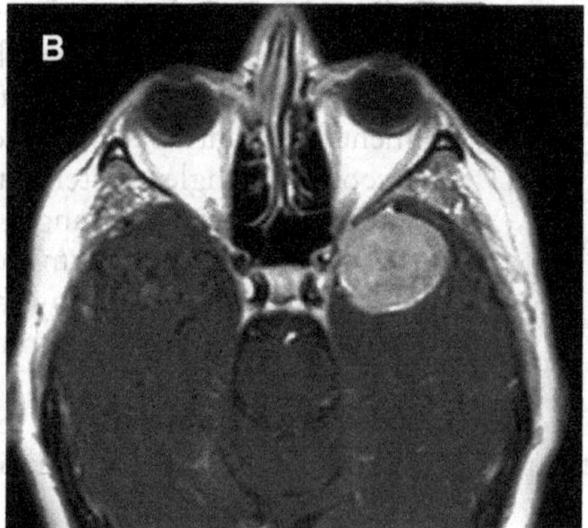

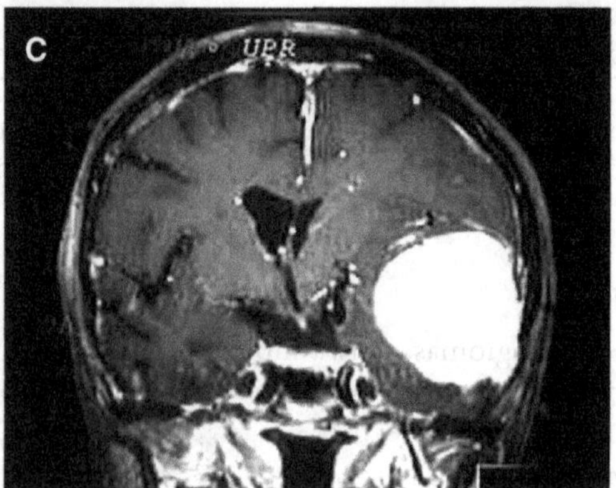

Fig. 2. T1-weighted+Gd MR images of meningiomas in the sphenoid wing. **A** Meningioma in the inner third of the sphenoid wing with optic nerve involvement. **B** Meningioma originating from and confined to the middle third of the sphenoid wing. **C** Pterional global meningioma in the outer third of the sphenoid wing

Cushing and Eisenhardt divided the sphenoid ridge into three approximately equal sections: deep, inner, or clinoidal; middle or alar; and outer or pterional [3]. They described two types of pterional lesions: meningiomas en plaque, which provoke hyperostosis of the greater wing; and global meningiomas, which expand within the crotch of the Sylvian fissure.

Inner third sphenoid wing- or clinoidal meningiomas (Fig. 2A) are characterized by involvement of the optic nerve (ON) early in their growth. Hyperostosis of the ACP is usually present, and there is partial or total encasement of the internal carotid artery and its branches. The tumor may also attach to the lateral wall of the cavernous sinus (CS) and/or invade it. Involvement of the CS may cause diplopia and facial hypoesthesia. Venous congestion, hyperostosis, and orbital extension may lead to exophthalmos.

Meningiomas confined to the middle third of the sphenoid ridge are rare (Fig. 2B), and usually represent extension of a clinoid or pterional lesion.

Meningiomas of the outer third or pterional section may be either global or en plaque. Pterional-global lesions behave as convexity meningiomas (Fig. 2C), which can become large and cause seizures, mass effect, and focal neurological deficits, with or without signs of intracranial hypertension. The en plaque lesions (Fig. 3), also known as spheno-orbital meningiomas, are characterized by hyperostosis of the sphenoid wing and orbital bone, causing exophthalmos. Tumor can also infiltrate the orbit, optic canal, CS, and base of the middle fossa. Visual deficits are not infrequent.

Petrous apex meningiomas (Fig. 4) can be considered as a type of petroclival meningioma originating in the anterior aspect of the petrous bone, me-

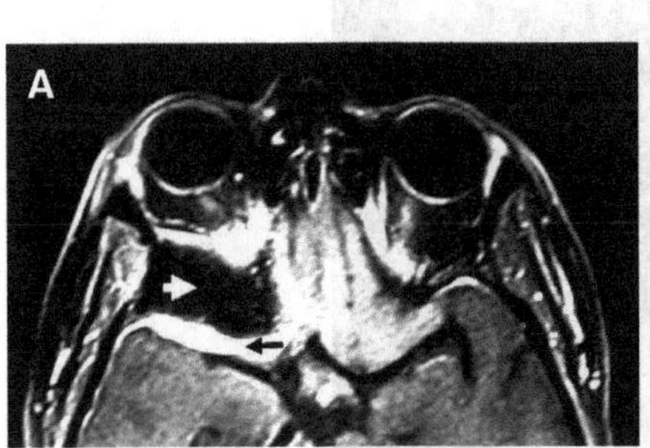

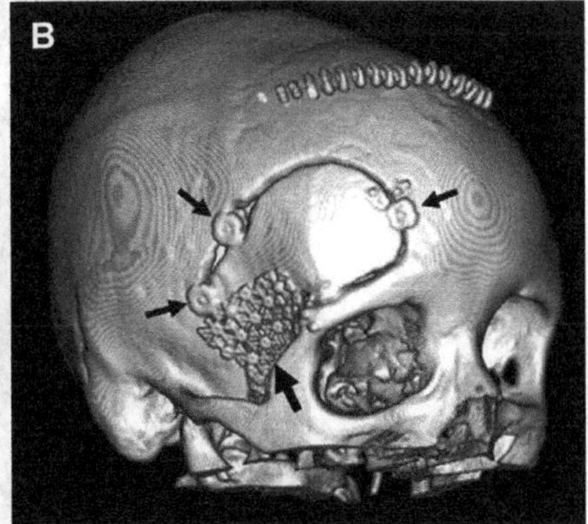

Fig. 3. **A** T1-weighted Gd-enhanced MR image of a spheno-orbital or en plaque meningioma. Note extensive bony hyperostosis (white arrow) and the enhanced plaque of the lesion (black arrow). **B** 3-D reconstruction of the craniotomy site showing closure using the Craniofix titanium clip (3 small arrows) (CF: Aesculap AG, Tuttlingen, Germany) and titanium mesh (large arrow)

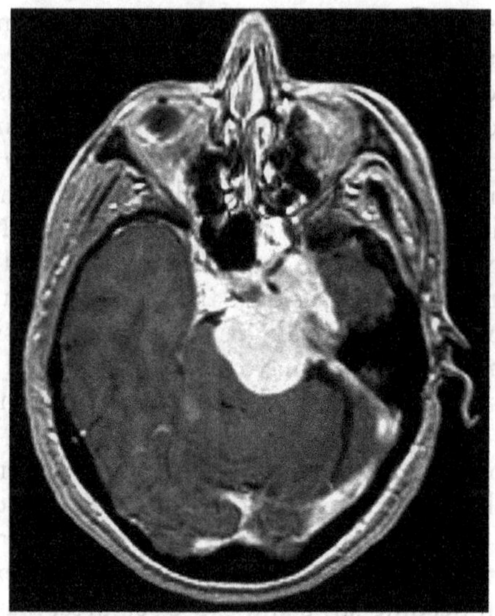

Fig. 4. T1-weighted Gd-enhanced MR image of a petrous apex meningioma

dial to the internal auditory canal. These tumors can be resected by an extended middle fossa approach with anterior petrosectomy and opening of the tentorium, as described by Kawase in 1991 [9].

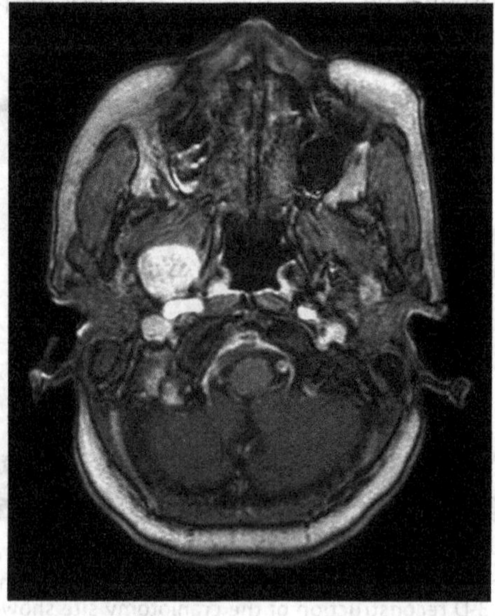

Fig. 5. T1-weighted Gd-enhanced MR image of a right trigeminal schwannoma arising from V3

3.2 Schwannomas

The schwannomas are benign tumors composed entirely of Schwann cells. They are the second most common extra-axial intracranial tumor, preceded by meningiomas. They constitute 5–10% of all intracranial neoplasms, and have a predilection for sensory nerves. The vestibular division of the eighth cranial nerve is the most common site of origin, followed by the trigeminal nerve. Schwannomas of the jugular foramen and the facial nerve are less frequent. Trigeminal schwannomas (Fig. 5) can originate from the cisternal segment of the nerve, from Meckel's cave, in the CS, and in the superior orbital fissure. The tumor can extend below the skull base through the foramen ovale. A dumbbell configuration with supratentorial (Meckel's cave) and infratentorial (cerebellopontine angle) components is not unusual.

3.3 Epidermoid and dermoid cysts

Intradural epidermoid and dermoid cysts are congenital developmental lesions composed of a layer of stratified squamous epithelium covered by an external fibrous capsule. Mesoderm elements (hair, sebaceous, and sweat glands) can be found inside the dermoid cysts. Epidermoid cysts, frequently called "pearly tumors" because of their gross external appearance, represent approximately 1.5% of all intracranial tumors. They grow slowly by desquamation of the epithelial cells and conversion to keratin and cholesterol crystals. They are usually located

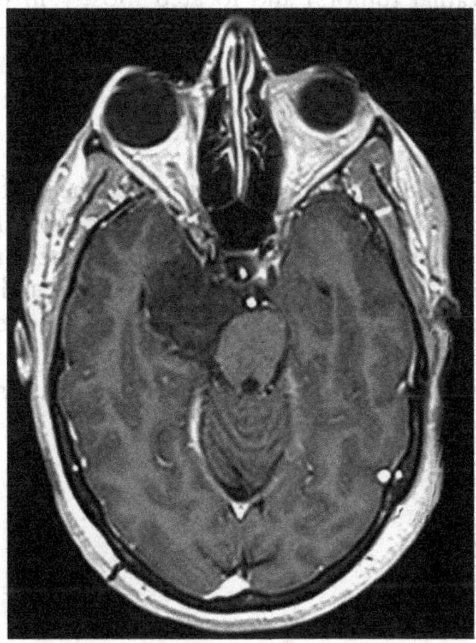

Fig. 6. T1-weighted Gd-enhanced MR image of an epidermoid in the parasellar region compressing the brainstem

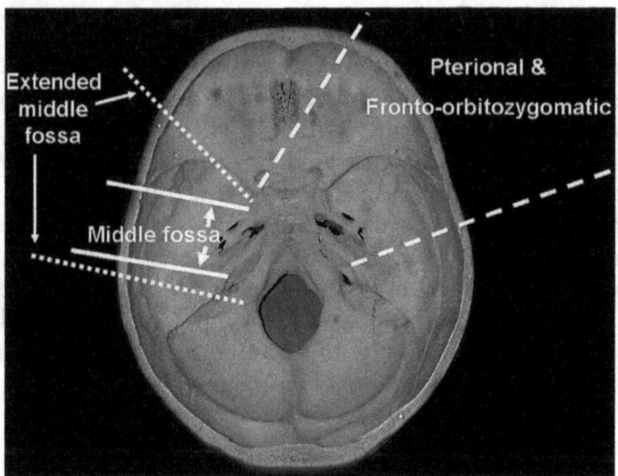

Fig. 7. Frequently used approaches for tumors of the middle fossa drawn on the skull base

in the cisterns of the cerebellopontine angle, supra- and parasellar regions, or the middle cranial fossa (Fig. 6). They can be differentiated radiologically from arachnoid cysts using MRI diffusion-weighted imaging. On T1-weighted MRI, epidermoid cysts demonstrate mild hypointensity, while dermoid cysts show marked hyperintensity. Dermoid cysts are less frequent than epidermoid cysts (0.3–0.6% of intracranial tumors) and located mostly in the posterior fossa. They can rupture into the subarachnoid space or inside the ventricles.

DECISION-MAKING

In order to obtain a successful outcome in the treatment of neurosurgical diseases, the decision-making process is based on indications for surgery and its timing. Choosing the best operative approach for a particular situation is as important as the choice of specific instrumentation and updated technology. Surgical approaches to deal with middle fossa tumors (Fig. 7) are chosen based in the location and size of the lesions. Other considerations will be the neurosurgeon's experience, the extent of resection sought, and the patient's expectations.

SURGERY

1. PTERIONAL APPROACH

1.1 Superficial planes

The pterional-transylvian approach is the most common and useful approach to deal with a wide range of lesions in the anterior, middle, and posterior cranial fossa. It is a classic approach, which was popularized by Yaşargil et al. [12], and can be modified according to the pathology into frontolateral or fronto-orbitozygomatic (FOZ) craniotomies (Fig. 8).

The patient is positioned supine with the head turned about 40° to the opposite side, and slightly extended. After positioning, the patient is securely

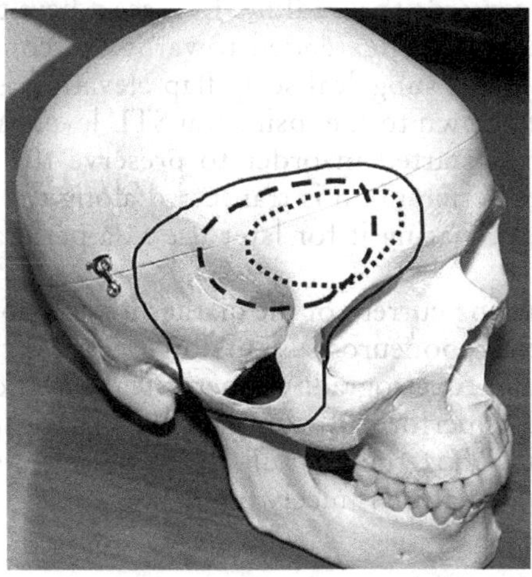

Fig. 8. The pterional approach (dashed line) and its frontolateral (dotted line) and fronto-orbital zygomatic (solid line) variants drawn on the skull surface

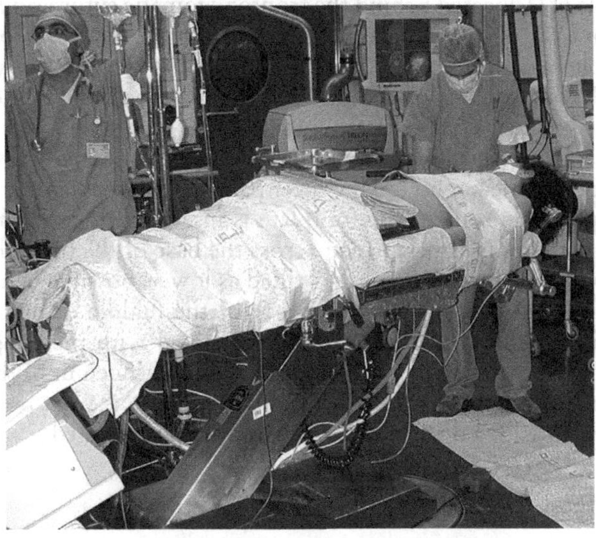

Fig. 9. The patient is firmly attached to the table with hip supports and plastic tape to enable tilting in the desired direction

attached to the table with plaster tape so that the table may be rotated in any direction (Fig. 9). For the frontolateral approach, the head is turned only about 20°. For expanded exposure, an orbitozygomatic osteotomy can be added.

The head is fixed to the operating table with the Mayfield three-pin headrest. The scalp incision starts inferiorly, just anterior to the tragus and behind the superficial temporal artery (STA). From here it runs superiorly behind the hairline towards the midline. In cases where the FOZ approach is to be used, the incision is extended towards the contralateral superior temporal line (STL). The subgaleal scalp flap elevation is sharply begun at the frontal convexity down to the ipsilateral STL level. At this point an interfascial dissection is started in order to preserve the frontal branch of the facial nerve. The pericranium is transected along the temporal line and elevated separately, preparing it for later use as a pericranial flap to cover the frontal sinus.

Next, with the cutting current of the diathermy, the posterior belly of the temporal muscle and its aponeurosis is cut down to the periosteum and parallel to the skin incision. A retrograde subperiosteal elevation of the temporal muscle from the STL is performed with the aid of a periosteal elevator, without any cauterization. Thus, the full bulk of the muscle is atraumatically elevated and its neurovasculature is nicely preserved.

1.2 Craniotomy

Two small diameter burr holes, just large enough to admit the craniotome footplate, are usually used to develop the bone flap. The first burr hole is the MacCarty keyhole [11], located behind the frontozygomatic suture, and the second is placed above the posterior part of the zygoma at the temporal fossa floor. A third burr hole may occasionally be necessary, and is located beneath the temporal line. No burr hole is placed in the forehead. The bone flap cut is made with the fluted router of a pediatric craniotome to minimize bone loss. From the temporal burr hole, the bone cut is directed across the temporal squama and the frontal bone to the keyhole. The lower part of the bone flap is cut using the same fluted pediatric router. The footplate is inserted into the temporal burr hole and the osteotomy is performed across the base of the bone flap towards the keyhole with the fluted router drill tilted as low as possible beneath the reflected temporal muscle, towards the floor of the middle cranial fossa. This usually eliminates the need for extra bone removal with the rongeurs upon completion of the craniotomy. The osteotomy is continued until the footplate is stuck at the lateral part of the sphenoid wing. Here, the last bone bridge is finally transected with a drill, and the free bone flap is elevated.

1.3 Frontolateral approach

The field of vision achieved with a more medially placed craniotomy, such as in the frontolateral approach, described by Brock and Dietz [1], can also be achieved with the pterional approach, by tilting the operating table in the desired direction.

1.4 Fronto-orbitozygomatic approach

Although variations of the orbitozygomatic approach have been used since the 1970s, it was popularized a decade later by Jane et al. [7] for the exposure of tumors of the lateral anterior cranial fossa and those in the orbit and retro-orbital regions.

The pterional approach will be used for the vast majority of tumors located in the anterior two thirds of the middle cranial fossa. In some circumstances, when a more basal approach is needed, an orbitozygomatic craniotomy may be necessary. We prefer to utilize the so called "two piece" orbitozygomatic craniotomy, which means that the pterional bone flap is elevated first, and then as a second, distinct step, the orbitozygomatic osteotomy is performed. This osteotomy will include the supraorbital rim, part of the roof and lateral wall of the orbit, and a portion of the zygoma.

1.5 Extradural stage

Meningiomas of the inner third of the sphenoid ridge, including clinoid meningiomas, frequently involve the ON, causing visual deterioration. They may also encase the internal carotid artery (ICA) and its branches, and induce hyperostotic thickening of the ACP. In many cases we prefer to begin with extradural drilling of the skull base to diminish tumor vascularization, to obtain early decompression of the optic nerve by opening its canal,

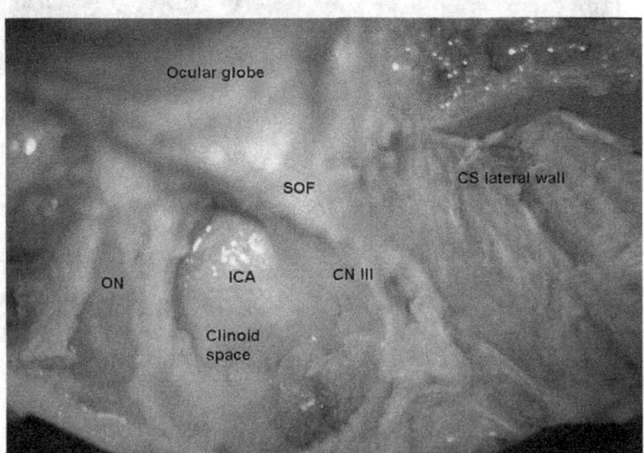

Fig. 10. Right side anatomical specimen after extradural drilling of the anterior clinoid process and opening of the optic canal and superior orbital fissure (*SOF*). The optic nerve sheath has been opened revealing the nerve (*ON*). Note the proximity of CN III to the internal carotid artery (*ICA*) in the clinoid space. The lateral wall of the cavernous sinus (*CS*) is clearly seen

and to identify the ICA in the clinoid space proximal to its encasement by the tumor. After the pterional bone flap is elevated, the microscope is brought to the surgical field. The dura mater covering the anterior and mid-

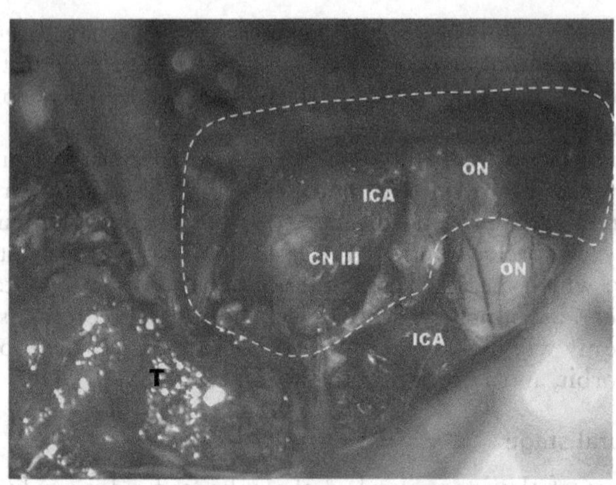

Fig. 11. Intraoperative view of a left inner third sphenoid wing meningioma after opening the dura mater. The area of extradural drilling is delineated by the broken line, showing the optic nerve (*ON*) after opening the canal, the ICA within the clinoid space, and CN III by transparence in the most medial aspect of the superior orbital fissure. Outside the broken line, the intradural portion of the ICA and ON are also seen, already dissected free from the tumor (*T*)

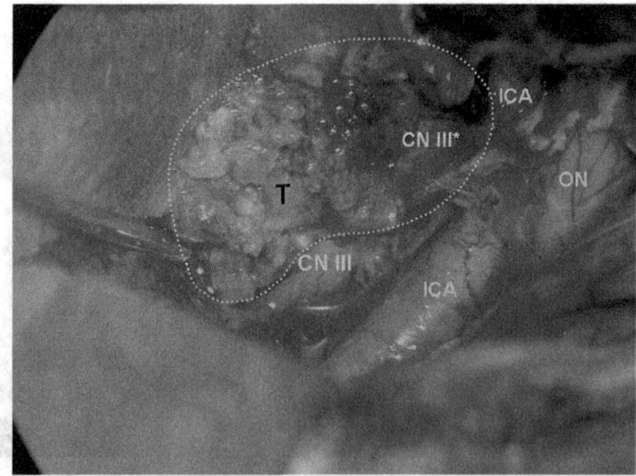

Fig. 12. Removal of the tumor has progressed toward the cavernous sinus (CS) with peeling of the outer layer of its lateral wall. The last piece of the tumor (*T*) is seen still attached to this layer. CN III is shown entering the CS, and then by transparence embedded in the deep layer of the lateral wall (*CN III**). The area of the CS is delimited by the dotted line

dle cranial fossa is elevated from the orbital roof and the lesser- and greater sphenoid ridges, under magnification. The meningo-orbital band is cut to facilitate further retraction of the dura mater, and the superior orbital fissure is exposed. An extradural clinoidectomy is performed, and the optic canal unroofed to expose the extradural ON (Figs. 10–12). Cutting and diamond drills accompanied by copious irrigation are used for this extensive drilling.

In cases of spheno-orbital meningiomas or meningiomas en plaque, there is a lot of hyperostotic bone that needs to be drilled away. The drilling includes the lesser sphenoid wing, the roof and lateral wall of the orbit, the edges of the superior orbital fissure down to the foramen rotundum, and the beginning of the superior orbital fissure. A partial clinoidectomy and unroofing of the optic canal are also performed. The intra-orbital extension of the tumor is removed, avoiding injury to the ocular muscles.

1.6 Dural opening and tumor removal

The dura mater is opened low and parallel to the skull base. An additional perpendicular cut is placed, following the Sylvian fissure. The fissure is opened, and CSF is released, exposing the tumor. Internal debulking will facilitate the dissection of the tumor from the vascular structures and optic apparatus. The falciform ligament is cut to complete exposure of the tumor and decompression of the ON. Meningiomas of the middle third of the sphenoid ridge will be managed in a similar manner, except that there is no need for either clinoidectomy or unroofing of the optic canal.

If the tumor is adherent to the lateral wall of the cavernous sinus, the outer layer of this wall can be peeled out together with the tumor, starting the cleavage plane anteriorly at the level of the superior orbital fissure, and advancing posteriorly.

2. SUBTEMPORAL APPROACHES

In this category can be included the classic middle cranial fossa approach and the transpetro-apical or extended middle cranial fossa approach.

2.1 Middle fossa approach

Hartley in 1892 [5], and Krause in the same year [10], independently described an anterior temporal craniotomy with extradural approach to the trigeminal roots and the gasserian ganglion for treatment of trigeminal neuralgia (TN). In 1900, Cushing [2] described total gasserian ganglionectomy for TN. House, in 1961, developed the middle fossa approach to reach the internal auditory canal (IAC) for the treatment of labyrinthine otosclerosis [6]. The approach is used for hearing preservation in cases of small vestibular schwannomas, and for removal of trigeminal and facial schwannomas.

The patient is positioned supine with the head turned towards the side opposite the tumor. A linear skin incision is performed anterior to the ear, extending from the zygoma to the parietal suture. The temporal muscle is cut and laterally retracted, and a temporal craniotomy flap reaching the skull base is tailored. Under the operating microscopy, the dura mater is elevated from the floor of the middle fossa in a posterior to anterior direction, with efforts to preserve the GSPN. The middle meningeal artery is cut at the level of the foramen spinosum. The arcuate eminence is identified, and lateral to it the tegmen tympani. In cases of vestibular schwannoma, the location of the IAC can be delineated with image-guided neuronavigation, and drilling can be started. In cases of trigeminal neurinoma, the tumor can be seen bulging through the dura, overlying Meckel's cave.

2.2 Transpetro-apical approach (extended middle fossa approach)

This approach, which consists of an anterior petrosectomy and tentorial incision, allows the removal of lesions that extend from the middle- to the posterior fossa, including the area of the petrous apex and superior clivus, to the level of the IAC. These lesions include meningiomas, chordomas, schwannomas, cholesterol granulomas, cholesteatomas.

The patient is positioned supine with the head rotated 60° to the side opposite the tumor, and extended. The skin incision is similar to that used for the pterional approach, but extended posteriorly to include more temporal bone in the craniotomy. This type of bone flap allows for extradural subtemporal drilling, as well as splitting of the Sylvian fissure for a better mobiliza-

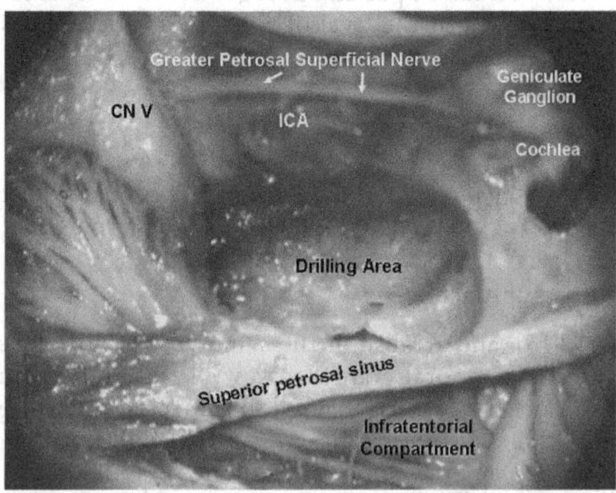

Fig. 13. Right-side anatomical specimen showing the area of drilling in Kawase's triangle for an extended middle fossa approach. The tentorium has been cut, revealing the infratentorial compartment

tion of the temporal lobe when needed. Sometimes a zygomatic osteotomy can be added. Drilling in the area of Kawase's triangle (see the anatomic description) (Fig. 13) and cutting of the tentorium provide access to the upper petroclival region.

HOW TO AVOID COMPLICATIONS

Despite many advances in surgery of the skull base, complications still occur. While mortality has been substantially reduced, morbidity remains significant. Some important considerations are worth noting here. Even experienced surgeons have complications; only those who do not operate have none. Be open minded, listen to your colleagues, and learn from their and your mistakes. Don't forget to put your ego to sleep when operating. Work in a team. Practice techniques in the anatomical laboratory.

As a first step in complication avoidance, the indications for surgery should be carefully analyzed, taking into consideration the patient's age and expectations; presumptive pathology; size, location, and natural history of the tumor; the extent of resection that may be achieved; and possibilities for adjuvant therapy. Although ideally the goal of surgery is gross total removal at the first attempt, in many patients this goal will not be achievable due to a high risk of morbidity. In these cases, leaving a small residual for imaging followup or radiotherapy may be the best option.

1. PLANNING

Resecting tumors of the central nervous system is based on the principle of atraumatic surgery. To achieve this goal, the surgeon must have a well-developed operative plan to optimize the use of the working corridors offered by the special anatomy of the brain and its surroundings. Although the best possible strategy is selected during preoperative planning, we must be prepared to deal with the unexpected. The choice of a surgical approach must accommodate the possibility of adverse situations, unforeseen difficulties, and related complications. Modern neurosurgery demands profound knowledge of anatomy, surgical skill, meticulous work, and honesty. The concept of minimally invasive surgery refers not only to a small skin incision and cranial opening, but to the use of basic principles of microneurosurgery in order to limit the damage to perilesional tissue.

The introduction of image-guidance to the neurosurgical armamentarium has provided a valuable tool for planning and performing neurosurgical procedures, allowing us to localize the anatomical boundaries of the tumor and recognize the neurovascular structures related to it. Since tumors of the skull base are attached to the dura mater and the bone, volumetric changes and shifting that occur while carrying out the surgical dissection are minimal when compared to those seen during the resection of intra-axial lesions.

2. POSITIONING, SKIN INCISION, AND CRANIOTOMY

Most middle fossa tumors are removed with the patient in a supine position, with the table slightly flexed and the head turned to the opposite side and extended. Care should be taken with fixation devices for the head. The homolateral shoulder should be elevated to avoid kinking of the neck veins and strain on the cervical muscles. Eyelids should be taped after protecting the eyes with lubricants, and bony prominences must be well padded. Pneumatic devices are applied to the lower extremities to avoid venous thrombosis, and the patient is securely attached to the table with several plaster tapes to allow for lateral tilting.

The skin incision should take into consideration the scalp vascularization and preserve the superficial temporal artery. Branches of the facial nerve crossing the zygoma to reach the frontalis muscle should not be injured. The temporal muscle is superiorly elevated without using cautery, to help maintain muscle trophism and improve the cosmetic outcome. A frontal pericranial flap is elevated separately and prepared for possible use during closure of the frontal sinus whenever it is transversed. In cases of a subtemporal approach, a temporal muscle flap is used to cover possible sources of CSF leak in the middle fossa floor. Reconstruction with vascularized pediculated flaps reinforced by application of fibrous glue is the best method to avoid leaking. If, despite these measures, there is a postoperative CSF leak, it usually will be controlled with a short period of spinal drainage.

To avoid the deleterious effects of excessive brain retraction, craniotomies are made low enough to reach the skull base, and bone drilling is frequently added. High speed drills are used with cutting and diamond burrs of different sizes. The skill to use these powerful instruments is developed in the laboratory during long hours of training. Overheating may damage cranial nerves, especially the optic nerve, and constant copious irrigation is needed.

3. INTRADURAL DISSECTION

After completing the extradural drilling, the dura mater is opened, and the intradural stage of the operation begins, usually with the splitting of the Sylvian fissure. CSF is released and sharp dissection of the middle cerebral artery and its branches is performed. The arachnoid of the Sylvian fissure should be opened in the frontal side, medial to the temporal veins. The ICA is dissected in the carotid cistern, and when necessary in the clinoid space. In cases of arterial encasement, angiography and balloon test occlusion will provide valuable information. Injury of the vessels during surgery may result in intra- or postoperative bleeding or infarction.

During resection of inner-third sphenoid wing meningiomas, the olfactory tract and optic and oculomotor nerves can be injured. Special attention is required when unroofing the optic canal and opening the superior orbital fissure.

In cases of a middle fossa approach (classical or extended), the dura elevation from the floor of the fossa may result in injury to the GSPN, resulting in loss of lacrimation. Traction of the geniculate ganglion or its injury during drilling will cause facial paralysis. Difficulties in closing the eye together with the absence of lacrimation result in severe keratitis and visual deterioration.

Drilling of the petrous apex can injure the petrous ICA, and result in profuse bleeding. Special care should be taken not to damage the cochlea.

The trigeminal ganglion and its branches are at risk in surgeries of the floor of the middle fossa and petrous apex, resulting in variable degrees of facial hypoesthesia, including loss of sensation in the cornea.

CONCLUSIONS

Neurosurgeons frequently deal with tumors of the middle fossa, of which meningiomas are the most common. Several surgical approaches may be used; the pterional approach and its variants are the mainstays in this anatomically complex area. Careful consideration of tumor characteristics, patient preferences, and personal experience are essential while planning surgical strategy in order to achieve a good outcome. Efforts should be made to achieve a complete removal at the first surgery when possible. A thorough knowledge of skull base anatomy and experience acquired in laboratories are prerequisites in order to minimize complications and limit surgical morbidity.

References

[1] Brock M, Dietz H (1978) The small frontolateral approach for the microsurgical treatment of intracranial aneurysms. Neurochirurgia (Stuttg) 21(6): 185-191

[2] Cushing H (1900) A method of total extirpation of the Gasserion ganglion for trigeminal neuralgia. J Am Med Assoc 34: 1035-1041

[3] Cushing H, Eisenhardt I (1938) Meningiomas: their classification, regional behavior, life history, and surgical end results. Charles C Thomas, Springfield, Ill

[4] Glasscock ME 3rd (1969) Middle fossa approach to the temporal bone. An otologic frontier. Arch Otolaryngol 90: 15-27

[5] Hartley F (1892) Intracranial neurectomy of the second and third divisions of the fifth nerve. NY State J Med 55: 317-319

[6] House WF (1961) Surgical exposure of the internal auditory canal and its contents through the middle, cranial fossa. Laryngoscope 711: 363-385

[7] Jane JA, Park TS, Pobereskin LH, Winn HR, Butler AB (1982) The supraorbital approach: technical note. Neurosurgery 11: 537-542

[8] Kawase T, Toya S, Shiobara R, Mine T (1985) Transpetrosal approach for aneurysms of the lower basilar artery. J Neurosurg 63: 857-861

[9] Kawase T, Shiobara R, Toya S (1991) Anterior transpetrosal-transtentorial approach for sphenopetroclival meningiomas: surgical method and results in 10 patients. Neurosurgery 28: 869-875; discussion 875-876

[10] Krause F (1892) Resection des Trigeminus innerhalb der Schädelhöhle. Arch Klin Chir 44: 821-832

[11] MacCarty CS (1959) Surgical techniques for removal of intracranial meningiomas. Clin Neurosurg 7: 100-111

[12] Yaşargil MG, Fox JL, Ray MW (1975) The operative approach to aneurysms of the anterior communicating artery. Adv Tech Stand Neurosurg 2: 113-170

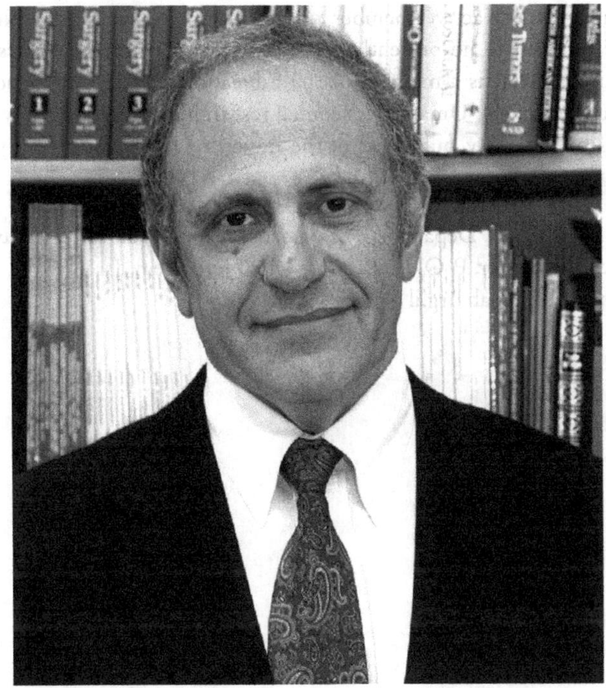

Felix Umansky

Felix Umansky is chairman of the Department of Neurosurgery at the Hadassah–Hebrew University Medical Center in Jerusalem. He completed his medical training at the Universidad Nacional de Rosario in his native Argentina, and his neurosurgical residency at the Beilinson Hospital in Tel Aviv, Israel, where he did joint research with world renowned anatomist and anthropologist Prof. Nathan Hillel. Their work in the neuroanatomy of the lateral wall of the cavernous sinus made a significant contribution to surgical approaches involving structures in this region.

Prof. Umansky completed fellowships at Massachusetts General Hospital under Prof. William H. Sweet, and at Henry Ford Hospital in Detroit, Michigan, U.S.A. under Prof. James Ausman.

In 1984, Prof. Umansky joined the Department of Neurosurgery at the Hadassah–Hebrew University Medical Center in Jerusalem. In 1993, he was named Chairman, and later Professor of Neurosurgery at the Hebrew University – Hadassah Medical School. Under his leadership, Hadassah has established the leading skull base practice in Israel, where meningioma incidence is among the highest worldwide, and participates in the care of over 1500 neurosurgical patients annually.

From 2005, Prof. Umansky has also been appointed as a staff neurosurgeon in the Department of Neurosurgery of Henry Ford Hospital.

Prof. Umansky is an active member of the World Federation of Neurosurgical Societies (WFNS), where he presently serves as Chairman of the Ethics and Medico-Legal Affairs, as well as a member of the Education and Training, and Skull Base Surgery Committees. Prof. Umansky's seminal research in neuro-anatomy and clinical experience has been widely published in the literature, and he frequently lectures in international meetings.

Contact: Felix Umansky, Department of Neurosurgery, Hadassah–Hebrew University Medical Center, P. O. Box 12000, 91120 Jerusalem, Israel
E-mail: umansky@hadassah.org.il

HOW TO PERFORM CENTRAL SKULL BASE APPROACHES

L. N. SEKHAR

INTRODUCTION

The central skull base may be defined as the spheno-clival and clival areas. Lesions involving this region may be intradural or extradural. Intradural lesions may be petroclival or lower clival/foramen magnum meningiomas, trigeminal or jugular foramen/hypoglossal schwannomas, or other benign tumors. Lesions involving the extradural area are predominantly chordomas, chondrosarcomas, cholesterol granulomas, adenoid cystic carcinomas, and some invasive pituitary tumors. Many specialized skull base approaches have been developed to deal with these lesions.

In this chapter, different approaches will be described. Approaches described in detail in other sections of the book will only be mentioned briefly. In general, the approaches may be divided into anterior approaches (transsphenoidal, transnasal endoscopic, transmaxillary, and transoral), antero-lateral approaches (fronto-temporal orbito-zygomatic, subtemporal transzygomatic with petrous apex resection, subtemporal infratemporal), and postero-lateral approaches (transpetrosal, and extreme lateral transcondylar).

DECISION-MAKING

Preoperative Studies. In addition to a neurological examination and a comprehensive physical examination, an audiogram is indicated whenever an approach through the temporal bone is contemplated. Most of the patients undergo an MRI examination, but a bone windowed CT scan will demonstrate the bony anatomy to help the surgeon. Whenever major arteries are affected by the tumor, a cerebral angiogram with demonstration of the collateral blood supply is performed. If the internal carotid artery is at risk, then an angiogram with ipsilateral carotid compression is performed with injection into the contralateral carotid artery, and the vertebral artery to demonstrate the collateral flow. This is adequate as long as the surgeon plans only a temporary occlusion, and a vascular repair or a bypass is performed in the event of a major arterial injury. When major venous sinuses are at risk, the venous phase of the angiogram must be carefully evaluated to examine the major venous sinuses, and their collateral circulation.

Keywords: skull base, central skull base approaches, microsurgery

Team Planning. Often, multiple approaches are possible to a lesion. The surgeon must be familiar with all of them. The final selection will be based on the location of the tumor, the areas of invasion, major arteries involved, the physical characteristics of the tumor (soft vs. hard), and the extent of resection (total, subtotal, or partial) planned. In some cases, the initial approach may not be adequate, and another approach may need to be performed in a different stage. In many cases, the services of a surgeon from another specialty (such as ENT or plastic surgery) may be needed in order to perform an approach, or the reconstruction. In addition, the patients will need to be under the care of a neuro intensivist postoperatively in a neurosurgical intensive care unit, with well trained neurosurgical nurses. Rehabilitation may be important for some patients after they leave the hospital.

Anesthesia and neuro-monitoring planning. In all patients, the anesthesiologist must strive to maintain an adequate blood volume and oxygenation during the case. The brain needs to be slack during the operation, and both diuretics and moderate hyperventilation may be used at the start of the operation. For extradural operations, this may be achieved by means of a lumbar drain (if the cisterns are open), or a ventriculostomy (if obstructive hydrocephalus is present). For intradural operations, cisternal drainage may be adequate, after the standard measures. For most procedures, total intravenous anesthesia using intravenous propofol is employed, to allow the monitoring of Motor Evoked Potentials (MEP). In addition to MEPs, the electroencephalogram, and SSEP (somatosensory evoked potentials) are monitored. The function of cranial nerves 5, 7, 8, 10, 11, and 12 are monitored as needed, when these nerves are involved by the tumor.

SURGERY

1. ANTERIOR APPROACHES

1.1 Transsphenoidal approach

The transsphenoidal approach is predominantly used for pituitary adenomas, which are intrasellar and suprasellar. The use of the endoscope (either primarily or as an assistive device) allows larger intracranial extensions to be resected. However, the purely endoscopic approach takes longer to perform, and is more difficult to learn. If excessive bleeding occurs, this can be a problem in the endoscopic approach, which may require a conversion to a microsurgical approach. The "extended transsphenoidal approach" allows the removal of tuberculum sellae meningiomas, which are encasing the carotid arteries.

For the microsurgical approach, the patients are placed supine and the head slightly tilted away from the surgeon (to the left for a right handed surgeon) with the neck in a slightly extended and in a pin-holder. We prefer to use intraoperative navigation, rather than the C arm fluoroscope in order to localize the anatomy. A sublabial approach is useful for very large tumors which have a considerable suprasellar extension, and may also be used in the "extended transsphenoidal approach" for meningiomas of the planum sphenoidale. If a sublabial approach is used, the upper lip is retracted and a transverse incision is made in the upper gingival mucosa after infiltration of the soft tissue with local anesthetic. Dissection is continued with a dissector to expose the cartilaginous nasal septum. The septal mucosa is separated from the septum. The nasal septum is then fractured from the bony septum (perpendicular plate of the ethmoid), and a nasal speculum inserted and opened exposing the anterior wall of the sphenoid. Under the microscope, the sphenoid sinus is then opened at the ostia with a Kerrison rongeur, or a high speed drill and widened laterally until the floor of the sella turcia is completely visualized. The floor of the sella is removed exposing the overlying dura, from one cavernous sinus to the other, and from the palnum to the dorsum sellae. For the removal of tuberculum sellae meningiomas, the planum sphenoidale must be removed with a high speed drill, in addition to the sellar floor.

The transnasal transsphenoidal approach is preferred for most pituitary tumors. The nasal mucosa is treated with cocaine pledgets to reduce the vascular congestion. A speculum is placed on one side of the nasal cavity, and under the microscope, the postero superior wall of the septum and the anterior wall of the sphenoid are reached, using the middle turbinate as the landmark. A small incision is made in the nasal mucosa and careful dissection of mucosa free from the cartilaginous nasal septum and then fractured laterally. A microdebrider may be used here to partially remove the middle turbinate to enlarge the access to ostia. From here on the sphenoidectomy proceeds as in the sublabial approach, exposing the sella and the dura. During the resection, endoscopic assistance may be used for the removal of laterally placed, and suprasellar tumor.

For closure, Duragen and alloderm are laid in the defect, tucked under the residual bone edges with a final layer of Bioglue. We then augment the closure with Nasopore packing. If an obvious CSF leak is encountered, a lumbar drain is placed in the operating room. If a large dura defect is created, an abdominal fat graft is harvested and placed within the sphenoid to augment the layer closure. A Foley catheter may be left inflated inside the sphenoid sinus, to keep the packing in place.

Currently, we often use an endoscopic transsphenoidal approach for pituitary tumors. However, for invasive tumors which involve the clivus extensively, a transmaxillary approach is preferred, because of the shorter, and wider exposure.

1.2 Transmaxillary/transfacial approach

This is an approach which is very good for extradural lesions in the midclivus, with slight extension to the upper clivus. Moderate extensions into the cavernous sinus and the pterygoid space can be easily dealt with. But this approach is not preferred when there is extensive invasion beyond these limits, or when there is extensive intradural invasion. The patient is positioned supine with the neck slight extended and head held in a Mayfield pin-holder. A sublabial incision is made preferred for this approach to maximize cosmesis, however a Weber-Fergusson incision can also be employed to approach this region. A sublabial incision is made in the upper gingival mucosa and subperiosteal dissection is carried forward superiorly towards the frontal-nasal suture and laterally towards pterygoid plates to expose the nasomaxillary region. Additional dissection of the periorbita of the inferior and medial orbit

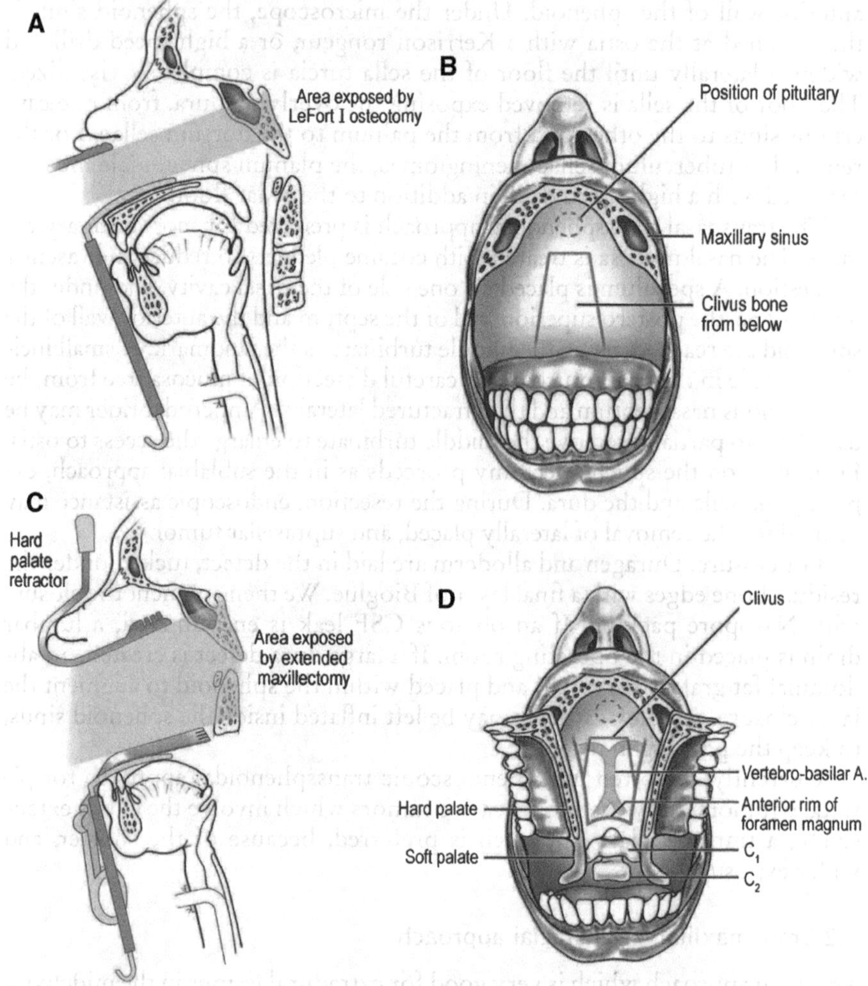

Fig. 1. **A** and **B** Transmaxillary approach. Upper and middle third of the clivus exposed with Lefort I osteotomy. **A** Lateral view. **B** AP view. **C** and **D** Extended maxillectomy. **C** Lateral diagram. **D** AP view

allows for further exposure of the nasomaxillary region. The lateral exposure is partially limited by the infraorbital foramen containing the nerve and blood vessels. A Lefort I osteotomy can be then performed to detach the maxillary bone flap to expose the necessary regions of the clivus and the infratemporal fossa (Fig. 1A, B). Titanium plates are placed before the osteotomy to secure a good alignment post operatively.

Once the lesion has been removed, if a dural defect is present, the defect is closed with an abdominal fascial graft and augmented with Duraseal, or bioglue. This is reinforced with a layer of abdominal fat graft followed by Duragen. This entire repair is held in place by Titanium mesh which is attached to the surrounding bone with titanium screws. The maxillary bone flap is reattached to the face with plates and screws. A lumbar drain is placed before the operation and used post-operatively for 3–5 days to prevent CSF leak.

For good accessibility to both clivus and craniocervical junction an extended maxillectomy approach can be used. This combines the Lefort I osteotomy with a midline incision of hard and soft palate (Fig. 1C, D). The initial incision is made like the transmaxillary approach; along the alveolar margin, extending to the molars on both sides and titanium plates placed in position similarly. Then a midline incision is made in the hard and soft palate and saw cut applied to hard palate between the upper incisors to allow flaps to wing laterally. A transpharyngeal retractor is applied to hold the palatal flaps along with the transoral retractors for adequate exposure to clivus and region below. This is particularly useful for extensive tumors and congenital anomalies producing basilar invagination. Closure is done as mentioned above for transmaxillary approach, but needs to be more meticulous to effect proper occlusion and functioning of the palate, making the surgery long and intricate.

1.3 Transoral approach

We rarely use this approach for tumors, since it becomes very limited in its lateral reach, which prevents the complete removal of tumors. It is a preferred approach for the resection of developmental and rheumatoid lesions of the C1 and lower clival area. The patient is positioned supine and the neck extended. The region of interest along the clivus will dictate the amount of extension of the neck (Fig. 2A, B). Once the oral retractor is placed, a longitudinal incision is placed in the posterior pharyngeal wall. The soft tissues are then retracted laterally to expose the nasopharynx and the adenoid pad. The mucosa of the nasopharynx is then open in the midline and elevated off the clivus. Superiorly, the dissection can be stopped at the junction of the hard and soft palate, however if needed the hard palate can be partially resected to transverse palatine suture. This will expose the posterior portion of the bony septum. Once the mucosa has been removed, the bony septum can then be resected to gain more exposure. Inferiorly, the anterior ring of C1 and C2 and also be easily exposed. Frequently, after the abnormal bone is resected, there

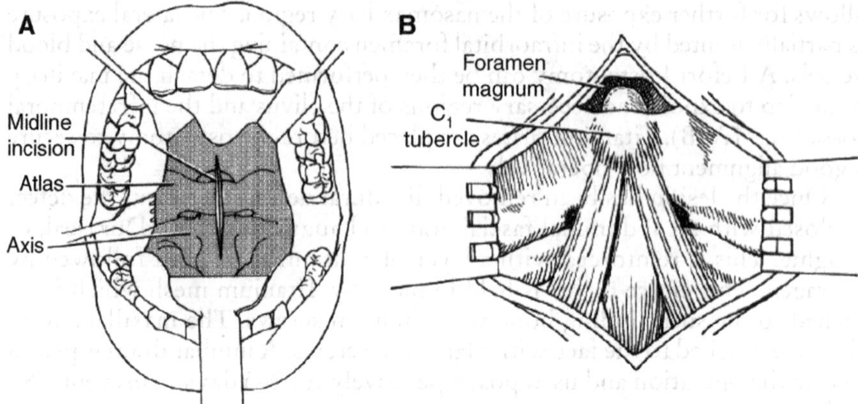

Fig. 2. Transoral approach. **A** Midline vertical incision with soft palate elevated to expose the posterior pharynx. **B** Exposed C1 tubercle with muscle and ligament attachment through the incision (courtesy Raven Press, from "Surgery of cranial base tumors" L. Sekhar, I.P. Janecka)

are hypertrophied soft tissues which have to be removed all the way to the dura mater. If there is entry into the dura, it must be repaired as previously outlined in the transmaxillary approach. The mucosa and the palate are closed in layers, and the patient is fed through a nasogastric tube until the mucosal layers are healed.

1.4 Extended subfrontal approach

The extended subfrontal approach (Fig. 3A–D) is used for lesions in the same areas as the transmaxillary approach. However, a much wider exposure is obtained, with the ability to remove intradural and cavernous sinus lesions and even repair the ICA in the event of an injury. The patient is in the supine position without a head turn, and the surgeon frequently rolls the patient from side to side, in order to visualize the opposite corner. This is thus referred to as an X shaped approach, and the decompression of the orbits is needed for this as well as to enhance the midline exposure, and to reduce the brain retraction.

A bicoronal incision is made well behind the hair line, and a pericranial falp is dissected, starting behind the incision. As one approaches the nasion, care must be taken to preserve the supraorbital and supratrochlear arteries, which is best done by getting into the galeal–frontalis layer. The supraorbital nerves are notched out and freed, if they lie inside a foramen. Dissection is done just inferior to the frontonasal suture and the periorbita is dissected bilaterally for a distance of approximately 3 cm. A low bifrontal craniotomy is then performed, without dural tears. The subfrontal dura is dissected from the roofs of the orbit bilaterally and if possible from the

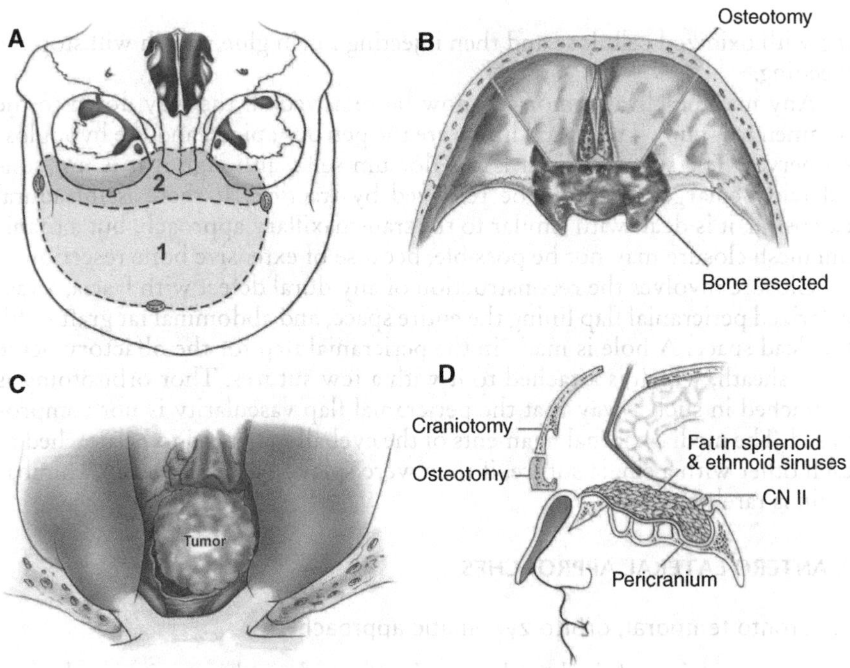

Fig. 3. Extended frontal transbasal approach. **A** Craniotomy. **B** Osteotomy. **C** Optic nerves unroofed and planum sphenoidale removed. Cavernous carotid artery unroofed and tumor resection begins. **D** Reconstruction of cranial base with free fat grafts and a pericranial graft

planum area, sparing the ethmoidal regions, under the microscope. CSF drainage from the lumbar drain is useful in this stage. In order to preserve olfaction, the entire cribriform ethmoidal plate is drilled away, preserving the dural sheath around the olfactory nerves. A bilateral orbitofrontal osteotomy is performed in a bat wing shaped fashion, encircling the olfactory dural sheath. The olfactory mucosa is then divided inside the nasal cavity, preserving it along with the olfactory dural sheath. This entire complex can then be retracted superiorly.

The next step is to decompress both optic nerves in their dural sheath, and removing the bone of the planum sphenoidale, and the sella turcica. The removal of the anterior clinoid process and the optic struts may be done if necessary. The bone is then removed from the body of the sphenoid, forming the medial wall of the cavernous sinus. Some of the petrous apex may also be removed in this fashion. The intracavernous ICA will be exposed extradurally at the posterior bend, horizontal segment, and the anterior bend. If the periosteum overlying the cavernous sinus or the intercavernous sinuses is open, profuse venous bleeding may occur. This is controlled by gently packing with oxidized cellulose and then injecting fibrin glue, which will stop the bleeding.

Any midline clival tumor can now be removed all the way down to the foramen magnum. The lateral limits are the petrous apices, and the hypoglossal nerves. The superior limit is the dorsum sella, although if it is not considerably enlarged, this can be removed by traction. If there is intradural extension, it is dealt with similar to the transmaxillary approach, but a titanium mesh closure may not be possible, because of extensive bone resection.

Closure involves the reconstruction of any dural defect with fascia, a vascularized pericranial flap lining the entire space, and abdominal fat graft to fill the dead space. A hole is made in the pericranial flap for the olfactory nerve dural sheath, which is attached to it with a few sutures. Thor orbitotomy is reattached in such a way that the pericranial flap vascularity is not compromised. The medial canthal ligaments of the eyeball may need to be attached to each other with a single suture, if they were splayed by the lesion. A lumbar drain is rarely needed.

2. ANTERO-LATERAL APPROACHES

2.1 Fronto-temporal, orbito-zygomatic approach

This approach is useful when there is significant lateral extension, and when the cavernous sinuses are involved in a significant way. The patient is positioned supine and the head turned 45° to the contralateral side with slight extension of the neck, malar eminence at the highest point (Fig. 4A–C), and fixed. An area in the abdomen or lateral thigh needs to be prepared for an autologous fat graft. Either a bicoronal or a pterional incision crossing midline is made behind the patient's hairline. The inferior portion of the incision lies in the skin crease anterior to tragus of the ear. Dissection to elevate the skin flap is carefully carried-out preserving the pericranium for repair of dura and/or frontal sinus. The dissection is carried anteriorly until the supraorbital nerve is encountered paramedially. Laterally, along the dissection of temporalis muscle occurs until the superficial temporal fat pad is encountered, and then an interfascial dissection would be required to elevate the skin flap anteriorly to preserve the frontotemporal banch of the facial nerve (Fig. 4C). A subperiosteal dissection is required along lateral orbit to expose the lateral orbit and inferiorly along the entire course of the zygoma. After the temporalis muscle is carefully elevated subfascially to preserve the underside, thin fascial layer of the temporalis muscle. The muscle is then retracted laterally. The craniotomy is done separately from the orbital osteotomy. A frontal-temporal craniotomy is then fashioned to include the ipsilateral anterior and middle fossa extending medially to the supraorbital notch.

The periorbita and the dura are then carefully dissected off the orbital roof and walls. Dissection of the frontal dura extends posteriorly to the superior

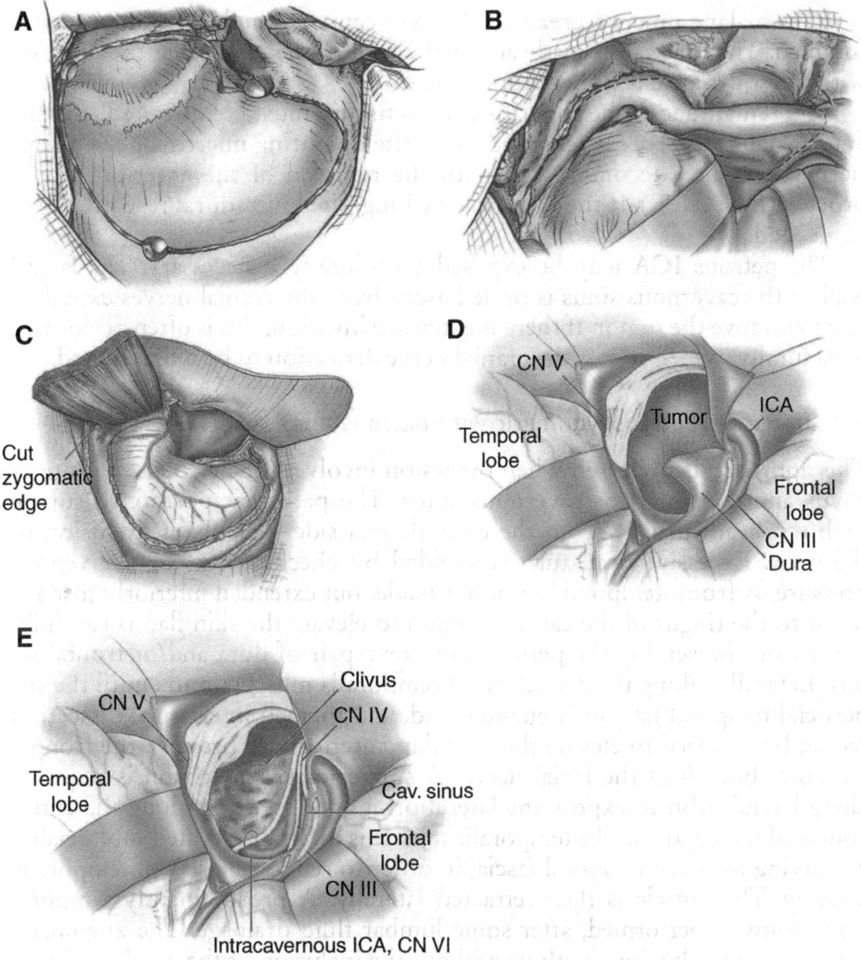

Fig. 4. **A** Frontotemporal transcavernous approach – osteotomy cuts for a standard OZO (orbitozygomatic osteotomy). **B** Osteotomy cuts in the orbital roof. **C** Final appearance after craniotomy and OZO. **D** Intradural exposure of tumor in the cavernous sinus. The sylvian fissure is split and lateral dural wall over tumor incised. **E** After removal of intracavernous tumor – cavernous sinus and clivus exposed. *ICA* Internal carotid artery

orbital fissure. Retractors are then placed to gently retract and protect the brain during the orbitozygomatic osteotomy. The medial cut is made lateral to supraorbital notch. Posteriorly the orbital osteotomy is made to preserve at least 2/3rds of the orbital roof to prevent enophthalmos, and anterior to the superior orbital fissure. Laterally, the osteotomy is made beginning of the inferior orbital fissure to the level of the zygomaticofacial foramen. A second lateral cut is made from the anterior, inferior edge of the zygoma to connect with the malar eminence, creating a "V" cut centered on the zygomaticofacial foramen. The final cut is made across the root of the zygoma at the junction with the squamosal temporal bone (Fig. 4B).

The remainder of the superior orbital fissure must be unroofed, and the anterior clinoid process removed using the operating microscope. The optic nerve is also decompressed with the removal of the anterior clinoid process (Fig. 4D, E). If the ACP is very long, then intradural resection may be needed.

The petrous ICA may be exposed extradurally if necessary. The lateral wall of the cavernous sinus is peeled away from the cranial nerves extradurally to remove the tumor. If there is extensive invasion, this is often performed intradurally, which allows the cranial nerve dissection to be more limited.

2.2 Subtemporal transzygomatic with petrous apex resection

This approach is preferred when the lesion involves the petrous apex, upper clivus and the posterior cavernous sinus. The patient is positioned supine with the head turned 70° to the contralateral side with slight extension of the neck. Excessive head turn is avoided by checking the jugular venous pressure. A frontotemporal incision is made, but extended inferiorly just anterior to the tragus of the ear. Dissection to elevate the skin flap is carefully carried-out preserving the pericranium for repair of dura and/or frontal sinus. Laterally, along the dissection of temporalis muscle occurs until the superficial temporal fat pad is encountered, and then an interfascial dissection would be required to elevate the skin flap anteriorly to preserve the frontotemporal branch of the facial nerve. A subperiosteal dissection is required along lateral orbit to expose the lateral orbit and inferiorly along the entire course of the zygoma. The temporalis muscle is carefully elevated subfascially, preserving the deep temporal fascia, in order to reduce the risk of temporalis atrophy. The muscle is then retracted laterally. A predominantly temporal craniotomy is performed, after some lumbar fluid drainage. The zygomatic osteotomy may be done with or without the inclusion of the condylar fossa, as dictated by the need for posterior exposure. If done without the condylar fossa, then the posterior cuts are made just anterior to the temporomandibular joint, and the anterior cuts lateral to the lateral wall of the orbit.

Any additional squamous temporal bone is resected piecemeal or as a single piece. Under the microscope, the middle fossa dura is elevated to expose the middle meningeal artery, greater superficial pertrosal nerve (GSPN), V3, and arcuate eminence of the petrous bone are identified. The middle meningeal artery and GSPN are cauterized and divided. From here the greater wing of the sphenoid is drilled to expose foramen ovale (lateral) and foramen rotundum (anterior). The dura overlaying V2 and V3 can be cut and elevated for added exposure medially along the petrous apex. Venous bleeding from the pterygoid plexus or the cavernous sinus is handled in the usual way, by gentle packing, and fibrin glue injection.

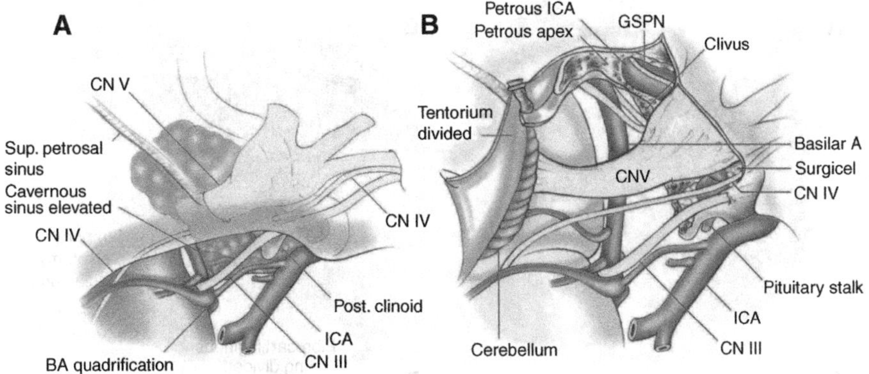

Fig. 5. A Subtemporal transzygomatic petrous apex resection with tumor lying in the cavernous sinus and extends to the level of the horizontal petrous internal carotid artery (*ICA*). **B** Exposed anatomy after tumor resection with this approach. *BA* Basilar artery; *GSPN* greater superficial petrosal nerve

From the exposure of the petrous apex, the petrous portion of the internal carotid artery (ICA) is identified at the junction of GSPN and V3 (Fig. 5A, B). The ICA is then unroofed anterior to the genu of the petrous ICA, which is medial to Eustachian tube. Once the carotid artery is identified, it can be skeletonized and freed from the surrounding bone. Mobilization of the carotid artery allows for further exposure of the apex. The petrous apex is removed with a high speed drill or the ultrasonic bone curette.

Once the bone is removed, the petroclival dura will be exposed. In order to expose the posterior cavernous sinus or the upper clivus, it is essential to open the dura mater, and to work between the fascicles of the trigeminal root inside the Meckel's cave, or by dividing the trigeminal ganglion between V2 and V3 (trans trigeminal approach).

Opening the dura of the medial wall of the cavernous sinus then exposes the dorsum sellae and the posterior cavernous sinus.

2.3 Subtemporal-infratemporal approach

The subtemporal-infratemporal approach is an inferior extension of the subtemporal transzygomatic with petroclival bone. A more extensive exposure of the mid and lower clivus is obtained, especially on the ipsilateral side. This is an ideal approach for some petroclival chondrosarcomas and cholesterol granulomas. The difference lies in performing an osteotomy of the zygoma with the condylar fossa, removing the Eustachian tube, and exposing and displacing the entire petrous ICA anteriorly.

The details of the approach are similar to the previous one until the zygomatic osteotomy (Fig. 6A, B). The dura mater is elevated over the condylar fossa extradurally. The temporomandibular joint capsule is opened and the

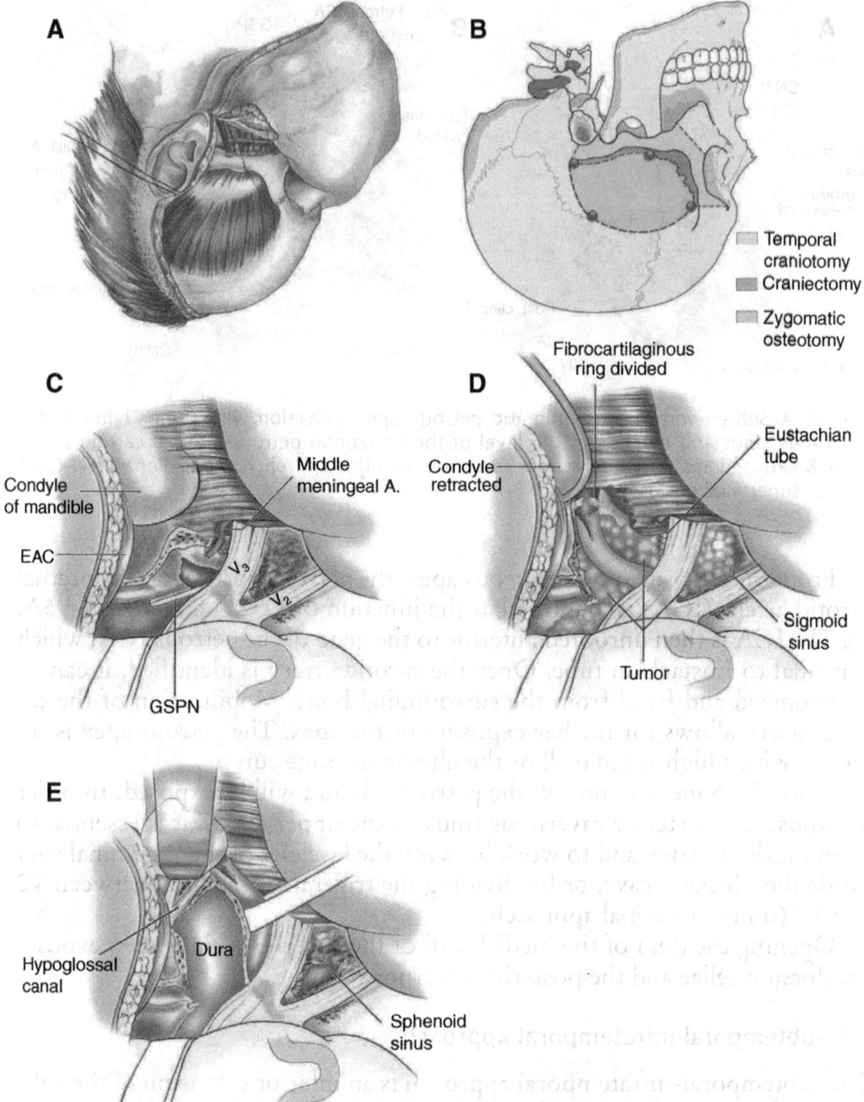

Fig. 6. Subtemporal infratemporal approach. **A** Incison. **B** Craniotomy and osteotomies. **C** After elevation of temporal lobe dura and division of middle meningeal artery and greater superficial petrosal nerve (*GSPN*) and partially exposed horizontal portion of the internal carotid artery (**D**). After incising the dura propria over the semilunar ganglion and V2 and V3.The sphenoid sinus is seen between V2 and V3. **E** Mobilization of petrous ICA from the ICA from the carotid canal

meniscus of the joint is depressed inferiorly. The middle fossa dura is elevated to expose the middle meningeal artery, greater superficial pertrosal nerve (GSPN), V3, and arcuate eminence of the petrous bone are indentified (Fig. 6C–E). The middle meningeal artery is cauterized and divided and foramen spinosum is packed with bone wax. The condylar fossa then is transilluminated to outline the entire fossa and the two cuts are made to include the entire fossa medial to the foramen of spinosum and the root of the zygoma. Care must be taken not to make the cuts too medially, to avoid damaging the facial nerve or the ICA.

After the horizontal segment of the petrous ICA is exposed by extradural dissection, the dissection is extended inferiorly by removing the tensor tympani muscle, the Eustachian tube, and the tympanic bone, unroofing the genus and the vertical segment of the petrous ICA. The ICA is dissected from the bony canal extraperiosteally. At the entrance to the carotid canal, there is a thick fibrocartilaginous ligament which has to be divided, and partially excised. Superiorly, the bone is removed medial to V3, and lateral to the petrous ICA. This will allow the complete mobilization of the petrous and upper cervical ICA (Fig. 6E).

Critical structures lie medially and posteriorly. The middle ear and the genu of the facial nerve lie superiorly and posteriorly, whereas the jugular bulb and the lower cranial nerves lie posteriorly and inferiorly to the petroclival region. Entry into the jugular bulb is dealt with in the usual manner with gentle packing, and if necessary by fibrin glue injection. Both ends of the Eustachian tube must be closed, the anterior end by packing oxidized cellulose and a suture, and the posterior end with a small fat graft.

If there is a dural defect, it is closed in the usual fashion with fascia and Duraseal, augmented with abdominal fat graft. Flow through the petrous ICA must be confirmed by Doppler flowmetry.

3. POSTERO-LATERAL APPROACHES

3.1 Transpetrosal (retrolabyrinthine, partial labyrinthectomy/petrous apicetomy (PLPA), translabyrinthine, and total petrosectomy)

This approach is used predominantly for intradural tumors such as petroclival meningiomas. However, when an extradural lesions such as a chordoma has an extensive intradural invasion, marked compression of the brain stem and encasement of the basilar artery, this approach would be preferred, since it allows these structures to be removed under direct vision.

A lumbar drain is in place. The preoperative angiogram must be carefully inspected to observe the venous sinuses and the vein(s) of Labbe. The patient is placed in a supine position with the head turned 70° to the contralateral side or in a park bench position if a limited mobility of the patient's neck is observed preoperatively. A U-shaped incision starting in the preauricular area (1 cm anterior to the root of the zygoma), curving up into the temporal re-

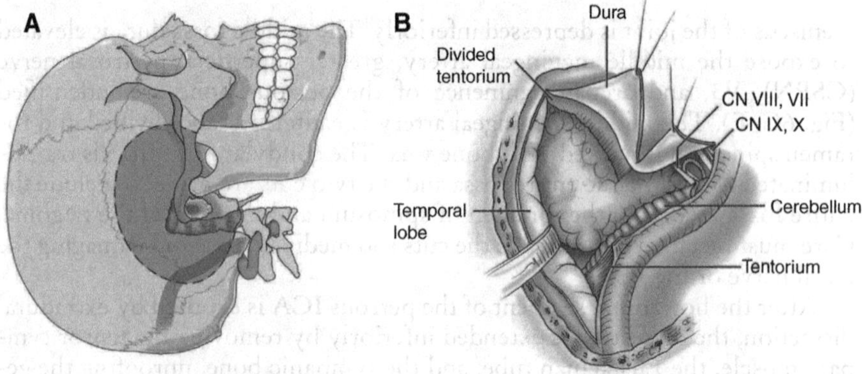

Fig. 7. A Lateral approach with PLPA (for trigeminal schwannoma). Temporal craniotomy zygomatic osteotomy and transpetrosal approach. **B** Tumor exposure after cutting the tentorium

gion, and extending retro auricularly to just below the mastoid tip is used (Fig. 7A). The posterior half to third of the temporalis muscle and some of the pericranium in the frontal region (temporofascial flap) is elevated separately and reflected inferiorly. The retrosigmoid muscles are reflected inferiorly. After draining some fluid from the lumbar drain, a mid and posterior temporal craniotomy is performed, extending at least 2 cm posterior to the projected transverse sigmoid junction. Following this, a retrosigmoid craniotomy is performed (if necessary) across the transverse sinus, down to the floor of the posterior fossa. Depending on the petrosal approach chosen to expose the presigmoid space; a radical mastoidectomy is required to expose the sigmoid sinus, superior, lateral, and posterior semicircular canal, the vestibular aqueduct, jugular bulb, and the facial nerve canal (Fig. 7B). In the PLPA approach, the posterior and superior semicircular canals are opened and waxed to prevent the loss of endolymph and hearing loss. They are then removed. A petrous apicectomy is then performed, working through this space. This provides more room than a standard retrolabyrinthine approach, particularly on the right side, where the sinus is often larger. In the translabyrinthine approach, the entire labyrinthine bone is removed to the level of vestibule along with the bone to the IAC.

A total petrosectomy approach is rarely used in order to gain a much better exposure of the brain stem. Here, the facial nerve is completely skeletonized from the cisternal segment to the stylomastoid foramen, and after dividing the GSPN, displaced postero inferiorly. The petrous ICA is displaced anteriorly, similar to the subtemporal-infratemporal approach. The remaining temporal bone is drilled away, sacrificing ipsilateral hearing. The jugular bulb and the lower cranial nerves are carefully protected.

Once the bony work is completed the dura opening starts with an incision in the presigmoid area beginning anterior and parallel to the sigmoid sinus and superior to the jugular bulb. This incision is then extended anteriorly until the superior petrosal sinus. A second dura opening occurs on the temporal side over the inferior temporal gyrus towards the superior petrosal sinus. The superior petrosal sinus is ligated and divided and the tentorium is then incised. Care must be taken to avoid the fourth nerve and superior cerebellar artery. Meckel's cave is then opened, with the control of the bleeding from the cavernous sinus as needed. The operation then proceeds with minimal brain retraction, working between cranial nerves 3–9.

For the closure of the transpetrosal approach, the mastoid air cells and the entrance into the middle ear are carefully closed with bone wax. Any dural defect is closed with pericranium or Duragen. The temporofascial flap is then rotated over the mastoidal area. Abdominal fat graft is used to fill any remaining defect posterior to the temporofascial flap. If the bone over the mastoid area has been removed by drilling, it must be replaced with titanium mesh, in order to prevent a depression in the area when it heals.

3.2 Extreme lateral transcondylar approach

This is the best approach for tumors in the foramen magnum upper cervical area which are anterior to the spinomedullar junction. The extreme latera approach has 6 variations, which are useful for neoplastic and vascular lesions of this area. We will only describe the partial transcondylar (used for foramen magnum meningiomas), and the complete transcondylar (used for extradural lesions such as chordomas) approaches.

The patient is placed in a lateral, park bench position with the lower arm placed in a cloth sling and the upper arm padded around a pillow. The head is held in a Mayfield pin holder with the head rotated slightly towards the surgeon, and neck flexed and extended laterally (Fig. 8A). A C-shaped incision extending from the superior temporal line posteriorly into the retroauricular region and into the lateral neck is used. The inferior extent of the incision will depend on the need to expose C2. The skin flap is reflected forward with the sternomastoid muscle, and the remaining muscles are elevated in layers. The next layer consists of the Splenius capitis, the next layer has the semispinalis capitis, the longissimus capitis and cervicalis, and the oblique and recti muscles. The occipital artery lies between the second and third layers (Fig. 8B).

A key step is to identify the vertebral artery (the second and third segments) from C2 to the foramen magnum. This is done under the microscope. It may be identified in the suboccipital triangle, between C2 and C1. The C1 lamina, the perivertebral venous plexus, and the C2 nerve are useful landmarks in its identification. Any bleeding from the venous plexus is handled by bipolar cautery, and fibrin glue injection. The foramen transversarium of C1 is completely unroofed, and the lateral third of the C1 lamina is removed. The VA can then be displaced medially.

A small retrosigmoid craniotomy is performed extending through the foramen magnum. A low mastoidectomy just posterior to the facial nerve is

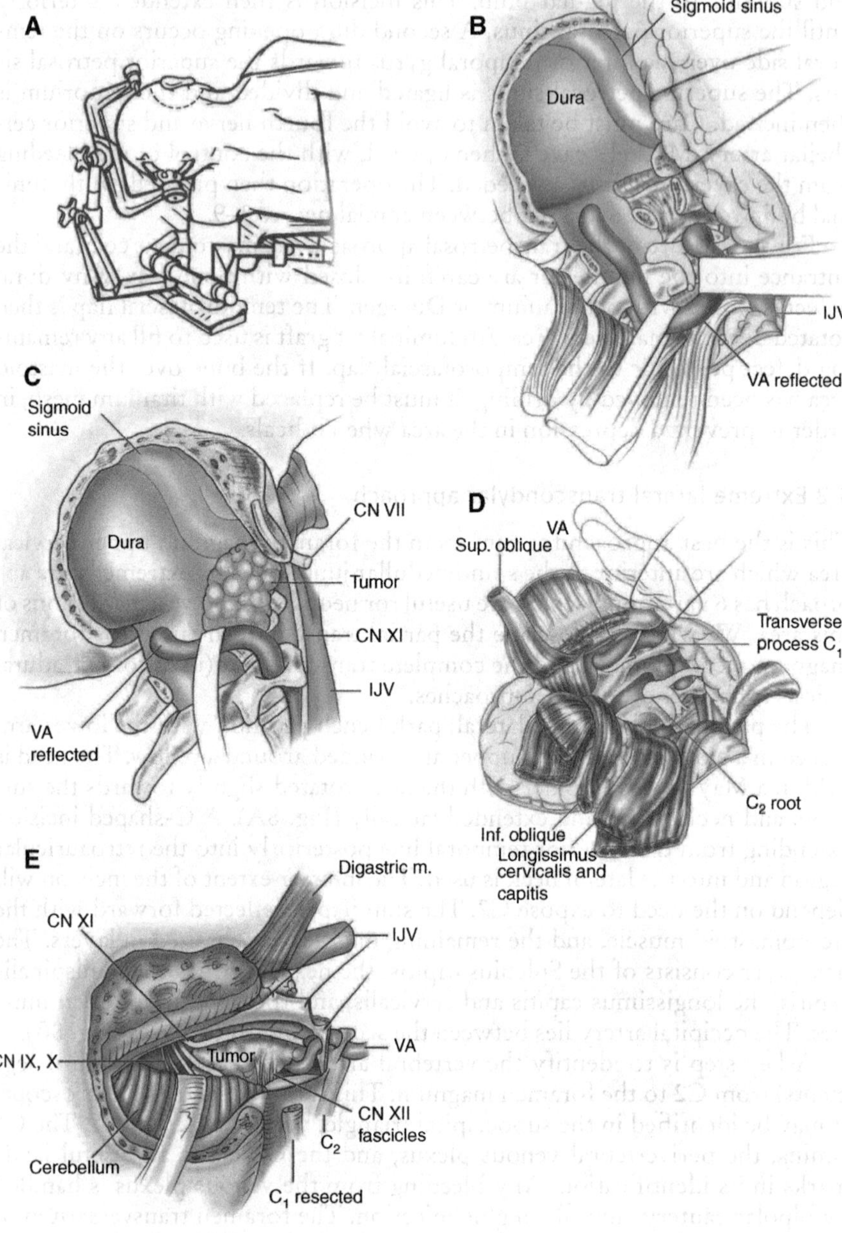
A
B
Sigmoid sinus
Dura
IJV
VA reflected
C
Sigmoid
sinus
Dura
CN VII
Tumor
CN XI
IJV
VA
reflected
D
VA
Sup. oblique
Transverse
process C_1
C_2 root
Inf. oblique
Longissimus
cervicalis and
capitis
E
Digastric m.
CN XI
IJV
VA
CN IX, X
Tumor
CN XII
fascicles
C_2
Cerebellum
C_1 resected

performed to expose the posterior edge of the sigmoid sinus, and to access the occipital condyle. Any bleeding from the condylar emissary vein is stopped with oxidized cellulose, and bone wax (Fig. 8C). This venous canal is also a marker to the hypoglossal canal which lies just inferior to it.

The posterior half of the occipital condyle, and the lateral mass of C1 including portions of the jugular tubercle are removed with a drill or ultrasonic aspiration which will expose the hypoglossal canal (Fig. 8E). For intradural tumors, removal of enough bone should be performed in order to have about 1 cm of dura exposed lateral to the entrance of the VA into the dura mater. The dural opening then is performed encircling the artery (Fig. 8C, D). The first dentate ligament and the C1 rootlets are divided, and tumor resection proceeds with no brain stem retraction. During closure, the resection bed is gently packed with autologous fat and dura primarily sutured if violated. Primary dural closure is usually impossible; a fascial or pericranial graft is used and supplemented with tissue glue, followed by autologous fat.

For extradural tumors, the entire occipital condyle and lateral mass of C1 are removed. Complete unroofing of the jugular bulb may also be helpful. Further inferior exposure can be achieved by unroofing the VA in the C2 foramen, and removing the lateral mass of C2. When a complete condylar resection is performed, a fusion procedure is needed. We prefer to delay this by about a week from the tumor removal. If possible, a bone graft may be placed from C2 to the clivus. The actual fusion is from the occiput to C2–3. using a preshaped titanium ring, screws into the occipital bone, and the lateral masses.

4. USE OF COMBINED/ALTERNATIVE APPROACHES

Extensive tumors may require the use of combined approaches in stages, usually in 2 and rarely in 3 stages.

HOW TO AVOID COMPLICATIONS

The key to complication avoidance is the use of the correct operative approach, anatomical knowledge, and expertise, which is gained by learning from one's and others' experience. Common complications include CSF

◄

Fig. 8. A Patient positioning and incision for a complete transcondylar extreme lateral approach. If combined with petrosal approach, then the patient is placed supine with head turned 45°. **B** Retrosigmoid craniotomy and C1 laminectomy have been performed. The VA (vertebral artery) has been mobilized medially. The occipital condyle can now be resected as needed for complete tumor removal. **C** Tumor resection commenced. **D** Relationship among the VA (vertebral artery), C2 dorsal root, C1 lamina and occipital condyle. **E** Extreme lateral partial transcondylar approach for a hypoglossal eschwannoma. Intradural exposure shows the location of hypoglossal schwannoma. *IJV* Internal jugular vein

leaks, cranial nerve palsies, infection, hematomas, vascular injuries, and rarely brain or brain stem injuries. Management of complications addresses recognition of the cause of the problem, and appropriate treatment.

Acknowledgement

Doctors Chong C. Lee, MD, PhD, and Dinesh Ramanathan, MD, TNS, are acknowledged as co-authors.

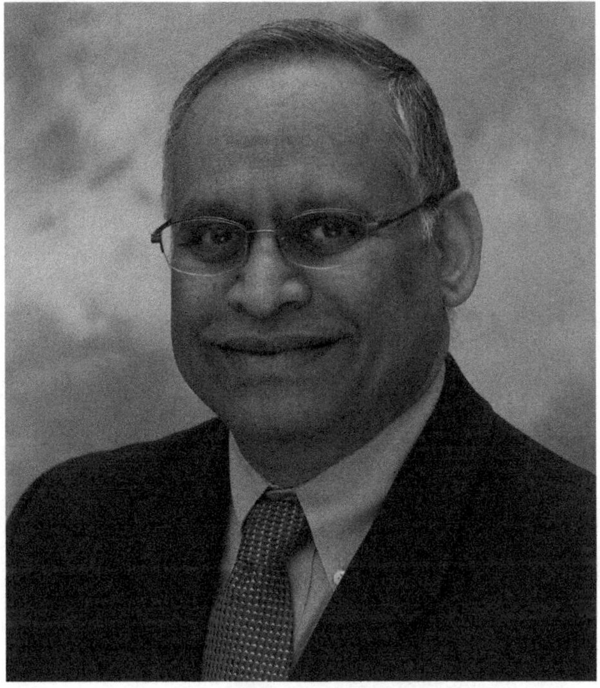

Laligam N. Sekhar

Laligam Sekhar is Professor and Vice-chairman at the Department of Neurosurgery, University of Washington, Seattle. He received his degrees in biology from the Loyola College (1967) and Vivekanada College (1968) of Madras University in India and obtained his M.B.B.S. in Medicine from Madras University in 1973.

He then pursued his training in neurology and neurosurgery at Cook County Hospital (Chicago, IL), the University of Cincinnati (OH) and then at University of Pittsburgh (PA). He trained briefly with Prof. M. Gazi Yaşargil and Prof. Majid Samii in neurosurgery.

Dr. Sekhar completed his residency in 1982 and after that he worked extensively in skull base surgery and pioneered numerous new techniques. He was appointed as Assistant Professor in the Department of Neurological Surgery at the University of Pittsburgh. In 1993 he became chairman of the Department of Neurological Surgery at George Washington University in Washington, DC. Dr. Sekhar has published, more than 200 peer-reviewed papers, 100 book chapters and 4 books.

Contact: Laligam N. Sekhar, Department of Neurosurgery, University of Washington, Harborview Medical Center, 325 Ninth Ave., Box 359924, Seattle, WA 98104-2499, USA
E-mail: lsekhar@u.washington.edu

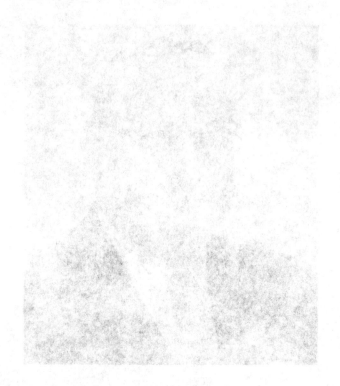

HOW TO PERFORM SELECTIVE EXTRADURAL ANTERIOR CLINOIDECTOMY

Y. YONEKAWA

INTRODUCTION

The anterior clinoid process is a part of the sphenoid bone overlying the optic nerve and the carotid artery taking a veer medially to the planum sphenoidale, anterolateraly to the sphenoid ridge and caudally to the optic strut. Partial removal of the process has been recommended for the surgical management of aneurysms of the internal carotid artery (ICA) at its proximal intradural part, already as early as in 1972 [11, 12, 19]. It was however only in 1993 that the method of systematic en bloc removal of the bone fragment including the whole anterior clinoid process (ACP), namely, selective extradural anterior clinoidectomy (SEAC) was carried out, which then was reported in 1997 [22]. With this method one may obviate the more invasive and time consuming technique of extensive orbital roof removal together with anterior clinoidectomy which had been applied in surgical treatment for parasellar and cavernous pathologies pioneered by Dolenc [2, 3]. In this chapter, advantages, indications, technical details and complications are clarified.

RATIONALE

The ACP is located at the medial end of the ala minor of the sphenoid bone and forms the lateral wall of the optic canal and the medial wall of the superior orbital fissure. The space gained by removal of the ACP by SEAC is called the clinoid space. Its floor makes the superior wall of the cavernous sinus. Removal of the ACP makes the operative field more spacious, which facilitates the handling of microsurgical instruments in the depth and allows to obtain much more illumination of the operating microscope. Incision of the lateral wall of the optic nerve sheath and partial or circumferential dissection of the distal dural ring of the internal carotid artery (ICA) after the SEAC enable easier further mobilization of the optic nerve and the ICA. This increased mobility of both structures enables radicality of procedures in the vicinity such as tumor removal or aneurysmal clipping with much more security. Opening of the cavernous sinus after the procedure enables surgical treatment of intracavernous pathology with complicated anatomy [7].

Keywords: skull base approaches, anterior clinoidectomy, microsurgery

Drilling away the posterior clinoid process and the upper clivus is helpful for clipping of lower lying distal basilar aneurysms [13, 18, 20, 21].

DECISION-MAKING

Indications of SEAC are as follows (Fig. 1): aneurysms at C2 portion, especially proximal C2, and at C3 portion, meningioma of the tuberculum sellae, pituitary adenoma, craniopharyngioma, aneurysms of the distal basilar artery with or without combination of extensive posterior clinoidectomy by opening the cavernous sinus at its postero-superior corner [22]. A high-flow bypass between the C4 and the C2 portion can be performed in combination with the anterior petrosectomy [6].

Furthermore, aneurysm surgery in the acute stage for the distal basilar artery can be better performed even in the presence of brain swelling by pterional approach combined with SEAC than by subtemporal approach, by gaining the clinoid space and by better CSF drainage via third ventriculostomy by opening the lamina terminalis [20, 21].

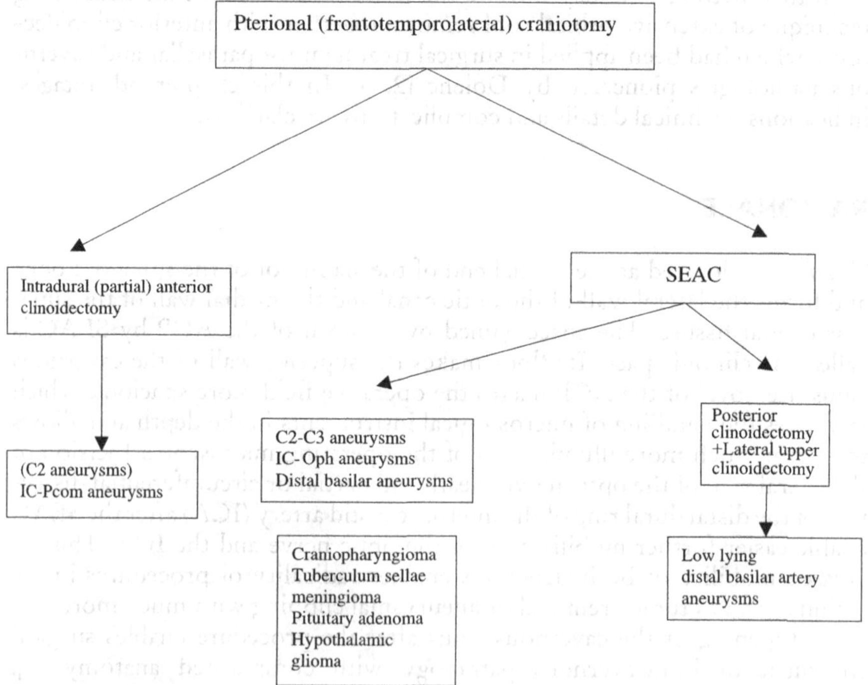

Fig. 1. Decision algorithm for anterior clinoidectomy. Although internal carotid-ophthalmic artery aneurysms are to be included with paraclinoid aneurysms (C2–C3), they are classified here separately in the traditional way

SURGERY

1. SELECTIVE EXTRADURAL ANTERIOR CLINOIDECTOMY (Fig. 2)

After having completed a pterional craniotomy, the sphenoid ridge is drilled away up to the lateral corner, the so-called frontotemporal dural fold (FTDF) (or orbitotemporal periosteal fold) [2, 5] of the superior orbital fissure (SOF), which might contain the lacrimal branch of the middle meningeal artery. Far medially extradurally towards the midline, one may reach the falciform fold of the optic nerve, which in our experience can be noticed in more than 80% of cases, so that one may postulate the course of the optic canal. Otherwise, this has to be checked after opening the dura by confirming the optic nerve. Careful drilling away with cutting burr of 2–3 mm is begun from the crossing point of the above mentioned FTDF of the SOF medioanteriorly so that the cutting or drilling line can cross over with that of the roof of the optic canal. With these two drilling procedures one may luxate the ACP and remove it en bloc. At that time, one has to pay attention to the following three points. (1) Compression or contusion to the optic nerve should be avoided. (2) The anesthesiologist should be informed and prepared for arhythmia or even for cardiac arrest for a while due to trigeminal nerve stimuli. We are doing topical application of procaine in order to alleviate the reaction. (3) There is profuse bleeding from the clinoid space. This bleeding is no direct bleeding from the cavernous sinus and can be controlled effectively with oxycellulose immersed in fibrin glue and a sponge for compression with slight head elevation.

If the en bloc removal is difficult, as in our experience it appears in around 30–40% of cases mostly due to a strong optic strut, the part of the strut should be drilled away carefully and once more the en bloc removal should be tried. If the process still cannot be removed, one has to doubt and check the bony connection of the ACP to the posterior clinoid process, although such situation is rare. The connection is to be cut by drilling away to complete the SEAC procedure. Sometimes the strategy of en bloc removal might have to be abandoned in case of more difficulty and the remaining part of the ACP has to be removed only by drilling away. After the removal, the optic strut can be still so strong that a considerable part remains between the optic nerve and the ICA. One has to drill away the part in order to get a spacious clinoid space for performance of further surgical procedures.

During this procedure one may encounter two paranasal sinuses. One are the ethmoid cells at the time of drilling away of the roof of the optic canal at its medial corner, so that one should remain just at the most medial corner of the canal and not exceed the limit. The other sinus, the sphenoid sinus, can extend into the ACP, around 8–10% after previous reports [10] and our experience, so that its mucous membrane can be exposed on ACP removal. In both cases, the mucous membrane is pushed back with Betadine-immersed oxycellulose and is treated afterwards with fatty tissue or muscle piece and

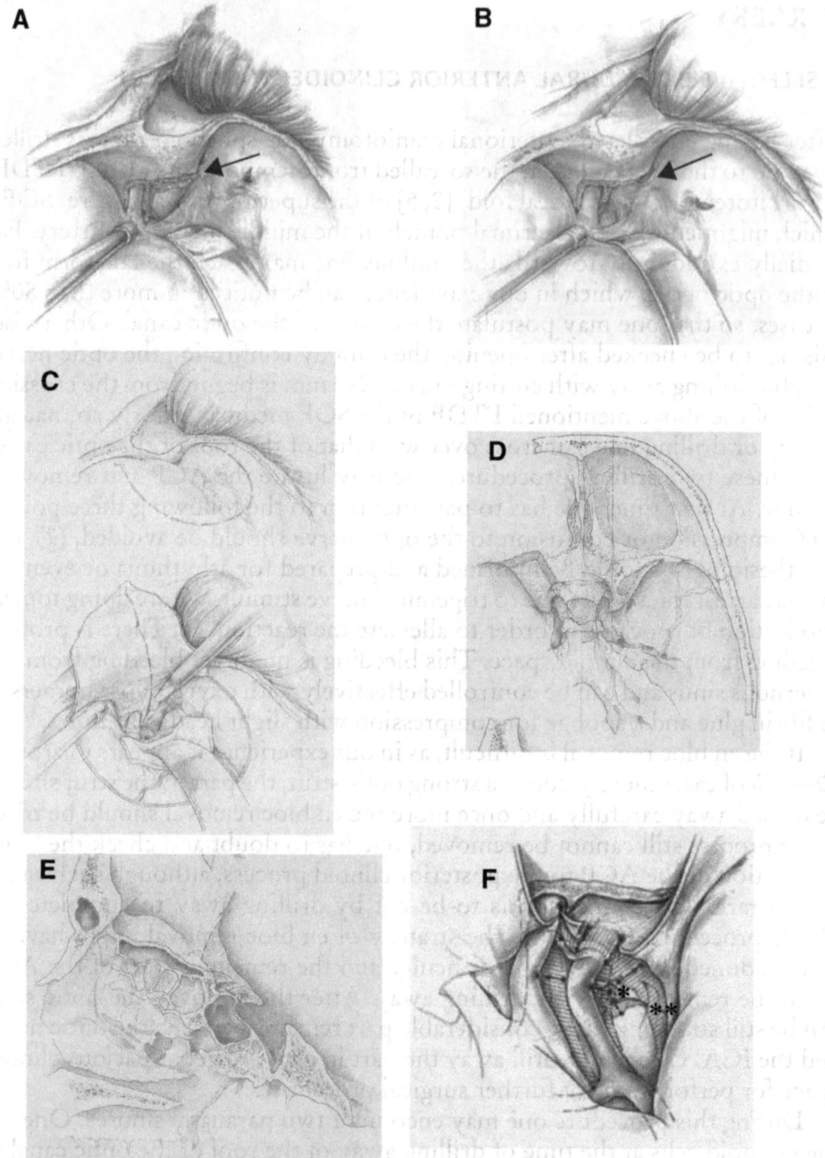

Fig. 2. Artist drawing of SEAC procedure. **A** Drilling lines of SEAC showing over the optic canal and over the FTDF (arrow). **B** Clinoid space obtained by en bloc removal of the ACP. **C** Additional dural incision for preparation of the clinoid space. **D** Axial view of the skull base showing the extent of SEAC and paranasal sinuses. **E** Paramedian sagittal view of the skull showing paranasal sinuses. **F** Overview after dural opening and dissection of the optic nerve and the carotid artery as described in the text. Note the posterior clinoid process and the distal basilar artery (*) in the depth medial to the oculomotor nerve (**)

fibrin glue. Contents of the superior orbital fissure (the ophthalmic nerve, oculomotor nerve, nasocilial nerve, abducens, trochlear nerve, superior ophthalmic vein, recurrent branch of the ophthalmic artery and lacrimal branch of the middle meningeal artery) are not exposed during the SEAC procedure. Lesions of the cavernous sinus can be accessed by opening the anteromedial triagle after Dolenc, but this is beyond the scope of this chapter so that the other chapter about this should be referred.

After dural opening in a curvilinear fashion, the proximal dural flap is cut again to the direction of the clinoid space. After having reached the distal dural ring of the ICA, one may extend the cutting line to the falciform fold over the optic nerve. Longitudinal incision on the optic nerve sheath at the lateral corner about 5 mm anteriorly makes mobilization of the optic nerve easier, so that the ophthalmic artery origin located at the mediosuperior corner of the ICA comes into view in case of usual intradural origin (around 85%). This procedure can be done only after the unroofing of the optic canal is done following the original SEAC method. The distal dural ring of the ICA is incised according to the need of ICA mobilization. This might have to be combined with opening of the cavernous sinus so that the bleeding from the opened sinus has to be filled with oxycellulose together with fibrin glue successively. By this increased mobilization of the optic nerve and the ICA, aneurysms of the C2–C3 segment can be managed successfully with a conventional clipping method, also those of the distal basilar artery with or without combination of an extensive posterior clinoidectomy (Figs. 3 and 4). Radicality of tumor removal of the parasellar and hypothalamic region is accomplished by this increased mobility of the structures [1, 15, 22].

In cases with potential risk of aneurysmal rupture at the time of clinoidectomy [9] even in SEAC, it is recommended to perform dissection of the cervical carotid artery beforehand for eventual temporary carotid ligation for its management.

2. INTRADURAL ANTERIOR CLINOIDECTOMY

Anterior clinoidectomy can be carried out after dural opening especially for the treatment of aneurysms of the internal carotid–ophthalmic or the internal carotid–posterior communicating artery, whose neck locates very near to or under the clinoid process [11, 19]. Intradural en bloc removal has been also reported [17]. Precise neuroradiological evaluation has been reported to enable prediction of the necessity of clinoidectomy, for example, in cases with the distance between the proximal aneurysmal neck and the carotid knee C3 being less than 1 cm in the lateral view of angiography [14]. One has to be careful only with slipping off the drilling burr onto the carotid and neighboring optic nerve, as they are without dural covering, which is not the case for SEAC.

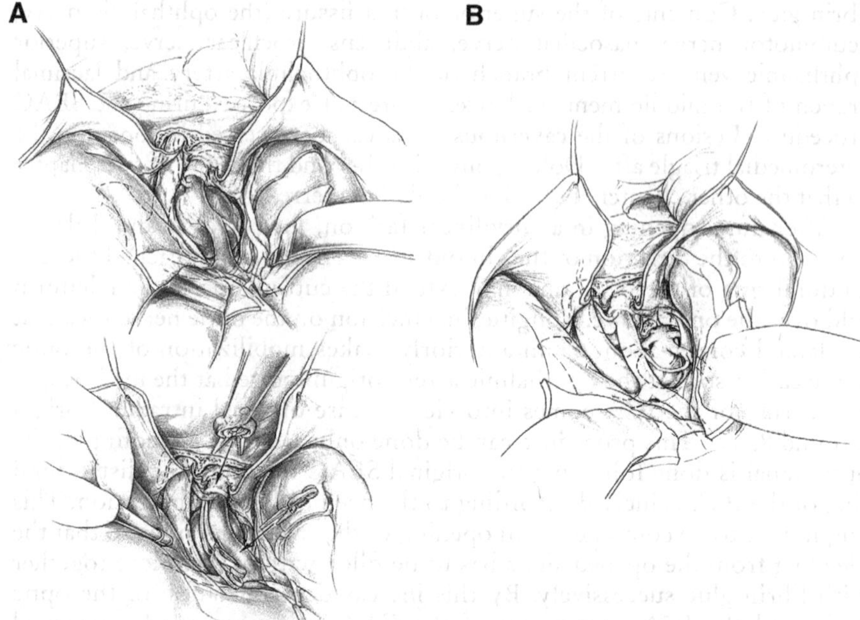

Fig. 3. Artist drawing of aneurysm neck clipping after SEAC procedure. **A** Large posterior wall aneurysm of the ICA-C2 portion. **B** Basilar bifurcation aneurysm.

3. POSTERIOR CLINOIDECTOMY

Combination of extensive posterior clinoidectomy with SEAC is effective for the surgical treatment of low lying distal basilar artery aneurysms; aneurysms of the basilar bifurcation, basilar SCA aneurysms and even upper basilar trunk aneurysms (Fig. 4) lying lower than the level of the posterior clinoid process at the lateral view of the angiogramm [4, 13, 16, 18, 20, 21]. After the procedure of SEAC and partial or complete circumferential dissection of the carotid dural ring for mobilization of the ICA, the dural canal of the oculomotor nerve is opened by cutting the dural sheath towards the proximal dural ring. This enables mobilization of the oculomotor nerve, so that the procedures for the extensive posterior clinoidectomy can be carried out smoothly and safely due to a widened working space. The dura over the posterior clinoid process and that over the posterosuperior cavernous sinus are incised to enable the procedure. Bleeding from the cavernous sinus is managed with fibrin glue-immersed oxycellulose. Drilling away of the clinoid and lateral part of the upper clivus can be done thus more safely with a burr drilling equipped with a diamond head and irrigation.

4. CLINICAL RESULTS AND COMPLICATIONS

SEAC was carried out in 214 cases during the period between September 1993 and May 2007 as are shown in Table 1. SEAC-related complications are

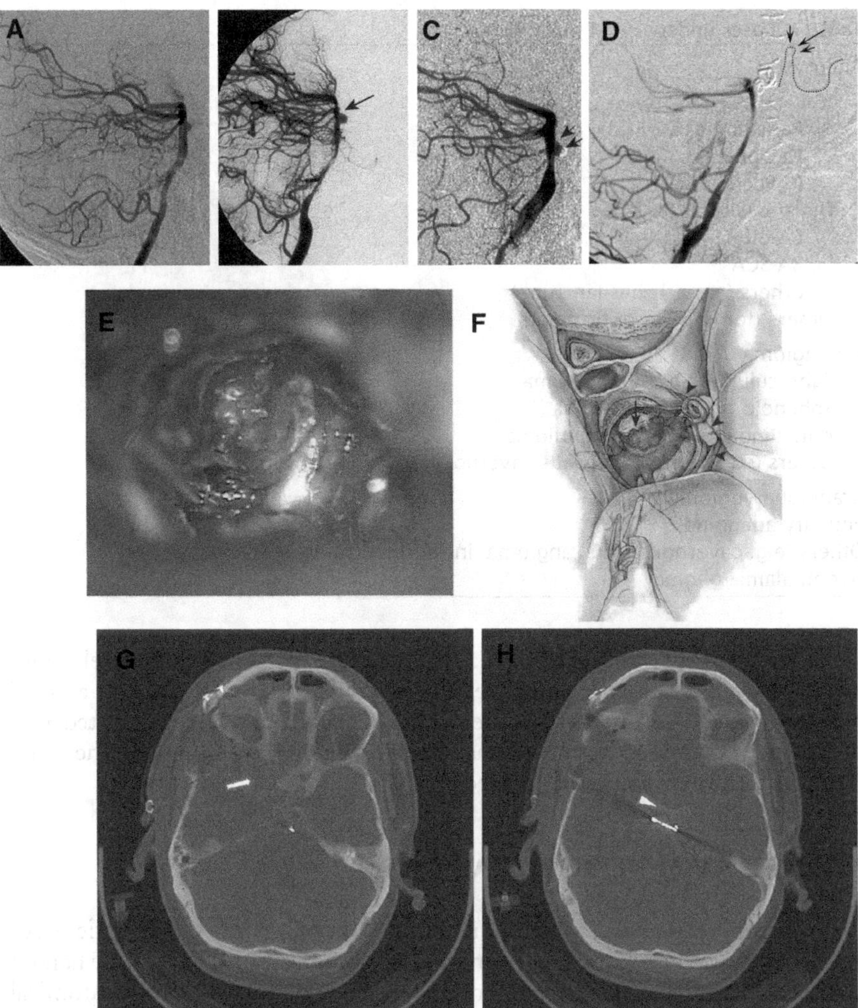

Fig. 4. A case of basilar trunk dissection aneurysm located lower than the level of the posterior clinoid process. **A** This small outpouching at the anterior wall of the distal basilar trunk was overlooked on day 0 digital substraction angiography (DSA) after subarachnoid hemorrhage. **B** Repeated DSA 5 days later revealed growth of the dissecting aneurysm (arrow), so that this was successfully coiled. **C** Coil compaction (double arrows) on the repeated DSA on day 17 after a rebleeding. **D** Follow-up angiography after the complete neck clipping. Notice the hight of the posterior clinoid process and sellar (triple arrows) drawn additionally. **E** Exposure of the dissecting aneurysm after SEAC and extended posterior clinoidectomy. **F** Artist drawing of the situation of **E**. Notice the drilled upper lateral clivus on the left side (arrow) and opened oculomotor nerve canal on the right (arrowheads). **G** This bone window CT indicates status after SEAC right (arrow) following a standard pterional craniotomy. **H** This slice CT shows the status after the posterior clinoidectomy and the lateral clivectomy (arrowhead). Notice the aneurysm clip to the dissecting aneurysm. The compacted coil can be seen between the clivus and the tip of aneurysm clip

Table 1. Cases underwent SEAC (*N*=214)

Aneurysms	
ICA	
Paraclinoid (C 2+C3)	25
IC-Oph	24
IC-Pcom	6
Distal basilar artery	
BA-bifur	44
BA-SCA	17
others (e.g. P1, basilar trunk)	4
Others (for ligation or trapping)	6
Meningioma	
Tuberculum sellae meningioma	18
Sphenoid ridge meningioma	10
Ant. clinoid process meningioma	10
Others (e.g. petroclival, sinus cavernosus)	8
Craniopharyngioma	18
Pituitary adenoma	13
Others (e.g. cavernous sinus angioma, intraorbital tumor)	9
Hypothalamic glioma	2

visual disturbances in 3 cases. One of them presented postoperatively with amaurosis which did not improve. Postoperative CT scan showed a small hematoma in the clinoid space. Persistent rhinorrhea was complicated in 4 cases; one was treated with transnasal repair plus V-P shunting and the other three with transcranial repair by recraniotomy.

HOW TO AVOID COMPLICATIONS

Major complications are, as before mentioned, compromise of the optic nerve and CSF rhinorrhea. For prevention of these complications, on the one hand it is important to have appropriate preprocedural expectation of the anatomical relationship of the optic nerve and the carotid artery by correct interpretation of findings of neuroimagings including status of pneumatization of paranasal sinuses. One should be familiar with their topographical anatomy along with their pathological deviation, as one is requested to work correctly very closely to these important structures. Opening of sinuses should be noticed without oversight and treated as mentioned above. On the other hand microsurgical training with cadaver dissection is therefore mandatory and it cannot be overemphasized to carry out the procedure very carefully avoiding direct mechanical injury and heat transmission of drilling by continuous saline irrigation. By trained hands, the procedure can be completed within 15–20 min.

Another thing to be cared is strong dural adhesion to the clinoid process in aged patients at the time of en bloc removal. In order to avoid inadvertent injury to the neighboring structures in such situation, the removal should be carried out with great care.

CONCLUSIONS

The anterior clinoid process covers part of the optic nerve and the internal carotid artery. On its removal, parasellar pathological processes such as tuberculum sellae meningiomas, craniopharyngiomas, paraclinoid aneurysms and upper basilar aneurysms can be managed surgically with more radicality and security. The removal can be done ideally by SEAC, which has some potential risk of injury to important structures so that it should be performed with good knowledge of topographical anatomy and by trained hands.

Acknowledgment

I am indebted to P. Roth for the work of illustrations.

References

[1] Andaluz N, Beretta F, Bernucci C, Keller JT, Zuccarello M (2006) Evidence for the improved exposure of the ophthalmic segment of the internal carotid artery after anterior clinoidectomy: morphometric analysis. Acta Neurochir (Wien) 148: 971-976

[2] Coscarella E, Baskaya MK, Morcos JJ (2003) An alternative extradural exposure to the anterior clinoid process: the superior orbital fissure as a surgical corridor. Neurosurgery 53: 162-167

[3] Dolenc VV (1985) A combined epi- and subdural direct approach to carotid-ophthalmic artery aneurysms. J Neurosurg 62: 667-672

[4] Dolenc VV, Skrap M, Sustersic J, Skrbec M, Morina A (1987) A transcavernous-transsellar approach to the basilar tip aneurysms. Br J Neurosurg 1: 251-259

[5] Froelich S, Aziz KMA, Levine NB, Theodosopoulos PV, van Loveren HR, Keller JT (2007) Refinement of the extradural anterior clinoidectomy: surgical anatomy of the orbitotemporal periosteal fold. Neurosurgery 61(5 Suppl 2): 179-186

[6] Fukushima T (1992) Operative technique of the skull base bypass. Jpn J Neurosurg 1: 41-47

[7] Inoue T, Rhoton AL Jr, Theele D, Barry ME (1990) Surgical approaches to the cavernous sinus: a microsurgical study. Neurosurgery 26: 903-932

[8] Khan N, Yoshimura S, Roth P, Cesnulis E, Koenue-Leblebicioglu D, Curcic M, Imhof HG, Yonekawa Y (2005) Conventional mirosurgical treatment of paraclinoid aneurysms: state of the art with the use of the selective extradural anterior clinoidectomy SEAC. Acta Neurochir Suppl 94: 23-29

[9] Korosue K, Heros RC (1992) "Subclinoid" carotid aneurysm with erosion of the anterior clinoid process and fatal intraoperative rupture. Neurosurgery 31: 356-360

[10] Mikami T, Minamida Y, Koyanagi I, Baba T, Houkin M (2007) Anatomical variations in pneumatization of the anterior clinoid process. J Neurosurg 106: 170-174

[11] Morgan F (1972) Removal of anterior clinoid process in the surgery of carotid aneurysm, with some notes on recurrent subarachnoid haemorrhage during craniotomy. Schweiz Arch Neurol Neurochir Psychiatr 111: 363-368

[12] Nutik SL (1988) Removal of the anterior clinoid process for exposure of the proximal intracranial carotid artery. J Neurosurg 69: 529-534

[13] Nutik SL (1998) Pterional craniotomy via a transcavernous approach for the treatment of low-lying distal basilar artery aneurysms. J Neurosurg 89: 921-926

[14] Ochiai C, Wakai S, Inou S, Nagai M (1989) Preoperative angiographical prediction of the necessity to removal of the anterior clinoid process in internal carotid-posterior communicating artery aneurysm surgery. Acta Neurochir (Wien) 99: 117-121

[15] Otani N, Muroi C, Yano H, Khan N, Pangalu A, Yonekawa Y (2006) Surgical management of tuberculum sellae meningioma: role of selective extradural anterior clinoidectomy. Br J Neurosurg 20: 129-138

[16] Seoane E, Tedeschi H, de Oliveira E, Wen HT, Rohton AL Jr (2000) The pretemporal transcavernous approach to the interpeduncular and prepontine cisterns: microsurgical anatomy and technique application. Neurosurgery 46: 891-899

[17] Takahashi JA, Kawarazaki A, Hashimoto N (2004) Intradural en-bloc removal of the anterior clinoid process. Acta Neurochir (Wien) 146: 505-509

[18] Yaşargil MG, Antic J, Laciga R, Jain KK, Hodosh RM, Smith RD (1976) Microsurgical pterional approach to aneurysms of the basilar bifurcation. Surg Neurol 6: 83-91

[19] Yaşargil MG, Gasser JC, Hodosh RM, et al. (1977) Carotid-ophthalmic aneurysms: direct microsurgical approach. Surg Neurol 8: 155-165

[20] Yonekawa Y, Khan N, Imhof HG, Roth P (2005) Basilar bifurcation aneurysms. Lessons learnt from 40 consecutive cases. Acta Neurochir Suppl 94: 39-44

[21] Yonekawa Y, Kaku Y, Imhof HG, Kiss M, Curcic M, Taub E, Roth P (1999) Posterior circulation aneurysms. Technical strategies based on angiographic anatomical findings and the results of 60 recent consecutive cases. Acta Neurochir Suppl 72: 123-140

[22] Yonekawa Y, Ogata N, Imhof HG, Olivecrona M, Strommer K, Kwak TE, Roth P, Groscurth P (1997) Selective extradural anterior clinoidectomy for supra- and parasellar processes. Technical note. J Neurosurg 87: 636-642

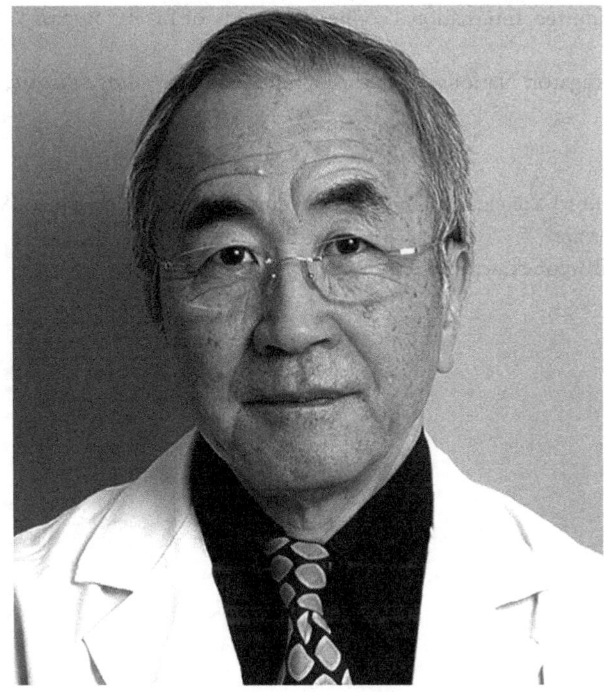

Yasuhiro Yonekawa

Yasuhiro Yonekawa is consultant neurosurgeon at the Klinik im Park, Zurich, and at the Kantonsspital Aarau
1939: Born in Tsu, Mie, Japan
1964: Graduation, School of Medicine, Kyoto University, Kyoto, Japan
1970: Resident, Department of Neurosurgery, University Hospital Zurich, Zurich, Switzerland
1973: Chief Resident, Department of Neurosurgery, University Hospital Zurich, Zurich, Switzerland
1981: Associate Professor, Department of Neurosurgery, Kyoto University Hospital, Kyoto, Japan
1986: Director, Department of Neurosurgery, National Cardiovascular Center, Suita, Osaka, Japan
1993: Director, Department of Neurosurgery, University Hospital Zurich, Zurich, Switzerland
2007: Emeritation, Department of Neurosurgery, University Hospital Zurich, Zurich, Switzerland

Executive committee, International cooperative study of EC-IC Bypass (1978–1985 NIH, USA)
Principal Investigator, National research committee of Moyamoya disease, Japan (1988–1992)

Contact: Yasuhiro Yonekawa, University of Zurich, Haldenbachstrasse 18, 8091 Zurich, Switzerland
E-mail: yasuhiro.yonekawa@usz.ch

HOW TO PERFORM APPROACHES OF THE ORBIT

J. C. MARCHAL

INTRODUCTION

There are several types of tumorous or pseudo-tumorous lesions affecting the orbit. The first historical stage was to make a coherent nosological approach of it. Often confused with the diagnosis and the treatment of tumorous proptosis, the first descriptions of tumors of the optical pathways and the optic nerve sheath are due to Antonio Scarpa (1816), who described a tumor of the optic nerve. Similarly, Jean Cruveilhier (1835) considered that meningiomas are tumors which do not belong to the central nervous system itself and must be distinguished from it. Albrecht von Graefe applied the same principle to tumors of the optic nerve. A. C. Hudson (1912) considered meningiomas of the optic nerve sheath as being separate from tumors of the optic nerve itself. However, it was Harvey Cushing [4], who provided the first accurate description of meningiomas as he distinguished meningiomas according to their origin from the arachnoid mater. He therefore dissociated orbito-sphenoidal meningiomas spreading the orbital content from meningiomas affecting the optic nerve sheath.

We can therefore understand why the neurosurgical approach to the orbit appeared only recently in the history of orbital surgery. The concept of the neurosurgical approach is directly linked to surgery of the craniofacial boundaries, and in this respect it should always be preceded by a multidisciplinary discussion. The concept of an endocranial approach was described and implemented by Durante (1887). Since then, retraction of the frontal lobe has been identified as the main obstacle to using this approach. Frazier (1913) partially resolved this technical difficulty when he suggested removing the superior orbital rim. Then came the work of Naffziger (1948), who established the specifically neurosurgical principles of the orbital approach, followed by Hamby (1964), who proposed the pterional approach for some of these lesions. In the 1960s and 1970s, plastic surgeons such as Converse, Mustarde, Stricker, and Tessier showed particular interest in craniofacial malformations, which gave new force to the aforementioned neurosurgical approaches as they added the notions of reconstruction and of volumetric reduction of the orbit to the existing notions of exocranial

Keywords: orbit, orbital approaches, tumor, pediatric neurosurgery

Table 1. Main orbital tumors in childhood in terms of histology and management[a]

Disease	Follow-up only	Biopsy	Chemo- or radiation therapy	Surgery
Optic nerve glioma	1 – clinical and MR imaging		2 – clinical worsening, avoid radiation therapy (NF1)	3 – resistant to chemotherapy, tumor spreading backwards
Plexiform neurofibroma	1 – clinical and MR imaging			2 – oculomotor and cosmetic considerations
Rhabdomyosarcoma		1	2 – after biopsy (bone marrow and/or tumor)	3 – checking MR findings at the end of treatment
Fibrosarcoma		1		2 – radical excision
Metastasis (neuroblastoma, Ewing's)			1 – according to histology	1 – primitive cancer unknown
Leukemia		1 – leukemia not diagnosed (chloroma)	1	
Teratoma				1 – radical excision
Dermoid cyst				1 – radical excision
Capillary hemangioma	1 – disappears spontaneously			
Lymphangioma	1 – clinical and MR imaging			2 – partial excision of cysts when growth spurts
Cavernous angioma				1 – radical excision
Fibrous dysplasia	1 – clinical and MR imaging			2 – oculomotor palsy, threatens optic nerves

[a] 1–3, steps in management

and endocranial approaches, and excision. These findings paved the way for surgical treatment of more complex lesions such as fibrous dysplasia and plexiform neurofibroma.

The history of neurosurgery reflects the difficulty of establishing a logical classification of the nature and origin of orbital tumors. These issues are still of concern today as specialists continue to face difficulties at the diagnosis stage [5], which can then lead to problems in choosing an appropriate strategy for treatment (Tables 1 and 2).

Table 2. Main orbital tumors in adulthood in terms of histology and management[a]

Disease	Follow-up only	Biopsy	Chemo- or radiation therapy	Surgery
Metastasis			According to histology	1 – primitive cancer unknown 2 – resistant to chemotherapy
Primitive lymphoma		1	2	
Optic sheath meningioma	1 – clinical and MR imaging			2 – if blindness of the eye
Spheno-orbital meningioma			2 – conformational radiation therapy following incomplete surgery	1 – excision (as complete as possible)
Schwannoma				1 – radical excision
Cavernous angioma				1 – radical excision

[a] 1–3, steps in management

RATIONALE

The traditional anatomy of the orbital content is extremely complex as it describes numerous muscular, nervous and vascular structures within a small volume. Although anatomy books cover the elementary physiology of vision and of oculomotricity, the complexity of these books is not sufficient when dealing with the more pragmatic requirements of microneurosurgery. Furthermore, orbital fat is an anatomical factor of even greater importance than blood as it impedes navigation as well as surgical positioning in the orbit. As a result of these two considerations, traditional anatomical description should be considered as a concept rather than as a surgical model. It is equally important, when considering the neurosurgical approach of the orbit, to keep in mind a certain number of key anatomical references.

1. DEFINITION OF "NEUROSURGICAL ORBIT"

Tumorous or pseudo-tumorous lesions of the neurosurgical orbit are those which concern the two posterior thirds of the orbit [2]. Tumors of the eyeball should therefore be excluded. The choice of an approach depends on several topographical factors: the position of the tumor in the coronal plane of the orbit; monitoring of the orbital content, and, in the event of a tumor of the bone cavity or muscular cavity; monitoring of the epidural space, monitoring the optic nerve (ON) in the orbit, in the optic canal, and in the subarachnoid spaces; an approach which allows excisions of possible extension to the temporal fossa, the maxilla, zygomatic, and the nasal region.

2. LATERAL ORBITAL RIM: ACCESSING THE TWO POSTERIOR THIRDS OF THE ORBIT

The anatomy of the anterior region of the orbit is formed by the suture of the zygomatic process of the frontal bone and the frontal process of the zygomatic bone. These two processes join backwards with the greater wing of the sphenoid bone. The frontal crest extends towards the rear on the parietal bone and bounds the lateral temporal fossa superiorly. By separating the periorbit from the medial aspect of the lateral wall of the orbit, and detaching the insertions of the temporal muscle at the anterosuperior region of the lateral temporal fossa, the surgeon can easily perform an orbitotomy which will remove the entire lateral wall of the orbit (in other words, the zygomatic process of the frontal bone and the frontal process of the zygomatic bone). From there the greater wing of the sphenoid bone is easily reached, and by removing the greater wing, the surgeon can access the superolateral region of the superior orbital fissure. Opening the periorbit superiorly towards the front provides access to the lachrymal nerve and to the lachrymal artery, running above the lateral rectus muscle and up to the lachrymal gland situated in the superolateral quarter of the orbit. The inferior oblique muscle is situated underneath the lateral rectus muscle. At the posterior part on the eyeball, the ON can be seen with the artery and the ciliary nerve. The ophthalmic veins can be seen at the rear of the eyeball.

3. ORBITAL ROOF: ACCESSING THE SUPERIOR PART OF THE ORBIT AND THE EXOCRANIAL AND ENDOCRANIAL OPTIC CANAL

The orbital roof can be easily separated from the dura of the inferior surface of the frontal lobe upwards and from the periorbit underneath. Once the orbital roof has been removed, it is possible to see, laterally across the periorbit in a posteroanterior direction, the frontal nerve, then the supra orbital nerve with the superior ophthalmic veins (Fig. 1). Medially from the frontal nerve, showing through an equally posteroanterior and medial direction, the trochlear nerve can be seen. These nerves are embedded in a substantial amount of periorbital fat, making dissection very delicate (Fig. 1). The incision of the periorbit can be made on either side of the frontal nerve, which rises above the levator palpebrae muscle–superior rectus muscle (LPM–SRM) complex. The retrobulbar part of the ON can either be exposed laterally or medially from the LPM–SRM. In order to reveal the ON, an incision should be made laterally on the periorbit, between the LPM–SRM and the LRM. At this point it is possible to see the lateral part of the ON [7], crossed over by the ophthalmic artery and the nasociliary nerve. The LRM is moved aside laterally with the abducens nerve, which penetrates into it at its me-

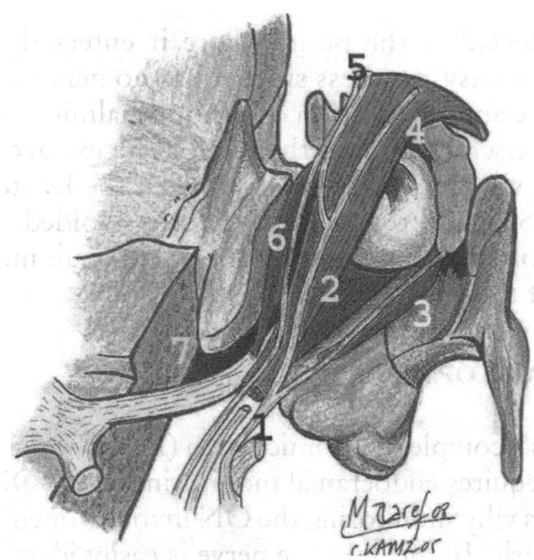

Fig. 1. Superior aspect of the right unroofed orbit. *1* Ophthalmic nerve (V), *2* frontal nerve (V), *3* lachrymal nerve (V), *4* supraorbital nerve (V), *5* supratrochlear nerve (V), *6* trochlear nerve (IV), *7* optic nerve (II)

dial aspect. Medially, by making an incision of the periorbit between the LPM–SRM and the medial surface of the superior oblique muscle, the entire intraorbital course of the ON is exposed and it is possible to make an incision into the common tendinous ring between the tendon of the SRM and the medial surface of the superior oblique muscle and to extend the visible part of the nerve towards the orbital apex (Fig. 2). The trochlear nerve must

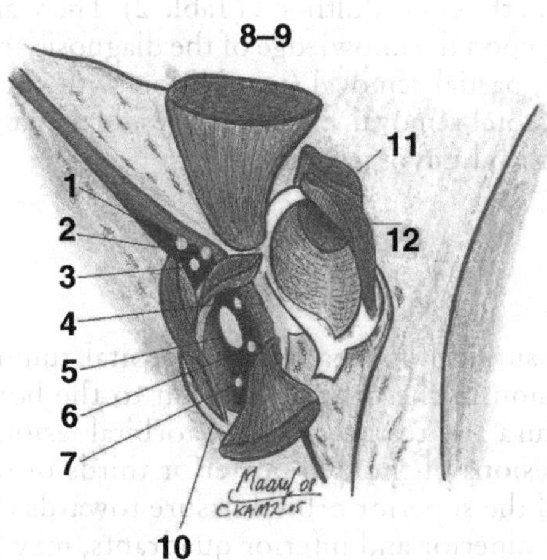

Fig. 2. Coronal section of the right orbital apex. *1* Lachrymal nerve (V), *2* frontal nerve (V), *3* trochlear nerve (IV), *4* abducens nerve (VI), *5* oculomotor nerve (III), *6* sympathic root of the ciliary ganglion, *7* nasociliary nerve (III), *8* and *9* levator palpebrae-superior rectus muscles, *10* common tendinous ring, *11* superior oblique muscle, *12* medial rectus muscle

therefore be protected at the point where it enters the oblique superior muscle. This area is easy to access since it has no nervous or vascular structure (except for the anterior section of the ophthalmic artery and the part of the trochlear nerve which crosses the LPM at its extraconical section). The central approach, which is performed between the levator palpebrae superioris muscle (LPSM) and the SRM, should be avoided as there is a risk to injure the nerve of the LPM (issuing from the oculomotor nerve) on the inferior surface of this muscle.

4. OPTIC CANAL AND OPTIC NERVE

The orbital apex is a complex anatomical area (Fig. 2) which, in order to be approached safely, requires endocranial monitoring of the ON and endo-orbital monitoring. This is why monitoring the ON involves opening the dura and the optic canal superiorly. In this way the nerve is easily identified at its endocranial exit of the optic canal in the optochiasmatic cistern. After drilling the roof of the optic canal, the superior surface of the ON up to the optic canal is situated between the LPM–SRM medially and the superior oblique muscle–medial rectus muscles superiorly and laterally. Laterally from the common tendinous ring, the lachrymal, frontal, and trochlear nerves are visible (Fig. 2).

DECISION-MAKING

In terms of histology and management, main orbital tumors in childhood (Table 1) differ from those in adulthood (Table 2). There are 4 indications for surgery depending upon the knowledge of the diagnosis and the course of the disease [5]: biopsy, partial removal (in addition with chemotherapy and/or radiation therapy), total removal, checking a residual image after chemotherapy (for example, rhabdomyosarcoma).

SURGERY

Choosing a neurosurgical approach to an orbital tumor depends on the location of the lesion in the orbit, extension to the bony structures, and extension to the dura and to the ON. Intraorbital lesions and intraconical and extraconical lesions of the two posterior thirds of the orbit which do not spread beyond the superior orbital fissure towards the rear, and which are situated in the superior and inferior quadrants, may be approached via a lateral orbital approach (schwannoma, cavernous angioma, and dermoid cyst, etc.) [1]. Lesions affecting the two posterior thirds in the medial quadrants with access to the orbital roof and to the dura require a frontal extradural approach. The subfrontal approach can be completed by opening the dura in order to gain access to the ON from its extracranial entrance into the optic canal up to its endocranial exit in the optochiasmatic cistern (optic nerve glioma, optic sheath meningioma). If approaching via the temporal maxilla-zygomatic area, a pterional approach is recommended (orbitosphenoidal meningioma, fibrous dysplasia). This pterional approach, although it does offer an excellent approach of the lateral rim and of the lateral walls of the orbit, will not be covered in this chapter as it is frequently performed as a preliminary to the lateral approach of the skull base for numerous pathologies.

1. LATERAL APPROACH

By this approach it is possible to avoid retraction of the frontal lobe [1]. The patient is in the supine position, with the head turned 30 to 40° on a head holder. The eyebrow should not be shaved off. The cutaneous incision follows the external orbital rim from the extremity of the eyebrow which stems from the zygomatic process (Fig. 3A). It is continued medially, either in the eyebrow or in a fold of the upper eyelid, thereby giving access to the superior orbital rim, and then continued in an S shape laterally and towards the rear in order to extend the zygomatic process. The incision is made right to the bone of the superior external orbital rim. The periosteum that lines the bony orbit is continuous with the periosteum of the skull's outer surface. The periosteum is detached upwards whilst the periorbit is carefully dissected from the medial surface of the lateral orbital wall downwards. Depending on requirements, the temporal muscle is detached from the anterior section of the temporal crest and the lateral orbital rim (Fig. 3B). The periorbit and the temporal muscle are protected on both sides of the lateral orbital rim with cottonoids. An osteotomy of the lateral orbital rim is performed using an oscillating saw. It is detached from the lateral orbital wall with a chisel (Fig. 3C). Excision of the lateral wall may be carried out using rongeurs or a drill. During this part of the operation, care must be taken to protect the periorbit, as any rupture into the operating field can hinder excision. If dealing with an intraconical lesion, the periorbit is opened above the raised area of the LRM, which is lowered carefully. The posterior part of the orbital globe is then accessible, as is the intraorbital section of the optic nerve because there are no important anatomical elements in the way. The only hindrance is the periorbital fat as it could block the surgical approach. It must be pushed aside and separated, and care must be taken not to remove it as this would cause bleeding.

By extending the incision outwards and backwards along the length of the zygomatic process, the surgeon gains easy access to both the lateral temporal fossa and the greater wing of the sphenoid bone (Fig. 3D). Extending the incision along the eyebrow or in an inward fold of the eyelid facilitates a small frontal craniotomy if the anatomy of the frontal sinus allows this. When the incision is extended inwards, care must be taken to avoid the supraorbital

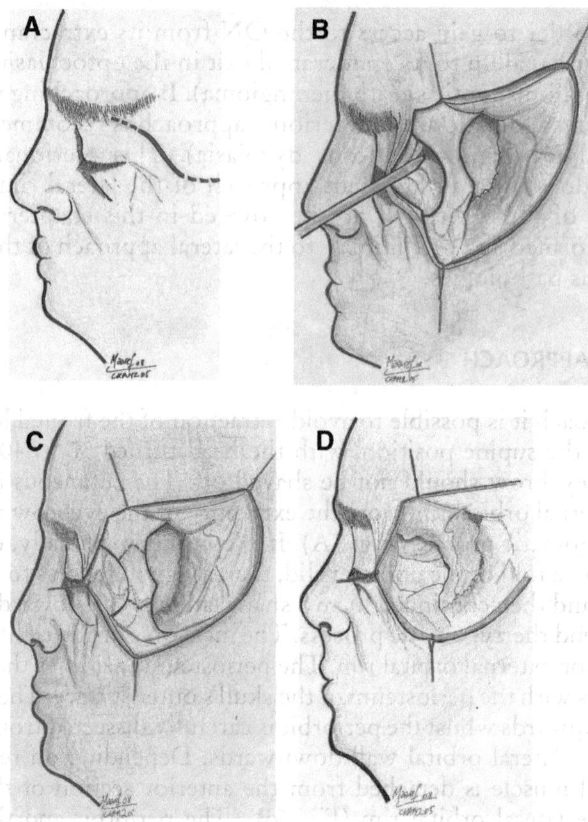

Fig. 3. **A** Cutaneous incision follows the external orbital rim from the extremity of the eyebrow. It is continued medially, either in the eyebrow or in a fold of the upper eyelid. **B** Periorbit is dissected from the medial surface of the lateral orbital wall downwards. Depending on requirements, the temporal muscle is detached from the anterior section of the temporal crest and the lateral orbital rim. **C** Osteotomy of the lateral orbital rim. **D** Access to the lateral temporal fossa and the greater wing of the sphenoid bone

nerve, which penetrates the orbit via the supraorbital notch at the junction between the first medial third and the two lateral thirds of the superior orbital rim; it is perpendicular to the surgical approach and must be opened up and pushed inwards. It is important to remember that there is a possibility of extension of the frontal sinus from the superior orbital rim or from the orbital roof. If only an orbitotomy of the lateral rim is performed, there is no risk of this. However, if one wishes to perform a medial extension and small frontal craniotomy (in order to reveal the dura and remove the orbital roof, for example), there is a risk. If extension occurs, it must be treated, as failure to do so may cause postoperative infection, which is often difficult to treat. The simplest solution is to fill the gap with fat or with muscle that is stuck with biological glue. The lateral orbital rim is laid down and osteosynthesis is performed using steel wires or screwed microplates.

2. SUBFRONTAL AND INTRACONICAL APPROACH OF THE ORBIT

2.1 Cutaneous incision, frontal craniotomy, and superior orbitotomy

The patient is in the supine position, with the head slightly extended and turned 10° opposite the side of the orbit to be explored. The bicoronal incision, skin flap and homolateral temporal muscle are bent back en bloc by detaching the periosteum directly from the bone situated on the pathological side. The superior insertions of the frontal muscle are progressively detached from the lateral temporal fossa, starting at the temporal crest during the folding of the skin flap towards the face. This detachment runs directly from the maxillary process of the frontal bone and the nasal bones medially and, laterally towards the zygomatic process of the frontal bone. Care must be taken to detach the anterior muscular insertions of the temporal muscle slightly towards the rear of the zygomatic process of the frontal bone, and to detach the latter as low as it is necessary to reveal the fronto-zygomatic suture. The supraorbital nerve is freed from its foramen or supraorbital notch: the nerve is accompanying its bony foramen, which is detached with a chisel and folded over downwards with the skin flap. Then, the periorbit is carefully dissected away from the inferior surface of the orbital roof, up to 2 cm. On the unaffected side, care must be taken to avoid injury to the temporal aponeurosis. A subcutaneous dissection can provoke paralysis of the frontal branch of the facial nerve. The frontal craniotomy can be confined to the vertical part of the frontal bone with or without the superior orbital rim. Removing the superior orbital rim can be carried out en bloc with the frontal craniotomy (Fig. 4), or in a second step, after lifting the frontal craniotomy (which is easier to perform on adults). A burr hole is made backwards from the zygomatic process

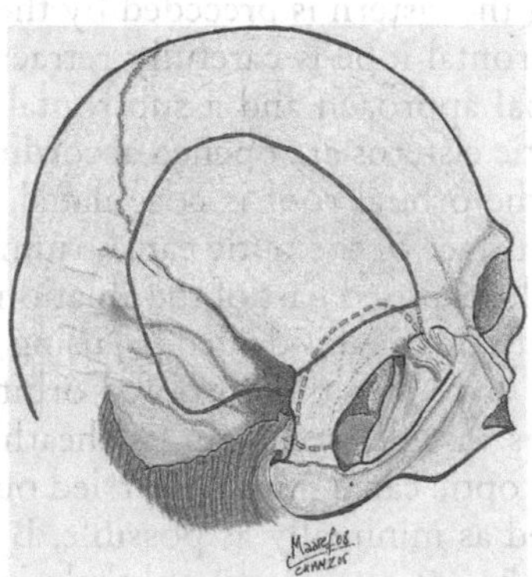

Fig. 4. Frontal craniotomy is confined to the vertical part of the frontal bone with (dotted line) or without (continuous line) the superior orbital rim

of the frontal bone, just under the crest of the insertion of the temporal muscle. After dissecting the dura, a rotative saw is used to cut the craniotomy along the lines (previously drawn on). The osteotomy of the superior orbital rim runs from the junction between the zygomatic process of the frontal bone and the frontal process of the zygomatic bone laterally and the medial third of the orbital roof. There is a risk, at this point, of entering the frontal sinus. Careful reading of the preoperative scan should prevent this to happen. If entering of the frontal sinus mucosa occurs, it must be sealed off in the manner described for the lateral approach. If the superior orbital rim is dissected en bloc with the frontal craniotomy, it is often necessary to end the craniotomy by separating the external orbitotomy with a chisel.

2.2 Unroofing the orbit

When the orbital rim has been pulled out, it is possible to remove the orbital roof [3] with a chisel, following a triangle at the anterior base. If the decision is made to leave the superior orbital rim in place, which is usual procedure when the frontal sinus spreads laterally, an orbitotomy is performed by perforating the roof with a perforator, then detaching it like a postage stamp. It is advisable to put it back at the end of the operation. This prevents the forming of a late post-operative meningocele and makes reoperation easier. It can be simply placed and fastened onto the periorbit in the final stages of the treatment.

2.3 Exposing the ON in the optic canal

When removing a tumor from the optic canal, from the sheath or the ON itself, it is necessary to expose not only the intraorbital part of the ON but also its course through the optic canal and the optochiasmatic cistern, as far as to the optic chiasm. This explains why the removal of the orbital roof must be completed by drilling the roof of the optic canal and opening the optochiasmatic cistern. Opening the cistern is preceded by the opening of the dura of the frontal lobe. The frontal lobe is carefully retracted following a midway axis between a pterional approach and a subfrontal approach. The optocarotid and optochiasmatic cisterns are opened according to microsurgical procedures. The dura of the orbital roof is coagulated, and then an incision is made on the superior surface of the optic canal, running parallel to the nerve and then joining with the exposed part of the ablation of the orbital roof. The superior surface of the optic canal is drilled [6] using a diamond ball which is carefully dampened so as to join the unroofed orbit. The surgeon must remember that the ON is vascularised from its sheath in a centripetal way so that the opening of the optic canal must be carried out minutely and the ON mobilized and dissected as minimally as possible. By carefully reclining the ON sheath laterally in the optic canal, the ophthalmic artery is exposed medially as it crosses the ON inferiorly. When it is necessary to cut the optic nerve, it is advisable to do so within the optic canal or at the point where it

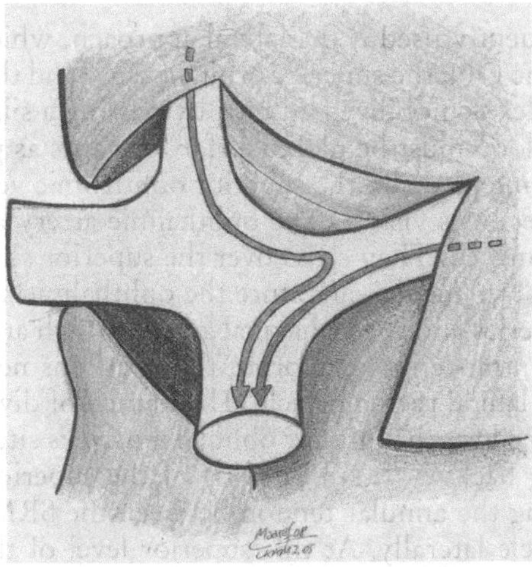

Fig. 5. Contralateral nasal fibers cross over at the optic chiasm and pursue a recurring course in the ON

exits the canal. In fact, the contralateral nasal fibers cross over at the optic chiasm and pursue a recurring course in the ON, so if cutting is desired, this contralateral nasal contingent must be spared to avoid the risk of contralateral hemianopia on the unaffected side (Fig. 5). In the event of an optic nerve glioma, there is no need to open the roof of the optic canal. Cutting the ON in the orbit, working backwards from the tumor and level with the endocranial opening of the optic canal, is quite sufficient. The residual part of the optic nerve situated in the canal is emptied on either side, using the cavitron ultrasonic surgical aspirator. Access to the superior orbital fissure completes this approach by drilling the anterior clinoid process laterally from the ON.

2.4 Intraconical exploration of the orbit

When the orbital roof is removed, the frontal nerve becomes visible in an anteroposterior axis through the orbit: this is the point at which to open the periorbit. An incision is made forwards, towards the rear from the orbital insertion of the LPM. Two further anterior and posterior incisions can be made perpendicularly to the first. There is a risk to injure the trochlear nerve on the posterior part of the incision of the periorbit, forwards from the optic canal, because from this angle the nerve is situated just inside the frontal nerve. Orbital fat, although it is considered as a predominant factor for the mobility of the oculomotor muscles, is in the way of all the intraconical approaches. However, its coagulation and retraction are essential to obtain a satisfactory view of the intraconical anatomical elements (Figs. 1 and 2). There are two ways of approaching the intraconical part of the orbit on either side from the LPM: the lateral approach and the medial approach.

The most frequently used is the lateral approach, which allows access to lateral lesions of the ON, the superior orbital fissure and the orbital apex. The LPM–SRM complex is mobilized en bloc by passing a silicone surgical loop underneath. This loop must be placed as far forwards as possible, under the muscles. By reclining medially the superior ophthalmic veins, the lateral surface of the ON becomes visible. The ophthalmic artery and the nasociliary nerve must be identified. They cross over the superior side of the ON laterally to medially. At its medial curvature the ophthalmic artery branches out into the ciliary arteries and the lachrymal artery, which are laterally reclined. Laterally to this entrance into the orbit, the abducens nerve runs along the medial side of the lateral rectus muscle. The branch of division of the oculomotor nerve destined for the inferior oblique muscle is situated at the level of the ON. Running backwards, an opening of the superior orbital fissure is feasible by dividing the annular tendon between the SRM medially and the lateral rectus muscle laterally. At this superior level of the superior orbital fissure the superior branches of division of the oculomotor nerve, the nasociliary nerve, and the abducens nerve are visible.

The medial approach runs between the oblique superior muscle medially and the LPM–SRM laterally. The ON is thus exposed across its entire length. The ophthalmic artery appears at the medial side of the ON after crossing it. An incision may be made to the common tendinous ring towards the rear, between the LPM and the SRM in such a way to expose the ON at the level of the apex. During the incision, care must be taken to protect the trochlear nerve because it is in an extraconical position.

The central approach should be avoided, except for limited and superficial surgery. As the LPSM overlaps the medial side of the SRM it is theoretically feasible to recline the LPSM medially and the SRM laterally. The frontal nerve is pulled away either medially with the LPSM or laterally with the SRM. The surgeon must remember that the trochlear nerve is in an extraconical position at this level; medial to the frontal nerve and in front of the ON sheath. This approach can be deleterious for the branch of division of the oculomotor nerve that innervates the LPSM and should therefore be undertaken with extreme care.

HOW TO AVOID COMPLICATIONS

1. AMAUROSIS

Worsening of preoperative visual deficiencies in the affected eye is a potential consequence of excessively brutal manipulation of the ON, of dissection which strips the ON sheath across its entire circumference, or of heating up of the ON during drilling of the optic canal. The nerve must therefore be handled very gently, and dissection of any tumor adjacent to the ON should not be carried out beyond its sheath. A diamond ball must be used for drilling the optic canal, and it should be abundantly dampened. Impairment of the visual field of the unaffected eye may be the result of either accidental injury of the optic chiasm or of the recurrent contralateral nasal contingent during cutting of the ON.

2. MOST COMMON POSTOPERATIVE OCULOMOTOR NERVE PALSIES

2.1 Postoperative ptosis of the upper eyelid

Postoperative ptosis of the upper eyelid is frequent when the LPM–SRM complex is mobilized. Normally any paralysis will improve within a few days or a few months, but may be permanent if the LPM has been separated from the SRM as a result of dissecting them too far posteriorly.

2.2 Postoperative diplopia

Injury to the abducens nerve may occur during dissection of the medial surface of the lateral rectus muscle. This may improve if it is followed up and given ophthalmic treatment, but sometimes it may require a further ophthalmic operation in order to restore tension of the LRM. The surgeon should therefore try to work above the superior rim of the LRM and avoid dissecting the medial surface too far forwards. Injury to the trochlear nerve can occur during incision of the periorbit as the nerve is in an extraconical position. As a result, it is particularly vulnerable during the medial intraorbital approach. The surgeon must therefore take great care when identifying these key anatomical points prior to making an incision on the periorbit. With this in mind, the frontal nerve is the most visible marker.

2.3 Other nerve injuries

Palsy of the frontal branch of the facial nerve can occur when dissection of the skin flap is performed subcutaneously instead of under the periosteum.

Anaesthesia in the supraorbital area can occur if the supraorbital nerve has not been freed from the supraorbital notch or foramen during dissection of the superior orbital rim. To resolve this, the nerve must be pulled with the skin flap.

2.4 Opening the frontal sinus: postoperative infections, cerebrospinal fluid leak

In patients less than ten years old, the frontal sinus is little developed, if at all; and in adults, it can pneumatize the entire superior orbital rim. Opening the frontal sinus is a major concern and can lead to severe postoperative infections: meningitis, epidural abscess, and osteitis of the bone flap. The best way to anticipate this complication is to know the particular anatomy of the patient's frontal sinuses. A preoperative CT scan will provide details on this anatomy better than those by MRI. An anti-pneumococcus vaccination should be performed prior to the surgical procedure. When a postoperative infection occurs, the surgeon should always keep this hypothesis in mind even when there is no evidence of frontal sinus entering during the craniotomy. A reoperation is required for these infected patients, in order to plug the frontal sinus. Antibiotics are required in case of meningitis or general infection prior to reoperation. If the patient has a local infection, surgery must be performed prior to administering antibiotics, in order to take a sample of pus or infected tissue for bacteriological culture.

CONCLUSIONS

The orbit is a narrow anatomical space which contains many highly functional anatomical elements. Tumors of the orbit are extremely varied in nature and require a multidisciplinary approach to treatment. Furthermore, etiologies in children are different from those in adults. Not all of them require surgery. This is why the patient's medical history, clinical tests, and preoperative imaging must be comprehensive. Neurosurgeons are primarily concerned with tumors affecting the two posterior thirds of the orbit, the ON, and those of the ON sheath. Tumors of the bony structures may require reconstruction, in which case it is often necessary to collaborate with a plastic surgeon during the procedure.

Acknowledgement

I thank Dr. Maaref of the Henri Poincare University in Nancy (France) for the realisation of the illustrations displayed in this chapter.

References

[1] Al Mefty O, Fox JL (1985) Superolateral orbital exposure and reconstruction. Surg Neurol 23: 609-613

[2] Benedict WL (1950) Diseases of the orbit. Am J Ophthalmol 33: 1-10

[3] Blinkov SM, Gabibov GA, Tcherekayev VA (1986) Transcranial surgical approaches to the orbital part of the optic nerve: an anatomical study. J Neurosurg 65: 44-47

[4] Cushing H, Eisenhardt TL (1938) Meningiomas: their classification, regional behaviour, life history and surgical end results. Charles C Thomas, Springfield, Ill, pp 250-282

[5] Marchal JC, Civit T (2006) Neurosurgical concepts and approaches for orbital tumors. Adv Tech Stand Neurosurg 31: 73-117

[6] Newman SA, Jane JA (1991) Meningiomas of the optic nerve, orbit, and anterior visual pathways. In: Al Mefty O (ed) Meningiomas. Raven, New York, pp 461-494

[7] Rhoton AL, Natori Y (1996) The orbit and sellar region: microsurgical anatomy and operative approaches. Thieme, Stuttgart, pp 208-236

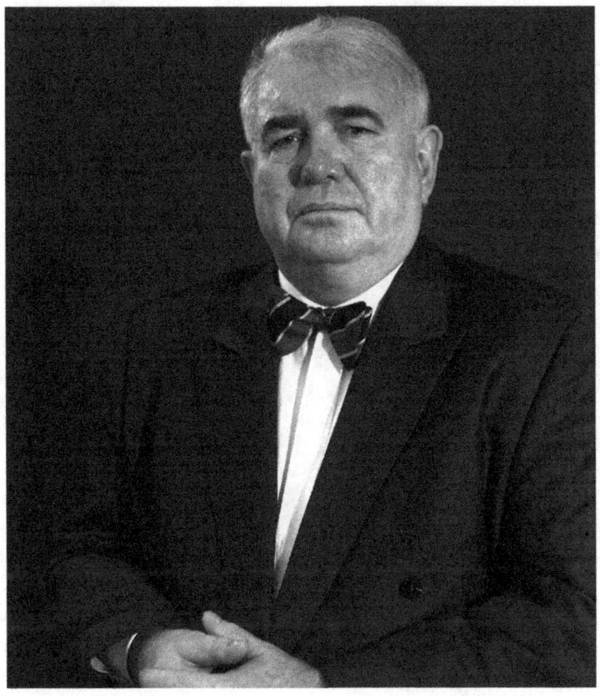

Jean Claude Marchal

Jean Claude Marchal is professor and head of the Unit of Pediatric Surgery at the Institute of Neurological Sciences in Nancy, France. He was born on 30 September 1950 in Nancy and there he began studying medicine in 1968. He wrote his PhD thesis on the subject of traumatic injuries of the craniofacial boundaries. He continued his career in Nancy, working in both the Adult Neurosurgical Department and as clinic manager at the Henri Poincare University. Having obtained his certificate in general surgery in 1982, he was appointed as professor of neurosurgery in 1986. From 1990 onwards he began to specialize in paediatrics as manager of the Pediatric Neurosurgical Unit in Nancy. From 1999 to 2000 he was visiting professor at Sainte-Justine Hospital at the University of Montreal. Jean Claude Marchal is also a passionate piano player with a keen interest in chamber music and abstains from partaking in any sporting activities whatsoever.

Contact: Jean Claude Marchal, Chirurgie Pédiatrique (Pôle Neuro. Tête et Cou),
Bâtiment des Neurosciences, Hôpital Central, 54035 Nancy Cedex, France
E-mail: jc.marchal@chu-nancy.fr

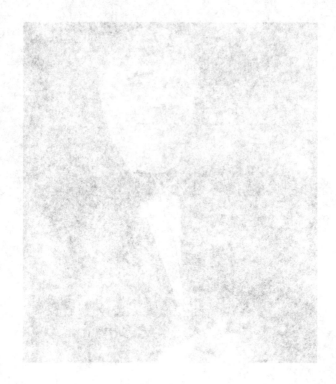

HOW TO PERFORM TRANSSPHENOIDAL APPROACHES

A. J. BASSO

INTRODUCTION

1. *The introduction of the surgical microscope* for the excision of pituitary adenomas by Jules Hardy in 1966 marked a new era in the treatment of hyperfunction clinical syndromes (namely, acromegaly, amenorrhea-galactorrhea or sexual impotence in men).

Considering that in most cases these syndromes are produced by a pituitary adenoma (sometimes a very small 0- or 1-grade intraglandular *microadenoma*), the contribution of neurosurgeons was essential for the understanding of their pathophysiology, which had historically been difficult to characterize.

During the 1970s, radioimmunoassay and immunohistochemistry were critical to accurately establish the type of pathological secretion of the anterior pituitary gland. CT scan and MRI in the 1980s led to in-depth anatomical knowledge of the lesion, its extension, and its relationships.

Determining adenoma aggressiveness, invasive ability and recurrence potential is a function of molecular biology, a specialty which over the last 10 years has provided pertinent, albeit insufficient information, through tumor marker examination. Nevertheless, thirty-five years of continuous progress translate into an almost complete control of the disease.

International experience over the last 30 years has proved that the transsphenoidal approach is the procedure of choice for the treatment of most pituitary adenomas. This surgical choice has become widespread basically because it constitutes a low-risk highly efficient procedure. Favorably enough, complications are relatively uncommon, averaging approximately 4% in institutions largely conducting pituitary procedures [32].

2. Late in the eighteenth century and early in the nineteenth century, *transcranial approaches for the treatment of pituitary tumors* were associated with a high mortality rate. Horsley's reported 20% mortality rate in a series of 10 patients was significantly better than the 50–80% mortality rate range reported by his colleagues. As a result of these high rates, surgeons believed that a transfacial approach to the sella turcica would be safer [28]. Thus, based on Giordano's experience with cadavers [28], Hermann Schloffer (Fig. 1) performed in Austria the first transsphenoidal pituitary tumor resection in 1907;

Keywords: pituitary adenoma, transsphenoidal approach, sella turcica, endoscopic surgery

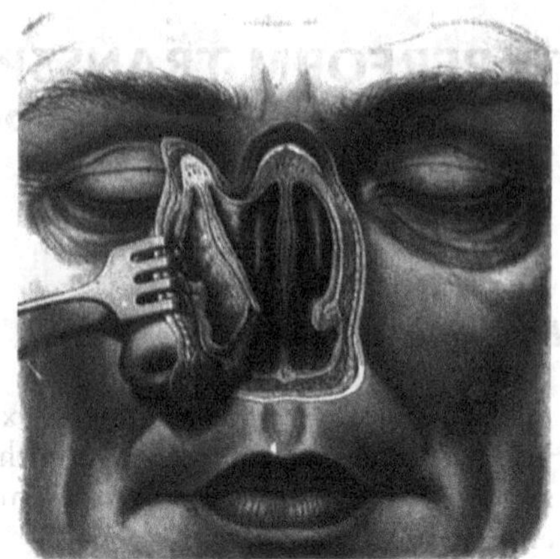

Fig. 1. Schloffer's first transsphenoidal approach

his technique involved first moving the nose en bloc to the right, then removing the nasal turbinates and septum, accessing and opening the anterior wall of the sphenoid bone and, lastly, once within the sphenoidal sinus, opening the floor of the sella turcica [33]. This technique was applied by other general surgeons, with many patients dying intraoperatively or postoperatively owing to meningitis [34]. For this reason, new techniques were subsequently developed. In 1909, Theodor Kocher, in Switzerland, proposed a submucous dissection and resection of the septum, sparing the nasal cavity; for this procedure, a complex nasal incision was required [25]. Submucous septal dissection and resection marked the beginning of lower extracranial approaches to the pituitary gland, since it afforded a reduced risk of infection and an easier midline orientation [27]. In 1910, Oskar Hirsch, an otorhinolaryngologist from Austria, described the endonasal transseptal-transsphenoidal approach [22]. Also in 1910, Albert Halstead, in Chicago, described the sublabial-gingival approach [14]. Harvey Cushing initially used the transcranial approach (8 subtemporal and 5 subfrontal approaches); however, since he achieved poor results, he adopted the transsphenoidal route [28], thereby becoming the first surgeon to perform a sublabial-gingival transsphenoidal approach to the pituitary gland [34]. He used the transsphenoidal approach between 1910 and 1925, operating on 231 patients with pituitary tumors, with a mortality rate of 5.6% (Fig. 2A, B) [20]. From 1929 onwards, however, Cushing abandoned the transsphenoidal route and came to favor the transcranial route. Norman Dott, a disciple of Cushing's, continued to perform the transsphenoidal approach in Scotland [27] and eventually introduced a speculum with a built-in light [32]. Gerard Guiot, from France, visited Dott in 1956 and learned the transsphenoidal technique from him [27]. That year, Dott performed 80 consecutive operations with the transsphenoidal approach, with no deaths [34]. In subsequent years, Guiot started to refine the transsphenoi-

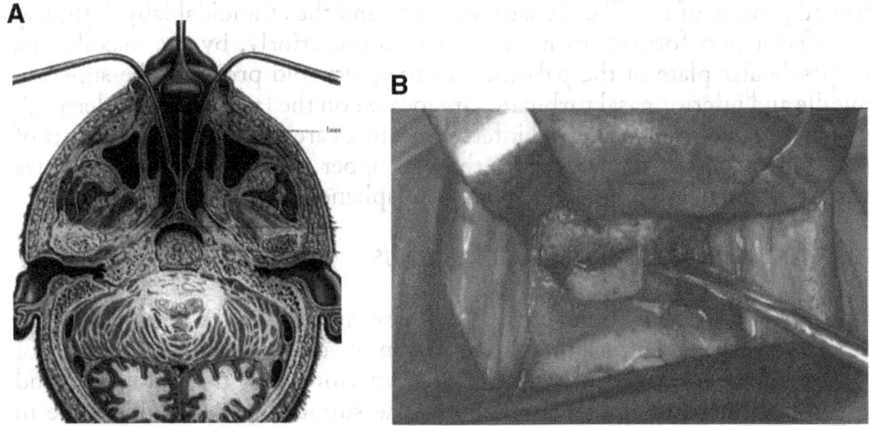

Fig. 2A, B. Cushing's sublabial rhinoseptal transsphenoidal approach

dal approach by introducing intraoperative radiofluoroscopy [16]. Driven by his pioneering spirit, Guiot applied the transsphenoidal approach to the treatment of craniopharyngiomas, clivus chordomas and parasellar lesions [28]. Jules Hardy, from Canada, learned this procedure from Guiot. In 1967, Hardy adopted the surgical microscope for this procedure [18], and in 1968, he introduced the concept of microadenoma (a patient with endocrine disorders with no enlargement of the sella turcica) [19].

The many years' of experience we gained next to Guiot and Hardy provided us with extensive practice in terms of these modern techniques. In 1969, we performed the first microsurgical transsphenoidal approach in South America [2].

Technological advances in endoscopy, neuronavigation and intraoperative MRI have been applied to transsphenoidal surgery in an effort to further lower the morbidity and mortality rates associated with the classic procedure [28].

RATIONALE

Rationale is based on surgical anatomy.

1. NASAL CAVITY

The nasal cavity, which comprises the first upper respiratory tract, is limited by the anterior cranial fossa superiorly, by the orbits and the maxillary sinuses laterally, and by the palate inferiorly. The nasal cavity is divided into two halves, left and right, by the nasal septum, which has a sagittal and middle location, and an anterior cartilaginous part and a posterior osseous part (perpendicular plate of ethmoid bone superiorly and vomer inferiorly). The lateral wall exhibits a superior part formed, from anteriorly to posteriorly, by the frontal process of maxilla, the lacrimal bone and the ethmoidal labyrinth, and an inferior part formed, from anteriorly to posteriorly, by the maxilla, the perpendicular plate of the palatine and the pterygoid process. The superior, middle and inferior nasal turbinates are located on the lateral wall, underneath which the superior, middle and inferior meatuses are found. The lower part of the cavity is comparatively wider than its upper part, and it communicates with the frontal, ethmoidal, maxillary, and sphenoidal sinuses.

2. SPHENOID BONE AND SPHENOIDAL SINUS

The sphenoid bone is found at the skull base, anterior to the temporal bones and the basilar part of occipital bone. Given the close contact of the body of the sphenoid bone with the nasal cavity inferiorly and the pituitary gland superiorly, the transsphenoidal route is the surgical approach of choice in most sellar tumors (Fig. 3) [30]. The body of the sphenoid bone is more or less cube-shaped and contains two large air sinuses that are separated by one or several septa; as a whole, this cavity is commonly called sphenoidal sinus. Form, size, degree of pneumatization, and number and location of septa in the sphenoidal sinus are highly variable. At birth, the sphenoidal sinus is a small cavity, which becomes pneumatized after puberty. With advancing age, the sphenoidal sinus enlarges as a result of bone wall resorption [30]. Therefore, depending on the level of pneumatization the sphenoidal sinus presents

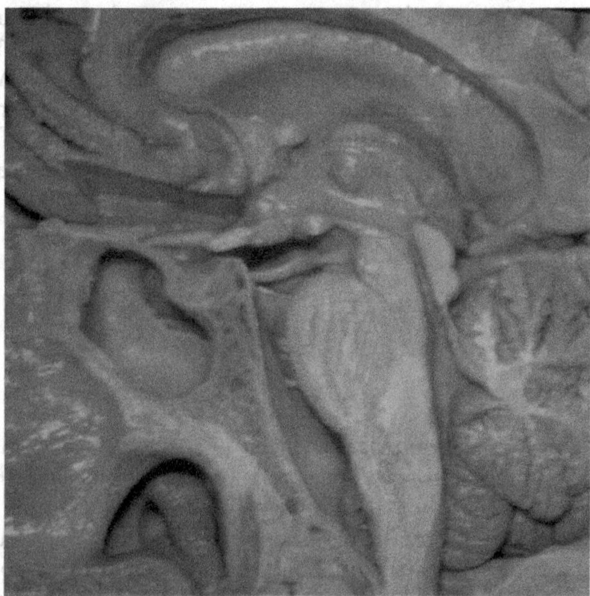

Fig. 3. Sellar-type sphenoidal sinus and sella turcica

one of three different patterns: conchal (absent sinus pneumatization), presellar (pneumatization is restricted to a vertical line parallel to the anterior border of the sella turcica) and sellar (pneumatization reaches the clivus). The sellar sphenoidal sinus is the most common pattern. The internal carotid artery abuts the lateral surface of the body of the sphenoid bone, and its course creates a channel on the bone, known as the carotid groove. The carotid groove produces lateral protrusions within the sinus at either side and below the sella turcica.

3. CAVERNOUS SINUS

The cavernous sinus is a paired structure placed on either side of the pituitary gland (Fig. 4). Each cavernous sinus has four walls formed by dura matter. The lateral, superior and posterior walls consist of two layers, the external layer, the so-called dura propria, and the internal layer, also known as periostal dura. Through the internal layer of the lateral wall course the oculomotor and trochlear nerves, and the ophthalmic division of the trigeminal nerve. The cavernous sinus medial wall comprises two segments. One is superior to the pituitary gland and the other is inferior to the lateral wall of the body of the sphenoid bone; different from the other walls, the medial wall has a unique, very thin dural layer, which could account for the lateral expansion of a pituitary adenoma. These four dural walls lodge venous blood contained in plexi, the internal carotid artery and its intracavernous branches, the abducent nerve, the sympathetic plexus, and fatty tissue. Both superior walls continue

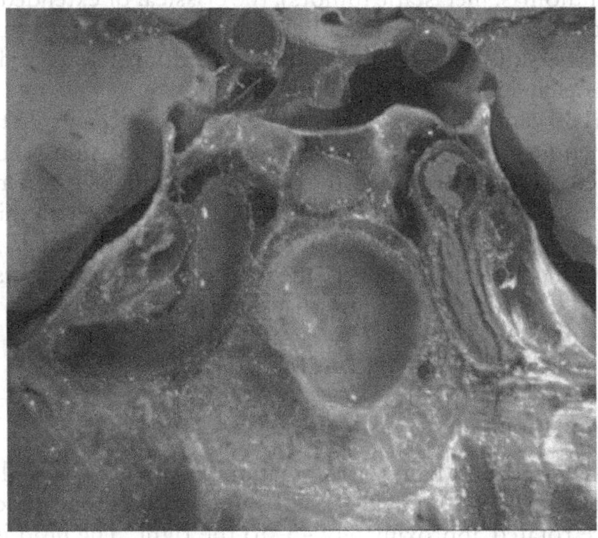

Fig. 4. Cavernous sinus

medially to form the diaphragm sellae. The diaphragm sellae is the roof of the sella turcica and wholly covers the pituitary gland but for a central opening through which the pituitary stalk courses. Occasionally, it may be a very thin structure, and thus proves not enough of a protective barrier for suprasellar structures during transsphenoidal surgery [30].

4. PITUITARY GLAND

The pituitary grand is a grayish-red body with transverse and anterior posterior diameters of 12 mm and 8 mm, respectively. The pituitary gland is formed by two different embryological and functional regions, i.e. anterior (adenohypophysis) and posterior (neurohypophysis) pituitary glands. The anterior pituitary gland comprises the anterior (glandular part or anterior lobe) and the intermediate part, and the posterior pituitary includes the posterior part (neural part or posterior lobe), the stalk and the median eminence [31]. The lower surface of the gland usually takes the shape of the sellar floor, whereas the lateral and superior margins have variable shapes since those walls are composed of soft tissue but no bone [30].

SURGICAL APPROACHES

1. TRANSSEPTAL-TRANSSPHENOIDAL APPROACH

Mainly indicated for sellar tumors (including adenomas, craneopharyngiomas, granulomas, metastatic tumors), the classical or extended transseptal-transsphenoidal approach is currently used for other types of tumors arising centrally at the skull base, such as clivus chordomas or chondrosarcomas, tuberculum sellae meningiomas, among others.

For nearly twenty years, i.e. since 1969, we have been using the transseptal-transsphenoidal approach through a sublabial incision from incisor to incisor, exactly as first described by Harvey Cushing. Postoperative rhinological, respiratory or cosmetic complications associated with this technique, which are minor indeed, prompted our abandonment at the end of the 1980s and replacement with the (modified) technique described by Oskar Hirsch, which we call lateral transseptal approach and describe below.

2. LATERAL TRANSSEPTAL APPROACH

2.1 Patient positioning

The patient is placed in a half-seated position (Fig. 5A, B), with the head resting on a horseshoe head-holder. The left shoulder lifted on a pillow, the head and neck are rotated approximately 45° to the right. The head is positioned with the nose in the "sniffing position", so that the zygomatic arch stays

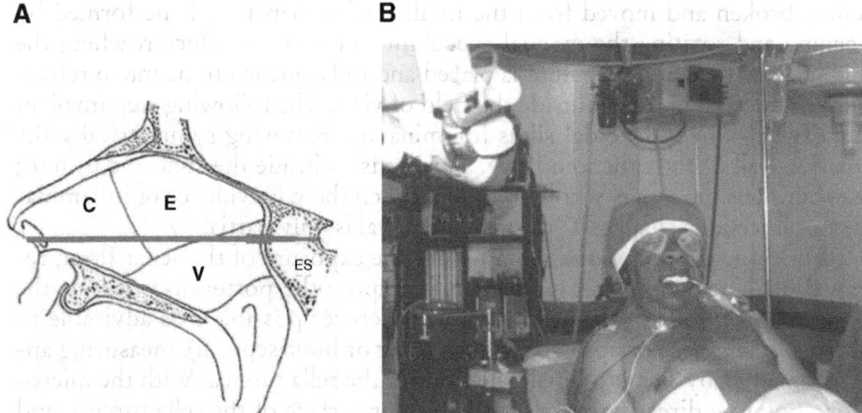

Fig. 5A, B. Patient placed in a half-seated position

flexed approximately 20° relative to the floor. Importantly, the head should be well fixed to the head-holder with adhesive tape in order to prevent any intraoperative movements. One major advantage of thte half-seated position is that it frees the surgical field from blood, since any kind of potential bleeding falls on account of gravity and does not interfere with the surgeon's view. The patient is given general anesthesia with endotracheal intubation, and to prevent blood ingestion, a pharyngeal packing is used.

2.2 Preparation

After occluding the eyes with adhesive tape, the nose, the nasal area and the gingival mucosa are prepped with antiseptic solution (Pervinox solution). When the tumor has a suprasellar extension, the lower right quadrant of the abdomen is also prepped to harvest a fat graft to pack the sella turcica after tumor excision in order to prevent the potential development of a cerebrospinal fluid (CSF) fistula.

Surgical drapes are then placed and the surgical microscope is positioned.

2.3 Surgical technique

As the surgical assistant (standing to the left of the surgeon) separates the lateral border of the right naris, the surgeon infiltrates the septal mucosa with 1% xylocain containing epinephrine and then performs a 1.5 cm long vertical incision through the septal mucosa. The septal mucosa is then separated from the nasal septum with the help of a dissector. This is an easily performed maneuver since the mucosa has been partially detached from the nasal septum with the aid of a previous xylocain infiltration. The dissection is continued deeply until reaching the proximity of the attachment of the perpendicular plate of the ethmoid bone and the vomer with the sphenoid body; at that point, the bone septum is broken and moved from the midline (this maneuver is performed by opening and rotating the manual speculum to the right). Once reaching the midline, an autostatic speculum is placed and fully opened to maintain retraction of the nasal mucosa outside the field of view. The following step involves identifying both sphenoidal sinus foramina and removing symmetrically the anterior wall of the sphenoid bone. This leads us inside the sphenoidal sinus; the thin sinus mucosa is wholly removed when there is evidence of inflammatory or infectious changes. Otherwise, removal is only partial.

When one or more bone septa hinder the exposure of the sellar floor, removal of these septa is required to fully expose the posterior aspect of the sinus and the floor of the sella turcica. Wherever possible it is advisable to obtain a small piece of bone (from the vomer or bone septum), measuring approximately 1 by 1 cm, to repair the floor of the sella turcica. With the microscope pointing directly to the anterior lower surface of the sella turcica, and with the help of a small chisel, the sellar floor is opened from midline to lateral, creating a 1.5 cm wide, 1 cm long window. When the lesion is a macroadenoma with sella turcica enlargement, the sellar floor will be extremely thinned or partially absent. Sellar dura mater may also be thinned owing to tumor growth. The next step involves a cruciate incision of the sellar dura up to the margins of the bone opening; this is done with a bayonet-shaped knife holder. In most cases, after opening the dura and as a consequence of intrasellar pressure, grayish tumor tissue is expressed and should be removed with punch forceps for pathology examination. The remaining adenoma is dissected with differently angled curettes, directed in all orientations, plus a surgical aspirator. As soon as the sellar cavity has been emptied, the suprasellar extension of the tumor will move downward spontaneously towards the sella turcica and as a result of normal intracranial pressure. If this does not happen, intracranial pressure may be increased by applying compression to both internal jugular veins. At the end of the tumor excision procedure, the surgeon should perform a thorough exploration of the whole cavity to check for complete removal of the lesion and preservation of the normal gland. It is at this point that endoscopic assistance becomes highly useful, using a 30°- or 60°-angulated view endoscope.

After correct hemostasis is achieved, the piece of bone previously taken from the vomer is used to cover the sellar bone defect and fixed with methylmethacrylate. Finally, the nasal septum is moved back to its normal position and both nares are packed.

3. ENDOSCOPICALLY ASSISTED MICROSURGICAL TRANSNASAL APPROACH

Endoscopic surgery, a minimally invasive and maximally effective procedure so defined after a modern conception of surgery, has also become widespread practice in neurosurgery in general and in pituitary surgery, in particular.

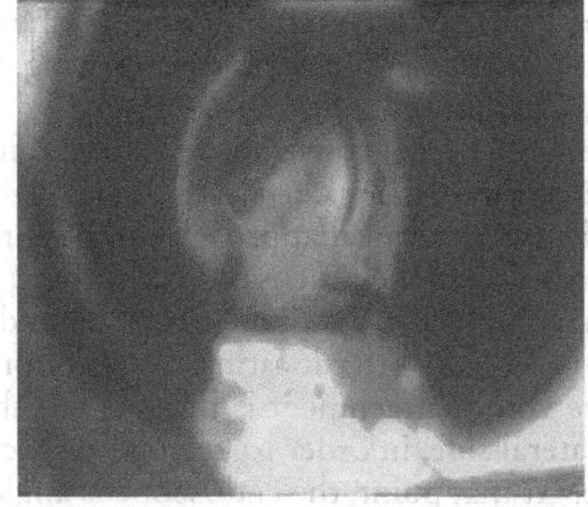

Fig. 6. Transnasal microsurgical approach

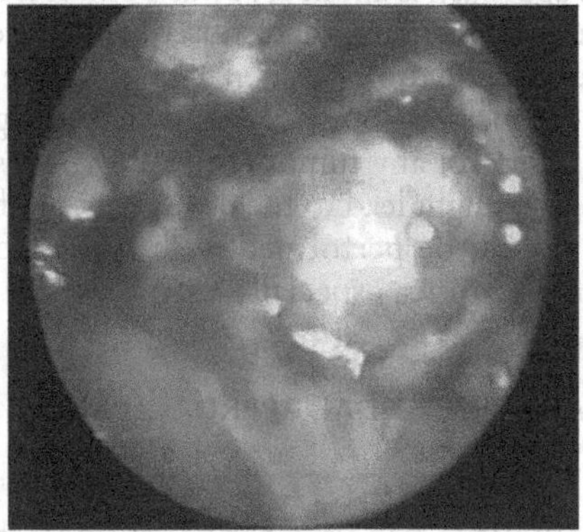

Fig. 7. Inspection of the sphenoidal sinus

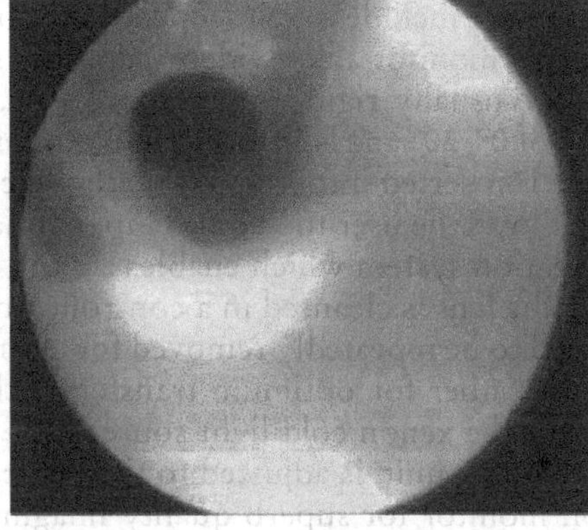

Fig. 8. Control of the intrasellar residual cavity

In fact, during the 1990s, several authors started to show interest in the possibility of exploiting the benefits of endoscopic viewing, i.e. lateral views and excellent lighting [3, 23], for transsphenoidal surgery.

The aid of an endoscope can prove very useful if added to classic transsphenoidal microneurosurgery (Figs. 6–8).

In these cases, the microsurgical approach can be directly transnasal, i.e. right-handed surgeons access the mucosa directly through the right naris to perform an incision anteriorly to and along the sphenoid ostium, at the level of the middle nasal turbinate. After locating the anterior aspect of the sphenoid bone body, the vomer attachment is broken and the septum displaced towards the contralateral side, in order to get a better view of the area with a surgical microscope. At that point, the endoscope is angled at 30° or 60° into the cavity for inspection of the sphenoidal sinus and recognition of bone indentations corresponding to the carotid arteries or optical nerves.

When this mixed approach is applied, at this point it is advisable to switch to the ordinary microsurgical technique and subsequently open the sellar floor and the dura and, then, excise the tumor. When adenomas are large in size it is important that the endoscope be relocated at the end of the procedure in order to observe the residual cavity for any tumor remnant, which should be completely excised, or openings that might lead to the development of a CSF fistula.

Finally, closure should be performed with an appropriate technique, in order to prevent complications, especially CSF fistula.

4. ENDOSCOPIC TRANSSPHENOIDAL APPROACH – SURGICAL TECHNIQUE

The endoscopic technique is also used for the surgical treatment of sellar lesions, as it precludes the use of intranasal specula while offering a 360° panoramic view of the area, thereby assisting in the recognition of all anatomic structures at nasal, intrasphenoidal, sellar and suprasellar levels [33].

Endoscopic equipment includes a telescope, optical fiber, a light source, a digital videocamera, a monitor and a video-recording system. Telescopes used in these cases are usually rigid, 4 mm in diameter, 180 mm long and offer angles of vision of 0°, 30° and 45° to suit the different surgical requirements. The telescope is inserted into a rigid sheath which provides protection to the unit and allows the user to handle it appropriately. The sheath is connected to an irrigation system which enables a clean vision through the whole procedure, as the lens is cleansed in a controlled manner and the endoscope does not need to be repeatedly removed for cleaning. The telescope is connected to optical fiber for optimum transfer of the quality lighting generated by means of the xenon cold light source. The digital video camera, preferably a three-chip unit, is adjusted to the telescope and connected to a high-resolution monitor for superb quality imaging. A digital video-recording system is used for surgery documentation.

The endoscopic and microsurgical approaches use surgical instruments of similar features, the only exception being that the endoscopic approach uses straight instruments rather than the bayonet-shaped instruments preferred in microsurgery [9].

During the sellar phase of the procedure, the endoscope can be immobilized by means of a mechanic fitting which is attached to the bed. This helps to get a stable picture of the surgical field and allows the surgeon to use both hands concurrently.

The monitor, the light source, the digital video camera and the video-recording system are placed behind the patient's head, all together as a full block, on a straight vision line towards the neurosurgeon, who stands to the right of the patient. The surgeon's assistant stands to the left of the patient, whereas the surgical nurse stays at the level of the patient's feet. Finally, the anaesthetist remains to the left of the patient's head (Fig. 9).

Under general anaesthetic, the patient's trunk is positioned at 15°, the head fixed to the head-holder and 10° lateralized to the right towards the neurosurgeon. Whether the head is flexed or extended will depend on the suprasellar extension of the lesion, though excessive flexion should be avoided in order to prevent the thorax from hindering suitable handling of the endoscope.

Five percent chlorhexidine is used for face and nasal cavity asepsis. Surgical drapes are then positioned leaving only the nose exposed. Epinephrine

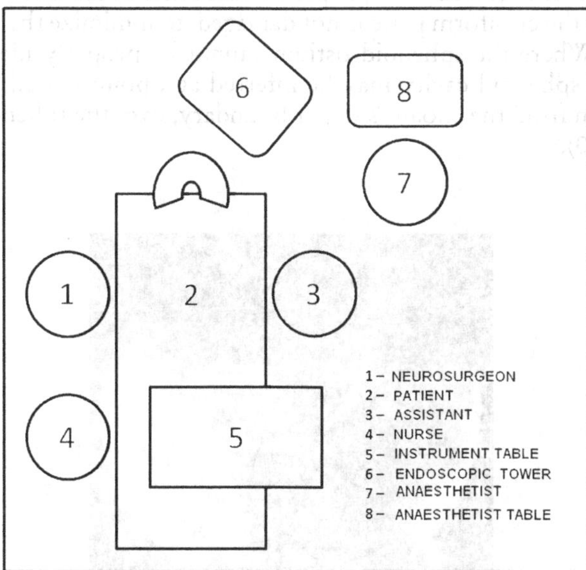

Fig. 9. Endoscopical team placement

solution (1:100000) is used for intranasal topicalization to assist in mucous decongestion for ease of procedure.

In this case, as in the microsurgical approach, three surgical phases are recognized: the nasal phase, the sphenoidal phase and the sellar phase [1, 6, 8, 13, 14, 24].

4.1 Nasal phase

This phase starts by angling the endoscope at 0° through the right naris. The anatomic structures in the nasal cavity are recognized, firstly by identifying the lower nasal turbinate laterally and the nasal septum medially. The middle nasal turbinate is the closest to the nasal septum. As the endoscope penetrates deeply along the floor of the nasal cavity, we reach the choana, which is bounded superiorly by the sphenoidal sinus, inferiorly by the soft palate, laterally by the lower nasal turbinate and medially by the vomer in the septum. At a rhinopharyngeal level, the Eustachian tube can be recognized. The endoscope must be then moved on superiorly between the middle nasal turbinate and the nasal septum towards the sphenoethmoidal recess. This can be quite difficult owing to the close proximity between the middle nasal turbinate and the septum, as already explained. Once at the level of the sphenoethmoidal recess, the sphenoid ostium can be identified, as it is the entry towards the sphenoidal sinus. When pneumatization of the sphenoidal sinus is significant, the ostium can be found more laterally behind the upper nasal turbinate and be thus difficult to identify. In these cases, partial removal of the upper nasal turbinate may be required for a proper visualization of the ostium, carefully ensuring that the cribiform plate is not damaged, to minimize the risk of CSF fistula [10]. Where the sphenoid ostium cannot be properly identified, the access to the sphenoid cavity may be inferred at a point placed at approximately 15 mm from the choana's upper boundary, over the sphenoethmoidal recess (Fig. 10).

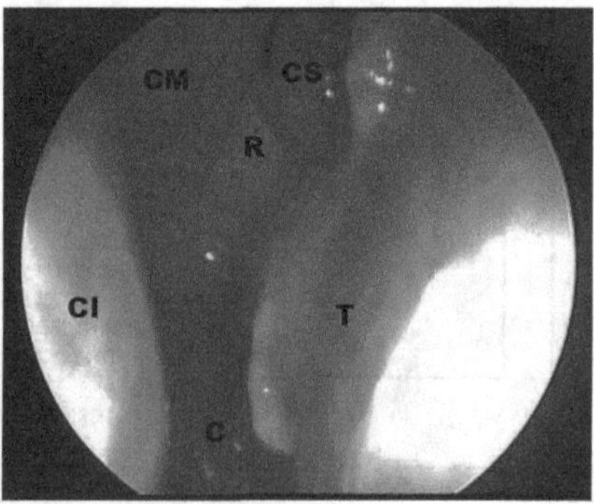

Fig. 10. Endoscopical view of the right nasal cavity

4.2 Sphenoidal phase

This phase is initiated by coagulating the mucosa in the sphenoethmoidal recess around the sphenoid ostium. This prevents insidious bleeding of the septal branches of the sphenopalatine artery. After coagulation, a longitudinal incision is made along the mucosa and up to the bone plane. The nasal bone septum, which is composed of the vomer inferiorly and the perpendicular plate of the ethmoid bone superiorly, is drilled apart from the anterior aspect of the sphenoid bone with a 4 mm drill, thereby exposing the complete rostrum of the sphenoid bone – and its typical keel-like shape – submucousally and bilaterally. Removal of the sphenoid rostrum is done by drilling or with rongeurs. The procedure starts at the level of the sphenoid ostia, which are taken as the upper boundary of the bone opening. Rostrum osteotomy must be widely performed inferiorly to allow enough room for the instruments required later for the sellar phase to slide through. The mucosa of the sphenoidal sinus can be partially excised to avoid impairing endoscopic view. As the endoscope descends deeply into the sphenoidal sinus, it should be possible to recognize the bone septa, and there should exist a correlation between endoscopic anatomy and imaging studies (MRI and CT scan). By removing the septa in the sphenoidal sinus, the endoscopically anatomical bone recesses of the posterior and lateral walls of the sinus will be largely exposed, especially in the case of sphenoidal sinuses with good pneumatization. The sellar floor can be recognized centrally, with the planum sphenoidale above and the clivus underneath. The carotid protuberance, the optic nerve protuberance and the optic-carotid recess in between the two protuberances can be recognized on each side of the sellar floor. All together, bone endoscopic anatomy resembles embryological anatomy of the fetal face, where the forehead corresponds with the planum sphenoidale, the eyes with the optic-carotid recesses, the eyebrows with the optic prominences, the cheeks with the carotid prominences, the sellar floor with the nose and the clivus with the mouth. When pneumatization of the sinus

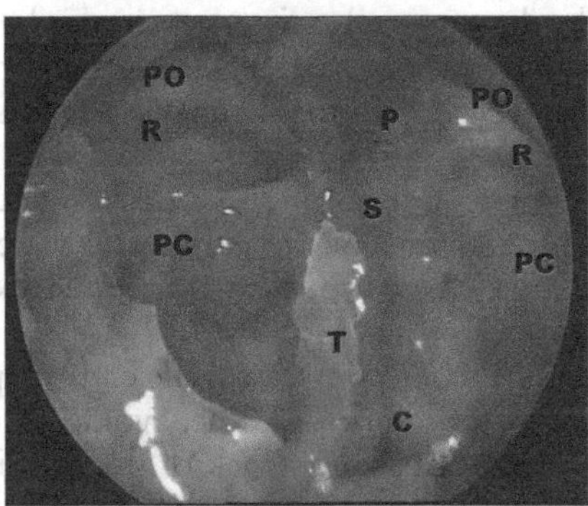

Fig. 11. Endoscopical view of the sphenoidal sinus

is not well developed, all these anatomic recesses may be absent. If this is the case, identification of the planum sphenoidale, the clivus and the carotid prominences should be enough to accurately establish the position of the sellar floor (Fig. 11).

4.3 Sellar phase

Once the sellar floor has been correctly identified, the endoscope is immobilized by means of a mechanic fitting. The sellar floor is drilled open or cut open with the aid of rongeurs, the extent of the opening depending on the type of lesion requiring treatment. After dural coagulation, whose purpose is to prevent potential bleeding of the (coronal) intercavernous venous sinuses, the dura is cut open in a linear or cruciate pattern to expose the sellar lesion.

After complete resection of pituitary microadenomas, there is no need to explore the sellar cavity with an endoscope, so hemostasis and reconstruction of the sellar floor can be initiated straightforwardly.

Resection of pituitary macroadenoma starts at the lower portion and proceeds on to the lateral extension of the adenoma to conclude on its upper portion. If resection would be initiated at the upper portion of the macroadenoma, the diaphragm selae might descend prematurely and visually obstruct resection of the rest of the adenoma. A Valsalva maneuver (usually by bilateral jugular compression) can be useful to allow the diaphragm sellae to go down, where spontaneous descent does not occur. This assists in the resection of any adenoma remnant that might have been left adjacent to the diaphragm.

Telescopes with 30° and 45° angulations prove very useful to explore the sellar cavity, especially because they enable recognition of the lateral and suprasellar extension of macroadenomas and their resection, when the diaphragm sellae has not descended adequately. They also assist in recognizing the pituitary gland more clearly, as this is usually thinned on the superior and/or posterior sectors of the sellar cavity. Where the diaphragm sellae is large or practically inexistent, the suprasellar cistern can be recognized as a thin arachnoid membrane with CSF content and must be taken as the resection limit. To avoid the risk of CSF fistula, the suprasellar cistern must not be damaged.

Hemostasis of the sellar cavity is performed in a manner like the microsurgical technique is carried out, applying hemostatic agents, coagulation or cotton compression for some minutes.

Reconstruction of the sellar floor in this situation does not differ from the microsurgical technique and must be carried out in a watertight manner where occurrence of CSF fistula is confirmed, in which case external postoperative lumbar drainage is also performed [7].

Once the procedure has been completed, the endoscope is slowly removed and the nasal septum replaced in the midline, avoiding contact with the middle nasal turbinate and the consequent risk of postsurgical synechiae. Nasal tamponade is not regularly applied, except when insidious bleeding of the nasal mucosa is confirmed.

HOW TO AVOID COMPLICATIONS

In general terms, the transsphenoidal approach is a safe procedure offering a low rate of complications when conducted by a well-trained team.

Interdisciplinary work is an important concept to be observed during perioperative care: the neurosurgeon, the anesthetist, the endocrinologist and the intensive care specialist must work closely to identify and prevent complications.

These can be classified as follows:

a) Surgery-related complications
b) Sodium and fluid balance disorders
c) Hormone hypersecretion or hyposecretion disorders

Surgery-related complications
Complications occur in <1% of the cases and are associated with anatomical manipulation during surgery [24, 25]. They can be immediate or mediate complications:

Immediate complications

a) Worsening of visual symptoms: Secondary to compression of the optical nerves during surgery or owing to the postoperative development of hematoma.
b) Injury of the intracavernous carotid artery.
c) Intracranial hematoma: Subdural, extradural or intraparenchymal.
d) Brain ischemia: Secondary to vascular injury.
e) CSF fistula.

Mediate complications

a) CSF fistula
b) Postoperative meningitis

We will focus exclusively on the diagnosis and management of CSF fistula because we have practically never encountered the above mentioned complications throughout our experience.

In patients who were treated with a transsphenoidal approach, CSF fistula diagnosis is established mainly when tamponades are removed. It is commonly confirmed by evaluating nasal secretion with blood glucose-measuring test strips. Once a fistula has been clinically diagnosed, prophylactic antibiotics should be avoided to prevent meningitis: this generates a selection of nosocomial bacteria which require broader-spectrum and longer-lasting therapies with antibiotics. These fistulae tend to close spontaneously in the course of 48–72 hours. If closure does not occur, however, a continuous lumbar drainage for 48–72 hours can be attempted. Radioisotope cisternography, metrizamide-enhanced CT scanning, intravenous gadolinium-enhanced MRI or even intrathecal gadolinium-enhanced MRI can be performed to confirm fistula closure. Surgical repair will be considered on the basis of the results obtained with these imaging methods.

CONCLUSIONS

Historically, the transsphenoidal approach to intracranial structures was applied to corpses in ancient Egypt for ceremonial reasons, as it was considered to be the best solution to extract encephalic remnants without aesthetically altering the skull or the face of the deceased who would be mummified.

Early in the twentieth century, truly pioneering otorhinolaryngologists and neurosurgeons ventured to approach sellar disease through the body of the sphenoid bone.

Advances in imaging (CT scan and MRI) coupled with the evident improvement achieved with the introduction of the surgical microscope, T.V. fluoroscopic control, neuronavigators and, lately, the endoscope and intraoperative MRI have granted the adequately trained surgeon such safety that morbidity and mortality rates in this respect stand practically at zero.

Our own series of transsphenoidal approaches over the last 35 years has comprised more than three thousand cases covering the intrasellar benign tumors (96% of pituitary adenomas, the remaining 4% being hypophysectomies, Rathke's pouch cysts, craniopharyngiomas, pituitary granulomas, clivus chondrosarcomas and chordomas, metastatic tumors, small meningiomas of the tuberculum sellae, etc.).

We have used alternative pterional or subfrontal approaches only in the event of tumors with lateral intracranial extension.

Acknowledgments

The author acknowledges his collaborators Santiago Gonzalez Abbati, MD, and Alvaro Campero, MD, for their support in the preparation of this chapter.

References

[1] Apuzzo MLJ, Heifetz M, Weiss MH, Kurze T (1977) Neurosurgical endoscopy using the side-viewing telescope: technical note. J Neurosurg 16: 398-400

[2] Basso A, Amezúa L, Guitelman A, Ghersi J, Molocznic I (1973) Síndrome acromegalique: choix de la technique chirurgicale. Neurochirurgie 19: 537-544

[3] Cappabianca P, Alfieri A, Colao A, et al. (2000) Endoscopic endonasal transsphenoidal surgery in recurrent and residual pituitary adenomas: technical note. Minim Invasive Neurosurg 43: 38-43

[4] Cappabianca P, Cavallo LM, de Divitiis E (2004) Endoscopic endonasal transsphenoidal surgery. Neurosurgery 55: 933-934

[5] Cappabianca P, Alfieri A, Thermes S, Buonamassa S, de Divitiis E (1999) Instruments for endoscopic endonasal transsphenoidal surgery. Neurosurgery 45: 392

[6] Cappabianca P, de Divitiis E (2004) Endoscopy and transsphenoidal surgery. Neurosurgery 54: 1043-1050

[7] Cappabianca P, Cavallo LM, Esposito F, Valente V, de Divitiis E (2002) Sellar repair in endoscopic endonasal transsphenoidal surgery: results of 170 cases. Neurosurgery 51: 1365-1372

[8] Carrau Ricardo L, Jho H-D, Ko Y (1996) Transnasal-transsphenoidal endoscopic surgery of the pituitary gland. Laryngoscope 106: 914-918

[9] Caton R, Paul FT (1893) Notes of a case of acromegaly treated by operation. BMJ 2: 1421-1423

[10] Ciric I, Ragin A, Baumgartner C, Pierce D (1997) Complications of transsphenoidal surgery: results of a national survey, review of the literature, and personal experience. Neurosurgery 40: 225-237

[11] Cushing H (1914) The Weir Mitchell lecture. Surgical experiences with pituitary disorders. JAMA 63: 1515-1525

[12] de Divitiis E, Cappabianca P, Cavallo LM (2002) Endoscopic transsphenoidal approach: adaptability of the procedure to different sellar lesions. Neurosurgery 51: 699-707

[13] de Divitiis E, Cappabianca P, Cavallo LM (2003) Endoscopic endonasal transsphenoidal approach to the sellar region. In: de Divitiis E, Cappabianca P (eds) Endoscopic endonasal transsphenoidal surgery. Springer, Wien New York, pp 91-130

[14] de Divitiis E, Cappabianca P (2002) Endoscopic endonasal transsphenoidal surgery. Adv Tech Stand Neurosurg 27: 137-177

[15] Frazier CH (1913) An approach to the hypophysis through the anterior cranial fossa. Ann Surg 57: 145-150

[16] Guiot G (1973) Transsphenoidal approach in surgical treatment of pituitary adenomas: general principles and indications in nonfunctioning adenomas. In: En Kohler PO, Ross GT (eds) Diagnosis and treatment of pituitary tumors. American Elsevier, New York, pp 159-178

[17] Halstead AE (1910) Remarks on the operative treatment of tumors of the hypophysis. With the report of two cases operated on by an oro-nasal method. Surg Gynecol Obstet 10: 494-502

[18] Hardy J (1967) Surgery of the pituitary gland, using the trans-sphenoidal approach. Comparative study of 2 technical methods. Union Med Can 96: 702-712

[19] Hardy J (1969) Transsphenoidal microsurgery of the normal and pathological pituitary. Clin Neurosurg 16: 185-217

[20] Henderson WR (1939) The pituitary adenomata. A follow-up study of the surgical results in 338 cases (Dr. Harvey Cushing's series). Br J Surg 26: 811-921

[21] Heuer GJ (1931) The surgical approach and the treatment of tumors and other lesions about the optic chiasm. Surg Gynecol Obstet 53: 489-518

[22] Hirsch O (1910) Endonasal method of removal of hypophyseal tumors. With a report of two successful cases. JAMA 55: 772-774

[23] Jho HD, Carrau RL, Ko Y, et al. (1997) Endoscopic pituitary surgery: an early experience. Surg Neurol 47: 213-222

[24] Jho HD, Carrau RL, Ko Y (1996) Endoscopic pituitary surgery. In: Wilkins RH, Rengachary SS (eds) Neurosurgical operative atlas. AANS, Park Ridge, pp 1-12

[25] Kocher T (1909) Ein Fall von Hypophysis-Tumor mit operativer Heilung. Dtsch Z Chir 100: 13-37

[26] Krause F (1905) Hirnchirurgie. Dtsch Klin 8: 953-1024

[27] Lanzino G, Laws ER (2001) Pioneers in the development of transsphenoidal surgery: Theodor Kocher, Oskar Hirsch, and Norman Dott. J Neurosurg 95: 1097-1103

[28] Liu JK, Das K, Weiss MH, Laws ER Jr, Couldwell WT (2001) The history and evolution of transsphenoidal surgery. J Neurosurg 95: 1083-1096

[29] McArthur LL (1912) An aseptic surgical access to the pituitary body and its neighborhood. JAMA 58: 2009-2011

[30] Rhoton AL Jr (2002) The sellar region. Neurosurgery 51(Suppl 1): 335-374

[31] Williams PL, Warwick R (1992) Gray anatomía, tomo II. Churchill Livingstone, Edinburgh

[32] Rosegay H (1981) Cushing's legacy to transsphenoidal surgery. J Neurosurg 54: 448-454

[33] Schloffer H (1907) Erfolgreiche Operation eines Hypophysentumors auf nasalem Wege. Wien Klin Wochenschr 20: 621-624

[34] Welbourn RB (1986) The evolution of transsphenoidal pituitary microsurgery. Surgery 100: 1185-1190

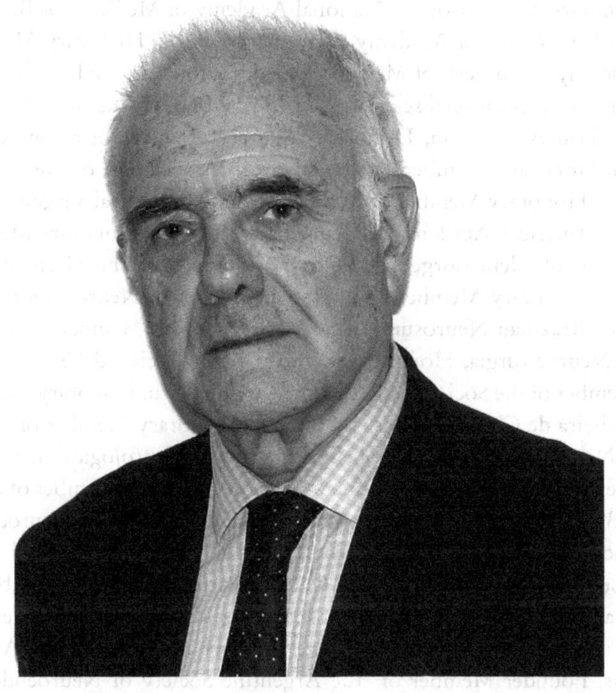

Armando J. Basso

Armando J. Basso is Director of the Neuroscience Institute and Professor emeritus of the Department of Neurosurgery at Buenos Aires University. Born in Buenos Aires, Argentine, married to Milva Peca, three daughters, Dana, Carla and Daniela, seven grandchildren. Doctor in Medicine and Diplome d'etudes approfondies (Ph.D.) in Neurophysiology, Université d'Orsay, France, 1968, Director of the Neuroscience Institute University of Buenos Aires, Clinical Research Director of the Consejo Nacional de Investigaciones Científicas y Técnicas (CONICET), Argentine, President of the World Federation of Neurosurgical Societies Foundation (WFNSF), Past President of the World Federation of Neurosurgical Societies (WFNS) 1993–1997, Honorary President of the World Federation of Neurosurgical Societies (WFNS), Chairman of the WHO (World Health Organization) Working Group on Neurosurgery, Past-President of the Latin American Federation of Neurosurgical Societies (FLANC), Past-President of the Asociacion Argentina de Neuro-Cirugía. Past-President of the World Federation of Skull Base Societies (President of the III International Skull Base Congress), President of the Argentine Stroke Society, eleven granted prizes in Argentine and Foreing Scientific Societies, Argentine National Academy of Medicine Award. Member of International Academies: Honorary Member of the National Academy of Medicine of

Belgium, Honorary Member of the National Academy of Medicine of Brazil, Honorary Member of the National Academy of Surgery of Perú, Honorary Member of the National Academy of Surgery of México. Societies: Honorary and Active Member of many national and international scientific societies: Honorary National Member of the Argentine Medical Association, Honorary Member of the Asociacion Argentina de Neurocirugia, Honorary Member of the American Association of Neurological Surgeons (AANS), Honorary Member of the Society of Neurological Surgeons. Honorary Member of the American Academy of Neurological Surgery, Honorary Member of the Japanese Society of Neurosurgery, Honorary Member of the German Society of Neurosurgery, Honorary Member of the Italian Society of Neurosurgery, Honorary Member of the Brazilian Neurosurgical Society, Honorary Member of the Academia Brasileira de Neurocirurgia, Honorary Member of the Sociedad Chilena de Cirugia, Honorary Member of the Sociedad de Neurocirugia del Peru, Honorary Member of the Sociedad Brasileira de Cirugia de Base do Craneo. Honorary Member of the Sociedad Boliviana de Neurocirugia, Member of the Congress of Neurological Surgeons, Member of the International Society of Pituitary Surgeons, Founder Member of the International Skull Base Study Group, Active Member of the Societe de Neurochirurgie de Langue Francaise, Active Member of the Sociedad de Neurocirugia del Uruguay, Active Member of the Colegio Argentino de Neurocirujanos, Active Member of Sociedad Argentina de Electro-encefalografía y Neuro-Fisiología Clínica, Active Member of the Sociedad Argentina de Biologia, Active Member of the Sociedad Argentina de Neurociencias, Founder Member of the Argentine Society of Neuroendocrinology, Founder and Active Member of the Argentine Neurosurgical Forum. Author of more than 140 papers of his specialty.

Contact: Armando J. Basso, MD, PhD, President of the WFNS Foundation, Director of Neurosciences Institute, Buenos Aires University, Ayacucho 1342, Buenos Aires 1111, Argentina
E-mail: armandobasso@aol.com

HOW TO PERFORM TRANSORAL APPROACHES

A. CROCKARD

INTRODUCTION

While transsphenoidal surgery was developed almost a century ago, it was the detailed anatomical studies, procedure, specific instrumentation and masterful teaching of Jules Hardy in Montreal in the 1960s that finally launched it as a standard neurosurgical procedure. Strange then, that an approach through an adjacent orifice met such (emotional) resistance, with fears of infection, bleeding and wound complications deterring many neurosurgeons. There had been isolated reports of removal of a bullet (Kanaval 1917) and tumors, but the technique did not come of age until ready access to neuroimaging defined clearly the anatomy and pathology of the ventral craniovertebral junction [5]. Again it has been the development of appropriate retractors and specific instruments which has allowed the procedure to be within the standard armamentarium of skull base and high cervical spinal surgeons. Pioneers in the field have been Arnold Menezes (Iowa), who put his early ENT training to good effect, and Hiroshi Abe (Sapporo). In the UK, it was a far-sighted orthopaedic surgeon, George Bonney, who successfully decompressed posttraumatic deformities at the atlantoaxial joint.

The term "transoral" covers a suite of surgical procedures in which the surgical instruments are passed between the lips to gain access to the clivus [5], ventral craniovertebral junction and the upper two or three cervical vertebrae. No single procedure will be suitable for all pathology; also the more extensive procedures such as the "open-door" maxillotomy [6] or "trans-mandibular transglottic" approach are best served by a team approach combining their individual skills. Their development is an important message to the modern surgeon, a move from the individual "surgical master" to the "premier league surgical team".

RATIONALE

The transoral family of surgical procedures are particularly indicated for ventral, midline, extradural pathology. They are contraindicated in lateral extra-

Keywords: skull base, posterior fossa tumors, microsurgery

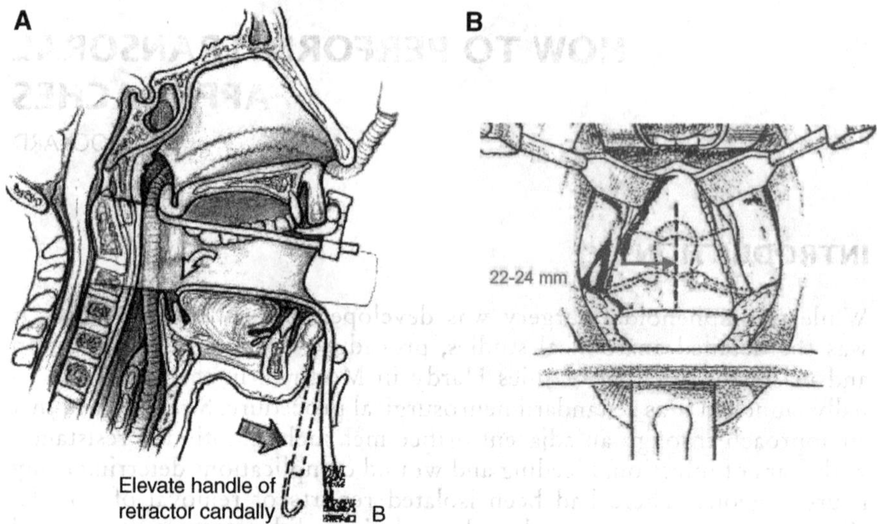

Fig. 1. The standard transoral approach. **A** Exposure of the arch of C1 and odontoid peg by elevation of the soft palate using the Crockard retractor. **B** A vertical incision in the mucosa over the anterior tubercles will expose C1 and C2

dural pathology and entirely intradural tumors and vascular abnormalities. However, small intradural extensions or a dural tear can be accommodated with careful preplanning (see below) [1, 5, 9].

Understanding the complex three-dimensional anatomy in the area is essential for positioning, surgical approach and complication avoidance. The normal clivodental angle is about 140° and with head on neck extension this can be increased. In basilar invagination, the angle may be 90° or less, and, without temporary mobilisation of the teeth and alveolar margins, will render the craniovertebral junction surgically inaccessible. There are no extradural arteries at risk in the "transoral" target area, which measures 22 mm between the vertebral arteries at the clivus and at the body of axis and below. At the level of the atlas, this bony area is double the distance (22–24 mm on each side of the midline, i.e., 48 mm in total).

The surgical key to the area is the anterior tubercle on the arch of C1; this is the anatomical and embryological midline and to this are attached the longus coli muscles (and between these muscles is the subaxial midline). Below the craniovertebral junction the mucosa and muscle layer slide over each other due to an alveolar layer and permit a 2 layer closure (see below). Surgical closure above the ventral foramen magnum is more difficult as the pharyngeal lining is osteomucosal with Sharpey's fibres firmly binding it to the bone underneath. There are also numerous venous intercommunications between the dural sinuses, the bone and the submucosal venous plexus. (The best way to control such bleeding is by elevation of the head above heart level and gentle prolonged pressure. Bipolar coagulation does not work.)

The craniovertebral junction's movements and stability depend on strong ligaments, the alar apical complex, the transverse ligaments of the occipito-atlantal and atlantoaxial joints. Surgical removal of any of these will demand that stability is carefully tested after a transoral procedure. In some conditions, e.g., rheumatoid atlantoaxial subluxations, the neuraxial compression exists because of instability and thus a planned stabilisation must be part of the surgical solution. Careful detailed three-dimensional imaging of the bone and soft tissue is essential in surgical planning (for example, 1 in 11 people have a very large vertebral artery which may "interfere" with a planned screw trajectory).

Image guidance surgery and endoscopic techniques will facilitate greatly all surgery in this area.

Brainstem monitoring (SSEP and MEP) before and during surgery will alert the surgical team as to impending problems during the procedure. However, patients with severe deformity with neuraxial compression of more than 30% will not have preoperative SSEP waveforms and thus peroperative monitoring of this will be fruitless [8].

DECISION-MAKING

Transoral surgery should be considered for midline ventral extradural pathology at the craniovertebral junction that is deforming or compressing the neuraxis and which cannot be alleviated by skull traction and realignment of the atlantoaxial joint.

Plain radiographs are insufficient and detailed CT and MR scanning essential; functional studies in flexion and extension are required. In advance of surgery there should be detailed knowledge of the pathology. If it is a "bony" problem such as the presence of translocation of the odontoid, any rotational element in the deformity and the quality of the bone of the lateral masses of the atlas and axis, then this information is essential. The vertebral foramina will alert the clinician to the path and size of the vessel which may be damaged by screw placement.

Image guidance is a great help but no substitute for rigorous preoperative investigations.

Vascular imaging is necessary for tumors, and tumor embolisation in some cases. A decision to remove a vertebral artery as part of the tumor surgery should not be made without first establishing that the patient has a complete circle of Willis. In some, a trial temporary balloon occlusion of the vessel in the conscious patient may be required (Table 1 and Fig. 2).

Table 1. Management of "transoral" patients

Pre op	Per op	Post op
Mouth opens more than 3 cm		
Bacteriology mouth swab		Repeat if wound inflamed
SSEP (MEP)		Repeat if deteriorate
Plain lateral radiograph of CCJ		To check for soft tissue swelling
Plain lateral radiograph of chest		To check for airway problem
Venous support stockings	Mechanical anti embolism	Venous support stockings
	Broad-spectrum antibiotic	Continue 24 hours
	Antiemetic	Continue 48 hours
	Hydrocortisone ointment	Continue 6 hourly 48 hours
	Nasotracheal tube*	Continue 24 hours
	Nasogastric tube*	Continue 5 days
		Nil orally 5 days
If a chance of a CSF leak	CSF lumbar drain (in position not opened unless a leak)	Remove if no leak 10–15 ml/hr for 5 days if leak Check CCJ instability
Open-door maxillotomy and transmandibular approach	Tracheostomy Percutaneous gastrostomy	As long as necessary

*Used only if swallowing intact – otherwise tracheostomy etc.

1. PATIENT MANAGEMENT

I bring this point up prior to description of surgery to emphasise the importance of a team approach in a Specialist Unit. While the surgical technique can and should be learnt in the laboratory, it is only a part in the management of these complicated patients. Timing of surgical intervention is critical and can only be carried out in a team used to long-term evaluation of these patients. For surgery, the anaesthetic team must be familiar with the management of the difficult airway and nasotracheal intubation [2, 3]; very few patients should require an elective tracheostomy. Intraoperatve electrical monitoring and image guidance need to be used regularly in a variety of surgical procedures to acquaint all the team for them to be of value in transoral surgery. A postoperative intensive care team well versed in the care of these patients is essential.

2. WHICH OPERATION FOR WHICH PATIENT?

There is a wide range of pathology which may be amenable, but surgical team's may use a variety of skull base procedures. Set out in Fig. 2 is the decision-making pathway for transoral surgery in anterior craniovertebral pathology.

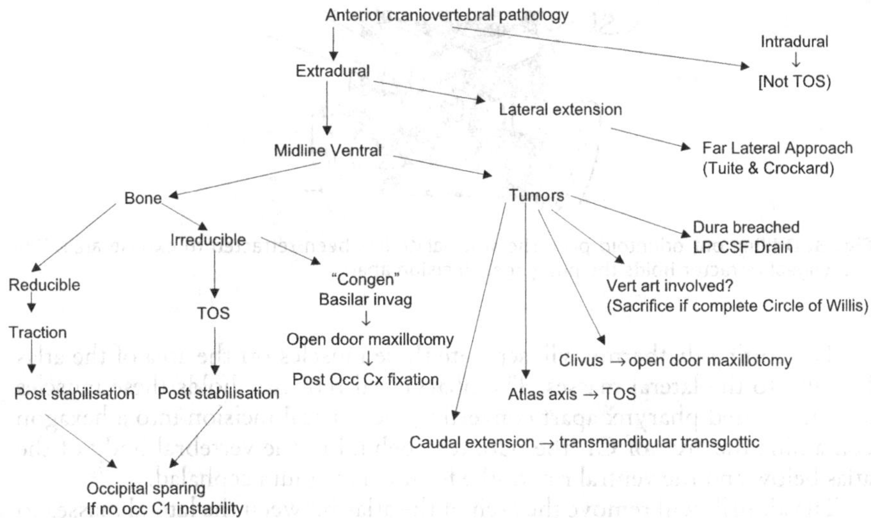

Fig. 2. Decision-making for transoral surgery for anterior craniovertebral pathology

SURGERY

1. A STANDARD "TRANSORAL"

The anaesthetised patient is secured supine on the table with head held in 3-pin head holder. The whole table is tilted 15–20° towards the surgeon; the head end of the table is titled 20° upwards. Image guidance is positioned and registered. The operating microscope provides best illumination and magnification for the procedure, although specific portions of the operations may be carried out with a flexible endoscope.

The transoral retractor (Coolman, Raynham, MD) is carefully positioned (after application of hydrocortisone ointment to the mucosal surfaces, lips and tongue). Great care is necessary to avoid "nipping" a portion of the tongue or lips between teeth and retractor. Meticulous attention to this will very significantly reduce postoperative swelling. All the instruments in the transoral set are sufficiently long and bayonetted to allow access to the depths of the wound. A long angled high-speed air drill is necessary.

The soft palate and the nasogastric and nasotracheal tubes are retracted to expose the posterior pharynx [1]. The anterior tubercle on the arch of C1 is identified by instrumental palpation. A 4 cm vertical incision over this will expose the atlantoaxial area after the pharyngeal wall has been infiltrated with lignocaine and adrenaline to reduce cut edge bleeding. Separate this layer off the prevertebral fascia and the longus coli muscles and bones.

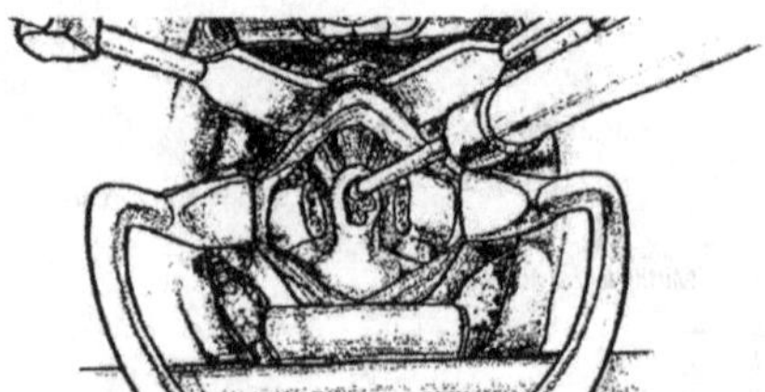

Fig. 3. Drilling out odontoid peg. The soft palate has been retracted to expose area. The pharyngeal retractor holds the pharyngeal incision apart

The cutting diathermy will separate these muscles off the area of the atlas laterally to the lateral masses. The pharyngeal retractor holds these muscles and the incised pharynx apart converting the vertical incision into a hexagon containing the arch of C1, the odontoid behind it, the vertebral body of the atlas below and the ventral rim of the foramen magnum cephalad.

The air drill will remove the arch of the atlas between the lateral masses to expose the odontoid, which in turn is hollowed out. During this manoeuvre the relative angle of the peg and the drill mean that the proximal position of the peg just below the transverse ligament may be the site of an unplanned penetration of the cortical bone and even the dura (Fig. 3). When the peg is thinned to a cortical shell, the latter is removed with the long 1 mm and 2 mm Kerrison upcuts along with the attached alar apical ligaments.

The transverse ligament is incised and removed to expose the cruciate ligament and any pannus in rheumatoid or pseudotumor of the elderly. The angled bayonetted blunt hook will separate these structures and the underlying dura which has usually a greyish blue colour. Adequate decompression can be verified by image guidance and prominent dural pulsations [1].

Wound closure is by 3/0 Vicryl on a round bodied needle angulated to convert the "C" to a "J" shape; two sutures to the muscles and four separate sutures to the pharyngeal wall. After the layered closure, fibrin thrombin "glue" is injected into the bony defect to fill the void and act as a haemostat.

2. "OPEN-DOOR" MAXILLOTOMY

This procedure was developed to gain access to the clivus in severe basilar invagination, e.g., osteogenesis imperfecta, or for a clival chordoma. It allows midline access from the pituitary fossa down to the base of the atlas; lateral extension is limited to the width of the clivus to prevent damage to the vertebral and carotid arteries and the lower cranial nerves.

Prior to this surgery, a percutaneous epigastric gastrostomy and a tracheostomy are necessary.

The superior alveolar bone above the level of the dental roots is exposed under the upper lip. Titanium miniplates are positioned in the nasal and pterygoid buttresses for postoperative fixations of the upper jaw. (To leave it till after

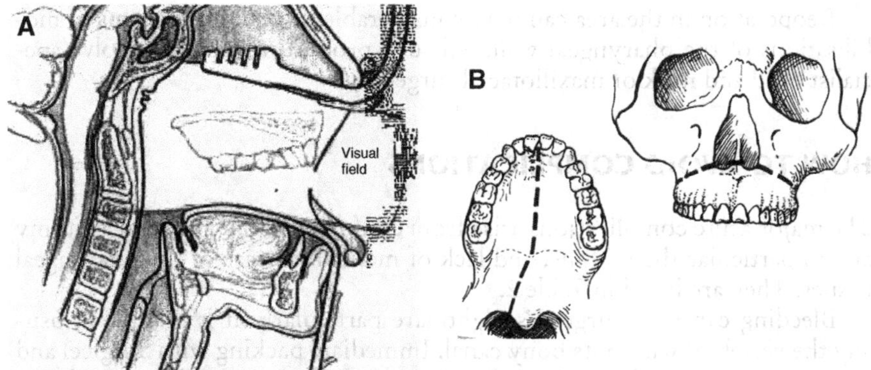

Fig. 4. The open door maxillotomy. **A** Area exposed. **B** Sawcuts for exposure

the maxillotomy will mean that the teeth are not in their exact preoperative position.) The plates are removed and carefully preserved till the end of the procedure. A Lefort III maxillotomy is effected using the reciprocating saw and the upper jaw down fractured into the mouth. A midline incision between the incisors across the alveolar margin, the hard palate and then the soft palate, will create the "open door" (Fig. 4). Both segments of the jaw depend on the blood supply from the vessels coming in from the pterygoid muscles. The front two teeth on each side may be denervated, but the author, in 20 years, has not seen major problems in these patients very ill with their presenting pathology.

3. TRANSMANDIBULAR TRANSGLOTTIC

In this procedure, a midline excision of the tongue back as far as the epiglottis and the mandible, coupled with a careful cosmetic incision across the lower lip will allow midline exposure caudad to C5. This is particularly useful in the staged excision of an extensive chordoma.

LONG-TERM RESULTS

Since 1983, I have been involved in over 560 cases for a wide variety of pathology. Over this period there have been changes in pathology. For instance, with the change in treatment of rheumatoid arthritis and particularly no steroids, the extreme odontoid translocations with and without pannus have become a thing of the past [4]. On the other hand more and more tumors in the area have been referred and this has resulted in more "open door" procedures (476 transorals, 74 open door, 20 transglottic and other).

The acute complications are listed in Table 2.

There are long-term problems associated with these procedures, the chief of which is nasal regurgitation especially of fluids and altered "nasal" speech.

Reoperation in the area can pose considerable difficulties in terms of mobilisations of the pharyngeal wall. All such procedures should involve specialist head and neck or maxillofacial surgeons.

HOW TO AVOID COMPLICATIONS

The major acute complications arise from confusion about the local anatomy and in particular the midline, and lack of meticulous care of the pharyngeal tissues. They are listed in Table 2.

Bleeding can be a surgeon's nightmare particularly if it is arterial, usually the vertebral within its bony canal. Immediate packing with Surgicel and bone wax will save the patient's life. It is virtually impossible to repair the vessel transorally, so control bleeding and request the interventional radiologists occlude the bleeding point. Following this it is most important to maintain good brain perfusion by keeping the systemic blood pressure normal or higher than normal.

Cerebrospinal fluid (CSF) leaks can lead to meningitis and a fatal outcome, so careful management is essential. The main preventative manoeuvre is to anticipate the possibility and have a lumbar drain in situ in those at risk (after the loss of a considerable amount of CSF it is practically impossible to establish a patient CSF line).

Table 2. Complication avoidance

Problem	Resolution
Access difficult	Pre-op mouth opening <3 cm. Increase head on neck extension
Irregular dentition	Pre-op manufacture "gum guard" to fit retractor
Where is midline?	Careful positioning, per-op X-ray, image guidance
Arterial bleeding	Surgeon not in midline
Venous bleeding	Surgical pack, "Head up" tilt table
Adequate decompression?	Image guidance
Possibility CSF leak	Lumbar CSF drain, Inserted during anaesthesia
"Accidental"	Lumbar CSF drain (after op)
	Multilayer closure, Surgicel, Fibrin glue
	Dural sutures will not work
Wound problems	Careful 2-layer closure, nil orally 5 days
Mouth and facial swelling	"Head up" position. Hydrocortisone ointment to mucosa (no systemic steroids)
Post-op swallowing	Re-intubate or change to tracheostomy
	If prolonged, tracheostomy or percutaneous gastrostomy
CVJ instability	Will require posterior fixation
Vertebral artery injury	Pack on op table → radiology → balloon occlusion (do not attempt transoral vascular repair)

In combination with lowering CSF pressure with regular lumbar drainage the wound should be closed very carefully and if necessary a rotation mucosal flap be used. Surgicel and fibrin thrombin glue injected into the space between the dura and soft tissue closure. It will be impossible to effect a watertight dural closure with dural sutures.

CONCLUSIONS

Transoral surgery provides a further weapon in the armamentarium of the skull base and upper cervical spine surgeon. It requires detailed anatomical knowledge and time spent in the surgical laboratory. It is not a procedure of the occasional operator.

That said it can produce an extremely satisfying clinical result for patient and surgeon.

References

[1] Bouramas D, Crockard A (2003) Anterior odontoid resection. In: Haher T, Merola A (eds) Surgical techniques of the spine. Thieme, New York, pp 10-15

[2] Calder I, Calder J, Crockard HA (1995) Difficult direct laryngoscopy in patients with cervical spine disease. Anaesthesia 50: 756-763

[3] Calder I. Anaesthesia and cervical spine disease. Anaesth Intens Care Med (in press)

[4] Casey ATH, Crockard HA, Bland JM, Stevens J, Moskovich R, Ransford AO (1996) Surgery on the rheumatoid cervical spine for the non-ambulant myelopathic patient – too much, too late? Lancet 347: 1004-1007

[5] Crockard HA, Johnston F (1993) Development of transoral approaches to lesions of the skull base and craniocervical junction. Neurosurg Q 3: 61-82

[6] Harkey HL, Crockard HA (1998) Transoral-extended maxillotomy. In: Dickman CA, Spetzler RF, Sonntag VFH (eds) Surgery of the craniovertebral junction. Thieme Medical Publishers, New York, pp 371-380

[7] James D, Crockard HA (1991) Surgical access to the base of skull and upper cervical spine by extended maxillotomy. Neurosurgery 29: 411-416

[8] May DM, Jones SJ, Crockard HA (1996) Somatosensory evoked potential monitoring in cervical surgery: identification of pre- and intraoperative risk factors associated with neurological deterioration. J Neurosurg 85: 566-573

[9] Tuite GF, Crockard HA (1997) Far lateral approach to the foramen magnum. In: Torrens M, Al-Mefty O, Kobayashi S (eds) Operative skull base surgery. Churchill Livingstone, New York, pp 333

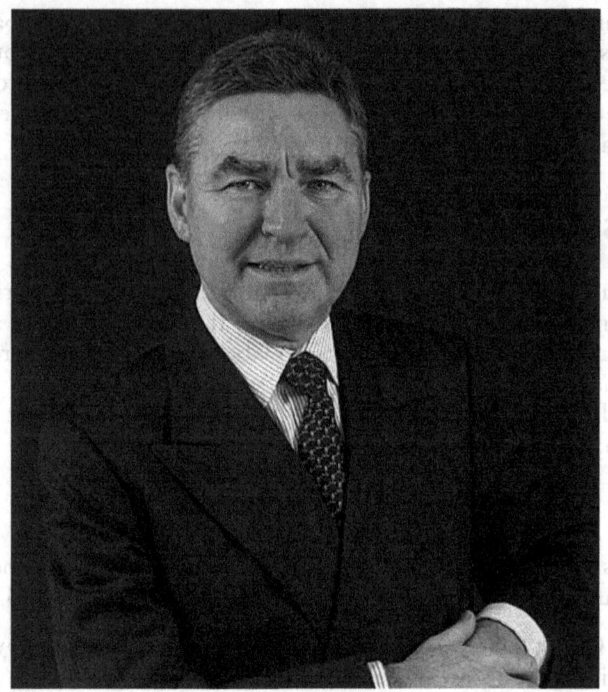

Alan Crockard

Alan Crockard is head of spinal surgery research unit, at the National Hospital for Neurology and Neurosurgery, London. He entered neurosurgical training in Belfast just as the civil disturbances began in 1969. He quickly became proficient in triage and haemostasis of gunshot injuries and was first to show the beneficial effects of controlled ventilation in head injuries. After research in London and Chicago, he was appointed to the National Hospital at Queen Square and there established a skull base and spinal referral practice. He carried out anatomical studies to establish new surgical access to these difficult areas and developed transoral instruments in 1983. Laterally he has devoted himself to teaching and anatomical masterclasses.

Contact: Alan Crockard, Victor Horsley Department of Neurosurgery, The National Hospital for Neurology and Neurosurgery, Queen Square, London WC1N 3BG, UK
E-mail: alan.crockard@uclh.nhs.uk

HOW TO PERFORM POSTERIOR FOSSA APPROACHES

J. J. A. MOOIJ

INTRODUCTION

The posterior fossa of the skull has always been considered a particular entity, from the beginning of the development of neurosurgery. This has to do with specific anatomical features, like the attachment of various muscle layers, the related irregular bony rims, the protuberantia externa (Inion), the mastoids, and within the skull barriers within the dura mater: the transverse and sigmoid sinuses. Inside the dural coverings, delicate structures of the central nervous system are hidden: the cerebellum, the brainstem, most of the cranial nerves, the vertebral arteries, the basilar arteries, their important branches, and the venous outflow system.

Surgery for pathologies in the posterior fossa started already in the 1890s, with Victor Horsley. All major founding fathers of neurosurgery have contributed to the development of surgery in this area: Cushing, Smith, Frazier, Krause, and De Martel, to mention the most important. In the beginning, surgery was done with the patient in a lateral position. A prone position became more popular with the development of a good head rest, the horse shoe type, by Frazier, and further developed by Cushing and Smith. Specific problems were immediately recognised, like abdominal pressure raise and concomitant haemorrhage risk. In 1905 Frazier performed the first operation with the patient in sitting position. De Martel propagated the sitting position and developed a special chair (1916). The risks for serious sequelae in the sitting position were recognised very soon, with pulmonary air embolism, syncope and shock. Therefore, the sitting position was not popularized in every centre. Instead, stepwise improvements in technique for other positions were developed. Generally four types of positioning have remained today: the prone position with variations; the lateral decubitus position with variations; the supine position with tilt and head rotation; and the sitting or semi-sitting position. Each has advantages and disadvantages, and certain preferences related to specific pathology and its localization within the posterior fossa. This will be dealt with in the next paragraphs of this chapter.

As is also true for neurosurgery in general, improvements in diagnostics, treatment techniques and operative results in posterior fossa surgery arose from the development of imaging (CT, MRI), the operative microscope,

Keywords: posterior fossa approaches, microsurgery, skull base

bipolar coagulation, CUSA, neuronavigation, and of course by improvement in anesthesiological and postoperative care.

Therefore, today surgery on pathologies in the posterior fossa can be as straightforward and safe as procedures in other places in the skull. There are, however, enough special aspects that warrant dealing with these in a separate chapter like this.

RATIONALE

1. SURGICAL ANATOMY OF THE POSTERIOR FOSSA

By "posterior fossa" is generally meant the most occipital and lower part of the skull. It is a compartment with a bony confinement consisting of the occipital and most caudal part of the cranial vault, extending from the midline to the mastoid processes on both sides. From there, bony thickenings, the pyramids containing the inner ear, converge medially to end in a basic bony structure, medially anteriorly located and called the clivus. The "roof" is formed by the tentorium, a dural double layer within the bony skull. Several openings in this rather closed compartment allow the content of the posterior fossa to be connected with other parts of the central and peripheral nervous system, and the body: (1) the opening in the tentorium, the hiatus tentorii, through which the upper brainstem and both fourth cranial nerves run; (2) the foramen magnum, an opening at the most basal side of the bony skull, allowing for the connection of the lower brain stem (medulla oblongata) with the spinal cord; and (3) numerous openings, foramina, for the cranial nerves, and the vessels that come in and go out [6]. On both sides of the foramen magnum, bony thickenings, called condyles, connect in a joint like fashion with the atlas, and thereby connect the skull as a whole with the vertebral column. Strong bands and ligaments, as well as many muscles, connect the lower part of the skull with the vertebral column and thorax, in a safe but flexible way. The attachment of the strongest muscles, the trapezius, the semispinalis, the splenium capitis and the sternocleidomastoid, lead to a curved ring that forms the upper border of the outside of the posterior fossa skull.

It is relevant to know that the suture between the occipital bone and the parietal bones, the lambda suture, reaches way above the borders of the posterior fossa.

On the inside, a dural layer is found, like in the rest of the skull. It covers the content of the posterior fossa, and folds within the skull to a double layer that covers the cerebellum, called the tentorium. In the middle part of this tentorium runs the straight sinus: a conduit connecting the vein of Galen to the connection of both transverse sinuses, the "confluens". The transverse sinuses are conduits within the dural layer following and forming the attachment of the tentorium to the inner skull. From their confluens, also called "Torcular", the sinuses run laterally to the petrous bone and bend caudally to

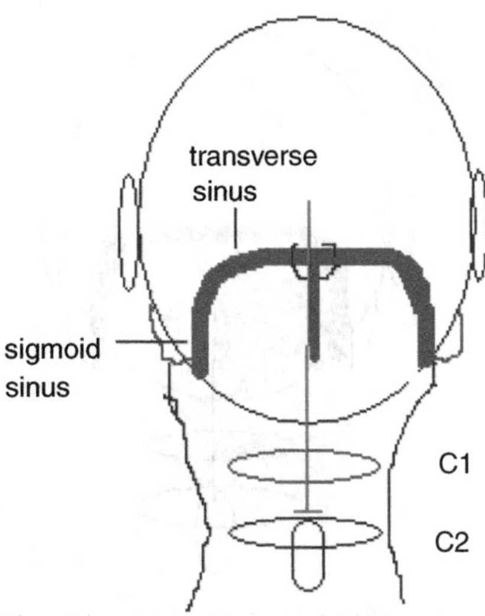

Fig. 1. Midline incision (red line) from above torcular (external protuberance) to upper rim of C2. In many cases an occipital sinus runs in the middle line from the confluence sinuum caudally

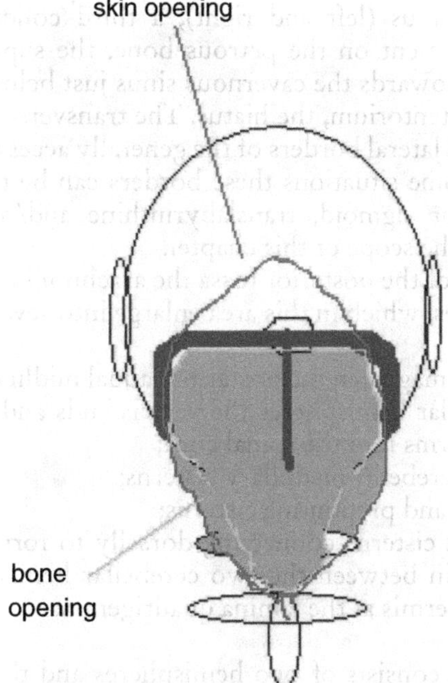

Fig. 2. Oval skin opening, bony opening up to transverse sinus, and showing beginning of sigmoid sinus. Middle part of atlas (C1) removed

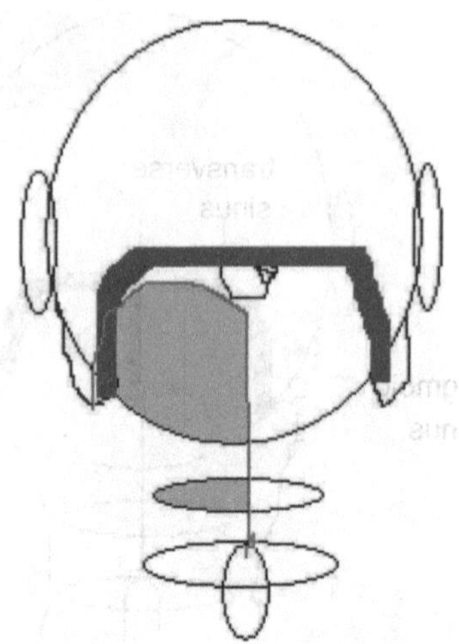

Fig. 3. Far lateral approach: less high up, but more caudally aimed at occiptal atlantoid junction, laterally

form the sigmoid sinus on both sides. They end through the jugular foramina in the jugular veins in the neck. At the site of transition form the transverse into the sigmoid sinus (left and right), a third conduit arises following the tentorial attachment on the petrous bone, the superior petrosal sinus. These sinuses run towards the cavernous sinus just below and laterally from the opening in the tentorium, the hiatus. The transverse and sigmoid sinuses form the upper and lateral borders of the generally accessible dura of the posterior fossa. For some situations these borders can be trespassed by special techniques: anterior sigmoid, translabyrinthine and/or transtentorial approaches, beyond the scope of this chapter.

Inside the dura of the posterior fossa the arachnoid layer is found. It contains the CSF spaces, which in this area enlarge into several cisterns:

- the cisterna magna, in the posterior caudal midline where between the two cerebellar hemispheres the vermis ends and the medulla oblongata transforms into the spinal cord;
- the lateral cerebello-medullary cisterns;
- the pontine and prepontine cisterns;
- the ambient cisterns connecting dorsally to form the quadrigeminal cistern, again between the two cerebellar hemispheres at the upper end of the vermis at the lamina quadrigemina.

The cerebellum consists of two hemispheres and the central connecting structure, the vermis. Detailed anatomical features can be found in neuroanatomical textbooks.

For the neurosurgeon a few aspects are specifically important: (1) The caudal part of both cerebellar hemispheres forms an appendage like extension, the tonsil. As a result of mass lesions, shifts may occur resulting in herniation of these tonsils into the foramen magnum with concomitant compression of the medulla oblongata and the spinal cord. (2) Laterally and more anteriorly, each hemisphere has an appendage near the lateral recess (opening) of the fourth ventricle, Luschka's foramen. This is called the flocculus, rather firmly attached to the dorsal and proximal part of the eighth nerve.

The cerebellum is connected to the brainstem by three major tracks on both sides, called brachium conjunctivum, brachium pontis and corpus restiforme. The most caudal part of the brain stem, the medulla oblongata, is reached directly caudally from the vermis. Between vermis and medulla opens the fourth ventricle through the foramen of Magendie. A thin covering form the velum medullare, and middle choroids plexus, is seen here. The anterior ("bottom") of the fourth ventricle is the pons, with some detailed elevations related to cranial nerve nuclei.

Seen from lateral or anterior, the pons is separated from the medulla by a sulcus, a helpful surgical landmark.

The cranial nerves XII–IV arise from the brainstem in the posterior fossa, at distinct and different places. They run through the arachnoid space to their specific foramina, which again are landmarks in surgical procedures. Again, detailed anatomical descriptions are beyond the scope of this chapter.

The most important veins to be considered in surgical approaches to the posterior fossa are, besides the already mentioned dural sinuses:

- the petrosal vein or veins, also called Dandy's vein, in the lateral pontine angle;
- the superior vermian veins, running dorsally from the upper vermis to the tentorium;
- the precentral cerebellar vein.

The arteries in the posterior fossa are:

- the vertebral arteries (VA) entering the posterior fossa through the dura on both sides of the foramen magnum, and joining into the basilar artery (BA) in front of the pons; before that, they give branches that form the anterior spinal artery;
- the posterior inferior cerebellar arteries (PICA), originating from the intradural vertebral arteries, looping around the XI–IXth nerves, the tonsils, and then branching to the choroid plexus and the medial cerebellar hemispheres;
- the anterior inferior cerebellar arteries (AICA), coming from the mid-basilar artery, running laterally and looping around the VII–VIIIth nerves before going to the middle portion of the cerebellar hemispheres;

- the superior cerebellar arteries (SCA), originating from the BA just caudally from the basilar bifurcation; the latter is lying just beyond the "borders" of the posterior fossa; the SCAs run on both sides over the upper pons, to the most cranial parts of the cerebellar hemispheres, and have a close relationship to the trigeminal and the trochlear nerves.

2. GENERAL ASPECTS OF PATHOLOGY AND PATHOPHYSIOLOGY IN THE POSTERIOR FOSSA

Surgical approaches to the posterior fossa are done for a variety of pathologies, details of which are found elsewhere in this book.

In general, surgery is done for:

- *tumors*
  - intrinsic tumors of the cerebellum
  - intrinsic tumors of the brain stem
  - tumors in the fourth ventricle
  - intrinsic tumors of the pineal gland/region
  - tumors of the cranial nerves (mostly vestibular schwannomas)
  - cerebellar metastases
  - extra axial tumors: meningeomas
    - superficial
    - petroclival
    - tentorial
    - foraminal
- *vascular lesions/problems*
  - aneurysms
  - arteriovenous malformations
  - fistulas
  - haemorrhage
- *neurovascular compression syndromes*
  - trigeminal neuralgia
  - hemifacial spasm
  - glossopharyngeal neuralgia
  - tinnitus-vertigo syndrome
- *infections (abscess, empyema)*
- *trauma (isolated posterior fossa trauma is seldom!)*

Symptomatology of these lesions is of course related to their localization, with or without impact on neurological function: it varies from cranial nerve dysfunction (deafness/dizziness in vestibular Schwannomas) to brainstem or cerebellar dysfunction, by distortion, compression or destruction.

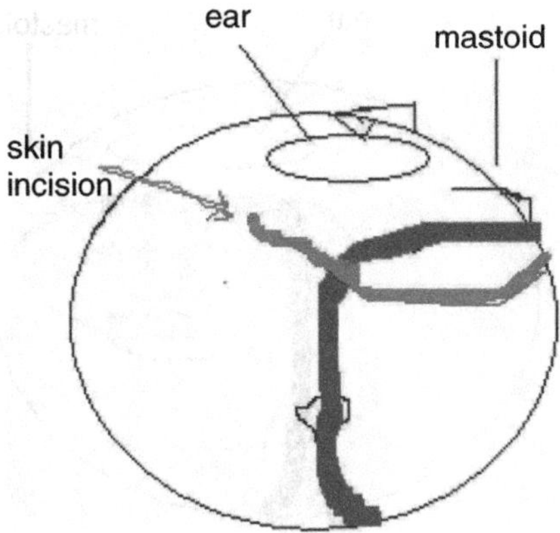

Fig. 4. Lateral position, retromastoid approach. Skin incision starts behind and a little above the ear, curving towards some crease in the skin of the neck

Besides local (intrinsic) neurological dysfunction, a general problem may arise which is pertinent to the posterior fossa: the relatively small and confined space leads easily to a rise in intracranial pressure with brainstem compression and dysfunction. This can result in loss of consciousness, disturbance of gaze and other oculomotor symptoms, and ventilation problems. Such a mechanism is seen especially in acute mass lesions like in cerebellar haemorrhage.

A separate and often concomitant mechanism is the interference of pathology in the posterior fossa with the circulation of the cerebrospinal fluid (CSF), resulting in acute hydrocephalus. It can be difficult to unravel the pathophysiological mechanism in a certain situation and to decide whether treatment of the hydrocephalus or of the mass lesion itself is preferable.

SURGERY

1. POSITIONING IN POSTERIOR FOSSA APPROACHES

It is well known that positioning of the patient for neurosurgical procedures is of paramount importance and may be decisive for the success of the surgery. This holds especially true for approaches to the posterior fossa.

There are four main positions to be considered [2, 4, 7, 8]:

- *Prone/Concorde*
- *Lateral decubitus/park-bench*
- *Supine with rotation of the head*
- *Sitting position*

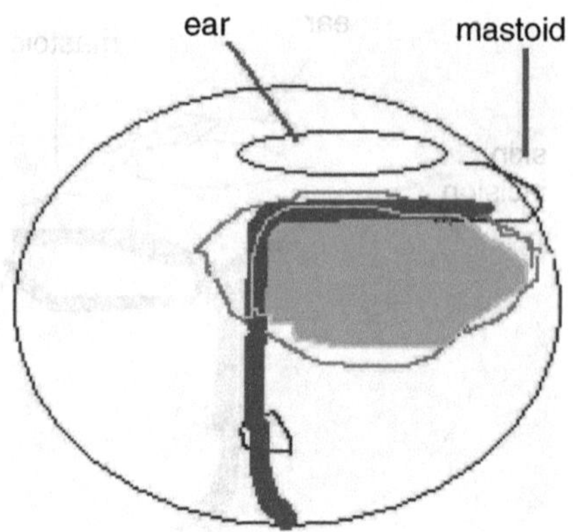

Fig. 5. Same as Fig. 4; oval skin opening (red line) bone opening reaching transverse and sigmoid sinus

1.1 Prone and Concorde position

These positions are predominantly used for pathologies where a midline approach is necessary. But also for a so-called far lateral approach, this position has some advantages above a lateral positioning (see next paragraphs). In the prone position, the patient is lying prone on the table with support to thorax, pelvis and legs. This support should leave the belly free. Therefore, a U-shaped cushion may be used under the thorax. The head is either supported by a horse-shoe cushion, or fixed in a Mayfield clamp. The latter is my favourite, and gives more freedom for flexion of the head with concomitant better exposure of the lower occiput and neck. Such exposure can be even more exaggerated by lifting the upper thorax and shoulders, and bending and lowering the head to a maximal flexion. That is what is called the "Concorde" position, a self-explaining name!

In such a position, the surgeon may stand from one side of the body looking from below towards the occipital region. Therefore, the head can even be angulated and tilted a little, according to the surgeon's preference. But, especially in the Concorde hyperflexion, the surgeon may work "upside down", standing and even sitting with the patient's head "in his/her lap". This is my favourite position for surgery on midline posterior fossa pathology in infants and young children.

1.2 Lateral decubitus and "park-bench" position

This approach is primarily used for unilateral entering of the posterior fossa: a paramedian approach for a cerebellar hemisphere lesion, or a retromastoid opening for pontine angle pathology, including VA and PICA aneurysms. Careful support for the thorax is necessary leaving some space for the

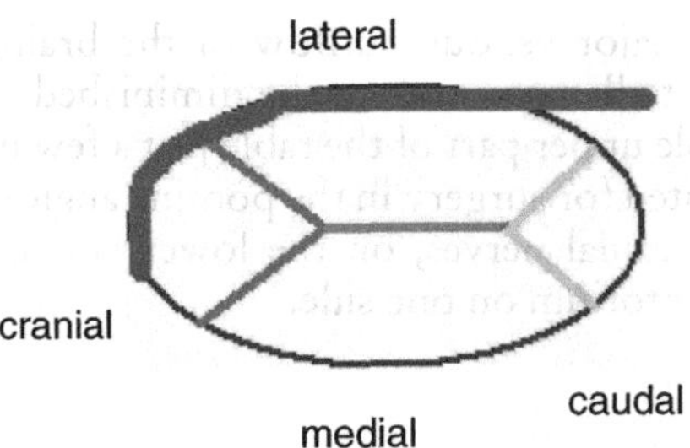

Fig. 6. See Figs. 4 and 5, concentrating on dural opening. This starts with a linear incision (red), followed by two caudal incisions (green), for a basal dural flap; now CSF can be drained, underneath the cerebellum. Last incisions are cranial (blue), making a triangular dural flap based on the transverse sinus. The lateral trapezoid flap (blue-red-green lines) is based on the sigmoid sinus and allows for maximal lateral approach along the cerebellum

underlying upper arm, with some flexion for the lower arm. Also the hips must be well-supported and fixed in this position, in order to avoid inadvertent sliding or rotation. Again, the head is held by a Mayfield clamp, the neck can be flexed as far as necessary and appropriate. The major advance is that rotation of the neck, with risks for kinking of the VA, and postoperative cervical vertebral and muscle pain, is avoided. The problem is primarily the underlying arm, with risks for compression of the brachial plexus. Another problem and risk may be some hypoventilation of the lower lung and postoperative atelectasis. This needs special attention, especially at the end of the surgery. After closing up, the patient should be rotated first to the supine position, ventilated well, and only extubated thereafter.

However, with some routine the lateral decubitus position can be fine and stable, especially for long lasting procedures in elderly patients.

The arm problem can be mitigated by letting the arm hang in a sling past the end of the table, with still good support for the thorax. Moreover, some rotation of the patient towards a more prone position is then easy and may be preferable. That is the "park bench" position.

1.3 Supine position with rotation of the head

For lateral pathology in the posterior fossa, a supine position with the head fixed in a Mayfield clamp and rotated to one side is sufficient. It is easier and much faster than the lateral (or park bench) position. Many patients can rotate the head far enough, but this should be tested in the awake situation preoperatively. In order to avoid too much rotation, and subsequent kinking of the VA, the thorax should be supported by an extra cushion on one side, thus rotating the body already quite a bit. Some flexion in the neck can be added, for better accessibility of the lower lateral part of the posterior fossa. The most important to avoid in this position, besides the already mentioned interference with the VA, is compression of the underlying jugular vein, which may be the major venous outflow of the brain. Venous congestion should be avoided at all costs, and can be diminished remarkably by lifting the head or the whole upper part of the table just a few degrees. This position is extremely well suited for surgery in the pontine angle (including petroclival meningeomas), on cranial nerves, on the lower lateral brain stem, and the cerebellum or the tentorium on one side.

1.4 Sitting position

As already mentioned in the first paragraph, in the beginning of posterior fossa surgery the sitting position became very popular. With table tilt and more bending in the hips, one can even lower the whole position towards a so-called semi-sitting position. Head fixation has been improved remarkably thanks to the Mayfield clamp, which can be mounted in front of the head with a U-shaped device fixed on the side bars of the operation table.

The advantages in this position are:

- Best overview for the upper cerebellum, the midline tentorium area, and consequently ideal for the supracerebellar infratentorial approach to the tectal and pineal area;
- CSF and blood drain outwardly, resulting in less need for (time consuming) suction compared to the other position;

The disadvantages are, however:

- risk for pulmonary air embolism: given the 10% chance for unknown patency of the cardiac oval foramen, there is even risk for air embolism in the cerebral circulation;
- sagging of the cerebellum, which needs retractor support;
- risk for cardiovascular instability during positioning; transverse cord lesions have been described;
- need for postoperative sitting position in the ICU for the first hours, with slow adaptation towards a more supine nursing position;
- fatigue for the surgeon in long lasting procedures, with his/her arms more stretched due to the longer working distance, depending on the building of the microscope (less angulation of the oculars on the microscope body).

The disadvantages can be overcome, when there is a strong preference for this position, related to the pathology to be treated. The following measures should be taken [1, 3, 4]:

- stockings or even G-suit for the legs;
- preoperative work-up to exclude a patent oval foramen;

- precardiac transthoracic Doppler probe, or, even better, transoesophageal cardiac Doppler equipment in place;
- intra-atrial catheter for immediate suction when air embolism is detected;
- pCO_2 measurement in the outflow channel of the ventilation tube is standard for anesthesia, but should get extra attention;
- good access to cervical area, in order to allow for jugular vein compression when air embolism occurs;
- alertness of the surgeon for any suspicion of air embolism, especially during the opening and closure: active communication with the anaesthetist, extensive and continuous irrigation of the surgical field, careful coagulation, and excessive waxing of all bony structures and rims.

It is clear that the sitting procedure adds risks to the surgery in the posterior fossa. Therefore, this position should only be used by an experienced team, that performs surgery in this position on a regular basis. It is only justified when the advantage outweighs the risks, as for example in the supracerebellar infratentorial approach to the pineal or tectal area.

2. STEPWISE PROCEDURES [5, 6, 8]

2.1 Midline approach

This procedure can be performed in the prone and in the sitting position.

Procedure after positioning, fixation, mounting electrodes for monitoring, and draping:

- Midline skin incision, from 2 cm above the external protuberance, to the palpable spinous process of C2.
- Loosening the skin from the underlying periost and muscle fascia for about 0.5 cm, important for easy closure.
- Continuation of midline incision with monopolar cutting and coagulation needle device; in the sitting position even more care is taken to coagulate any little vessel, under lots of irrigation and with regular jugular compression in the neck, see paragraph on sitting position. In the upper and lower part of the incision, the midline can be found and followed very easily, which helps in finding the right place in and underneath the fascia to separate the muscle bundles on both sides of the midline.
- The periost of the occipital bone is scraped to both sides, with the muscles attached. For a very large opening to both sides, it may be preferable to cut the muscles horizontally on both sides (0.5 cm caudally from their attachment, for better closure), but in my experience

this is hardly ever necessary with a fine linear midline incision that goes up highly enough.

- The extra cranial muscle work is finalized by freeing the upper part of the C2 spinous process, then coming to the atlas, from below and from above, and subsequently scraping the periost from the back of the atlas to both sides, beginning in the midline. This last part is done with knife and scissors, followed by sharp small dissector, in order to avoid inadvertent damage to dura and/or vertebral artery so easily done with the cutting needle!
- Once enough of the occipital bone and the atlas is freed, visible and accessible, definite retractors are placed. However, during the microscopical part of the surgery these retractors may form obstacles for smoothly bringing in and out microsurgical instruments. Therefore, we prefer to retract the muscles with sutures connected to rubber bands, or any type of fish hooks. So, the operation field is as flat as possible, making the surgery easier.
- The next step is the bone work. Decision on which technique to use is determined by age and local anatomical features. In children, and adults with a rather flat occipital bone, we make two burr holes on either side of the midline, just under the presumed position of the underlying transverse sinus. The holes are connected by drilling with a small burr head, and then the bone is cut from the burr holes caudally in a curved way using the craniotome. This is an osteoplastic technique, allowing for replacement of the bone at the end of surgery.
- In adults with thick bone, and/or irregularities, as well as in cases where the above technique encounters some (adhesion) problems, we use again the two burr holes, but continue with the Leksell rongueur. A piecemeal (osteoclastic) removal of the occipital bone results, more time consuming but sometimes safer than the method described before.
- Once the dura has been freed, one has to decide whether the opening is wide enough: for high located lesions it is mandatory to remove the bone until the first 3–5 mm of the transverse sinus are visible, allowing for better dural retraction upwards. In cases with significant mass lesions, and subsequent chance of already existing tonsillar herniation, the atlas should be removed in its middle 2–2.5 cm, upfront, before the dura is opened.
- Classically, one might prepare for a supratentorial burr hole, in order to have access to the ventricle for tapping CSF. In my experience I have hardly ever needed such an access: either the patient had already some CSF diversion because of a clinical emergency situation preoperatively, or the intraoperative situation could be easily handled by some table tilt or anaesthesiological measures, followed by rapid opening of one of the suboccipital cisterns as soon as the dura was opened.

- The next step is dural opening. The classical Y opening over both hemispheres, with the "long leg" of the Y in the midline as far down as necessary (so even to the upper rim of C2), is still my favourite. However, in some 10% of the cases, the midline dura contains ("hides") a sinusoidal remnant, the occipital sinus. The surgeon should be prepared to encounter this venous conduit. There are several methods to solve the problem: the incision can be made more lateral, parallel, with a straight crossing at the higher point of the sinus and suturing it at both sides of the cut; or stepwise opening and suturing – or clipping with hemoclips – can be performed, with some additional bipolar coagulation. The latter method is especially preferable when that sinus is rather wide, which is sometimes the case.
- Adjuvant dural incisions towards the lateral side, more caudally starting from the Y's long leg, may be helpful for a maximal overview.
- Since this approach is primarily chosen for midline or near midline pathology, the next step is to identify the fourth ventricle. The classical splitting of the vermis is not necessary in most cases: careful preparation (from now on under microscopic magnification) of the arachnoid, in particular between cerebellar hemisphere and vermis, allows lifting of the caudal end of the vermis. When more space is wanted, a subtle splitting of the velum medullare posterius on one side is sufficient in most cases. For further details of handling the intradural pathology one should read the chapters dedicated to these.
- Closure is done very carefully. The arachnoid cannot always be closed separately, which is less important here than for example in the spinal cord region. But the dura should be closed as watertight as possible, without causing compression. The latter might be the case when there is swelling of the cerebellum after removal of only relatively small pathology. In such a situation, a duroplasty should be performed, preferably with natural material: fascia from within the operative field, or even fascia lata, for which access should have been prepared in the draping procedure. There are many commercial products now for dural replacement, which may work fine. In our experience, body's own material still works best! Of course such closure may be supported by fibrin glue sealing. The latter never resists a real CSF outflow under a certain pressure, though!
- Replacement of bone, over an epidural gelatine layer or other haemostatic material, may be helpful in controlling haemostasis, but is not absolutely necessary. We never fixate the bone, but use it only as a support between the layers.
- The deep and superficial muscles can be approximated in two layers, over which the fascia should be closed separately in a tight fashion. Here the advantage of the subcutaneous loosening at the beginning becomes obvious, resulting in more freedom for handling this closure.

- Next, subcutis and skin are closed, with interrupted and a running suture, respectively. A drain is placed only rarely, and should never replace careful haemostasis!
- A tight (compressing) bandage is hardly possible in this area, and actually not necessary.
- It should be stressed once more that in the sitting position the closure can be more time consuming, with again attention for any kind of venous openings (jugular compression, waxing the bone etc.).
- When surgery was performed in the prone position, the patient is turned supine while still intubated, well ventilated in this new position and only extubated thereafter. After a sitting position procedure, the patient should be awakened and extubated in the sitting position. Then, postoperative surveillance in the ICU should be with the patient sitting, slowly (over many hours) changing towards a supine situation.

2.2 Variants of the midline approach

For a so-called far lateral approach, we use also the prone position. After full exposure, the table (with the patient well fixated to it) may be tilted and/or turned as far as necessary and acceptable.

- The procedure starts as the standard midline opening, but the skin incision turns to one side at its upper extension, bending just behind the mastoid process, and ending there. This is called a hockey-stick incision.
- After undermining the skin a little, the muscle layers are cut with the diathermic needle, at the upper rim just under the attachment to the nuchal line on one side. Skin and muscles are detached from the bone in one layer, with a sharp dissector and diathermia.
- Retraction is done again with fish hooks and/or sutures with rubber bands.
- Now the occipital bone should be visible from a little over the midline, to one side with exposure of the lateral mastoid. Caudally the rim of the foramen is exposed, low laterally the digastric groove and the occipital part of the condyle. The atlas is freed as was described before, but more to one side, where it forms the atlanto-occipital joint.
- The resulting working space allows for more bone removal laterally, as far as is found necessary for the specific surgery at hand.
- Bone work is done as described before; special handling of the vertebral artery, freeing it from C2 and C1, can be part of this procedure.
- The dural incision is now over one cerebellar hemisphere ending in the cervical area just above C2; a separate incision reaches as far later-

ally as possible, allowing for triangular dural flaps and a wide opening over the lateral medulla.
- Closure is straightforward and follows the same principles as described before.

2.3 Retromastoid craniotomy/craniectomy

With a well performed retromastoid approach one can access the whole lateral part of the posterior fossa, from the foramen magnum caudally to the hiatus tentorii cranially. We use it for all pontine angle tumors, petroclival tumors, neurovascular compression syndromes, lateral pontine pathologies, and VA and PICA pathology (f.e. aneurysms).

We position the patients mostly supine with shoulder support and rotation of the head fixed in a Mayfield clamp (see before).

Stepwise procedure for retromastoid approach:

- After positioning and mounting of electrodes for monitoring (when appropriate), shaving, prepping and draping, an incision is made, starting 1.5 cm above and behind the upper ear, following the curvature of the ear and ending some 2 cm under and behind the palpable mastoid process.
- The skin is undermined in its upper part (for easy closure), then fascia-periost and muscles are cut by monopolar needle diathermia. The occipital artery is always encountered and needs careful coagulation and cutting.
- Sharp dissection of the muscles from the bone – with some emissaria veins to be controlled with bone wax – results in a bony area of 4 × 4 cm, which of course can be modified and enlarged in one direction or the other.
- Laterally, the first cm of the mastoid should be visible, as well the digatric groove behind and caudally to it. We free the bone till it shows the horizontal (= vertical in this position!) plane, the lowest part of the lateral occipital bone.
- Retraction is done with fish hooks and sutures with rubber bands, resulting in a flat operation field.
- We generally start with one burr hole in the upper part of the bone exposure, which is always near or on the transverse sinus. We never feel the necessity for neuronavigation at this stage.
- Depending on the thickness of the bone, we now make a flap with two curved lines, using the craniotome and starting from the burr hole. If that is awkward and difficult, we drill part of the outer layer of the bone and use rongueurs, turning a planned craniotomy into a craniectomy; bone pieces and bone dust are saved in order to be used at closure.
- The bone opening is widened with some drilling or rongueurs to such an extent that the transverse and sigmoid sinuses are visible for at least

3 mm at the edges of the craniotomy. This allows for better retraction of the dura.

- Two problems are always encountered, but can be handled easily: the major emissaria vein in this area comes from the upper sigmoid sinus; it can be coagulated, but sometimes a small tear is unavoidable which can be covered by some haemostatic agent (surgicel, gelfoam). Furthermore, some mastoid air cells are almost always opened when adequate bony exposure is pursued. These air cells should be covered and closed very carefully with bone wax. We do it always before opening of the dura, and again after its closure.
- Because of the drilling, the operative field may have become quite dusty by now! Irrigation and additional draping is very adequate for providing a nice surgical field.
- The dura is opened. For most pathologies we do this with a standard order of incisions: first, a straight incision in the middle of the exposed dura, parallel to the mastoid. From there a triangular flap is prepared caudally, by two cuts.
- At this time, the smallest retractor or dissector is used to lift the caudal cerebellum and reach for the lateral cerebellomedullary cistern. Optimal access is obtained when the bony opening has indeed reached the flat part of the occipital bone. CSF comes out, sometimes after some minimal arachnoid perforation with a forceps. Waiting and draining carefully allows the cerebellum to sink adequately, after which no retractor is needed anymore for the rest of the procedure.
- Now the last dural opening is made with two cuts to the upper part, resulting in an upper dural triangle, based on the transverse sinus. The trapezoidal dural flap that is based on the sigmoid sinus is now tagged with two sutures as far laterally as possible; the triangular flaps may be tagged as well.
- The more medial part of the dura, as well as the cerebellum, are covered with thin gelfoam.
- The microsurgical part of the procedure should start now: lateral from the already fallen down cerebellum the arachnoid cisterns are reached. They are opened on purpose, after which more CSF can be drained and adequate exposure of the pathology at hand is obtained. See again the dedicated chapters.
- Closure starts with running sutures for dural closure; many times this seems inadequate in the beginning, but after a first run, additional suturing will bring the dural rims together in most cases.
- Pieces of muscle or gelfoam in fibrin glue may help finalize a watertight closure.
- The bony rims and opened mastoid cells are waxed again. The epidural surface is covered by thin layers of gelfoam, on which the bone, bony pieces and/or bone dust is applied.

- Muscle layer are adapted, after which a tight closure of the fascia takes place. Here, especially at the upper part of the incision, the subcutaneous preparation payes off, enabling a watertight closure of the fascia.
- The subcutaneous tissue is adapted with 3–4 stitches, and the skin is closed with a running suture.
- No drains are necessary, a simple skin drape is used, over which a compressive bandage is applied for 3 days.

2.4 Variation: the paramedian approach

For some pathologies that are located strictly in one cerebellar hemisphere, the surgeon might want to use an "intermediate approach", which is between the midline and the retromastoid (lateral) approach. The difference with the retromastoid is a more straight incision, parallel to it and halfway the midline and the mastoid area. There is no necessity to go so caudally in that approach, and the procedure is literally straight forward, allowing for an adequate opening of just a part of the lateral half of the occipital bone. It is not felt necessary to analyse such an approach again in a stepwise fashion.

HOW TO AVOID COMPLICATIONS

The most frequent complications of the approaches to the posterior fossa as such are:

- infection
- haematoma
- CSF leakage subcutaneously
- CSF leakage to oropharynx through mastoid and middle ear
- air embolism.

Infection prevention is pursued by meticulous sterility, avoiding necrosis by too heavy coagulation, and perioperative broad spectrum antibiotics (cephalosporine), a bolus before skin incision, and at 3 and 6 hours, when surgery takes that long.

Haematomas should be prevented by careful haemostasis, blood pressure control, and awareness of preoperative coagulation status of the patient (history, medication).

CSF leakage can occur intradurally, through the internal meatus when this is drilled open (in acoustic neuroma surgery); but more frequently, and related to any posterior fossa approach, by a not watertight dural closure. CSF can leak to the subcutaneous area only, or even come out through the skin. Or it can find its way through the opened and insufficiently waxed mastoid cells, given rise to rhinorrhoea.

As said before, avoidance is by optimal closure of dura and mastoid cells; or by plugging the internal meatus. In some 10% of cases even in the most experienced hands some CSF leakage occurs. Prompt treatment by a lumbar external CSF drain for some 3–5 days is generally adequate, and in case of significant subcutaneous CSF collections, by concomitant puncture of that and installment of a blood patch. We have used the latter only very seldom, though.

The problem of *air embolism* is already discussed before, in the paragraph on the sitting position. By adequate preparation of the patient, the installation of the right equipment (catheters, Doppler probes), and awareness of the risks by surgeon, anaesthetist and personnel, air embolism cannot be prevented in every case, but the sequaelae can and should be reduced to a safe minimum.

References

[1] Cucchiara RF, Black S (1993) Anesthetic considerations. In: Apuzzo MLJ (ed) Brain surgery: complication avoidance and management. Churchill Livingstone, New York, pp 1597-1608

[2] Goodkin R, Mesiwala A (2004) General principles of operative positioning. In: Winn HR (ed) Youmans neurological surgery, 5th edn, vol I. Saunders, Philadelphia, pp 595-621

[3] Hodge CJ, Primrose D (1993) Physiological considerations. In: Apuzzo MLJ (ed) Brain surgery: complication avoidance and management. Churchill Livingstone, New York, pp 1569-1596

[4] Leonard IE, Cunningham AJ (2002) The sitting position in neurosurgery – not yet obsolete! Editorial. BJA 88: 1-4

[5] Mohsenipour I, Goldhahn W-E, Fischer J, Platzer W, Pomaroli A (1994) Approaches in neurosurgery. Georg Thieme, Stuttgart, pp 107-125

[6] Seeger W (1978) Atlas of topographical anatomy of the brain and surrounding structures. Springer, Wien New York, pp 428-435, figs 205-258

[7] Tew JM, Scodary J (1993) Surgical positioning. In: Apuzzo MLJ (ed) Brain surgery: complication avoidance and management. Churchill Livingstone, New York, pp 1609-1620

[8] Yaşargil MG (1996) Microneurosurgery, IVB microneurosurgery of CNS tumors. Georg Thieme, Stuttgart, pp 58-65

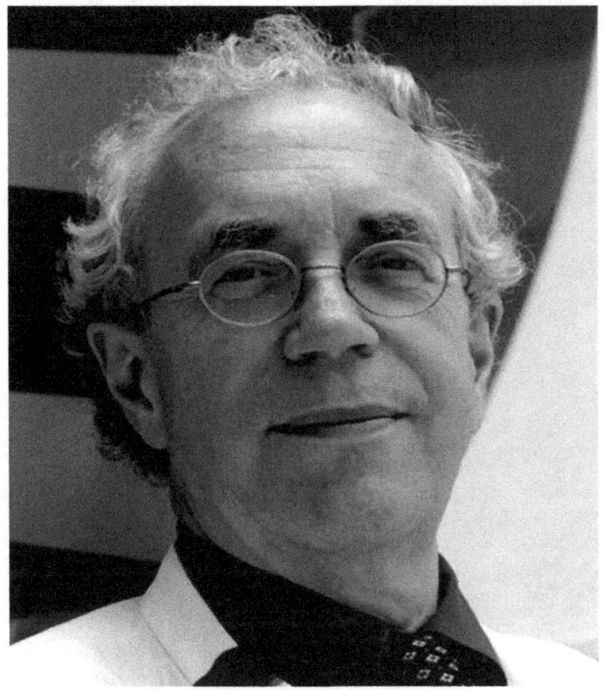

Jan Jakob A. Mooij

Jan Jakob A. Mooij is Professor and Chairman at the Department of Neurosurgery, University Hospital, UMCG Groningen. Born in 1945. After his medical education at the State University of Groningen, PhD programme in Neuropharmacology, thesis in 1976. Training in Neurosurgery, at Groningen University, Dept. of Neurosurgery (with Prof. Dr. J. W. F. Beks). Assistance residency training at the Department of Neurosurgery in Zürich with Prof Dr. G. Yaşargil (1982). Junior staff neurosurgeon at Dept. of Neurosurgery, University of Amsterdam, 1982. Returning to Groningen end of 1982. Assistant Professor from 1987 onwards. Neurosurgical observer and research fellow at Barrow Neurological Institute, Phoenix (AZ), U.S.A. (Prof. Dr. R.F. Spetzler) 1992. Chairman of Dept. of Neurosurgery, University Hospital Groningen, since 1993. Training Committee EANS, member 1997–2003, chairman 2003–2007, vice-president 2007–. Main interests: aneurysm surgery, neuro-oncology, neurovascular compression syndromes, training and education in neurosurgery.

Contact: Jan Jakob A. Mooij, Department of Neurosurgery, University Hospital UMCG Groningen, Hanzeplein 1, 9713 GZ Groningen, The Netherlands
E-mail: j.j.a.mooij@nchir.umcg.nl

HOW TO PERFORM TRANSPETROSAL APPROACHES

T. KAWASE

INTRODUCTION

The middle fossa transpetrosal approach was originally developed by King in 1970, and so-called "extended middle fossa approach", which was combined with middle fossa craniotomy and translabyrinthine approach [6]. The method was mainly applied to acoustic tumors, but it was indicated to clival lesions by Hakuba et al. [2].

An advantage of this approach is low risk of cerebellar damage to access more laterally to the brain stem. The disadvantages were sacrifice of hearing and venous complication (venous thrombosis of vein of Labbe and sigmoid sinus). Al-Mefty used this approach for more number of the petroclival meningiomas, by preservation of acoustic structures (posterior transpetrosal approach) [1]. In 1985 and 1994, Kawase reported the anterior transpetrosal approach for basilar trunk aneurysms and petroclival meningiomas by selected resection of petrous apex [3–5]. The clival lesions were accessed by the shortest way to the area anterior to the internal auditory meatus (IAM) without sacrifice their hearing. In this chapter the anterior and posterior transpetrosal approaches are described.

DECISION-MAKING

The anterior transpetrosal approach (ATP) is indicated for petroclival or prepontine lesions, such as meningiomas, chordomas or epidermoids. It is absolutely indicated for petroclival tumors showing extention into the middle fossa and Meckel's cave, such as dummbell type trigeminal neurinomas, or petroclival meningiomas showing middle fossa extension. Prepontime epidermoids over the midline or with supratentorial extension are indicated for this approach. Basilar trunk aneurysms or low positioned basilar top aneurysms are indicated for clipping by this approach. The maximal surgical field is limited in the area of foramen ovale anteriorly, oculomotor nerve superiorly, mid clivus inferiorly, internal auditory meatus posteriorly and contralateral abducens nerve medially (Fig. 1A).

Keywords: skull base tumors, transpetrosal approaches, minimal-invasive neurosurgery

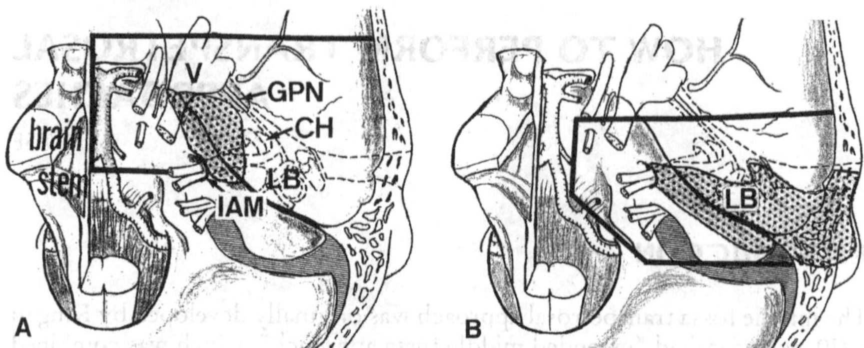

Fig. 1. A Anterior transpetrosal approach. **B** Posterior transpetrosal approach. Site of pyramid resection (dotted) and the surgical field (broad line). *GPN* Greater petrosal nerve, *CH* cochlea, *LB* labyrinth, *IAM* internal auditory meatus, *V* trigeminal nerve

The posterior transpetrosal approach (PTP) is indicated for large cerebellopontine angle (CPA) tumors such as meningiomas, or vestibular schwannomas (Fig. 1B). By combination with the ATP (combined petrosal approach), it can be indicated for large petroclival meningiomas extending posterior to the internal auditory meatus.

Patient's hearing can be preserved in the patient whose semicircular canals be preserved by otological technique.

Compared to the lateral suboccipital approach, the benefits are as follows: (a) No retraction damage to the cerebellum and cranial nerves from VII to XI, (b) easy access to the tumor extended into the middle fossa and Meckel cave, (c) dried surgical field during tumor removal by devascularization of tumor feeders of middle meningeal and tentorial arteries, (d) no surgical blindness to anterior brain stem and basilar artery. The disadvantage is a surgical limitation to the lower clivus and jugular area.

Compared to the subtemporal-transtentorial approach, the benefits are as follows: (a) lower risk of injury to the temporal bridging veins by the epidural access, (b) deeper observation below the trigeminal nerve. The disadvantage is longer operation time for resection of the pyramid.

SURGERY

1. SURGICAL INSTRUMENTS AND PREOPERATIVE PREPARATION

Sugita's hooked retractors and tumor retractors (Mizuho-Ika Co., Tokyo, Japan), surgical drill with twist tips of 5 and 3 mm in diameter and with a diamond tip of 2 mm, ultrasonic aspirator and evoked-potential monitoring system.

A spinal drainage tube is inserted before surgery. For large tumors with presumed risk of herniation, a ventricular drainage tube is inserted in the trigone, instead of the spinal drain.

2. OPERATIVE TECHNIQUES AND HOW TO AVOID COMPLICATIONS

2.1 Anterior transpetrosal approach

The patient is positioned in supine with a shoulder pillow, and the head is fixed completely laterally with slight vertex down.

1) Craniotomy. After scalp incision above the auricule, the temporalis fascia, which is used for closure, is dissected from the muscle with its pedicule inferiorly. The temporalis muscle is reflected anteriorly. Root of zygoma, external auditory meatus, and squamous suture are confirmed for orientation of the craniotomy site. The craniotomy is made along the squamous suture with 3 burr holes (Fig. 2). The inferior margin is drilled until the bone window is flushed to the floor of the middle fossa.
2) Exposure and resection of petrous apex. Dura mater is dissected and elevated from the temporal bone, using hooked retractors after drainage of cerebrospinal fluid. Anatomically important points, such as arcuate eminence, petrous ridge, foramen spinosum are confirmed. The middle meningeal artery (MMA) is coagulated and cut. The periosteal dura, adhesive to the greater superficial petrosal nerve (GSPN), is cut to preserve the nerve (Fig. 3A). Epidural venous bleeding around

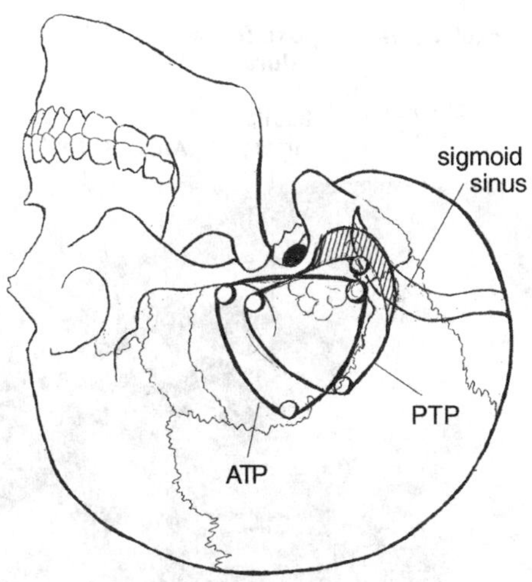

Fig. 2. Craniotomy site. *ATP* Anterior transpetrosal approach, *PTP* posterior transpetrosal approach, with partial mastoidectomy (shaded)

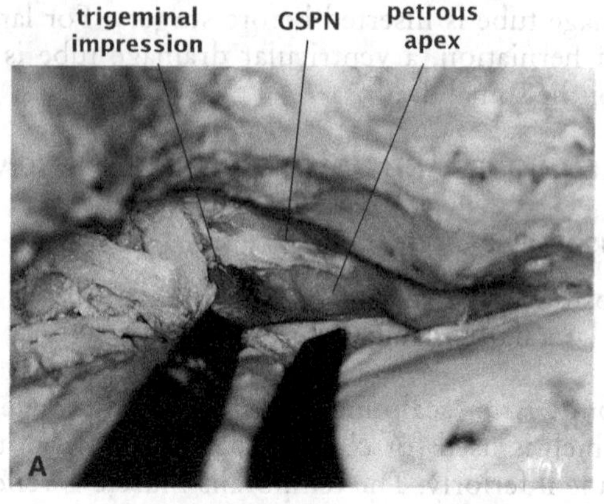
trigeminal impression
GSPN
petrous apex
A

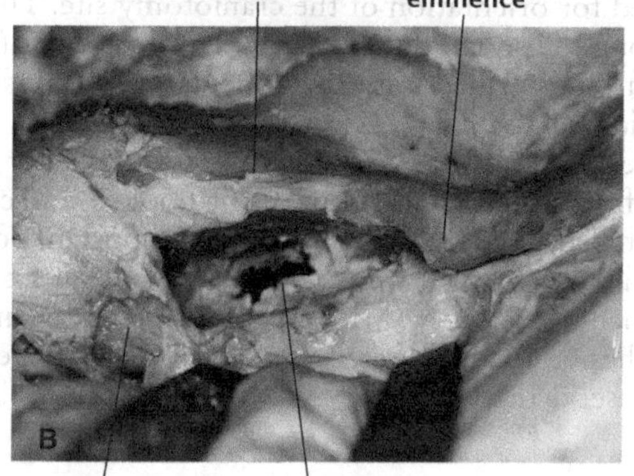
GSPN
arcuate eminence
B
Meckel's cave
post. fossa dura

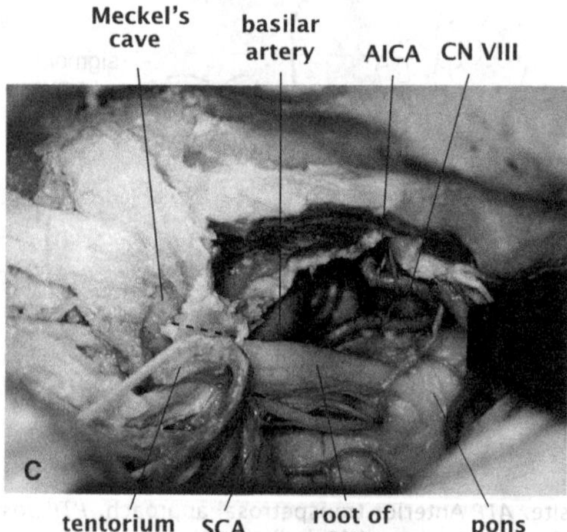
Meckel's cave
basilar artery
AICA
CN VIII
C
tentorium
SCA
root of CN V
pons

MMA is controlled by head up position and insertion of surgicel balls.

3) Lateral margin of the drilling is delineated medial to the GSPN and arcuate eminence. The triangular bone is resected until the posterior fossa dura is confirmed (Fig. 3B). The carotid artery and auditory structures are not exposed within the space. Take care not to break dural bulging of the internal auditory meatus (IAM) located postero-inferior margin of the triangle, and not to resect the bone above the geniculate ganglion of the facial nerve, located superficially on an extension line of the GSPN, to spare injury of the facial nerve. Overdrilling toward clivus may injure the abducens nerve in Dorello's canal.
4) Dural incision. Incision of the middle fossa dura is started from 2 cm lateral to the superior petrosal sinus (SPS), and extended in T shape along the SPS. After incision of the dura on the posterior fossa, the SPS is ligated with suture twice and incised. Incision of the tentorium is extended until the tentorium is cut completely. Take care not to injure the trochlear nerve at the tentorial notch. Both sides of the tentorial leaflets are reflected and retracted with tapered retractor, then the tumor and root of the trigeminal nerve are exposed (Fig. 3C). The course of the trigeminal nerve varies depending to the tumor origin.
5) Opening Meckel's cave and detachment of feeders from the Orifice of Meckel's cave, where the trigeminal nerve enters, is confirmed and incised anteriorly for 1 cm along the superior margin of the nerve, then the trigeminal nerve can be mobilized. The tumor in Meckel's cave is removed. The main tumor feeders originated from the tentorial artery are commonly located medial to the orifice of Meckel's cave. They are coagulated after the trigeminal nerve is mobilized inferiorly.
6) Removal of the tumor. Internal tumor decompression can be made using ultrasonic aspirator, without active bleeding from the tumor. The tumor attachment is gradually detached from the duramater. Margin of the tumor is retracted toward the tumor base with a tumor retractor, then the cranial nerves and arteries engulfed in the tumor appear in the surgical field. The tumor retraction makes dissection of cranial nerves and vessels easier, by increasing the peritumoral space and decreasing their overstretching. Possibility of the retraction technique may be one of the advantages of this approach (Fig. 4). Even if the tumor bulk is larger than the surgical field, it can be removed safely by this technique.

   The abducens nerve, courses medial to the tumor, must be cared and separated from the tumor.

Fig. 3. A Right pyramid is exposed epidurally (cadaver). Greater superficial petrosal nerve (*GSPN*) is preserved by periosteal dura remaining on it. Trigeminal nerve is exposed for anatomical understanding. **B** Resection of petrous apex is medial to GSPN and arcuate eminence. **C** After incision of the dura and tentorium. The basilar trunk is seen. Trigeminal nerve can be mobilized by cutting the dura on the cave (dotted)

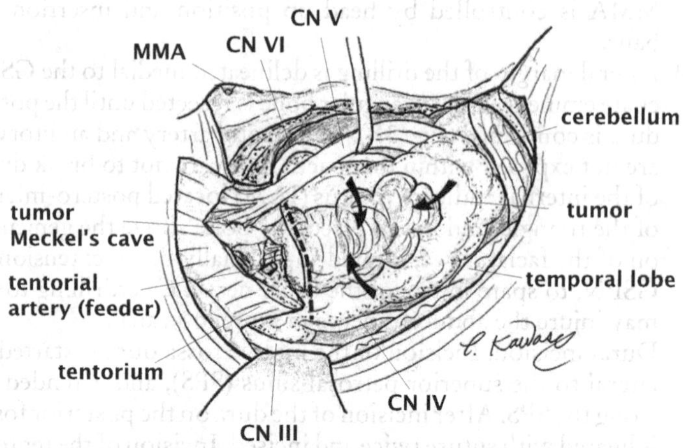

Fig. 4. Surgical illustration of right ATP. The tumor feeder (tentorial artery) is cut and trigeminal nerve is mobilized from the tumor. The tumor is decompressed and retracted toward the tumor attachment

Presence or absence of encased brain stem perforators and tumor invasion into the cavernous sinus may influence on the tumor radicality. In case of perforator encasement, the tumor surface must be remained in 2–3 mm thickness. Amputation of the tentorial leaflets may increase the tumor radicality.

7) Closure of the dura is not possible, and CSF leakage is prevented by following double barrier technique:

   (a) A piece of abdominal fat is transplanted on the exposed air cells of the pyramid and craniotomy and fixed with fibrin glue.
   (b) The fat is wrapped with a pediculed temporalis fascia and the fascia is sutured with dura mater. Accumulated subdural air is removed to prevent pneumocephalus. The bone flap is replaced and fixed with titanium plates. Artificial bone is not necessary. A subcutaneous drain is inserted. The spinal drain tube is kept for a few days for emergency drainage in a case of CSF rhinorrhea.

2.2 Posterior transpetrosal approach

The patient is positioned laterally with the head rotated 20° prone. The upper body is elevated 20° to decrease venous congestion.

1) Craniotomy. A U-shaped scalp incision is made around auricule preserving a perocranial flap underneath. The craniotomy is made more posterior to that of the ATP, and partial mastoidectomy is made by drill thereafter until the sigmoid sinus is exposed (Fig. 5).
2) Petrosectomy. Mastoid air cells are drilled out until the antrum is opened. By further bone resection antero-medially the surgeon will

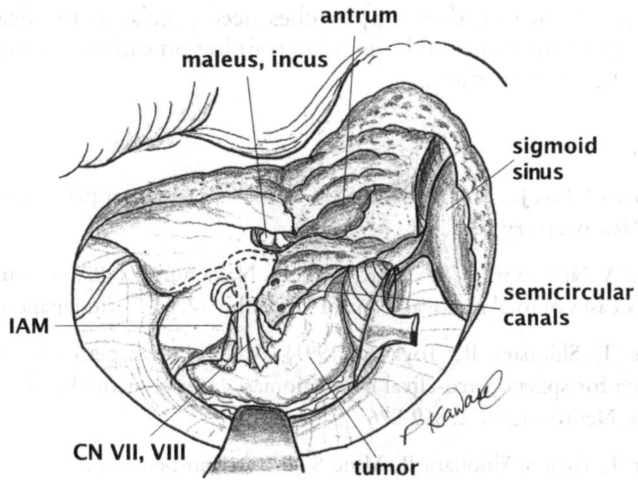

Fig. 5. Surgical illustration of cerebello-pontine angle tumor operated by PTP

meet a consistent bone which contains auricular organs, semicircular canal and labyrinth. Hearing preservation is depending on the resection of the organic bone or not. Location of the IAM is suspected medial to the anterior semicircular canal. It is safer to open the posterior wall and superior wall second to spare injury to the facial nerve. Never open the funds of IAM because the facial nerve courses superficially at this point. It is medial to the maleus, and the tympanic cavity can be opened to find the maleus.

3) Dural incision and tumor exposure. Method of the dural incision is similar to that of the ATP. The tentorial incision is made on the IAM, after double ligation of the superior petrosal sinus.

   In the vestibular neurinomas, the facial nerve is widened and stretched. It commonly course on the anterior surface of the tumor being identified by the facila monitoring. In the case of CPA meningiomas, it is not rare to preserve hearing, and the auditory monitoring (ABR) should be prepared.

4) Closure. Even by using two layers, abdominal fat and pericranial flap, complete closure of CSF leakage cannot be achieved, and a small piece of fat is inserted in the orifice of Eustachian tube, located anterior to the maleus.

CONCLUSIONS

By the two types of the transpetrosal approach, petroclival and CPA tumors can be removed without over retraction of the cerebellum, brain stem and cranial nerves. However, those approaches need precise anatomical knowledge of the temporal bone, and operative training on cadaver is requested to the surgeon before operation.

References

[1] Al-Mefty O, Fox JL, Smith RR (1988) Petrosal approach for petroclival meningiomas. Neurosurgery 22: 510-517

[2] Hakuba A, Nishimura S, Tanaka K, Kishi H, Nakamura T (1977) Clivus meningioma: six cases of total removal. Neurol Med Chir 17: 63-77 (in Japanese)

[3] Kawase T, Shiobara R, Toya S (1991) Anterior transpetrosal-transtentorial approach for sphenopetro-clival meningiomas: surgical method and results in 10 patients. Neurosurgery 2: 869-876

[4] Kawase T, Toya S, Shiobara R, Mine S (1985) Transpetrosal approach for aneurysms of the flower basilar artery. J Neurosurg 63: 857-867

[5] Kawase T, Shiobara R, Ohira T, Kanzaki J, Toya S (1996) Developmental patterns and symptoms of petroclival meningiomas. Neurol Med Chir 36: 1-6

[6] Shiobara R, Ohira T, Kanzaki J, Toya S (1989) A modified extended middle cranial fossa approach for acoustic nerve tumors. J Neurosurg 68: 358-365

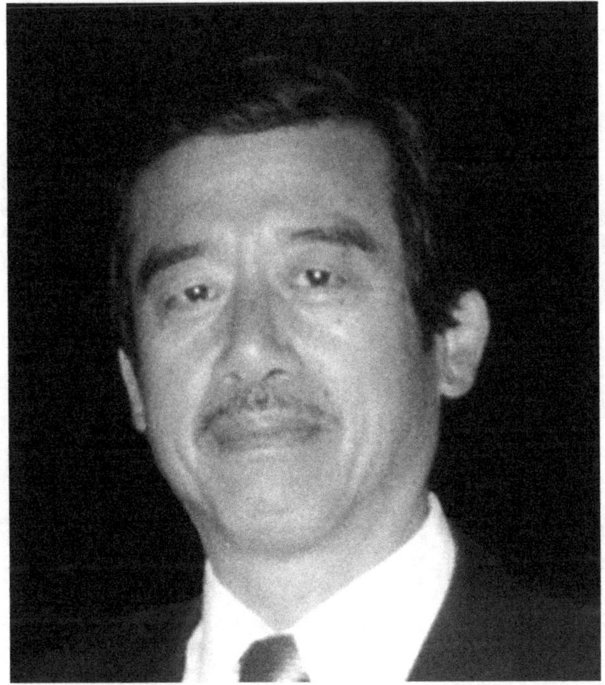

Takeshi Kawase

Takeshi Kawase is Professor and Chairman of the Department of Neurosurgery, School of Medicine, Keio University, Tokyo, Japan. He was born in Tokyo in 1944, is married and has two sons. 1970, graduate Keio University, Tokyo; 1977, neurosurgical board; 1978, oriented to cerebrovascular diseases at Mihara Memorial Hospital; 1983, oriented to skull base surgery at Keio University; 1990, assistant professor, Keio University; 1996, professor and chairman, Keio University; 2001–2003, vice president of Keio University Hospital; 2002, chairman of the WFNS Committee of Skull Base Surgery; 2005, president of the 64th Annual JNS Congress. His hobbies are drawing and outdoor sports such as mountaineering, skiing, sailing, driving, and golf.

Contact: Takeshi Kawase, Department of Neurosurgery, School of Medicine, Keio University, 35 Shinanomachi, Shinjuku-ku, Tokyo 160-8582, Japan
E-mail: kawase@sc.itc keio.ac.jp

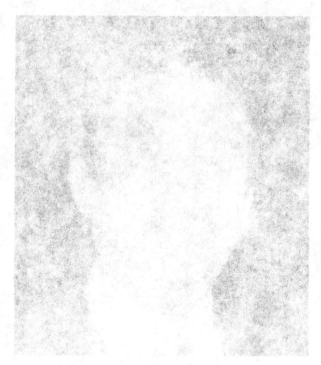

VASCULAR LESIONS

PRINCIPLES OF MICRONEUROSURGERY FOR SAFE AND FAST SURGERY

J. HERNESNIEMI

INTRODUCTION

Microneurosurgical anatomy and principles of microneurosurgery are the essence of neurosurgical training. Apart from basic theoretical knowledge, a competent neurosurgeon should be trained to be capable of operating in small and often narrow and deep gaps. Their aim should be to perform minimally invasive procedures in almost bloodless fields. Prof. Yaşargil emphasized that profound knowledge of the microneurosurgical anatomy is acquired in cadaveric laboratories, and gentle handling of cerebral arteries and veins is acquired by performing microvascular anastomoses in rats and mice [11]. Both training facilities could be – admittedly with considerable effort – installed in many hospitals to support a variety of microsurgeons. However, cadaveric dissections may be deemed impossible for cultural, religious, economical, or other reasons (Fig. 1).

The training of residents is inevitably at odds with the precious operation room (OR) time better spent by senior neurosurgeons. Some senior neurosurgeons may wish to begin the operation, whereas in other practices, the residents routinely open under supervision. One learns to play violin only by playing. Watching the mentor's performance helps to create one's own mental framework on what is reasonable in the microneurosurgical anatomy of the skull and brain. The more one knows, the more one sees old and true wisdom. When one's own proprioception is forming, exchanging ideas and experience with others during training courses and visits is important – discussing and observing one's own videos are fruitful. Scrutinizing videos of experienced microsurgeons is extremely helpful; like a present to the younger generation [2]. And with recent technological advances it is even easier to obtain these multimedia training means online, when one is thousands of kilometers away.

This review of the basics is distilled from the Helsinki and Kuopio Neurosurgery practices in Finland, as well as from the author's experience of approximately 10,000 operations, and to encourage young neurosurgeons of the world – most of them working with limited resources – to continue to improve their microneurosurgical skills to best serve their patients.

Keywords: microneurosurgery, vascular malformations, aneurysms

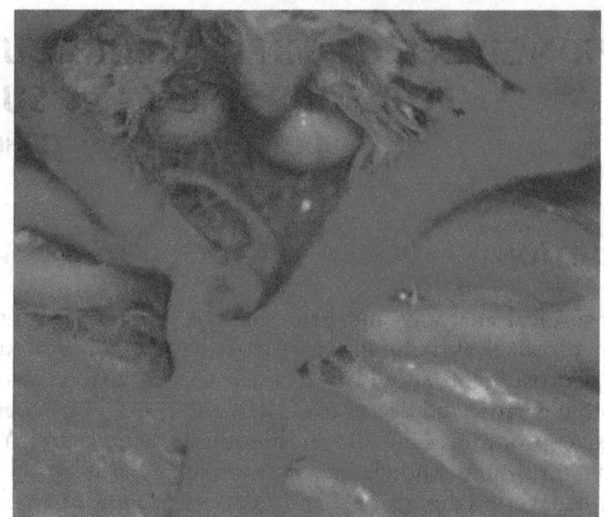

Fig. 1. A beautiful cadaveric microdissection view from the posterior part of Circle of Willis

OPERATION ROOM

Professional team work is an essential part of microneurosurgical operations. All the members of the operating team should be well-trained and able to work in harmony. The architecture and design of the OR should be based on maximum usage of space despite the technical equipment. Real-time images from the microscope, endoscope, and operation light camera in properly placed monitors allow the staff, residents, medical students, and visitors to appreciate the teamwork and follow the steps of the surgery. The atmosphere of the OR should support the conduct of the surgery. Traffic in and out, irrelevant talking, and unnecessary noises must be avoided. The neurosurgeons in action may prefer minimal talking, just exchanging a few words on the anatomy in hand, and encouraging words when difficulties are anticipated. Intraoperative music should suit the entire team (Fig. 2).

In the event of an emergency, such as aneurysm rupture, all action in the OR should calm down to support the neurosurgeons.

1. POSITIONING

Positioning is the first, and one of most important, steps in neurosurgical operations. Positioning of the patient should be planned by the surgeon, together with the other members of the team. Creating a comfortable and practical working positions for the neurosurgeons, anesthesiologist, and scrub nurse is of great importance. However, maximal moving ability for the oper-

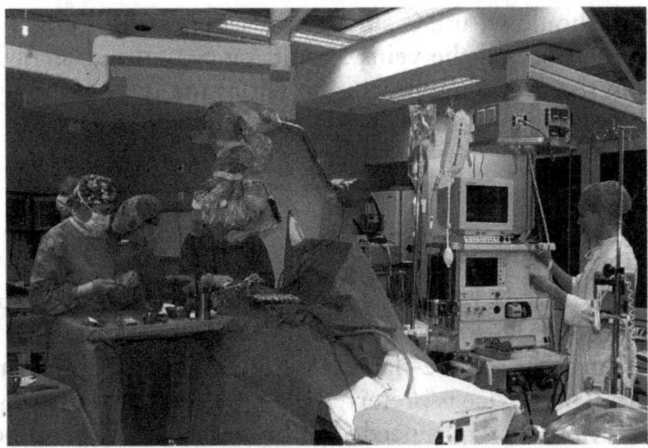

Fig. 2. General view of an operation room in the newly renovated operation theatre in Helsinki with more than 3000 yearly operations

ating neurosurgeon should always be kept in mind. Protection of the eyes, nose, ears, skin, extremities, nerves, blood vessels, and airways must be routine. All pressure areas and vulnerable nerve compression points should be protected with cushions and pads. To facilitate venous outflow and reduce venous blood pressure and, obviously, to prevent venous oozing, the author recommends the patient's head be elevated approximately 20 cm above the cardiac level. This principle is valid for most craniotomies, and is an effective way to have a clean and bloodless field. Accurately securing the patient's body and head provides the ability to quickly and safely tilt and/or rotate the operating table according to the surgeon's needs. The main principle in positioning of the head and body is to create a comfortable working angle (usually downward and somewhat forward) for the neurosurgeon. The head should be positioned so that gravitation helps to pull brain tissue away from the trajectory.

Positions used routinely in the practice of neurosurgery include supine, prone, semi-sitting, sitting, and lateral (park bench). However, these positions may be tailored and individualized for each patient, and according to localization and extent of the lesion and patient's medical status and general condition.

In the park-bench position for lateral posterior supratentorial and infratentorial approaches (used frequently by Dr. Drake), the upper shoulder is pulled away with strong adhesives to gain area, and spinal drainage (used routinely) helps produce a slack brain.

In the sitting position (e.g., in the supracerebellar infratentorial approach to the pineal region), the patient is secured by various cushions, the upper body by a vacuum cushion, and two fingers should fit between the manubrium and jaw to avoid too much flexion of the head. To prevent air embolism, the patient should wear a G suit at a pressure of 30–40 cm H_2O. Starting from the skin incision, all the veins should be coagulated meticulously and compression on the neck (jugular compression) may be a good way to demonstrate an open vein. Monitoring of the end-tidal CO_2 and Doppler is essential.

2. HEAD FIXATION

The patient's head should be fixed with three or four pins in a head frame. A Sugita head-fixation device is based on a four-pin fixation. It has the advantages of good skin and a muscle-flap-retraction system, as well as a system for brain retractors. This device is preferred in instances when a strong retraction of the skin-galea-muscle flap is needed or brain retractors are to be used. The Mayfield-Kees three-pin-head frame is more flexible with its one additional joint. This device is considered in the sitting, park-bench, and prone positions when linear skin incisions are used; here, a curved skin retractor is extremely useful.

No instruments or retractors should be constantly fixed immediately above the craniotomy, as they may accidentally cause injuries. Pin-fixation sites of the frames, as well as the arch and counter arch of the Sugita frame, should allow total access to the operative field and not prevent free movements of the neurosurgeon's hands, instruments, or the operating microscope. The position of the head should not compromise the arterial and venous flow in the neck. The head should not be turned too much, the cervical spine not positioned in extreme in any direction, and the trachea not overstretched or twisted. In temporal, parietal, and lateral occipital approaches, the park-bench position helps to avoid compression of the jugular veins. Fixation of the endotracheal tube by adhesives instead of a tape around the neck provides more safety during the positioning. After head fixation, further adjustments of the patient's position should be performed en bloc with the operation table.

3. NEUROSURGEON'S POSITION

After the patient is positioned and head and body fixed perfectly, the neurosurgeon should adjust his/her position continuously. To perform microneurosurgical operations in so-called "deep and narrow gaps," of vital importance is to have a good angle of vision. To have the maximum ability of being mobile around the operative field, the standing position is preferred by the author in majority of operations. The capability to use the mouthpiece effectively to focus and move the operation microscope to different directions should always be emphasized. Lifting or lowering and tilting of the operation table can provide further visual access to the operative field (Fig. 3). The neurosurgeon also may adjust the height by 3–4 cm by high-heeled clogs (by wearing them or not). Platforms are seldom necessary. Sitting might be more comfortable,

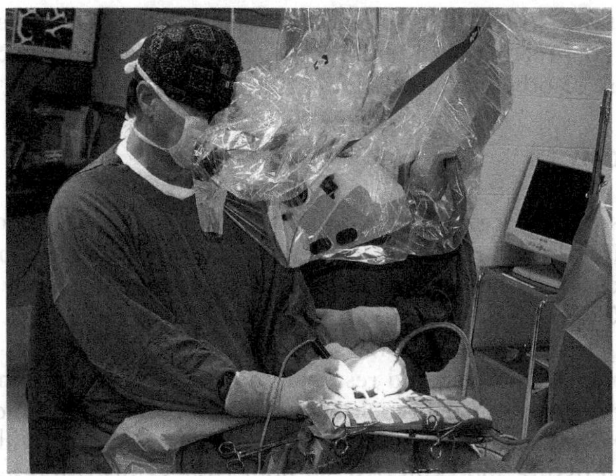

Fig. 3. Operating position preferred by the author. Using the mouthpiece to move the operating microscope, T-shape forearm support device and simultaneous performance of so-called "multifunctional right and left hands of the surgeon" are demonstrated

but reduces mobility. Sitting is preferable in certain instances; e.g., during the extracranial-intracranial bypass operations when the operative area is small and angle of vision does not have to be changed.

SURGERY

1. NAVIGATION

Preoperative planning and mental conduction of the entire procedure also should include ideas on unforeseen findings and occurrences – the art of dealing with them is achieved by experience. Cranial openings should be exactly placed and not larger than necessary, but sufficiently large to not endanger the safety of the operation. Neuronavigation is routine in many practices, and intraoperative imaging may become so in the future. However, it could be helpful to study the neuro-images carefully to identify landmarks such as the earlobes, coronal and lambdoid sutures, inion, sylvian fissure, central sulcus by the inverted omega hand area, confluens sinuum, straight and transverse sinuses, and others. However, neuro-navigators may not be available because they are too expensive for the institution. Quite frankly, to know neuroanatomy well is by far more important than to own and use a navigator. Careful measurements among the landmarks, the lesion and intended trajectory can usually be transferred to the scalp with acceptable accuracy. Many approaches, such as the opening to the cerebral aneurysms and most extraparenchymal brain tumors, are so dense with anatomical landmarks that no neuronavigation is needed, just operative experience. With experience, the surgeon can go directly to the cerebral aneurysm without widely opening the sylvian fissure or other structures [3, 7, 10].

2. CRANIOTOMY

The author's preference is to shave the scalp minimally and then wash and prepare it carefully. To reduce bleeding, infiltration of the incision line by a mixture of local anesthetic and vasoconstrictive agents is recommended. For more than 20 years, a single-layer flap is considered to be the most appropriate, especially for approaches to frontal and middle cranial fossae. This makes the procedure safe and fast, and results in no risks of temporal muscle atrophy or injury to the upper branch of the facial nerve. Furthermore, a good retraction system, such as Sugita frame fish hooks, provides a wide exposure of the sylvian fissure and skull base without large skull-base resections and, simultaneously, controls the scalp and muscle bleedings, which are swiftly dealt with by bipolar coagulation [3, 4].

It is possible to perform many craniotomies by only one burr hole and then to cut the bone flap with a craniotome. However, an additional burr hole may be necessary in the elderly in whom the dura can be adherent to the bone. A special curved dissector designed by our technician is useful for adequate dissection of dura. Detachment of the major dural sinuses can be achieved by placing the burr holes over them rather than laterally.

The author prefers high-speed electric microdrills because they are light, easy to use, fast, and safe. High-speed drilling is performed under the operating microscope. The burr is moved exactly by the right hand – some prefer both hands to avoid slipping – while controlled by proprioception, vision, and the right foot pedal. This interplay should be trained at cadaveric work. Important is to remove all coverings and cottonoids in and around the drilling area, as they can be caught by the drill and damage surrounding structures by windmill action. Only diamond-tipped burrs are used near eloquent structures. A bone-biting ultrasound aspirator is excellent for delicate removal of the skull base, and is safer than drilling.

Bleeding from the bone may be a problem while drilling. Drilling with diamond burrs without irrigation (hot drilling) controls such bleeding efficiently, but copious irrigation between drillings is necessary to avoid heat injury. Injection of fibrin glue or gelatin matrix–thrombin sealant also stops oozing. Injection of glue is the best and fastest way to stop some bleedings in the skull base or the cavernous sinus.

3. OPERATING MICROSCOPE

Stereoscopic vision, magnification, improved illumination, and counterweighted balance that allows the mouthpiece control constitute the essential assets of the present operating microscope. The neurosurgeon also should be familiar with the common types of mechanical and electrical failures of his/her preferred microscope. Counter-weighting provides an essentially weightless optic unit of the microscope that can be effortlessly, continuously, and quickly moved, adjusted, and focused with the mouthpiece, as was originally designed by Prof. Yaşargil. Mouthpiece control efficiently eliminates interruptions and liberates both hands for continuous operative work, which results in smoother conduct of surgery and reduced operation time (see Fig. 3). Insulated, electrical-heating cables around the oculars prevent fogging of the oculars – a truly helpful device. After removal of the bone flap, everything should be performed under the operation microscope, from the high-speed drilling of the bone to the last stitch of the skin. For the residents-in-training, closing the entire craniotomy under the operation microscope is the most efficient way to become familiar with the microscope. Several supporting features can be added to the present microscopes such as the image guidance and display over the operative field, or the fluorescence-based angiography and resection control. These costly additions, however, also increasingly require special technical skills in the OR to adjust and maintain the machinery.

4. MICROSURGICAL INSTRUMENTS

It should be emphasized again that a minimal array of microinstruments may reduce the number of instrument changes and operation time (Fig. 4). Some microinstruments have a single shaft (e.g., suction, dissectors), and others two

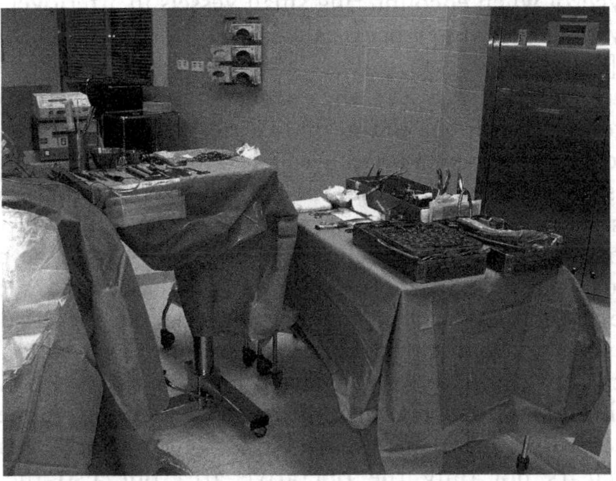

Fig. 4. Minimal array of microneurosurgical instruments reduces the number of changes and operation time

shafts (bipolar forceps and scissors), and also combined (Perneczky microinstruments). The bipolar forceps, suction, and dissector are the instruments used most frequently by most of the surgeons. The handle is designed to provide a steady and balanced grip. The two-shaft instruments, such as bipolar forceps and microscissors, are provided by a definite area to hold the instruments and control the opening and closure of the tips. The array of microinstruments should allow this hand position by various lengths such as very short, medium, long, and very long – more so with the two-shaft instruments. Fingertips should not obstruct the visual working channel. To minimize the fatigue and prevent the physiological tremor of the hands, use of mobile, bendable, and adjustable T-shaped forearm support designed by Prof. Yaşargil is highly recommended.

The bipolar forceps and suction are the multifunctional right and left hands of a right-handed neurosurgeon, respectively. The bipolar forceps can be used to dissect arachnoid planes, separate membranes, macerate tumor tissue inside solid tumors for suction, and even sharply cut glioma tissue when coagulation is applied. Malis forceps series are preferred by the author. These forceps are available in three to four different lengths, with two types of tips: sharp for delicate coagulation (Malis 20 or lower); and dissection and blunt for most of the work, stronger coagulation, manipulation of tumors, and coagulation of the aneurysm wall (Malis 25). Curved or angled-tip forceps are of assistance in awkward areas, such as the olfactory groove, or in cutting the tentorium or the falx. When coagulating small central nervous system vessels, it is important not to pinch them but to apply a delicate open-close and to-and-fro movement on the vessel trunk. This technique, together with the lowest effective coagulation power, copious irrigation, and careful cleaning of the tips by the scrub nurse, helps to prevent sticking of the tips. Swabbing the tips with glycerol when encountering small vessels in arteriovenous malformations may be helpful, and what is called "dirty coagulation" by using some brain tissue [8].

The suction is used for suction, retraction, and dissection. The distal shaft may gently retract the brain, cranial nerves, vessels, and aneurysms much more quickly than by adjusting self-retaining retractors. The strength of suction is controlled by sliding the thumb over the three holes in the handle. Mrs Dianne Yaşargil has introduced a suction tube pinch screw controlled by the scrub nurse. The OR staff also should be prepared to quickly adjust the strength of suction or run the second suction when needed. The suction tube should be of good-quality silicon rubber, light, and flexible so as not to disturb free movement of the left hand. Preferably, a set of suctions of three to four different lengths, each with two to three diameters, should be used. The tips of the suction should be checked regularly because drilling may cause sharp edges. The author's usual saying is: "irrigation clears not only the operative area but also the operator's mind."

5. COTTONOIDS

Cottonoids – or superior future materials – are used to protect the cortex and brain tissue, cranial nerves, arteries, and veins, in particular, when suction is applied. The dura is opened under the operating microscope with a cottonoid between the cortex and short scissors. Cottonoids can be used as soft expanders of the sylvian fissure or the interhemispheric space, or between the cortex and dura. Small ones serve as dissectors to separate small arteries from adjoining structures (e.g., in aneurysm, cavernoma, or meningioma surgery).

During tumor debulking, large ones support the walls of tumor cavity while preventing venous oozing by compression. To control bleeding from small arteries or veins, a cottonoid is placed over the vessel under the suction tip, which clears the field for coagulation by bipolar forceps tips. The author prefers those without identification threads, which require careful removal before closure. A cottonoid left unnoticed between the cortex and dura may cause reactive masses that resemble meningioma in neuroimaging.

6. OPENING OF THE ARACHNOID AND BRAIN RETRACTION

Much of microneurosurgical dissection is performed sharply. A circular, semi-sharp arachnoid blade, such as that introduced by Prof. Yaşargil, is used by many neurosurgeons. In our hands, a pair of short jeweler's forceps has proved to be efficient in opening the most superficial arachnoid membrane around a tumor or over the sylvian fissure. Dissection of the arachnoid cannot be performed without a perfect knowledge of cisternal anatomy [11].

Water-jet dissection, as first introduced by Dr. Toth in Budapest [9], is less known, but is the most elegant and inexpensive technique in microneurosurgery. First, the arachnoid is penetrated while viewing the venous anatomy. Then saline is injected repeatedly into the subarachnoid space of the fissural anatomy by a hand-held syringe to expand it more widely. Water dissection has been used safely and routinely in the opening of the sylvian fissure and interhemispheric space, as well as in dissection of meningiomas, cavernomas, metastases, abscess walls, and large and giant aneurysms in thousands of patients.

When the neurosurgeon is well-trained to use the suction and bipolar forceps for gentle retraction of the brain, no other retractors are needed. First, the bipolar forceps is retracting for the suction to release cerebrospinal fluid, and then the suction tip is mainly retracting to make space for the bipolar forceps and other instruments. In experienced hands, left- and right-hand instruments constantly and unconsciously change roles as microretractors, according to the demands of the microneurosurgical anatomy in the hand. By changing the retracting force between suction and forceps, one is going step-by-step (crawling), for example, under the frontal lobe. The bipolar forceps, when opened, can be used as a self-retaining retractor on the cortex protected by a cottonoid. Notably, the subtemporal approach toward a basilar tip aneurysm, for example, cannot be performed without self-retaining retractors and broad Aesculap-type retractors instead of the narrower Sugita-type retractors – the latter are preferred in other circumstances [4]. Brain injury caused by any retraction depends on the force, area of pressure, and time of exposure.

CONCLUSIONS

While appreciating our own neurosurgical performance, the following questions may come in mind: Who are the most capable of clipping cerebral artery aneurysms of our wives or husbands, or of removing craniopharyngiomas of our children?

When unsure, you should go to the place where you want these operations to be done. Visiting other departments increases the collection of different techniques and tricks. Consider the population size that departments serve. Consider also the following questions: What happens in undeveloped countries where benign tumors may reach gargantuan sizes before diagnosis? What are the standards for outcome and acceptable risks of complications [5, 6]?

Microneurosurgery is indebted to those who are totally devoted to their work, but find time to share their experience with the next generation [1, 11]. modern microneurosurgery will increasingly cover huge populations, such as the mega-cities of China, and there will be considerable opportunities for experience in cases that Western departments encounter only a few times a year. A single idea to be adopted in the OR is worthy to bring one out of their world-wide, well-known center. Buy a flight ticket, west or east, to pick up good tricks from other places.

Acknowledgments

The author thanks his own patients, staff, and the flow of critical fellows and visitors who have helped me to do better surgery with the rather moderate resources of a small country.

References

[1] Drake CG, Peerless SJ, Hernesniemi JA (1996) Surgery of vertebrobasilar aneurysms. London, Ontario experience on 1767 patients. Springer, Wien

[2] Hernesniemi J (2001) Mechanisms to improve treatment standards in neurosurgery, cerebral aneurysm surgery as example. Acta Neurochir Suppl 78: 127-134

[3] Hernesniemi J, Ishii K, Niemela M, et al. (2005) Lateral supraorbital approach as an alternative to the classical pterional approach. Acta Neurochir Suppl 94: 17-21

[4] Hernesniemi J, Ishii K, Niemela M, et al. (2005) Subtemporal approach to basilar bifurcation aneurysms: advanced technique and clinical experience. Acta Neurochir Suppl 94: 31-38

[5] Hernesniemi J, Koivisto T (2004) Comments on the impact of the International Subarachnoid Aneurysm Treatment Trial (ISAT) on neurosurgical practice. Acta Neurochir (Wien) 146: 203-208

[6] Hernesniemi J, Nimelä M, Karataş A, et al. (2005) Some collected principles of microneurosurgery: simple and fast, while preserving normal anatomy: a review. Surg Neurol 64: 195-200

[7] Kivisaari RP, Porras M, Öhman J, et al. (2004) Routine cerebral angiography after surgery for saccular aneurysms: is it worth it? Neurosurgery 55: 1015-1022

[8] Kuhmonen J, Piippo A, Vaart K, et al. (2005) Early surgery for ruptured cerebral arteriovenous malformations. Acta Neurochir Suppl 94: 111-114

[9] Nagy L, Ishii K, Karatas A, Shen H, Vajda J, Niemela M, Jaaskelainen J, Hernesniemi J, Toth S (2006) Water dissection technique of toth for opening neurosurgical cleavage planes. Surg Neurol 65: 38-41

[10] Niemela M, Koivisto T, Kivipelto L, et al. (2005) Microsurgical clipping of cerebral aneurysms after the ISAT study. Acta Neurochir (Suppl) 94: 3-6

[11] Yaşargil MG (1996) Microneurosurgery. Georg Thieme, Stuttgart

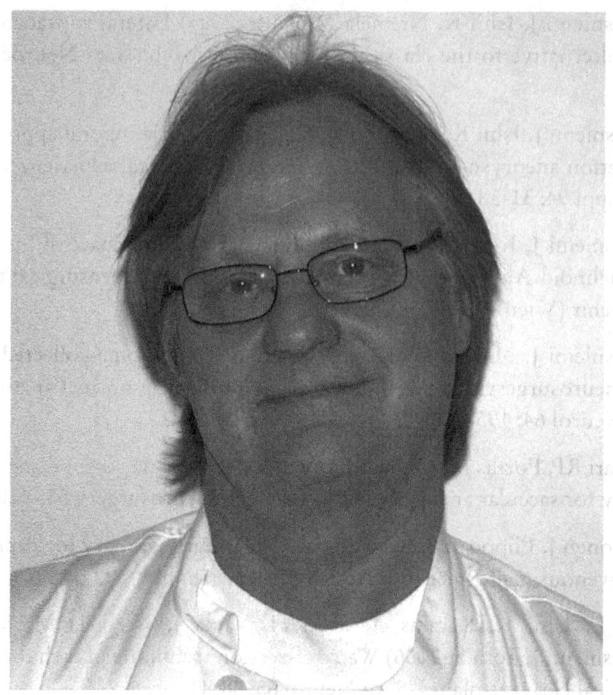

Juha Hernesniemi

Juha Hernesniemi is Professor and Chairman, Department of Neurosurgery, University Central Hospital of Helsinki, 1997–. He was born in a small village of Kannus, Finland, in 1947. High school in Ruovesi, Finland 1966, Medical school at the University of Zürich, Switzerland, Dr.med. Zürich 1973. Specialist in neurosurgery, Helsinki, 1979, Ph.D., Helsinki 1979. Associate Professor Kuopio 1987, Senior Physician and Co-Chairman Kuopio 1980–1997. Study periods at 20 foreign neurosurgical centers, including Profs. Yaşargil and Drake. Personal microsurgical experience: 10,000 operations including more than 3500 cerebral aneurysms and AVMS, more than 2500 brain tumors. Visiting Professor at many universities, more than 150 original articles, more than 100 reviews and text book chapters. Two short stories on childhood memories.

Contact: Juha Hernesniemi, Department of Neurosurgery, Helsinki University Central Hospital, Topeliuksenkatu 5, 00260 Helsinki, Finland
E-mail: juha.hernesniemi@hus.fi

SURGICAL MANAGEMENT OF INTRACRANIAL ANEURYSMS OF THE ANTERIOR CIRCULATION

C. RAFTOPOULOS

INTRODUCTION

The international literature reports a prevalence of intracranial aneurysms (ICA) of around 1000 per 100,000 persons, with 85% of the ICA located on the anterior circulation around the circle of Willis, 45% of which are on the anterior communicating artery [3, 25]. The highest incidence of ICA in the population is at around 55–60 years of age.

The risk of an ICA rupturing is around 1% per year and so, ruptured intracranial aneurysms (RIA) have an incidence of around 10 per 100,000 population [9, 19]. The rupture rate increases from 0.05 to 10% depending on the size of the aneurysm, varies according to the location of the aneurysm with a higher risk for locations on the posterior communicating artery and the posterior circulation [25], increases in patients who have a history of smoking (relative risk: 1.5), and decreases with the patient's age. Active smoking seems to play even a more important role in the occurrence of RIA with an odds ratio of up to 5.0. RIA are 1.6 times more common in women than in men [9]. If not occluded, around 15% of these RIA will re-rupture within the first two weeks with 4% within the first 24 h leading to the patient's death in the majority of cases. Therefore, in case of rupture, an ICA should be occluded endovascularly or surgically within 72 h [5]. Despite improvement in all aspects of management, an RIA remains a "catastrophic" event with a poor outcome, i.e., death or significant neurological deficit, in about 75% of cases [5].

It is, therefore, important to be aware of the main risk factors for the presence of an unruptured intracranial aneurysm (UIA) [18]. Risk factors include: a positive family history (at least two first-degree relatives with a subarachnoid hemorrhage [SAH] gives a relative risk of 6.6); alcohol (relative risk of 300 g/week: 5.6); autosomal dominant polycystic kidney disease (relative risk: 4.4); hypertension (relative risk: 2.8); and smoking (relative risk: 1.5–5). In our unit, we suggest that all patients less than 65 years of age with a family history of RIA or autosomal dominant polycystic kidney disease should be screened for UIA. The alcoholic risk factor is much more difficult to evaluate and to apply.

Keywords: aneurysm, anterior circulation, microsurgery, vascular malformation

The physiopathology behind the formation of an ICA is complex but appears to be essentially acquired, with genetic and environmental factors [22]. ICAs are characterized anatomically by a partial or complete disappearance of the middle muscular layer. They often herniate into the subarachnoid spaces so that when they rupture they cause a subarachnoid hemorrhage (SAH). Sometimes ICAs are enclosed within the brain and will first be responsible for an intraparenchymal hematoma. Hemodynamic stresses play a particular role in the formation of ICAs especially at specific locations around the circle of Willis [22]: the anterior communicating artery accounting for 45% of all ICAs, the internal carotid artery 20%, and the middle cerebral artery 20%. ICAs can be associated with various diseases affecting tissue elasticity, including autosomal dominant polycystic kidney disease, fibromuscular dysplasia, Ehlers-Danlos syndrome type IV, and Marfan syndrome. Smoking also appears to be related to ICA occurrence and particularly to RIA occurrence in women. This associated risk seems to decrease rapidly with smoking cessation [2].

RATIONALE

The history of the treatment of ICA, which now essentially comprises either coil embolization or surgical clipping, has been dominated by the work of just a few individuals. The major improvement in the surgical treatment of ICA came with introduction of the surgical microscope [5]. The first description of a microscope to help neurosurgeons in occluding ICA was made by Pool and Colton in 1966, but it was Yaşargil who really developed the technique providing exhaustive accounts of his experiences in a series of publications [7, 26–29]. Coil embolization with electrothombosis and coil electrolytic detachment was first reported by Guglielmi in 1991 and represented the second revolution [6] in the treatment of ICA but further discussion of this technique falls outside the scope of this chapter.

For optimal surgical management of ICA, three areas must be extensively studied and mastered. The first area is the surgical anatomy of the intracranial vessels and their surroundings, a good knowledge of which is an absolute prerequisite for managing ICA. Here, atlases of clinical brain-anatomy and, in particular, those written by Yaşargil or Lang focusing on the skull base and its related structures, provide a major source of information [8, 27]. The second area which must be watched and studied is the international literature focusing on the surgical treatment of ICA, in particular publications dealing with the surgical technique of ICA occlusion, wrapping or bypass [4, 7, 12, 21, 28, 29]. The third area is modern imaging techniques for ICA, in particular 3D rotational angiography and an original software with an adapted hardware, named Dextroscope (Volumes Interactions, Bracco, Singapore). The Dextroscope allows the user to see a 3D virtual reality multimodal head with its intracranial vessels, the brain and the skull base in whatever surgical position the neurosurgeon chooses. This interactive technology enables neurosurgeons to perform as many virtual neurosurgical approaches as they want, thus preparing themselves for the different structures and particular orientation of these structures that may be met during the surgical procedure.

A good knowledge of various aspects of vascular-related neurophysiology is also required. One of the most important facets is a correct understanding of the literature dealing with the brain ischemia process so that the key technique of temporary clipping of a parent vessel can be used appropriately [12]. The vascular neurosurgeon should also be aware of the neurophysiology behind arterial vasomotor function and the inflammatory reaction involved in SAH vasospasm with its highest risk between the 3rd and 10th day post-rupture.

DECISION-MAKING

The first step leading to diagnosis of an ICA is often clinical. For UIA, we distinguish three types of situation: incidental, symptomatic, or associated with a previous RIA. The discovery of incidental ICA is currently made by computed tomography (CT) or magnetic resonance (MR) angiography when investigating headaches, associated diseases or a positive family history of ICA. Symptomatic UIA can be associated either with a mass effect syndrome on a second or third cranial nerve or a transient ischemic stroke related to emboli originating from within the ICA. These symptoms support treatment of the related UIA. For RIA, the main symptom is an explosive – "as never

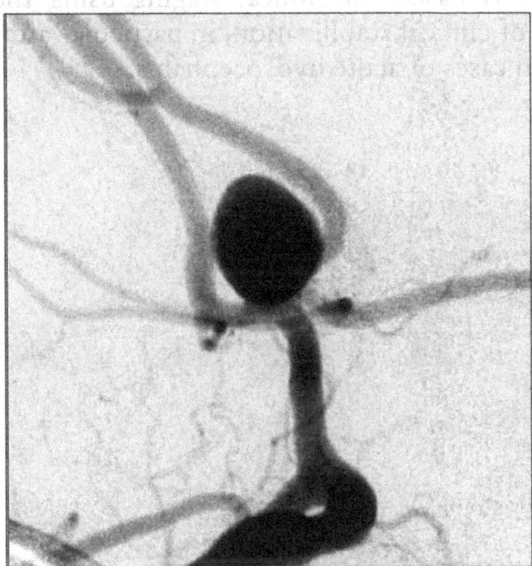

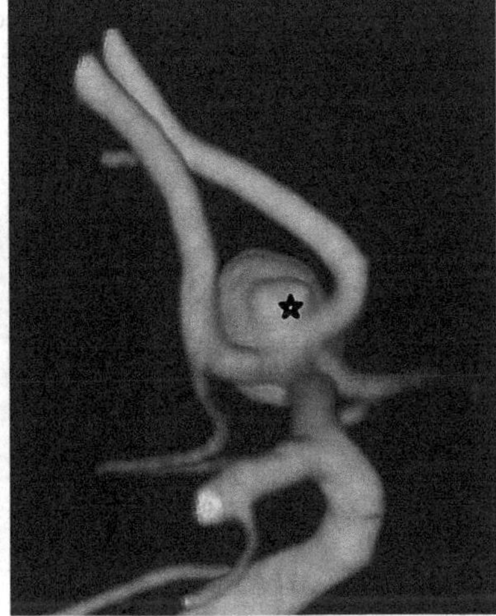

Fig. 1. Anterior communicating artery aneurysm showed by a catheter and a 3D angiograms. Note that the 3D angiogram shows additional details as the presence of two ecstasies (*)

before" – headache often followed by a meningeal syndrome. When the first rupture remains minimal, it can go unrecognized and followed later by a massive catastrophic hemorrhage. This first minimal hemorrhage is appropriately called "warning leak" and must be early recognized [5]. For RIA, we use a clinical score, the World Federation of Neurological Surgeons (WFNS) score, which is based on the Glasgow Coma Scale score (Fig. 1).

When a SAH is suspected, a CT scan should be performed first and two features evaluated. The first feature is the quantity of blood in the subarachnoid spaces, associated or not with blood in the ventricular system or in the brain itself. The quantity of blood is scored according to the *Fisher scale*: Grade I, no blood; grade II, blood in the subarachnoid spaces with a thickness of less than 1 mm; grade III, blood thickness equal to or greater than 1 mm; grade IV, intraparenchymal clot or intraventricular clot without or with little blood in the subarachnoid spaces. The presence of blood in the lateral ventricles represents an additional risk for developing vasospasm with cerebral ischemia (odds ratio: 4.1). The second feature which must be evaluated is the presence of acute hydrocephalus which can be subtle in the first few hours and occurs in about 20% of RIA. Late identification of this complication can be fatal.

The next step in a patient with a SAH is to assess the underlying cause using one of the following three techniques: CT angiography, MRI angiography, or the gold standard, catheter angiography. Currently, all our patients undergo at least catheter angiography with 3D rotational angiography (Fig. 1), the results of which are introduced into the Dextroscope to give the neurosurgeon a 3D view of the aneurysm from different possible surgical positions. Preoperative assessment is based on clinical staging using the WFNS scale (Fig. 2) after a period of clinical stabilization, in particular after placement of ventricular drainage in cases of acute hydrocephalus.

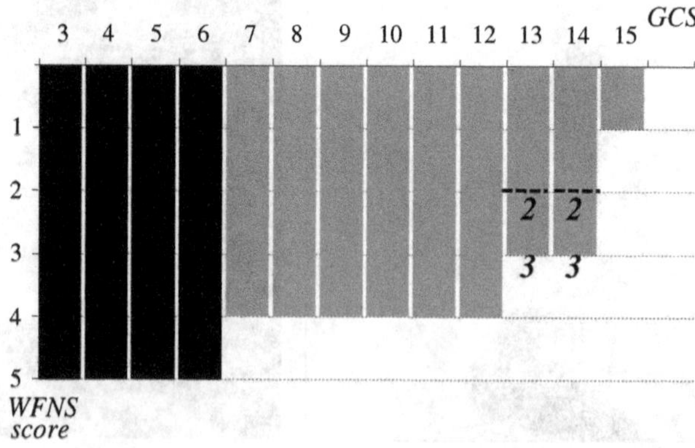

Fig. 2. World Federation of Neurosurgical Societies (WFNS) score for subarachnoid hemorrhage (SAH). This score is based on the Glasgow Coma Scale (GCS, 15 to 3). There are 5 possible WFNS scores, five being the worst. The WFNS score is 3 when there is a motor deficit

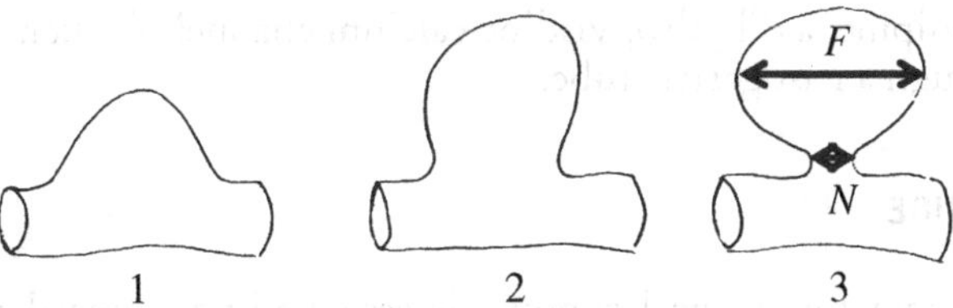

Fig. 3. Fundus-to-neck (F/N/) ratio. Coil embolization is recommended for case 3 with a F/N ≥ 2.5. Surgical clipping is recommended for cases 1 and 2

In the 21st century, all ICAs should be managed in centers with a multidisciplinary team, including at least an interventional radiologist and a vascular neurosurgeon. For UIA, we inform the patient about the controversy surrounding whether or not to treat such aneurysms, particularly those smaller than 7 mm [1, 10, 24]. However, in my group, we recommend treatment in all patients less than 65 years of age or if there is an associated risk, such as a previous RIA, a family history, or an associated disease, such as autosomal polycystic kidney disease. For RIA, we nearly always recommend immediate treatment at least by coil embolization to occlude the aneurysm fundus. The treatment we recommend follows the following algorithm: coil embolization is considered first for all ICAs not associated with an intraparenchymal hematoma and with a fundus-neck (F/N) ratio equal to or greater than 2.5 (Fig. 3) or located on the posterior circulation or for a patient with a poor WFNS score of 4 or 5. If there is an intraparenchymal hematoma or if the endovascular approach is deemed too difficult by the interventional radiologist (tortuous vessels, atheromatosis or fibromuscular dysplasia), if the aneurysm neck is 4 mm or more and not controllable by a stent, or if the F/N ratio is <2.5 for an anterior circulation aneurysm, surgical clipping is recommended. In patients with poor aneurysm geometry for embolization, especially in those with a poor clinical state (WFNS 4 or 5), we recommend at least a partial endovascular occlusion, followed by surgical clipping if necessary when the patient has recovered. Clip placement is also recommended where embolization has resulted in incomplete occlusion with increasing size of residual aneurysm six months or more after the endovascular procedure [17]. The residual aneurysm must be large enough to allow the placement of a clip.

SURGERY

1. PREOPERATIVE CARE

The day before surgery, all patients have three shampoos with a 7.5% iodine solution, receive a laxative and start to wear Kendall socks (Tyco Healthcare Group). To reduce the risk of developing vasospasm, patients with SAH are given nimodipine, a dihydropyridine calcium channel blocker, orally, if necessary through a nasogastric tube.

2. PROCEDURE

Our equipment for surgical clipping is essentially composed of a balanced microscope (OPMI Pentero, Zeiss), a high speed drill motor with curved tubes (Midas Rex, Medtronic), bipolar forceps with integrated water irrigation (Codman, Johnson and Johnson), Rhoton micro-instruments (Aesculap), and Perneczky clips, made initially by von Zeppelin and now by Adeor (Adeor Medical Technologies) [13]. The revolutionary design of these clips with the forceps passing inside the clip's posterior branches allows the surgeon to have a much better view of the aneurysm morphology and its surroundings and improved possibilities of using temporary clips and of removing the clips to relocate them in a better position.

For brain protection during surgery, all patients are kept normotensive, mildly hypothermic (32–33°C) and with a burst-suppression EEG. In a RIA, we also ask for cerebro-spinal fluid lumbar drainage and perfusion of an osmotic agent before opening the dura mater.

The majority of ICA of the anterior circulation are accessed by a pterional approach avoiding the fronto-temporal branch of the facial nerve [29]. The skull opening of 4–5 cm in diameter is perfectly centered on the sphenoid ridge for middle cerebral artery or internal carotid artery aneurysms. In anterior communicating artery aneurysms, the bone flap is extended slightly onto the frontal area just above the frontal crest. Using this approach, it is essential that the lateral part of the sphenoid ridge is completely removed to minimize brain retraction.

Once the dura mater is opened, we protect the cortex around the lateral fissure with an oxidized cellulose hemostat, such as Surgicel (Ethicon, Johnson and Johnson), and cottonoids and open the lateral fissure using a surgical blade to access the subarachnoid spaces. We then progress inside the lateral fissure separating the frontal lobe from the temporal lobe using forceps and micro-scissors to cut the arachnoid adhesions. A maximum of these arachnoid adhesions must be cut to allow gentle minimal retraction of the frontal and temporal lobes without impeding the brain microcirculation. Perfect hemostasis, in particular of venous origin, must be achieved and maintained.

Once the dissection approaches the ICA, the neurosurgeon will determine, depending on various factors, including experience, the type of ICA, and the existence of a SAH, whether or not to temporarily occlude the parent vessel(s). Our *protocol* for temporary occlusion is the following: less than 10 min for patients in mild hypothermia and with burst-suppression EEG; if any additional temporary occlusion is required, we always use a reperfusion period of at least 5 min between two temporary arterial occlusions of less than 10 min [14–17]. So far, using that protocol, no patient developed any permanent deficit related to parent vessel temporary occlusion. In presence of an ICA impacted into the brain, we perform a delicate subpial dissection most of the time under temporary occlusion. To facilitate clip placement, we frequently reshape the aneurysm and its neck by using *mild electrocoagulation*, always under temporary parent vessel occlusion to avoid aneurysm rupture. Once the aneurysm neck is perfectly visible and separated from all surrounding vessels, the most suitable Perneczky clip is chosen.

In unclippable aneurysms, such as, for example, blister aneurysms, we try to use a *wrap-clip technique* consisting of a piece of knitted fabric (knitted polyester with bovine collagen, Hemashield, Boston Scientific, USA) wrapped around the aneurysm and its parent vessel and fixed tightly using a clip. If this technique is not possible because of efferent vessels or the depth of the operating field, we then use small elongated pieces of cotton placed around the aneurysm and the parent vessel. This last procedure should only be used in exceptional circumstances due to its undemonstrated efficacy.

Once the clip is placed on the aneurysm's neck, we check that no small vessels are compromised by the clip, that the aneurysm is completely occluded, and, finally, that the parent vessel retains a normal diameter. For this check, a small Zini mirror is sometimes used which allows the neurosurgeon to examine hidden aspects of the aneurysm's neck. For ICA with a large neck, for large or giant ICA, and for ICA located in the paraclinoid area, somatosensory evoked potentials are used [17]. Stable somatosensory evoked potentials for more than 10min are always used to check the adequate vascularization of the explored area. So far, we have never used intraoperatively Doppler, catheter angiography or indocyanine green video angiography.

In patients with an SAH, we remove as much blood as possible. To wash the subarachnoid spaces at the end of surgery we use at least one liter of physiologic solution. For about 10 years from 1996, we administered 2mg tissue plasminogen activator (tPA) through a lumbar intrathecal catheter every 12h, for a maximum of 4 days, and 4mg into the peri-aneurysmal area just before wound closure. tPA was used only if there was no intraparenchymal hematoma or another unsecured UIA. Unfortunately, the price of this drug and the lack of incontrovertible data to support its use in such conditions led us to abandon it even though our positive experience favored another randomized controlled study.

Closure is an essential aspect of surgery, particularly from an esthetic point of view. Particular attention is taken to perfectly fixed the bone flap and to replace all the bone that has been removed with a methyl-methacrylate cement and to perform a perfect muscle reinsertion.

3. POSTOPERATIVE CARE

The postoperative care period is dominated by maintaining a normal circulating blood volume with a normal arterial blood pressure and by monitoring for potential complications, such as vasospasm or chronic hydrocephalus. If the patient is receiving nimodipine, this can induce hypotension which must be corrected immediately. In the presence of clinical vasospasm confirmed by Doppler (positive predictive value: 63%) or perfusion CT with CT angiography (positive predictive value: 90%), triple-H therapy is implemented. If the clinical signs do not resolve with treatment, catheter angiography should be performed, followed by angioplasty if possible and by injection of papaverine when necessary.

In case of chronic hydrocephalus, we first try to control it by performing three lumbar punctures on consecutive days, removing 40 ml of cerebrospinal fluid each time. If this treatment is not sufficient, we place a ventriculo-peritoneal drainage under neuronavigation.

4. RESULTS

The short-term results after surgical clipping of ICA are summarized in Fig. 5. Regarding UIA, we have just reported our experience (two centers: St-Luc, Brussels and Bicètre, Paris) with 238 UIA in 176 patients (only one on the posterior circulation): all patients in this group achieved a good Glasgow Outcome Score (grade IV or V, Fig. 4) with only 1.7% having *slight* permanent morbidity and no mortalities. When considering permanent morbidity, Solomon reported a rate of 0% for small aneurysms and of 6% for large ones [20]. In our series, 25% of the 238 UIA were large or giant and their surgical treatment was not associated with permanent morbidity. For RIA, we published a preliminary personal series in 2000 of 26 consecutive RIA deemed not accessible to coil embolization: in 81% of the cases a good GOS was achieved and in 89% there was complete aneurysm occlu-

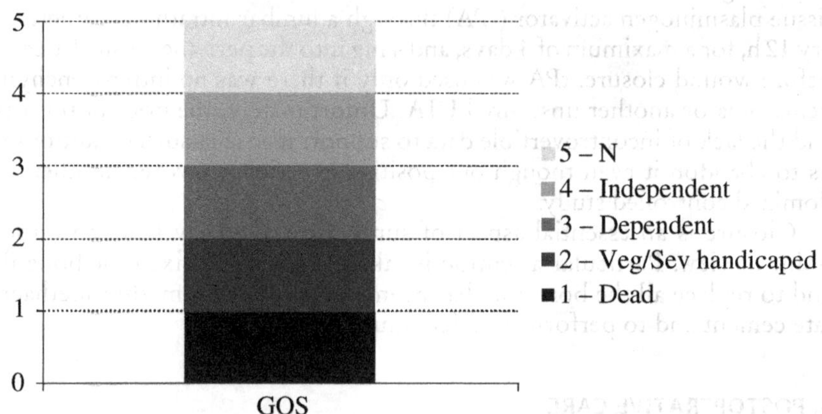

Fig. 4. Glasgow Outcome Scale. Outcome scale with five scores. A score of five corresponds to a normal clinical status. Score of two corresponds to severe (sev) handicap or a vegetative state

	UIA	RIA	
n	238[a]	141[b]	1055[c]
Good GOS (%)	100	74.5	69
CO (%)	95	90.8	82
Near CO (%)	2.5	6.3	12

Fig. 5. Short-term results after surgical clipping. [a] 238 unruptured intracranial aneurysms (UIA) in 176 patients as reported by Aghakhani et al. in 2008. [b] Number of ruptured intracranial aneurysms (RIA) clipped between 1996 and 2007 in St-Luc University Hospital Brussels by myself or my senior collaborator, Dr G. Vaz. [c] Number of RIA surgically clipped and reported by the International Subarachnoid Trial (ISAT) in 2005. Good GOS: Glasgow Outcome Scale score of 5 or 4. *CO* Complete occlusion. *Near CO* Nearly complete occlusion, i.e., residue less than or equal to 5% of the initial aneurysm volume

sion [16]. This series has now expanded to include 141 RIA deemed not accessible to an endovascular procedure and thus surgically more difficult; our results (two neurosurgeons) show a good GOS in 74.5% with aneurysm complete occlusion in 90.8% and near complete occlusion in 6.3% (Fig. 5). We stress that the rate of good outcome for patients with a good pre-operative clinical grade (WFNS 1-3) was even better at 88%. In 2005, the International Subarachnoid Aneurysm Trial (ISAT) reported on the surgical treatment of 1555 RIA with 69% good GOS and a lower rate of complete aneurysm occlusion of 82% [11].

Considering the long-term results obtained with surgical clipping of ICA (Fig. 6), in 2001, Tsutsumi et al. reported on 112 clipped ICAs with a

	Tsutsumi et al. (2001)
n	112
If CO	2.4%
If NCO	7.1%
De novo	8%

Fig. 6. Long-term results after surgical clipping. Percentage of aneurysm regrowth at a mean interval of 9 years after surgery. In a series of 112 patients with a clipped aneurysm, the rate of regrowth depends on the quality of clipping occlusion. In complete occlusion (*CO*), the rate of regrowth was 2.4%. In nearly complete occlusion (*NCO*), the rate of regrowth was 7.1%

mean interval from surgery of nine years. These authors observed a 2.4% rate of regrowth for completely occluded ICA, 7.1% regrowth for nearly completely occluded ICA, and 8% de novo ICA [23].

HOW TO AVOID COMPLICATIONS

The best way to avoid complications in the surgical treatment of ICA is first to acquire enough experience in brain surgery and particularly in vascular neurosurgery. In the 21st century, surgical ICA should only be treated by brain neurosurgeons with enough experience in vascular neurosurgery. The second essential requirement is the existence of a multidisciplinary group comprising an (preferably two) interventional radiologist(s) and a (preferably two) vascular neurosurgeon(s). Neuro-anesthesiologists, critical care physicians and nurses specially trained in the management of this very challenging pathology should also be involved.

CONCLUSIONS

In 2008, we believe that surgical clipping remains the gold standard treatment for ICA of the anterior circulation with a F/N ratio <2.5, especially in young patients without SAH or with a good preoperative clinical grade.

References

[1] (1998) Unruptured intracranial aneurysms – risk of rupture and risks of surgical intervention. International study of unruptured intracranial aneurysms investigators. N Engl J Med 339: 1725-1733

[2] Anderson CS, Feigin V, Bennett D, Lin RB, Hankey G, Jamrozik K (2004) Active and passive smoking and the risk of subarachnoid hemorrhage: an international population-based case-control study. Stroke 35: 633-637

[3] Atkinson JL, Sundt TM Jr, Houser OW, Whisnant JP (1989) Angiographic frequency of anterior circulation intracranial aneurysms. J Neurosurg 70: 551-555

[4] Deruty R, Dechaume JP, Lecuire J, Bret P, El OA (1976) Microsurgical treatment of a series of intracranial subtentorial arterial aneurysms. Neurochirurgie 22: 227-238

[5] Drake CG (1981) Progress in cerebrovascular disease. Management of cerebral aneurysm. Stroke 12: 273-283

[6] Guglielmi G, Vinuela F, Dion J, Duckwiler G (1991) Electrothrombosis of saccular aneurysms via endovascular approach. Part 2: Preliminary clinical experience. J Neurosurg 75: 8-14

[7] Krayenbuehl HA, Yaşargil MG, Flamm ES, Tew JM Jr (1972) Microsurgical treatment of intracranial saccular aneurysms. J Neurosurg 37: 678-686

[8] Lang J (1995) Skull base and related structures. Schattauer, Stuttgart

[9] Linn FH, Rinkel GJ, Algra A, van GJ (1996) Incidence of subarachnoid hemorrhage: role of region, year, and rate of computed tomography: a meta-analysis. Stroke 27: 625-629

[10] Mitchell P, Gholkar A, Vindlacheruvu RR, Mendelow AD (2004) Unruptured intracranial aneurysms: benign curiosity or ticking bomb? Lancet Neurol 3: 85-92

[11] Molyneux A, Kerr R, Stratton I, Sandercock P, Clarke M, Shrimpton J, Holman R (2002) International subarachnoid aneurysm trial (ISAT) of neurosurgical clipping versus endovascular coiling in 2143 patients with ruptured intracranial aneurysms: a randomised trial. Lancet 360: 1267-1274

[12] Ogilvy CS, Carter BS, Kaplan S, Rich C, Crowell RM (1996) Temporary vessel occlusion for aneurysm surgery: risk factors for stroke in patients protected by induced hypothermia and hypertension and intravenous mannitol administration. J Neurosurg 84: 785-791

[13] Perneczky A, Fries G (1995) Use of a new aneurysm clip with an inverted-spring mechanism to facilitate visual control during clip application. Technical note. J Neurosurg 82: 898-899

[14] Raftopoulos C (2005) Is surgical clipping becoming underused? Acta Neurochir (Wien) 147: 117-123

[15] Raftopoulos C, Goffette P, Vaz G, Ramzi N, Scholtes JL, Wittebole X, Mathurin P (2003) Surgical clipping may lead to better results than coil embolization: results from a series of 101 consecutive unruptured intracranial aneurysms. Neurosurgery 52: 1280-1287

[16] Raftopoulos C, Mathurin P, Boscherini D, Billa RF, Van BM, Hantson P (2000) Prospective analysis of aneurysm treatment in a series of 103 consecutive patients when endovascular embolization is considered the first option. J Neurosurg 93: 175-182

[17] Raftopoulos C, Vaz G, Docquier M, Goffette P (2007) Neurosurgical management of inadequately embolized intracranial aneurysms: a series of 17 consecutive cases. Acta Neurochir (Wien) 149: 11-19

[18] Rinkel GJ (2005) Intracranial aneurysm screening: indications and advice for practice. Lancet Neurol 4: 122-128

[19] Schievink WI (1997) Intracranial aneurysms. N Engl J Med 336: 28-40

[20] Solomon RA, Fink ME, Pile-Spellman J (1994) Surgical management of unruptured intracranial aneurysms. J Neurosurg 80: 440-446

[21] Spetzler RF, Carter LP (1985) Revascularization and aneurysm surgery: current status. Neurosurgery 16: 111-116

[22] Stehbens WE (1989) Etiology of intracranial berry aneurysms. J Neurosurg 70: 823-831

[23] Tsutsumi K, Ueki K, Morita A, Usui M, Kirino T (2001) Risk of aneurysm recurrence in patients with clipped cerebral aneurysms: results of long-term follow-up angiography. Stroke 32: 1191-1194

[24] Weir B (2002) Unruptured intracranial aneurysms: a review. J Neurosurg 96: 3-42

[25] Wiebers DO, Whisnant JP, Huston J III, Meissner I, Brown RD Jr, Piepgras DG, Forbes GS, Thielen K, Nichols D, O'Fallon WM, Peacock J, Jaeger L, Kassell NF, Kongable-Beckman GL, Torner JC (2003) Unruptured intracranial aneurysms: natural history, clinical outcome, and risks of surgical and endovascular treatment. Lancet 362: 103-110

[26] Yaşargil MG (1996) Clinical considerations, surgery of the intracranial aneurysms and results. Georg Thieme, Stuttgart

[27] Yaşargil MG (1996) Microsurgical anatomy of the basal cisterns and vessels of the brain. Georg Thieme, Stuttgart

[28] Yaşargil MG, Fox JL (1975) The microsurgical approach to intracranial aneurysms. Surg Neurol 3: 7-14

[29] Yaşargil MG, Reichman MV, Kubik S (1987) Preservation of the frontotemporal branch of the facial nerve using the interfascial temporalis flap for pterional craniotomy. Technical article. J Neurosurg 67: 463-466

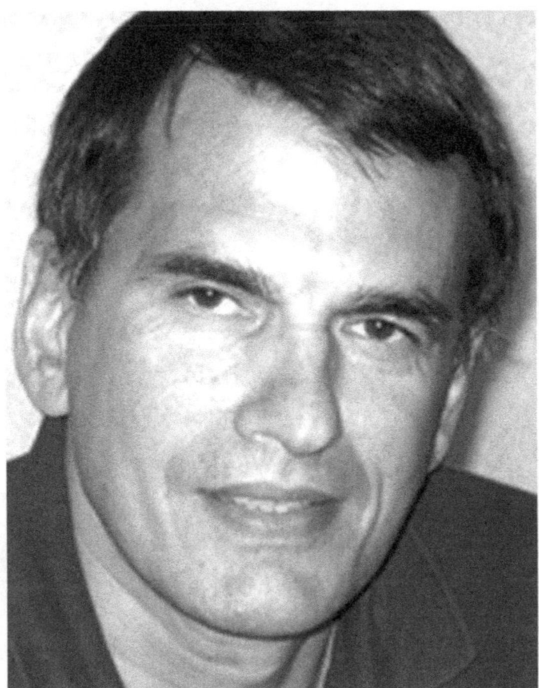

Christian Raftopoulos

Christian Raftopoulos is chairman of the new Department of Neurosurgery of University Hospital St-Luc in Brussels. Born in Africa (in former Belgian Congo) in 1958 (Belgium mother, Greek father). From 1978 to 1980, student-researcher in the neuroanatomy laboratory of Prof. M. Gerebtzoff (University of Liège, Belgium). 1983, diploma of medical doctor (University of Liège). 1989, diploma of neurosurgery (Free University of Brussels). 1994, Ph.D. in neurosurgery related to the normotensive hydrocephalus (Free University of Brussels). 1998, first implantation of a self-sizing cuff electrode around a human optic nerve. 1999, Mont Blanc summit climbing. 2000, full academic professor at the Université Catholique de Louvain. 2000 to 2006, General Secretary of the Société de Neurochirurgie de Langue Française. 2002, opening presentation at the American Association of Neurological Surgeons (Chicago, USA) about the surgical management of intracranial aneurysms. 2003, nominated as Master Neurosurgeon by the Congress of Neurological Surgeons (USA). 2005, co-director of the Center for Management of Pharmacological Refractory Epilepsy at the Université Catholique de Louvain. 2006, co-developer of a new operative suite with an intraoperative MRI at 3.0 T. 2007, creation of a surgical planning laboratory (Radionix, BrainLab, Dextroscope).

Contact: Christian Raftopoulos, Neurosurgical Department, Clinique Universitaire Saint Luc, Université Catholique de Louvain, Av. Hippocrate 10, 1200 Brussels, Belgium
E-mail: christian.raftopoulos@uclourain.be

INTRACRANIAL ANEURYSMS IN THE POSTERIOR CIRCULATION

K. LINDSAY

INTRODUCTION

Aneurysms of the posterior circulation have always proved a challenge to the neurosurgeon. In 1948, Schwartz reported a successful trapping of a large basilar artery aneurysm, but Drake, in 1961 was the first to report direct surgical repair of a ruptured basilar aneurysm in 4 patients [6]. He concluded that "direct surgical attack was feasible and worthwhile under exceptional circumstances, when life was threatened by repeated haemorrhages". With the introduction of the operating microscope, improved micro-instruments and clips and advances in neuro intensive care, surgical repair of such aneurysms became the accepted norm, but outcome figures for repair if basilar tip and trunk aneurysms were always worse than for repair of aneurysms in the anterior circulation. As a result, with the introduction of coil embolisation in the 90s, early series of endovascular treatment always included a high proportion of posterior circulation aneurysms. In many centres (including Glasgow) an endovascular approach has become the first line of treatment for such aneurysms and standard coiling has been supplemented by the possibility of balloon remodelling or stenting. Despite this management approach, a proportion of the patients still require direct surgical repair due to technical failure or repeated coil impactions.

RATIONALE

The International Study of Unruptured Intracranial Aneurysms (ISUIA) found that posterior circulation aneurysms are more likely to rupture than those in the anterior circulation [11]. Over a five year period, aneurysms over 6 mm diameter carry at least a 15% risk of rupture. This compares to 2.6% for those in the anterior circulation.

If rupture occurs, the chance of sudden death from a ruptured posterior circulation is double that of anterior circulation aneurysms and a smaller proportion of patients reach a neurosurgical unit. A community-based study reported that posterior circulation aneurysms constitute 18% of all docu-

Keywords: aneurysms, posterior circulation, vascular malformations, microsurgery

mented ruptured aneurysms, whereas in hospital based studies the instance of posterior circulation aneurysms varies from about 5 to 10% [9].

The goal of aneurysm repair, whether for ruptured or for unruptured aneurysms is to obliterate the aneurysm fundus and to preserve flow in adjacent vessels. For posterior circulation aneurysms, particularly those around the basilar tip, preservation of the thalamo-mesencephalic perforators is crucial.

DECISION-MAKING

A wide variety of operative approaches exist and the surgeon must select the most appropriate for the aneurysm site and size. An angiogram combined with bone imaging reveals important anatomical features, of value not only in determining the optimal approach but also in indicating the operative risks. Note the height of the aneurysm neck in relation to the posterior clinoids and the size and direction of the aneurysm fundus. Rotation of a 3-D digital or CT angiographic image provides an ideal method of assessing the width of the aneurysm neck and the optimal direction of clip application. Selection of approach also depends on the preference and individual experience of the surgeon.

In considering the optimal approach it is convenient to subdivide posterior circulation aneurysms into three sites (Fig. 1).

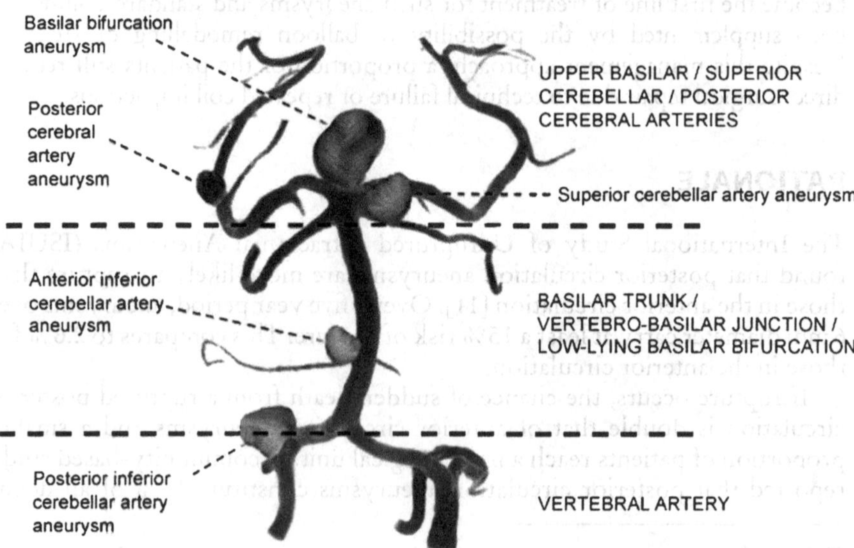

Fig. 1. Sites of posterior circulation aneurysms: three levels for operative approach

1. UPPER BASILAR/SUPERIOR CEREBELLAR/POSTERIOR CEREBRAL ARTERIES

1.1 Basilar bifurcation aneurysms

Operative repair at this site risks damage to perforators supplying the midbrain and thalamus. These arise from P_1, a few millimetres from the bifurcation but some may arise directly from the basilar artery and adhere to the posterior surface of the fundus.

The *subtemporal approach* described by Drake [7] is particularly suited for posteriorly projecting or low lying basilar bifurcation aneurysms (Fig. 2). Posteriorly projecting aneurysms carry a greater risk of operative complications because of the direct relationship with the perforating vessels; for these aneurysms a subtemporal approach improves visualisation and provides the safest approach. The wider the aneurysm neck, the greater the need to clip the aneurysm parallel to the plane of the adjacent vessels, particularly if the neck engulfs part of the posterior cerebral artery. This is only feasible with the subtemporal approach. Note the height of the neck in relation to the posterior clinoid. The higher the basilar bifurcation, the greater the amount of temporal lobe retraction required if the subtemporal approach is used.

The *transsylvian pterional approach* favoured by Yaşargil et al. [12] reduces such retraction, but access may still be difficult for aneurysms lying >10 mm above the posterior clinoids particularly if the internal carotid artery is also short (<10 mm) (Fig. 2). In such instances removal of the zygoma with

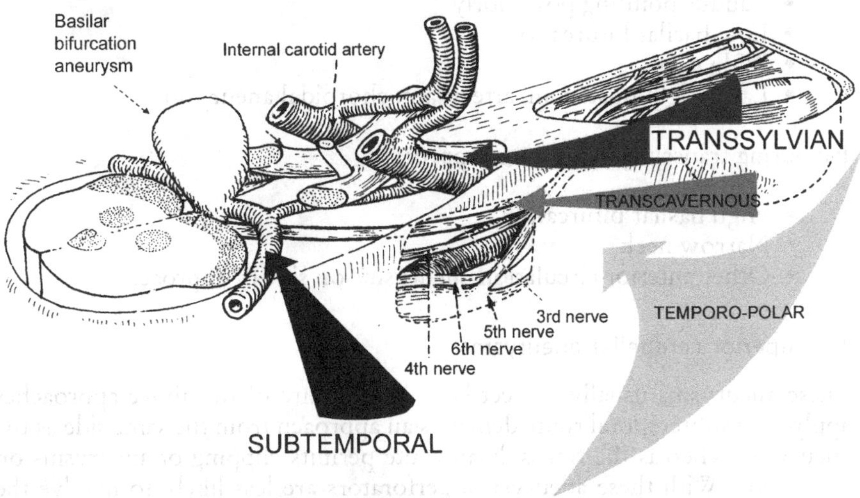

Fig. 2. Approaches to basilar bifurcation aneurysms (Adapted from Lindsay and Bone. Neurology and Neurosurgery Illustrated, 4th edn. Churchill Livingstone)

or without the lateral orbital margin may permit a steeper trajectory with less retraction. The transsylvian pterional approach also provides good exposure of both posterior cerebral vessels, but has the disadvantage of preventing direct visualisation of the perforators lying behind the aneurysm fundus. This route has the added advantage of permitting clipping of any anterior circulation aneurysms on the same side, but aneurysms arising at either the posterior communicating or anterior choroidal origins may hinder access to the basilar bifurcation.

The *temporo-polar approach* or "half and half" approach combines both routes. By changing the direction of temporal lobe retraction, the surgeon can approach from a more anterior or lateral direction as required (Fig. 2). Aneurysms lying *below* the posterior clinoids preclude a transsylvian pterional approach, unless this is combined with the trans-cavernous route described by Dolenc et al. [5]. Day et al. described an extradural trans-cavernous approach after removing the zygoma with or without the orbital rim [4]. This extradural technique preserves the temporal tip bridging veins and permits temporo-polar access to basilar apex aneurysms lying below the level of the posterior clinoids. The author has always favoured the subtemporal approach for low-lying aneurysms, believing this to be a simpler technique and allowing transtentorial extension if required (see below).

Basilar bifurcation aneurysms lying >10 mm below the posterior clinoids may require one of the approaches detailed in the next section.

Procedure selection for basilar bifurcation aneurysms
Favouring subtemporal approach:

- Fundus pointing posteriorly
- Low basilar bifurcation
- Wide neck
- Large right post. com. artery/ant. choroidal aneurysm

Favouring transsylvian pterional approach:

- High basilar bifurcation
- Narrow neck
- Other anterior circulation aneurysms on side of approach

1.2 Superior cerebellar aneurysms

These aneurysms usually project laterally and any of the above approaches apply. The subtemporal route demands an approach from the same side as the aneurysm, whereas the transsylvian route permits clipping of aneurysms on either side. With these aneurysms, perforators are less likely to involve the neck or the fundus, but the 3rd nerve is often closely adherent and must be dissected off the neck before clipping.

1.3 Posterior cerebral artery aneurysms

Aneurysms arising anterior to the midbrain (on either P_1 or P_2) can be approached either via the subtemporal, the trans-sylvian pterional or the temporo-polar route. Those lying in the ambient cistern arising from the P_2 segment require a subtemporal approach. For aneurysms arising from the most distal P_3 segment either an occipital interhemispheric approach or a posterior subtemporal approach will suffice. Occlusion of the distal posterior cerebral artery beyond the origin of the midbrain perforators or of the posterior choroidal artery seldom causes a permanent visual defect.

2. BASILAR TRUNK/VERTEBRO-BASILAR JUNCTION/LOW LYING BASILAR BIFURCATION

As with bifurcation aneurysms, the most important feature is the *height of the aneurysm neck* in relation to the posterior clinoid process and the clivus as seen on the lateral angiographic views.

The *subtemporal transtentorial approach* described by Drake [6] permits access to aneurysms extending down to 25 mm below the posterior clinoid process – in some as low as the vertebrobasilar junction (Fig. 3). Aziz et al. noted the variation in height of the posterior clinoids and suggested that the floor of the sella turcica provided a more accurate guide [2]. These authors recommended that approaches from above permitted access no lower than

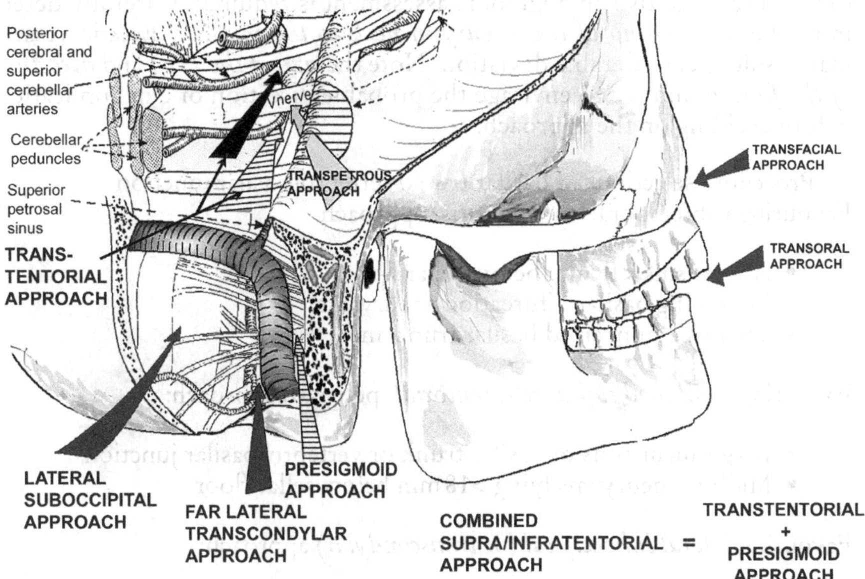

Fig. 3. Diagrammatic view of approaches to the basilar trunk, vertebro-basilar junction and vertebral artery (tentorium cerebelli omitted)

18 mm from the sellar floor. This may or may not include aneurysms of the vertebrobasilar junction since this varies considerably from one patient to another. Kawase et al. described an extradural *transpetrosal approach* where the petrous edge is drilled off between the internal auditory meatus inferiorly, the cochlea postero-laterally and the trigeminal ganglion anteriorly, however the narrow bony opening restricts the operative field (Fig. 3, light grey arrow) [8]. The same technique can also be adopted during an intradural transtentorial approach if a more anterior trajectory is required.

Alternatively aneurysms at the vertebrobasilar junction and on the basilar trunk can be approached from below. The standard lateral suboccipital route would require considerable cerebellar and brainstem retraction to reach the midline and seldom affords sufficient exposure, particularly for large aneurysms. A *combined supra-infratentorial (petrosal) approach* provides a wide view of the basilar trunk and vertebrobasilar junction. This combined approach minimises the extent of pontine and cerebellar retraction and shortens the distance to the aneurysm.

The *transclival approach* either through a *transfacial* route or a *transoral* route avoids brain stem and cranial nerve retraction (Fig. 3). However such techniques present significant hazards – the operative corridor is long and narrow and the lateral exposure usually extends only 5 mm from the midline. Anteriorly pointing aneurysms could rupture when opening the dura and the problems of postoperative CSF leaks persist despite the availability of modern tissue glues.

The selected approach often depends on the surgeon's preference, but careful pre-operative angiographic assessment is required. Carefully determine the *relationship of the aneurysm neck to the midline.* Ectatic vessels may result in considerable deviation. Note the *size of the neck* and *direction of the fundus* and try to envisage the probable direction of clip application before deciding on the approach.

Procedure selection for basilar trunk/vertebro-basilar junction
Favouring subtemporal transtentorial approach:

- Aneurysms <18 mm below sellar floor
- Low lying basilar bifurcation aneurysms
- Small/medium sized basilar trunk aneurysms

Favouring *combined supra-infratentorial* (petrosal) approach:

- Large aneurysms of basilar trunk or vertebro-basilar junction
- Midline aneurysms lying >18 mm below sellar floor

Favouring *lateral suboccipital* (or *transcondylar*) approach:

- Small aneurysms of basilar trunk or vertebro-basilar junction
- Aneurysms lying >18 mm below sellar floor

- Anteriorly arising/tentorial origin of a dominant vein of Labbé on side of approach

3. VERTEBRAL ARTERY

Most vertebral aneurysms arise at the origin of the posterior inferior cerebellar artery (PICA), but the height of this origin is variable ranging from the level of the foramen magnum to the vertebro-basilar junction. Rarely aneurysms lie extracranially – arising at the level of the anterior spinal artery or from a very low PICA origin. The height of the aneurysm to the midline should be determined from the lateral view of the angiogram and the distance from the midline from the AP/Towne's view. The standard *lateral suboccipital approach* usually provides sufficient access for most of these aneurysms, but for those lying more medially and nearer the vertebro-basilar junction a *far lateral transcondylar approach* may be required. This route improves access to the hyoglossal and jugular region and by creating a more caudal to rostral trajectory, provides a shorter route to the midline (Fig. 3).

SURGERY

1. OPERATIVE TECHNIQUE

1.1 Subtemporal approach

The patient is placed in the lateral position with the head slightly elevated and held horizontal in 3-pin fixation. A linear or curvilinear incision extends upwards from 1 cm anterior to the tragus. A 4 cm diameter bone flap is centred in line with the temporo-zygomatic junction, the surface landmark of the basilar artery. CSF drainage and mannitol aid retraction of the temporal lobe, but care is required to avoid damaging bridging veins, in particular the vein of Labbé. Access requires about one finger's breadth between the brain and the bone edge. Retraction of the retractor *tip* continues until the tentorial edge is identified. If venous bleeding occurs, temporarily ease retraction and if necessary, place some surgicel over the site of bleeding. Stitching back the edge of the tentorium (avoiding damage to the 4th nerve which runs just under the tentorial edge) improves access to the interpeduncular fossa. Look for the 3rd nerve lying under the arachnoid and open the double layer of arachnoid between this and the 4th nerve (Fig. 4A). Following the superior cerebellar artery medially leads to the basilar artery, the bifurcation and posterior cerebral vessels (Fig. 4B). Usually the 3rd nerve is retracted superiorly, but when the bifurcation lies above the level of the posterior clinoid it may be necessary to open the arachnoid above the nerve. Before clipping, it is important to identify the

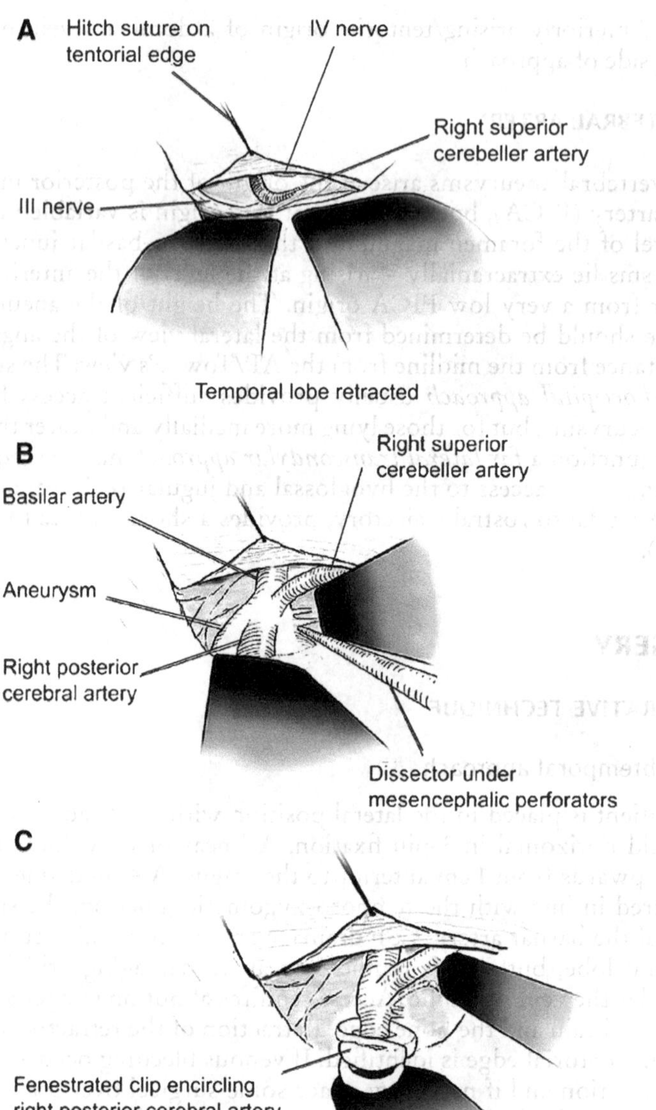

Fig. 4. Subtemporal approach to basilar bifurcation aneurysm

left posterior cerebral artery and the thalamo-mesencephalic perforators arising from P_1 and from the posterior surface of the basilar artery and to separate these from the aneurysm neck and fundus. The disadvantage of the subtemporal approach is the difficulty in visualising P_1 and the associated perforators on the left side, particularly with large aneurysms. Changing the microscope angle, working in front of the aneurysm and if necessary compressing the fundus, help the surgeon identify these vessels. Application of a temporary clip makes manipulation of the aneurysm sac safer and easier. Anteriorly projecting aneurysms tend to lie free from perforators and carry least risk during clipping. Superiorly and posteriorly projecting aneurysms usually require a fenestrated clip to encircle the right posterior cerebral artery and occasionally the 3rd nerve (Fig. 4C). The clip length should only extend to the distal edge of the neck, otherwise it may occlude perforators arising from the left P_1. Again a temporary clip reduces the intraluminal pressure and the chance of the clip slipping down on to the bifurcation. If this occurs place a second clip above the first and then remove the first. Large aneurysms may require several clips to prevent the fundus refilling. After clipping it is essential to re-inspect the vessels on each side and ensure that none are included in the clip. When the basilar bifurcation lies below the level of the posterior clinoids, proximal control may be harder to achieve with temporary clips. Preoperative insertion of an inflatable balloon into the basilar artery provides an alternative method of temporary basilar occlusion.

1.2 Transsylvian pterional approach

First described by Yaşargil et al. [12]. The patient is positioned with the head in 3-pin fixation, slightly elevated and rotated at about 45°. Through a pterional craniotomy, the arachnoid overlying the optic nerve and Sylvian fissure is widely opened. By retracting the frontal lobe, internal carotid artery and middle cerebral vessels medially and the temporal lobe laterally, and following the posterior communicating artery posteriorly back to its junction with the posterior cerebral artery, the basilar artery and bifurcation is approached from an antero/lateral direction. In most instances the route extends between the internal carotid/middle cerebral arteries and the 3rd nerve. Thereafter dissection continues either lateral to the posterior communicating artery or medially between the branches of its perforators. Dividing the posterior communicating artery between liga clips may improve access; this carries little risk provided that this vessel is not the dominant source of filling of the right posterior cerebral artery. Yaşargil et al. originally described the option of a route between the optic nerve and the carotid artery, but this is rarely required. The advantage of this antero-lateral approach is the ease of identification of the left posterior cerebral artery. Perforators can be separated easily from the neck of small aneurysms before safely clipping the neck, but for larger aneurysms, retraction of the fundus may be required to identify perforators running from the posterior surface of the basilar artery. From this route, basilar aneurysms are normally clipped across the plane of the vessels without the need of a fenestrated clip. As with the subtemporal approach temporary clipping can minimise dissection risks and reduce intraluminal pressure before clip application.

1.3 Subtemporal transtentorial approach

Position the patient as for a standard subtemporal approach. The temporal craniotomy is sited more posteriorly, centred above the mastoid. Considerable caution is required during retraction to avoid damaging the vein of Labbé. The tentorial edge is exposed and the tentorial layers are diathermied and divided parallel to the petrous ridge from near the junction of the petrosal and transverse sinus to the tentorial hiatus, to a point behind the dural entry of the 4th nerve. By stitching back the tentorial edge, the surgeon looks down the medial wall of the petrous bone. Aneurysms lying up to 20 mm below the posterior clinoids can be approached on the *medial* side of the trigeminal nerve (Fig. 3 black arrow); those lying more than 20 mm below require an approach *lateral* to the trigeminal nerve (Fig. 3, white striped arrow). Retraction of both the nerve and the pons may help identify the aneurysm neck. Rather than using a temporary clip, control may be achieved by inserting an indwelling non-detachable balloon catheter pre-operatively. If possible the aneurysm should be clipped in the plane of the vessels.

1.4 Combined supra-infratentorial (petrosal) approach

As described in detail by Al-Mefty et al., the patient is positioned in the lateral position with the head held horizontal in 3-pin fixation. In addition to a large temporo-occipital bone flap, a mastoidectomy permits a presigmoid retrolabyrinthine route to the posterior fossa [1, 3]. The temporal dura is opened and the superior petrosal sinus divided between clips just before its junction with the transverse sinus (Fig. 3). The dural opening is extended in front of the sigmoid sinus opening into the posterior fossa. Dividing the tentorium alongside the petrous ridge as described above and retracting the sigmoid sinus and cerebellum posteriorly and the temporal lobe superiorly, provides an extensive exposure. The 5th, 6th, 7th and 8th cranial nerves lie between the surgeon and the basilar artery/vertebro-basilar junction; all are at risk of damage during aneurysm dissection and clipping.

1.5 Lateral suboccipital approach

The patient is positioned semi-prone (or lateral), with the head held in 3-pin fixation and square to the shoulders and the chin tucked in to tighten the nuchal ligament. Through a paramedian excision the occiput and the atlas are exposed. The craniectomy extends from the midline to the edge of the transverse/sigmoid sinus and includes a rim of foramen magnum. For low-lying aneurysms, to gain proximal control, the vertebral artery can be exposed extracranially in the sulcus arteriosis as it crosses the arch of C1, before penetrating the dura. On opening the dura, the cerebellar tonsil is retracted medially to expose the vertebral artery, bridged by the lower cranial nerves. After opening the arachnoid layer and taking care to minimise any retraction of the nerves, the vertebral artery is followed rostrally until the origin of the PICA. Alternatively PICA may be easily identified running around and under the tonsil and this can be followed down to its origin and the aneurysm. Large aneurysms, or aneurysms lying near the vertebrobasilar junction may require the additional access gained by extending the bone removal as described below.

1.6 Far lateral transcondylar approach

The craniectomy is extended laterally using a high speed drill around the rim of the foramen magnum, deroofing the sigmoid sinus and jugular bulb, and removing up to a third or even a half of the occipital condyle (Fig. 3). After opening the dura, division of the dentate ligament may improve exposure of a laterally situated aneurysm. As with the above approach, it is often necessary to work between the branches of the lower cranial nerves to reach the aneurysm neck; this requires extreme care to avoid permanent nerve damage. If a large jugular tubercle masks the aneurysm neck, this can be removed with the air drill. In general, the larger the aneurysm and the nearer to the midline, the greater the need to extend bone removal in a lateral direction. This minimises cerebellar/brainstem retraction, shortens the distance to the midline and allows clip application from a trajectory more in line with the vertebral artery.

2. RESULTS

For the last 10 years coil embolisation has been used as the first line approach for most aneurysms of the posterior circulation. To obtain data on surgical outcome uninfluenced by the introduction of endovascular techniques, I return to results of an audit from 1989 to 1993 showing 3 month outcome of 66 patients undergoing clipping of a posterior circulation aneurysm (Table 1). Even during this period, 6 patients were treated with interventional techniques and they have been excluded from the table. Of the 66 patients, 2 presented with 3rd nerve palsies and 4 had incidental aneurysms. The remainder all suffered a subarachnoid haemorrhage. Patients with post-operative cranial nerve palsies alone were not categorised as disabled. Although numbers at each site are small, it is evident that surgical repair of basilar bifurcation aneurysms carries the highest mortality and morbidity with 2 deaths and 3 patients with severe disability. Patients in the severe disability category all sustained perforator damage.

Table 1. Results of surgical repair of posterior circulation aneurysms 1989–1993

	Good recovery	Moderate disability	Severe disability	Death	Total
Basilar bifurcation	25	4	3	2	34
Superior cerebellar	10	3	0	0	13
Posterior cerebral	2	0	0	0	2
AICA	3	0	0	0	3
Vertebro-basilar junction	2	0	0	0	2
PICA	9	2	0	1	12
Total	51	9	3	3	66

AICA Anterior inferior cerebellar artery, *PICA* posterior inferior cerebellar artery

HOW TO AVOID COMPLICATIONS

1. VENOUS INFARCTION

All subtemporal and petrosal (combined supra/infratentorial) approaches risk damage to the vein of Labbé. In about 50% of patients, occlusion will lead to venous infarction. If bleeding occurs, do not try to coagulate; ease back on retraction and pack with surgicel if necessary. A pre-operative CT venogram may help identify the relative importance of this draining vein and its position of entry into the transverse sinus. A dominant vein of Labbé entering the sinus immediately adjacent to the petrosal sinus or draining through a tentorial venous lake may be a reason to avoid the petrosal approach.

2. PER-OPERATIVE ANEURYSM RUPTURE

Temporary clipping of the proximal vessel (applied for 5 min, with 5 min reperfusion) may reduce the risk of aneurysm rupture during dissection and aid manipulation of the sac and identification of perforators and adjacent vessels, particularly with large aneurysms. The reduction in intraluminal pressure within the aneurysm sac allows optimal positioning of the aneurysm clip. For large basilar trunk or low lying bifurcation aneurysms, access to the proximal vessel may be difficult, if not impossible, particularly when approached from above. *Temporary endovascular occlusion* with a non-detachable silicone balloon inserted via a femoral catheter for 5-min periods provides a useful method of control. After clipping and deflating the balloon, the catheter permits intra-operative angiography to ensure accurate clip position with preservation of surrounding vessels. Over the last 30 years several authors have recorded the use of circulatory arrest in the treatment of giant intracranial aneurysms. These techniques permit up to

60 min of total circulatory arrest, thus helping both the dissection and clipping of such technically difficult aneurysms.

3. VESSEL OCCLUSION

It is essential to ensure that clip application does not constrict or occlude either proximal or distal vessels. A microdoppler probe can provide a guide to patency, but intraoperative angiography if available is a more certain method. Neither technique will show perforator occlusion. Only punctilious surgical technique can minimise this complication, particularly around the most vulnerable site at the basilar bifurcation.

4. CRANIAL NERVE DAMAGE

With the subtemporal approach to the basilar bifurcation about two thirds of patients sustain 3rd nerve damage. Most recover fully but in ¼ of those, some damage persists. The transtentorial approach to the basilar trunk risks damage to the 4th, 5th and 6th nerves and the combined petrosal approach also risks damage to the 7th and 8th nerves. Infratentorial approaches may damage the lower cranial nerves, particularly when dissecting and clipping PICA aneurysms. Great care and delicacy is required when retracting these nerves to gain access. Damage can lead to potentially fatal aspiration pneumonia.

CONCLUSIONS

Most centres now use coil embolisation as the first line approach for the treatment of posterior circulation aneurysms. Despite major advances in endovascular techniques over the last decade including balloon remodelling and coiling combined with the insertion of horizontal and "y" stents, a proportion of patients still require direct operative repair. Before proceeding to operation, careful evaluation of the angiographic findings is essential to indicate the optimal approach. Individual surgical preference and experience with a particular route may be the ultimate deciding factor. Where possible the surgeon should avoid complex skull base approaches. Simplicity often provides the safest option.

References

[1] Al-Mefty O, Fox JC, Smith RR (1988) Petrosal approach for petroclival meningiomas. Neurosurgery 22: 510-517

[2] Aziz KMA, van Loveran HR, Tew JM, Chicoine MR (1999) The Kawase approach to retrosellar and upper clival basilar aneurysms. Neurosurgery 44: 1225-1236

[3] Bowles AP, Kinjo T, Al-Mefty O (1995) Skull base approaches for posterior circulation aneurysms. Skull Base Surg 5: 251-260

[4] Day JD, Giannotta SL, Fukushima T (1994) Extradural temporopolar approach to lesions of the upper basilar artery and infrachiasmatic region. J Neurosurg 81: 230-235

[5] Dolenc VV, Skrap M, Sustersic J, Skrbec M, Morina A (1987) A transcavernous-transsellar approach to the basilar tip aneurysms. Br J Neurosurg 1: 251-259

[6] Drake CG (1965) Surgical treatment of ruptured aneuyrsms of the basilar artery. Experience with 14 cases. J Neurosurg 23: 457-473

[7] Drake CG (1979) The treatment of aneurysms of the posterior circulation. Clin Neurosurg 26: 96-144

[8] Kawase T, Toya S, Shiobara R, Mine T (1985) Transpetrosal approach for aneurysms of the lower basilar artery. J Neurosurg 63: 857-861

[9] Schievink WI, Wijdicks EFM, Piepgras DG, Chu C-P, O'Fallon WM, Whisnant JP (1995) The poor prognosis of ruptured intracranial aneurysms of the posterior circulation. J Neurosurg 82: 791-795

[10] Sugita K, Kobayashi S, Takemae T, Tada T, Tanaka Y (1987) Aneurysms of the basilar trunk. J Neurosurg 66: 500-505

[11] Wiebers DO, Whisnant JP, Huston J 3rd, et al. (2003) Unruptured intracranial aneurysms: natural history, clinical outcome and risks of surgical and endovascular treatment. Lancet 360: 1267-1274

[12] Yaşargil MG, Antic J, Laciga R, Jain KK, Hodosh RM, Smith RD (1976) Microsurgical pterional approach to aneurysm of the basilar artery. Surg Neurol 6: 83-91

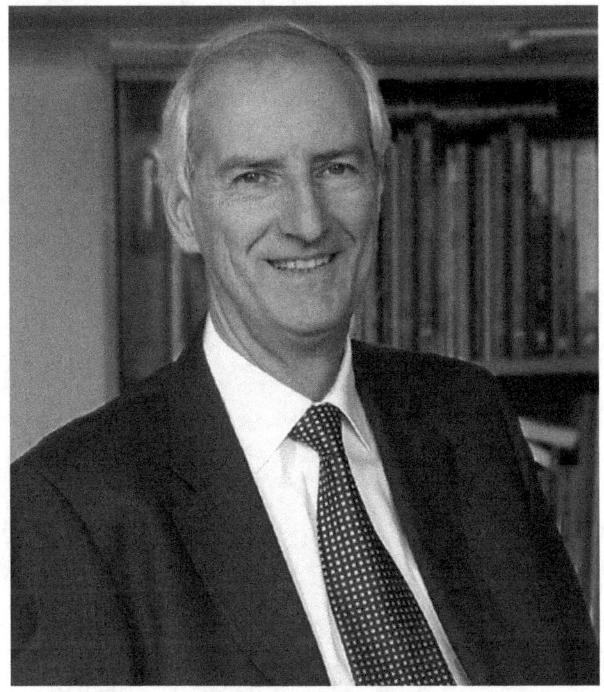

Ken Lindsay

Ken Lindsay is Consultant Neurosurgeon at the Institute of Neurological Sciences, Glasgow. He completed a PhD in Neurophysiology in 1975 before training in Neurosurgery in Glasgow under Bryan Jennett and Graham Teasdale. In 1981 he was appointed to a consultant post at the Royal Free Hospital in London and moved to his present post in Glasgow in 1988. There he extended his clinical and research interests in cerebral aneurysms and became responsible for managing all patients with posterior circulation aneurysms in the West of Scotland.

He became Chairman of the Specialist Advisory Committee in Neurosurgery, the committee responsible for standards of training throughout the UK from 1996 to 1999. From 1999 to 2001 he was Vice President (Surgical) of the Royal College of Physicians and Surgeons of Glasgow. He chaired the European Association of Neurosurgical Societies (EANS) Training Committee from 1999 to 2003 and was President of the EANS from 2003 to 2007. He is currently Chairman of the Joint Residency Advisory and Accreditation Committee (JRAAC) of the EANS/UEMS.

Contact: Ken Lindsay, Department of Neurosurgery, Southern General Hospital, 1345 Govan Road, Glasgow G51 4TF, UK
E-mail: ken.lindsay@ggc.scot.nhs.uk

GIANT ANEURYSMS

S. KOBAYASHI

This chapter has been written with collaboration of Prof. K. Hongo.

INTRODUCTION

Giant intracranial aneurysms (GAs) are the most difficult kind of intracranial aneurysms to treat. They present with subarachnoid hemorrhage and/or space occupying signs; they can also produce thromboembolic phenomena manifested by transient ischemic attacks or remain asymptomatic for many years. Their surgical treatment has been attempted by various renowned surgeons including Drake [1], Yaşargil [15], Sundt [12], Sugita et al. [11] and Spetzler et al. [10], all of them using innovative microneurosurgical techniques, and all of them with successes and failures. Recent development of bypass surgery techniques [2, 4] and endovascular treatment [14] have increased treatment options and improved surgical outcome for patients harboring GAs. Management options for surgery including deep hypothermia and cardiac standstill [7] are often instrumental. This chapter deals with the goals of treatment, surgical considerations, standard surgical techniques and complication avoidance.

RATIONALE

1. By definition, GA measures 25 mm or more in diameter and they represent approximately 3.5% of all intracranial aneurysms. It is known that the probability of rupture is higher than in smaller ones, and approximately 25% of GAs present with subarachnoid hemorrhage. The rate of rebleeding has been found as high as 18.4% at 14 days after admission [5]; observation after hemorrhage can lead to fatal outcome.
2. The goals of treatments of GAs are basically twofold; one is to prevent rupture and two to relieve the mass effect, if present. GAs are located either in the anterior or posterior circulation. In the anterior circulation, they are most common in the internal carotid artery followed by the middle cerebral artery, while in the posterior circulation the vertebral artery is most often involved. Occlusion of a GA is made by clipping with multiple clips or trapping the portion of

Keywords: vascular malformation, giant aneurysms, microsurgery the parent artery harboring the aneurysm with or without bypass surgery. Decompression of the thrombotic bulk of a GA is effected as necessary. When occluding a GA, special care should be taken to preserve perforating arteries. Knowledge of collateral circulation is important when trapping the aneurysm.

3. It is of great importance to know the anatomy of the parent artery and its branching and/or perforating vessels, especially regarding to their relation to the local skull base. There are particular cases such as the proximal internal carotid, in which cavernous sinus anatomy must be taken into account. In GAs of the posterior circulation, it is mandatory to know the topographic brainstem anatomy in addition to the vascular anatomy.
4. Current endovascular therapies, when properly selected and applied, can provide a lower-risk therapeutic modality, but do not provide results that are as durable as current surgical techniques [13], and do not represent an ideal solution.

DECISION-MAKING

1. DIAGNOSTIC STUDIES

1.1 Neurological symptoms and signs

- Asymptomatic GAs are incidentally found on brain CT or MRI taken for other purposes such as for headache, ischemic stroke or brain check-up screening.
- Subarachnoid hemorrhage causes symptoms ranging Hunt and Hess Grade 1.5. Often massive hemorrhage occurs with surrounding intracrebral hematoma.
- Mass signs are related to the location of GAs. For instance, a GA in the internal carotid artery can cause symptoms such as visual symptoms, cavernous sinus signs and hypopituitarism GAs in the vertebral artery cause brainstem compression with long tract signs and lower cranial nerve symptoms such as dysphagia, dysarthria and hoarseness. GAs at the basilar artery bifurcation can cause bilateral oculomotor pareses and hydrocephalus [6].
- Thromboembolic phenomena commonly manifest as transient ischemic attacks or infarction with its corresponding neurological deficits.

1.2 CT and MRI

- Location of the GA and its mass effect are well seen on the CT and MRI. MRA is obtained non-invasively and useful to see the aneurysm and involved arteries. Post-contrast CT or MRI provides information regarding intra-aneurysmal thrombosis. 3-D CT is especially useful for observing the interrelation of the aneurysm and surrounding arteries from different perspectives, which is instrumental in designing the surgical approach.

1.3 Angiogram

- Despite recent refinement of CT and MRI technology, angiography still has an important place in studying perforating arteries and dynamic flow and collateral circulation.
- Balloon occlusion test is useful in determining safety of trapping procedure [13]. However, efficacy of the balloon occlusion test is not totally guaranteed.

2. INDICATIONS

Which patients should be candidates for surgical treatment of GAs (Fig. 1).

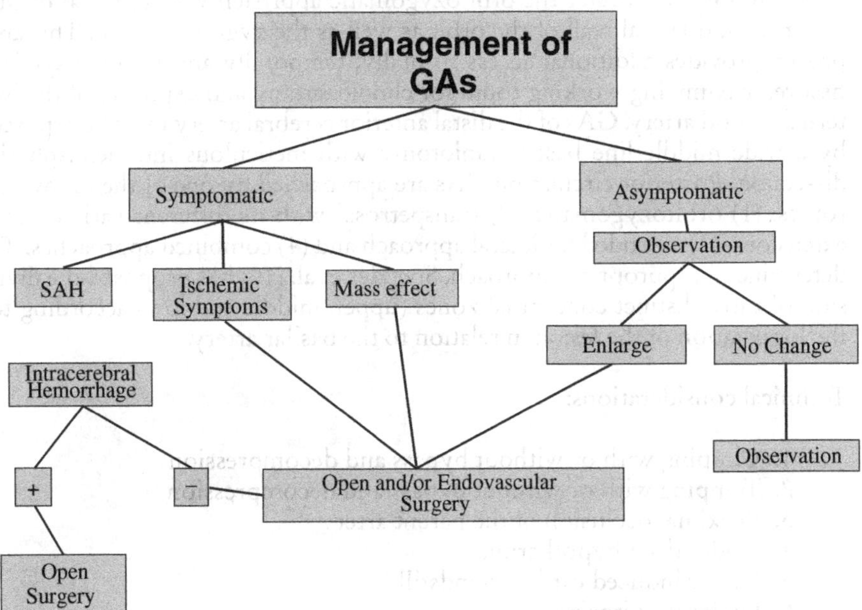

Fig. 1. Algorithm for the management of GAs. Asymptomatic patients should be followed by close observation until the presence of clinical symptoms or enlargement on radiological periodic examination; symptomatic patients must be treated via open surgery in case of rupture with the presence of intracerebral hemorrhage or via open surgery and/or endovascular treatment in case of other symptoms. *SAH* Subarachnoid hemorrhage

SURGERY

1. CEREBRAL PROTECTION

In GA surgery, temporary occlusion is usually required. Therefore, it is of vital importance to consider the neuroprotective measures such as intravenous infusion of mannitol and/or barbiturates (thiopental) with electroencephalographic burst suppression as a landmark; they are most effective when administered before periods of temporary occlusion. Patients can also be kept mildly hypertensive when a prolonged temporary clipping is expected [10].

2. OPERATIVE TECHNIQUE

The approaches for GAs are usually chosen under the same criteria as for non-GAs, considering always the need of proximal and distal control with minimal cerebral manipulation. For anterior circulation GAs, the pterional craniotomy with drilling of the lesser wing of the sphenoid bone and removal of the squamosal portion of the temporal bone, provides enough surgical working space. Some authors [10] prefer the orbitozygomatic approach with removal of the rim, roof and lateral wall of the orbit as well as the zygomatic arch. This approach provides additional access frontally, temporally and into the sylvian fissure, maximizing working room for clinoidectomy and exposure of the internal carotid artery. GAs of the distal anterior cerebral artery must be exposed by a wide middle-line based craniotomy with meticulous interhemispheric dissection. Posterior circulation GAs are approached by one of the following routes: (1) orbitozygomatic, (2) transpetrosal with its different variants and extensions, (3) extended far lateral approach and (4) combined approaches. To determine the appropriate approach, Spetzler et al. [10] has proposed the division of three distinct conceptual zones (upper, middle and low) according to the localization of the lesion in relation to the basilar artery.

Technical considerations:

1. Clipping with or without bypass and decompression
2. Trapping with or without bypass and decompression
3. Proximal occlusion of the parent artery
4. Under deep hypothermia
5. Under induced cardiac standstill
6. Under monitoring
7. Under temporary occlusion of the parent artery.

In order to occlude the aneurysm, clipping procedure is the most common and ideal, whereby long (ultra-long) clips or multiple clips are used. When

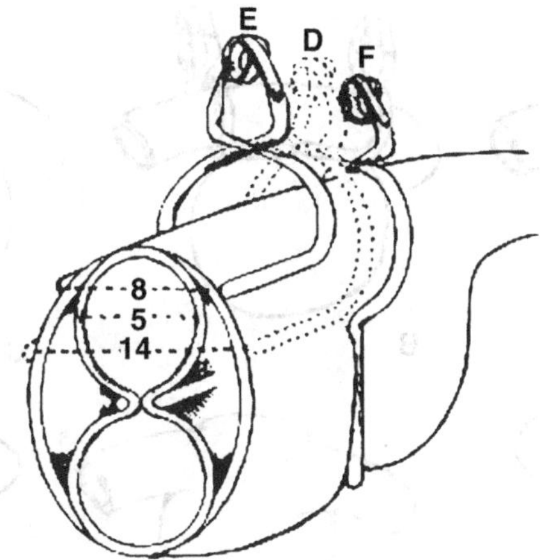

Fig. 2. Parent artery reconstruction with multiple clips. As the maximum opening distance of ring clip is not enough to prevent stenosis, it is recommended therefore to use first a straight ring clip to reduce the size of aneurysm and then one or two angled ring clips to completely close its neck. (The indicated distances are given in millimeters.) Modified from Sugita K (1985) Microneurosurgical atlas. Springer, Berlin Heidelberg, p 135

the aneurysmal neck of a GA is reconstructed, an ample volume of the neck portion of the aneurysm should be left on the side of the parent artery in order to avoid stenosis, because the neck is wide with thick wall. Special attention should be paid when using angled ring clips, because they do not open as wide as straight ones (Fig. 2).

There are several methods to occlude the neck with multiple clips and it is important to know them before undertaking surgery (Fig. 3).

Trapping procedure is used often for GAs of the internal carotid and vertebral artery, and less frequently for those in the middle and anterior cerebral artery. In a rare special case of basilar GA, trapping can be performed combined with bypass, after meticulous preoperative hemodynamic analysis.

Bypass procedure has become a useful addition to either clipping or trapping of GAs. The superficial temporal artery (STA) has shown to provide a sufficient collateral flow and is best used for restoring the distal middle cerebral artery flow. For an internal carotid artery GA, high flow bypass using the radial artery is often necessary [4].

For GAs of the posterior circulation, it is mandatory to study angiographically the patency of the posterior communicating arteries, as well as the relation between the lesion and the anterior inferior cerebellar artery and/or posterior inferior cerebellar artery. All these measures are followed in order to prevent brainstem infarction and to plan an accurate revascularization procedure.

When a high flow bypass is necessary, radial artery graft is preferred, because its diameter fits better with the recipient vessel, and this avoids the

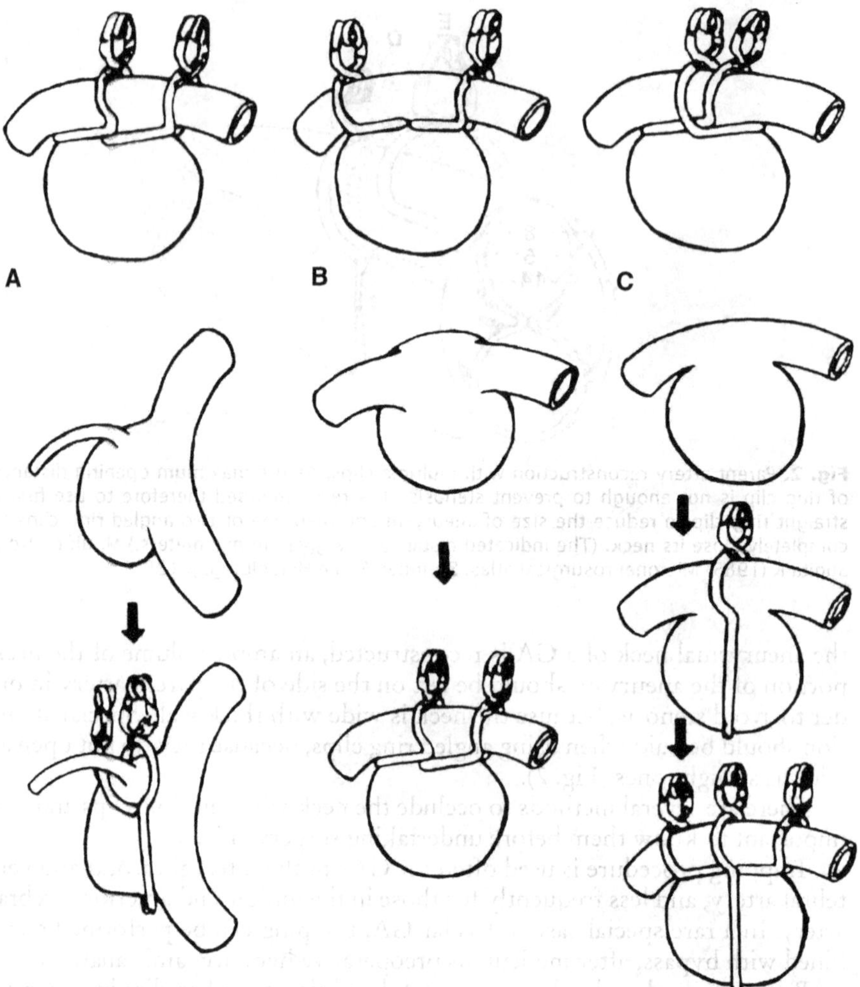

Fig. 3. *Top*: Multiple clipping, a method in which the aneurysm neck is occluded with more than two clips, includes many variations. Tandem clipping (**A**) and counterclipping (**B**, **C**) are commonly used for large or giant internal carotid aneurysms. Counterclipping can be carried out in facing (**B**) or crosswise fashion (**C**). *Middle and bottom*: Diagrammatic representation of formation clipping as branch artery formation (*left*), parent artery formation (*middle*) and aneurysm formation (*right*). (Modified from Kobayashi S, Tanaka Y, Apuzzo MLJ (1993) Brain surgery. Complication avoidance and management. Churchill Livingstone, New York, pp 833–843.)

presence of turbulent flow that has been observed with the saphenous vein grafts [4].

Despite the great importance of these revascularization procedures in the management of posterior circulation GAs, it is not to underestimate the

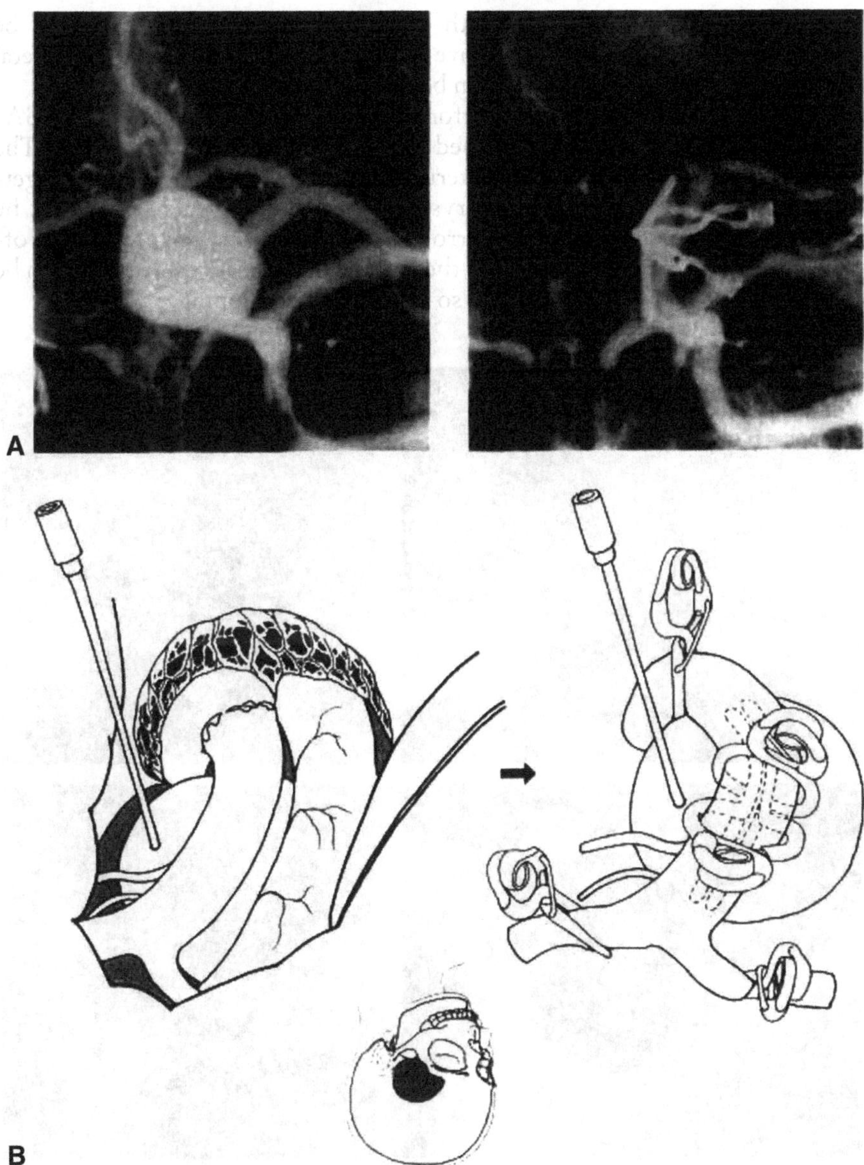

Fig. 4. ICA aneurysm clipped under temporary trapping without bypass. **A** Pre- and postoperative anteroposterior angiograms showing a giant aneurysm of the left internal carotid artery. A ring clip with blades bent to the left and a right-angled ring clip are applied with care to keep the original curve of the parent artery. **B** Schema of the operation in this case. Temporary clipping and suctioning of blood from the aneurysm reduce the aneurysm tension before application of permanent clips. (Modified from Kobayashi S, Tanaka Y, Apuzzo MLJ (1993) Brain surgery. Complication avoidance and management. Churchill Livingstone, New York, p 834.)

technical difficulties associated with its performance [2], and they must be taken into account in the preoperative plan. Even when considerable collateral flow is present, a bypass surgery can be used as an insurance procedure [3].

Decompression should be performed in thrombotic or sclerotic GAs causing mass signs. This is performed at the time of clipping or trapping. The aneurysm mass is debulked by internal decompression till the capsule gets thin enough to be soft (endoaneurysmectomy). The capsule should not be removed unnecessarily because surrounding arteries and perforators are often adherent to the outer surface of the capsule. Endoaneurysmectomy can be performed in the neck region only so as to facilitate clipping.

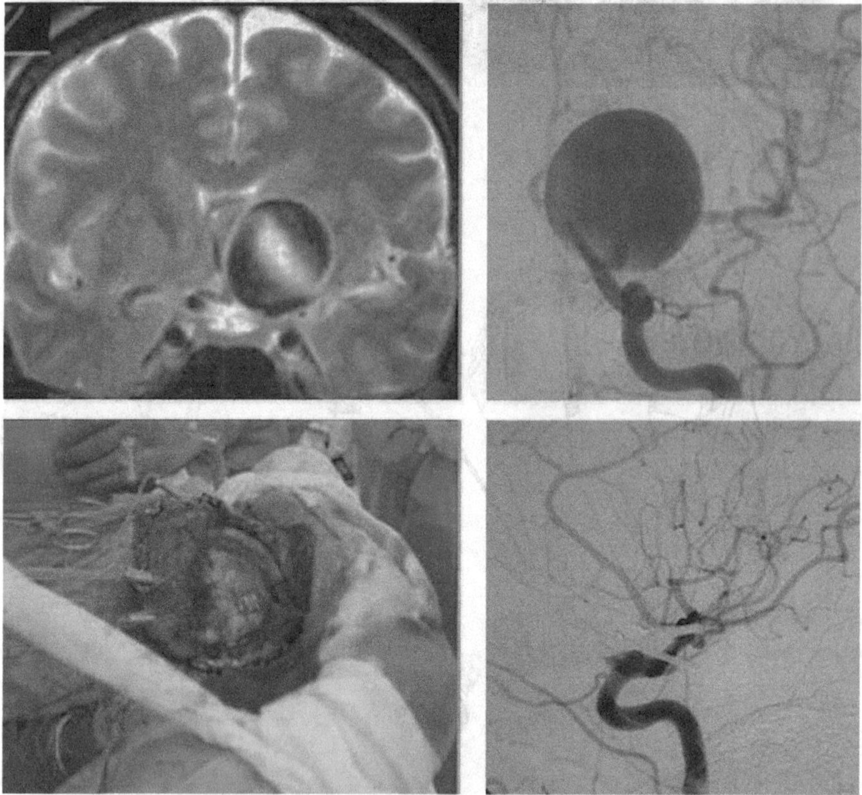

Fig. 5. ICA aneurysm clipped under temporary bypass with radial artery graft (**A** coronal MRI image; **B** preoperative anterior-posterior view of the left carotid angiogram). After exposure of M2, the patient's arm was raised (**C**) and a radial artery-M2 end to side anastomosis was made. The ICA was then trapped between the ophthalmic artery and the anterior choroidal artery, while the radial artery-M2 bypass was kept open. The aneurysm was then punctured and clipped with straight and ring clips (**D** postoperative lateral view of the left carotid angiogram). The bypass was closed: The radial artery was re-positioned to its original site at the wrist. Postoperative course was uneventful

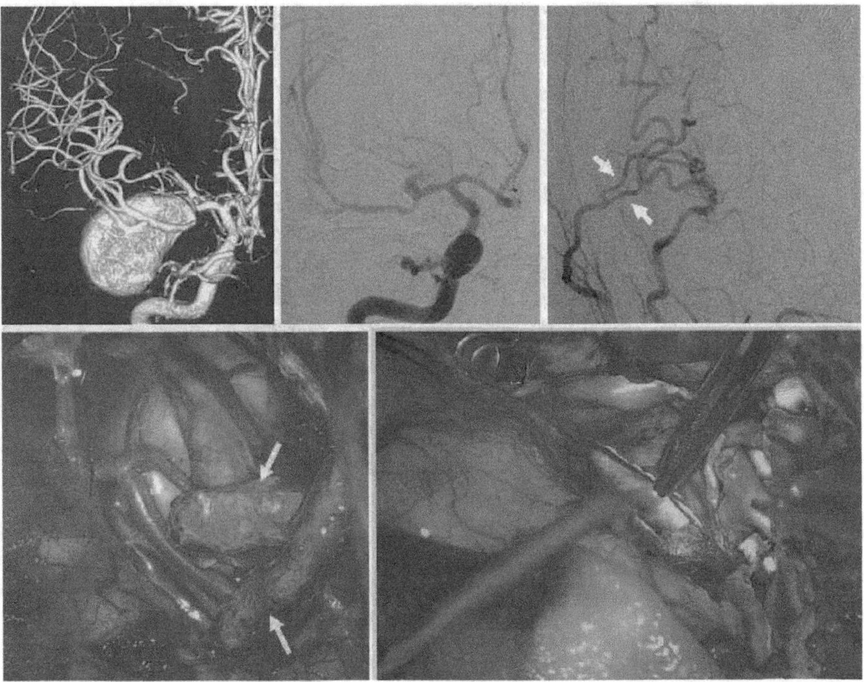

Fig. 6. MCA aneurysm clipped under STA-MCA bypass. (**A** Preoperative 3-D angiogram.) Through a pterional approach, the sylvian fissure was widely opened and a double end-to-side STA-MCA bypasses (superior and inferior trunks) were performed. (**D** Intraoperative photograph, arrows indicating STAs). The aneurysm was temporarily trapped, dissected and opened to remove thrombus, and it was obliterated with two clips in counterclipping fashion (**E**). (**B**, **C** Postoperative angiograms, showing respectively the occluded aneurysm with intentionally left small neck and patent double bypasses.) The patient was discharged without neurological deficits

Coil embolization is being used more in recent years, however, its long-term results have not been proved better than clipping [14]. Especially, coil compaction and incomplete embolization seem to be problematic. It is often chosen for basilar bifurcation GAs because of the technical difficulties by open surgery.

Illustrative cases.

- Internal carotid artery GA (Figs. 4 and 5).
- Middle cerebral artery GA (Fig. 6).
- Vertebral artery GA (Fig. 7).

3. LONG-TERM RESULTS

Despite the complexity of its treatment, GAs have a poor prognosis if left untreated, because most of GAs continue to enlarge, regardless of the

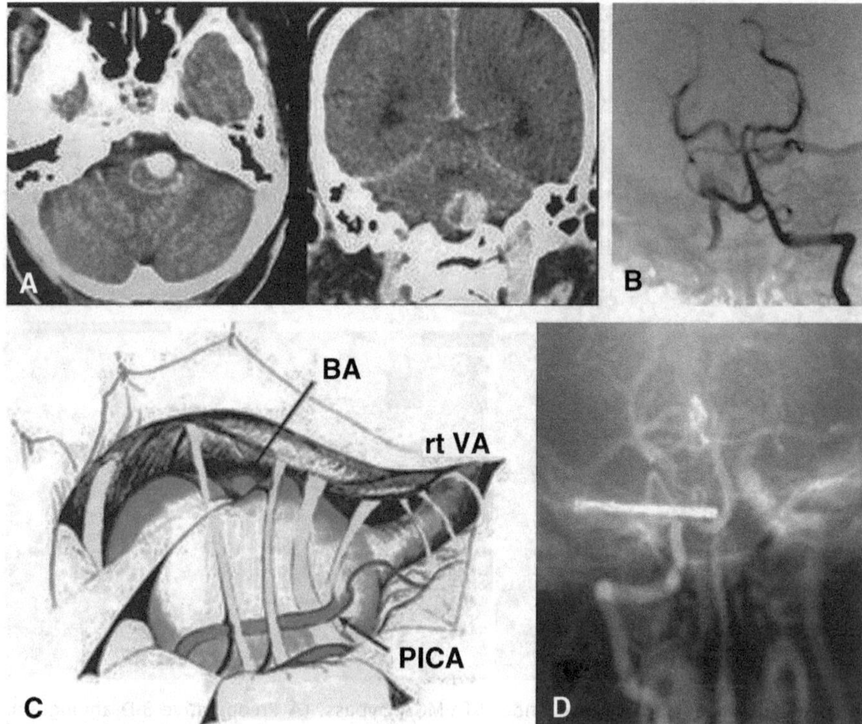

Fig. 7. VA-PICA partially thrombosed aneurysm, clipped under temporary trapping. Preoperative CT (**A**) and angiogram (**B**) showing a 26mm, partially thrombosed VA-PICA aneurysm. **C** Schematic view of the operative field. Under temporary trapping, partial thrombectomy was performed and the aneurysm was occluded with a single ultra-long clip. **D** Postoperative angiogram showing total occlusion

presence or absence of symptoms, and the risk of rupture increases during observation. Surgery reduces mortality from 31 to 4% compared with the conservatively treated patients [8].

HOW TO AVOID COMPLICATIONS

1. INTRAOPERATIVE RUPTURE

Prevention of intraoperative rupture starts before surgery by obtaining a 3-D image of the lesion and its topographic anatomy, which helps designing the surgical approach and clipping the aneurysm.

During surgery, sharp arachnoidal dissection is mandatory to free uninvolved cerebral lobules, and to carefully access through the cisterns to the parent artery. Once the proximal artery is freed from all arachnoidal tension points, dissection is followed proximally until the aneurysm neck is reached. In this point, it is of great importance to avoid tension to the aneurysm dome and to work as far as possible from the rupture point. There are some cases in which temporary clipping is needed, such as in some SAH cases, where arachnoidal plane is difficult to visualize because of thick hemorrhage, or in cases where the aneurysm is embedded in neural tissues, and its manipulation may cause tension with imminent rupture. In these cases one should strongly consider revascularization procedures, in order to maintain an adequate distal flow. This decision is made according to the preoperative analysis and intraoperative findings, depending on the expected time of ischemia and the possibility to restore flow through the parent artery after its occlusion.

2. CEREBRAL INFARCT

The complexity of these lesions provides a very high risk of postoperative cerebral infarction due to damage to perforators during dissection, inadvertent clipping of branches, failure to reconstruct properly the parent artery or prolonged temporary clipping without adequate alternative flow. Another possibilities leading to cerebral infarction are failure of bypass because of a tight anastomosis or because of the presence of thrombus inside the graft. Qualitative assessment of patency is easily made intraoperatively by micro-Doppler sonography. Exact confirmation by intraoperative angiography is of great value. A method gaining popularity in recent years is the Indocyanine Green Angiography (ICG) which is simple and provides real-time information on the patency of arterial and venous vessels, including small and perforating arteries (<0.5 mm) and the aneurysm sac [9].

3. CEREBRAL CONTUSION

In order to deal with GAs, a wide approach must be selected, one that permits clear visualization of proximal and distal vessels as much as surrounding venous and neural structures with minimal manipulation of nervous tissue [10]. Modern cranial base surgery techniques for approaches and proximal vascular control are invaluable tools to prevent excessive retraction and tension over brain tissue. When retracting the brain, it should be intermittently released as one practice for temporary arterial occlusion. Compromising veins should be avoided as much as possible, as venous congestion facilitate brain edema and contusion by retraction.

CONCLUSIONS

Symptomatic GAs are surgically treated best by clipping or trapping with bypass as necessary. Other methods of treatment include intravascular treatment. Asymptomatic GAs should carefully be observed and at a certain point, they should be treated as they would likely enlarge and eventually lead to rupture.

Acknowledgement

We thank Drs. Tetsuyoshi Horiuchi and Francisco Hasslacher for their cooperation in preparing this paper.

References

[1] Drake CG (1979) Giant intracranial aneurysms: experience with surgical treatment in 174 patients. Clin Neurosurg 26: 12-95

[2] Evans JJ, Sekhar LN, Rak R, Stimac D (2004) Bypass grafting and revascularization in the management of posterior circulation aneurysms. Neurosurgery 55: 1036-1049

[3] Hongo K, Horiuchi T, Nita J, Tanaka Y, Tada T, Kobayashi S (2003) Double-insurance bypass for internal carotid artery aneurysm surgery. Neurosurgery 52: 597-602

[4] Kamiyama H, Kazumata K, Kobayashi S (2005) Neurosurgery of complex vascular lesions and tumors. Thieme, New York, pp 338-345

[5] Khurana VG, Piepgras DG, Whisnant JP (1998) Ruptured giant intracranial aneurysms. Part I: A study of rebleeding. Neurosurg Focus (4)1: E1

[6] Kobayashi S (2005) Neurosurgery of complex vascular lesions and tumors. Thieme, New York, Chapters 3–7, 9–11, 14, 16, 19–21

[7] Mack WJ, Ducruet AF, Angevine PD, Komotar RJ, Shrebnick DB, Edwards NM, Smith CR, Heyer EJ, Monyero L, Connolly ES Jr, Solomon RA (2007) Deep hypothermic circulatory arrest for complex cerebral aneurysms: lessons learned. Neurosurgery 60: 815-827

[8] Nakase H, Shin Y, Kanemoto Y, Ohnishi H, Morimoto T, Sakaki T (2006) Long-term outcome of unruptured giant cerebral aneurysms. Neurol Med Chir (Tokio) 46: 379-384

[9] Raabe A, Beck J, Gerlach R, Zimmermann M, Seifert V (2003) Near-infrared indocyanine green video angiography: a new method for intraoperative assessment of vascular flow. Neurosurgery 52: 132-139

[10] Spetzler RF, Riina HA, Lemole GM Jr (2001) Giant aneurysms. Neurosurgery 49: 902-908

[11] Sugita K, Kobayashi S, Tanaka Y, Okudera H, Ohsawa M (1988) Giant aneurysms of the vertebral artery. Report of five cases. J Neurosurg 68: 960-966

[12] Sundt TM (1990) Surgical techniques for saccular and giant intracranial aneurysms. Williams & Wilkins, Baltimore

[13] Van Rooij WJ, Sulzewski M, Metz N, Nijssen P, Wijnalda D, Rinkel G, Tulleken C (2000) Carotid balloon occlusion for large and giant aneurysms: evaluation of a new test protocol. Neurosurgery 47: 116-122

[14] Wehman JCh, Hanel RA, Levy EI, Hopkins LN (2006) Cerebral aneurysms: endovascular challenges. Neurosurgery 59(Suppl 3): 125-138

[15] Yaşargil MG (1984) Microneurosurgery, vols I and II. Thieme-Stratton, New York

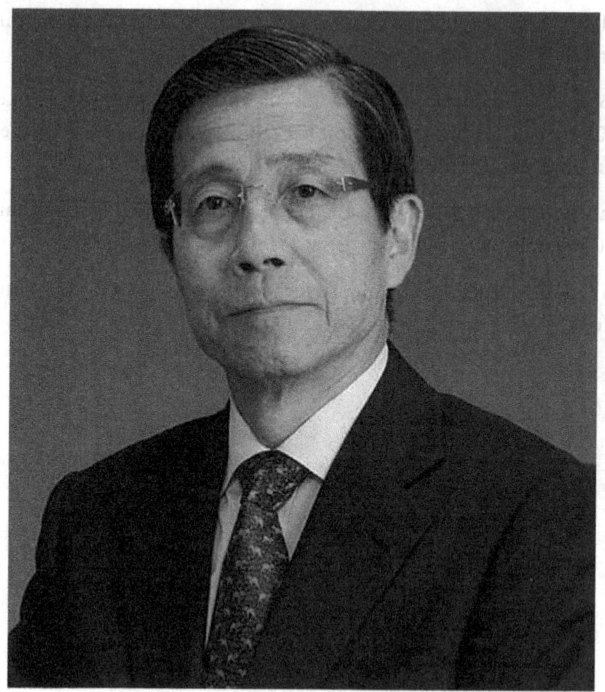

Shigeaki Kobayashi

Shigeaki Kobayashi is Director of the Stroke and Brain Center and of the Medical Education and Research Center at the Aizawa Hospital, Matsumoto.

Education: Shinshu University School of Medicine, 1957–1963; Residency in Neurosurgery at Mayo Clinic, 1965–1971.

Degrees: M.D. from Shinshu University, 1963; Master of Science in Neurological Surgery, Mayo Graduate School of Medicine, 1971; Ph.D., Neurosurgery, Shinshu University Graduate School of Medicine 1977.

Certificate: American Board of Neurological Surgery, 1971; Japanese Board of Neurological Surgery, 1971; Board of the Japan Stroke Society, 2003.

Professional and academic appointments: Professor and Chairman, Department of Neurosurgery, Shinshu University, School of Medicine, 1988–2003; Professor Emeritus, Shinshu University, 2003; Director, Stroke and Brain Center & Director, Medical Education and Research Center, Aizawa Hospital, 2006; Mayo Clinic Alumni Association Professional Achievement Award, 2005.

Scientific Societies membership (main only): Japan Neurosurgical Society (president 2001–2002, honorary president 2003); Japanese Congress of Neurological Surgeons (president 1977–1988, honorary member 2003); Japanese Society on Surgery for Cerebral Stroke (president 1996); American Association of Neurological Surgeons (member since

1971); Congress of Neurological Surgeons (member, Executive Committee 1992–1994); International Society for Neurosurgical Instrument Inventors (founding president 1995); World Federation of Neurosurgical Societies (treasurer 1997–2001, 2nd vice president 2001–2005, honorary president 2005); American Academy of Neurological Surgeons (corresponding member 1998–); Society of Neurological Surgeons (honorary member 2001–); Japan Stroke Society (Executive Committee member 1997–2007); Japanese Society of Acoustic Neuroma (president 1995).

Honorary memberships and professorship: honorary member, Brazilian Society of Neurosurgery; honorary professor, Hebei Medical University, China; honorary member, Neurosurgical Society of Taiwan (R.O.C.); honorary member, Italian Neurosurgical Society; honorary member, Japan Neurosurgical Society; honorary member, Japanese Congress of Neurological Surgeons; honorary member, Japanese Society of Skull Base Surgery; honorary member, Japanese Society for Computer in Neurosurgery; honorary member, Japanese Society on Surgery for Cerebral Stroke; honorary member, Conference on Neurosurgical Tools and Techniques.

Co-editor for scientific journals (present and past): Journal of Clinical Neuroscience (co-editor), Neurosurgery (international advisory panel), Neurologia medico-chirurgica (Tokyo) (review board), Surgical Neurology (consulting editor 1996–), Neurological Research (international editorial board), Minimally Invasive Surgery (advisory board), Skull Base Surgery (editorial board), Neurological Surgery (Tokyo) (advisory board), Acta Neurochirurgica (panel of reviewers), Japanese Journal of Neurosurgery (panel of reviewers), Techniques in Neurosurgery (editorial board), Operative Techniques in Neurosurgery (editorial board), Contemporary Neurosurgery (editorial board), Turkish Neurosurgery (international board), Zentralblatt fur Neurochirurgie (international advisory panel).

Medals and awards: HiVision Award '89, HDTV Promotion Society of Japan (for introducing HDTV in medicine), 1989; Kenneth Jamiesen Lecture and Medal, Australasian Neurosurgical Society, 1994; Nikkei BS Prize of the Year 2000: Development of Minimally Invasive Surgery for Brain Tumors and other Lesions; Japan Society of Mechanical Engineers Award (for robotics and mechatronics) 2002; Kanto Neurosurgical Conference Annual Distinguished Service Award 2002; Japan Robotics Society Award (for developing neurosurgical robotics), 2003.

Fields of professional interests: cerebrovascular surgery, brain tumor surgery (especially meningioma, acoustic neurinoma, etc.), skull base surgery, general neurosurgery; developing neurosurgical instruments; image analysis and surgical simulation; robotics in neurosurgery; microsurgical anatomy, cerebral circulation research (cerebrovascular innervation and physiology).

Contact: Shigeaki Kobayashi, Medical Research and Education Center, Aizawa Hospital, Honjo 2-5-1, Matsumoto 390-8510, Japan
E-mail: sub0305@wa2.so-net.ne.jp

ARTERIOVENOUS MALFORMATIONS OF THE BRAIN

R. C. HEROS

INTRODUCTION

Arteriovenous malformations (AVMs) are vascular abnormalities consisting of a number of direct connections of arteries and veins without a normal intervening capillary bed. AVMs are generally thought to be congenital, but they frequently grow during childhood, adolescence, and young adulthood. It is rare for them to grow significantly in the more mature adult. The most common presentation of intracranial AVMs is intracerebral hemorrhage closely followed by seizures. Other patients with AVMs present with headache and other signs of increased intracranial pressure and infrequently, with a progressive focal neurologic deficit which we generally attribute to a vascular steal, but which may well be due to venous hypertension in the territory of the veins draining the AVM.

Although the general orientation of this handbook is surgical, I will spend some time discussing issues relating to decision making which are extremely important and difficult with these lesions. I will also provide a short discussion of embolization and radiosurgery which are modalities of treatment that are frequently presented as "alternatives" to the patient but I will try to make the point that for each patient, there is only one best alternative and the different modalities of treatment should not be presented as interchangeable. Finally, I will discuss surgery, its results and its complications. While I will allude briefly to general surgical technique, most of the emphasis will be on the surgical approach to AVMs in different locations.

DECISION-MAKING

1. NATURAL HISTORY

It is obvious that a good understanding of the natural history of a disease is essential in the process of decision making. Fortunately, we have several very good studies in the literature that give us robust data about the natural history of both AVMs that present with hemorrhage and those that have never

Keywords: cerebral arteriovenous malformation, surgery of cerebral AVMs, intracranial surgery

bled. One of the most important and earliest studies was reported by Graf et al. [4] who reported a 2–3% risk of hemorrhage in patients that had never bled from their AVM. In the group of patients that presented with hemorrhage, the risk of re-hemorrhage over the first year was 6% and subsequent to that, the risk was 2% per year. Brown et al. reported an annualized hemorrhage rate of 2.2% in patients that presented with hemorrhage [2]. Likewise, Crawford et al. reported a hemorrhage rate of 2% per year but in this particular series, the risk for those patients that presented with hemorrhage was 36% over a ten year period as compared to 17% in patients that had never bled [3]. In an excellent study with a 23.7 year average follow-up, Ondra et al. found that in patients that presented with hemorrhage, the annualized bleeding rate during follow-up was 3.9%; for patients that presented with seizures, the rate was 4.3% per year and for those that were asymptomatic or had other symptoms, the rate was 3.9% per year [14].

In summary, it appears that patients with cerebral AVMs bleed at a rate of approximately 2–4% per year and that rate of bleeding in most studies is similar whether the patient has ever bled or not although patients that present with hemorrhage have about twice the risk of re-bleeding during the first year. It appears clear then that unruptured cerebral AVMs have a much greater annual rate of bleeding than unruptured aneurysms although of course, the consequences of a hemorrhage from an aneurysm are worse than those of a hemorrhage from an AVM; the latter hemorrhages result in significant morbidity in approximately 25–30% of the patients and they result in death in approximately 10% of the patients [1].

2. THE PATIENT

Factors related to the patient are extremely important in the decision making process with cerebral AVMs. The most important of these factors is, of course, the age. Age is the most important determinant of the number of future years at risk for a hemorrhage and in addition, it is also a very important factor influencing the ability of the patient to tolerate a prolonged difficult operation and to achieve a satisfactory recovery from any neurologic deficit that may occur from surgery. For the same reasons, the patient's general medical condition must be taken into account. The clinical presentation of the patient and the neurologic condition at the time of presentation are also very important factors. For example, if a patient has a fixed neurologic deficit which would be the deficit expected from resection on an AVM in a particular region of the brain, the surgeon may be more inclined to recommend surgery. The occupation and lifestyle of the patient are also important considerations. Even a modest speech deficit may be intolerable to a teacher or a lawyer whereas a visual field cut that may be well tolerated by most patients may be intolerable to a pilot or a truck driver. The psychological reaction of the patient to the knowledge that he/she has an AVM must also be taken into consideration.

Some patients are simply devastated by the thought that they have a lesion that could bleed at any time whereas others can go on with a perfectly normal life in spite of that knowledge.

3. THE AVM

Clearly, the size, configuration, pattern of arterial feeding and venous drainage and location of the AVM are extremely important factors to consider in the decision making process. To help the neurosurgeon estimate the surgical risk, a number of classifications have been developed including the one we use most frequently today, which is the Spetzler-Martin Grading Scheme. This classification simplifies the estimation of the surgical risk by considering the size of the AVM, its location and the presence of deep venous drainage which is an objective indicator of whether the AVM extends to or involves deeper portions of the brain. Although these classifications are helpful, particularly in terms of reporting and comparing results, there is no classification that can take into account all the different variables that the experienced surgeon must consider in estimating surgical risk. Factors such as the presence of deep perforating arterial supply, the location of the venous drainage, the configuration of the nidus (compact vs. diffuse), etc. would be difficult to account for in any classification. It can truly be said that no AVM is exactly like any other which adds to the importance of a very individualized, patient by patient, decision making process.

4. THE SURGEON

Finally, it should be obvious with these difficult lesions that the surgeon's experience with AVMs is an extremely important factor. Furthermore, the availability of the different modalities of treatment at the center in question as well as the understanding by the surgeon of proper use of adjunctive or alternative treatments such as embolization and/or radiosurgery is of paramount importance. In my opinion, it should be an experienced neurosurgeon that gives the ultimate advice to patients with cerebral AVMs as to what treatment is best for them. The experience of that neurosurgeon should not be limited to surgical excision but should also include knowledge of the indications, efficacy and complications of embolization and radiosurgery as stated above. With this experience, the neurosurgeon is in the position to give to the patient proper advice as to what would be the optimal treatment for him which may be conservative therapy, radiosurgery, surgical excision with or without embolization, embolization alone or a combination of these modalities. It is my firm opinion that it is the ethical responsibility of that surgeon to give to the patient in a straight forward manner, his opinion as to what would be the best treatment for that particular patient with that particular AVM without any ambiguities or hesitation unless the surgeon really does not know, in which case it may be prudent to refer the patient to a more experienced colleague. It does not seem fair to present the patient with a plethora of statistics and then tell the patient that it is "his decision" and that the surgeon will not make that decision for him. Of course, the patient will ultimately make the decision as to whether or not to accept the recommendation of the surgeon but he is entitled to have the benefit of the clear expert opinion that he is seeking.

TREATMENT MODALITIES

1. RADIOSURGERY

Unquestionably, radiosurgery, which was developed and is currently used mostly by neurosurgeons, has made a tremendous impact in the treatment of AVMs. It is clear that radiosurgery, as currently performed by a variety of techniques, is a very effective treatment for small AVMs, generally 3 cm or less in diameter. My colleagues and I have reviewed this topic in detail [1, 11] and have concluded that the average obliteration rate over a period of 2–3 years for AVMs treated with radiosurgery is somewhere between 60 and 80%. That rate appears to be closer to the higher figure for very small AVMs and decreases as we treat larger AVMs. The rate of clinically significant complications directly attributable to radiosurgery (radiation necrosis) is somewhere between 3 and 6% depending on whether the treated AVM involves an eloquent area of the brain or not. The morbidity of treating lesions in very critical regions such as the brainstem and the internal capsule may be substantially higher.

Obviously the great advantage of radiosurgery, in addition to its minimal invasiveness, is that it can be used for lesions that because of their deep and critical location would carry unacceptable surgical morbidity. The obvious disadvantage of radiosurgery, which is of course critical, is the uncertainty of cure (complete obliteration) and the fact that it generally takes between one and three or four years for compete obliteration to occur if it is going to occur at all. It has been clearly established that during this "latent" period of incomplete obliteration, the risk of hemorrhage is identical to the natural history of the disease [11]. In other words, the patient remains at the same risk that he was before treatment in terms of the probability of hemorrhage until the AVM is completely obliterated by radiosurgery. There are a few reports of late hemorrhage after angiographically proven complete obliteration and there are also reports of histologically proven patency of some of the components of the AVM after angiographic obliteration [8]; however, considering the very large number of patients that have been treated over the last 20 years with radiosurgery, it is fair to conclude that once angiographic obliteration has been demonstrated, the risk of a future hemorrhage after radiosurgery is extremely small and practically negligible.

2. EMBOLIZATION

Endovascular embolization of AVMs was also pioneered by a neurosurgeon, A. Luessenhop. Subsequently, many of our colleagues, particularly in neuroradiology, have improved and continue to improve these techniques. Unquestionably, preoperative embolization has made it feasible to operate with considerable safety, cerebral AVMs that were clearly inoperable or at least not operable without substantial morbidity, in the days before embolization. The issue then is not whether preoperative embolization facilitates surgical excision, which unquestionably it does, but when it should be used. If embolization could be carried out without morbidity, every neurosurgeon would choose preoperative embolization for essentially all AVMs. However, it is clear from our recent review of the literature on embolization, that the morbidity of embolization is still substantial [1]. For example, Taylor et al. reported in 2004 a 6.5% permanent morbidity and a 1.2% mortality per embolization procedure [16]. Other modern series from excellent centers have reported similar morbidity rates. With these morbidity rates, it is clear that preoperative embolization should not be used only to facilitate the surgery but rather it should only be used when in the judgment of the experienced surgeon, the combined morbidity of the embolization plus the surgery after embolization would be less than what the expected morbidity of the surgery would be if it were carried out without embolization. Additionally, I strongly believe that preoperative embolization should be carried out under the direction of the operating surgeon in order to optimally facilitate surgery and reduce morbidity. For example, with a large temporal AVM, there is no need to embolize superficial middle cerebral feeders to which the surgeon would have ready access during the early operative stages. Rather, it would be much more important to embolize deep feeders from the posterior cerebral artery to which the surgeon may not have early access without significant retraction of the temporal lobe and risk of damage to bridging veins. Likewise, the difference between safe and unsafe surgical resection may be determined by the ability of the endovascular surgeon to occlude critical perforating vessels to which the surgeon would not have ready access (Fig. 1).

Another critical issue is whether and when to recommend embolization as the primary and only therapeutic modality. There is no question that in very competent hands, when the patients are properly selected by a very experienced endovascular surgeon, a relatively high rate of obliteration can be achieved; however, even in the best hands, that rate of complete obliteration does not seem to exceed 40% of those lesions where total obliteration was thought to be possible by the interventionist [17]. The rate of complete obliteration by embolization is much lower, generally between 5 and 15%, when considering all AVMs that are embolized rather than those that are specifically selected for embolization because complete obliteration was thought to be possible [1]. The real issue is whether obliteration by endovascular surgery

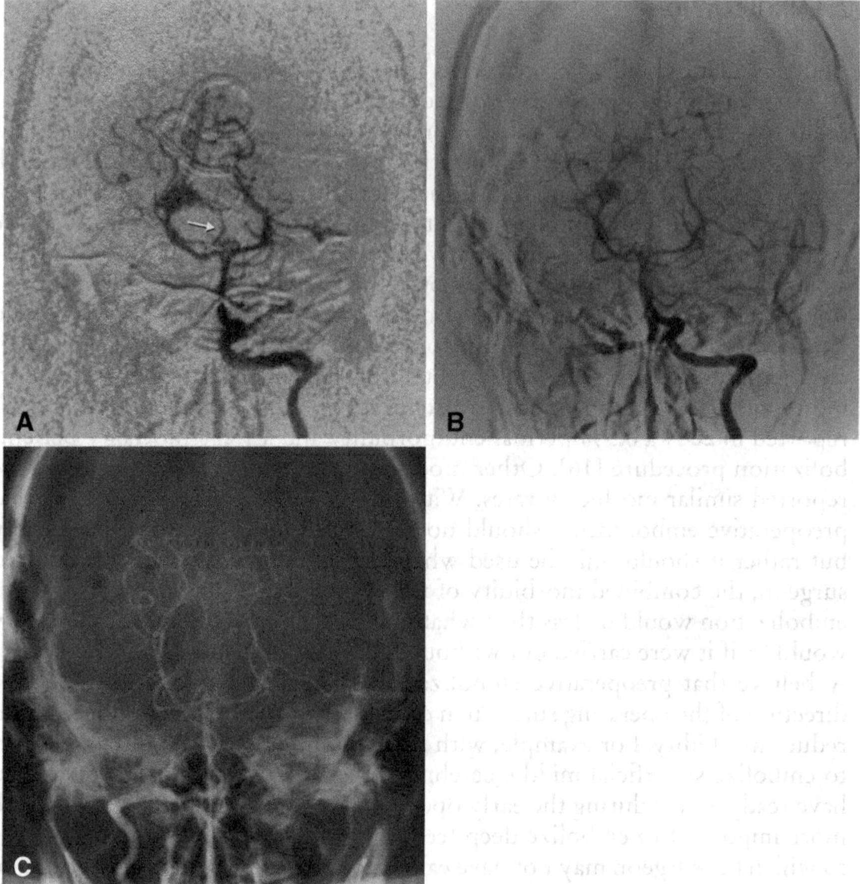

Fig. 1. Small thalamic AVM with large thalamoperforating feeder. **A** Anteroposterior (A-P) vertebral injection. Note large perforating feeder to the deep portion of the AVM (arrow). **B** A-P vertebral injection after successful embolization of large thalamoperforating feeder. **C** Postoperative A-P vertebral injection. The lesion was completely removed through a subtemporal approach

can be achieved with lower morbidity than the estimated surgical morbidity of microsurgical excision of those lesions, which are generally smaller AVMs with a limited number of arterial feeders.

When considering embolization as an "alternative" form of treatment, it should be kept in mind that, as our recent review has clearly indicated to us, the natural history in terms of risk of future hemorrhage is not changed at all for the better and may be changed for the worse (increased risk of hemorrhage) in those AVMs that are less than completely obliterated by embolization [1]. In other words, "palliative" embolization does not seem to improve the natural history of AVMs and it carries a significant morbidity;

therefore, it is only rarely, in my opinion, indicated. The exception is in cases that present with a progressive neurologic deficit due to steal, increased intracranial pressure from venous hypertension, intractable epilepsy which frequently can be improved by palliative embolization and intractable focal headaches that can be improved by obliteration of large dural feeders. It is also reasonable to consider palliative embolization in patients that present certain angiographic features such as stenosis of the main venous outlet, intranidal fistulas and aneurysms, aneurysms in feeding vessels, etc. who may be presumed to be at higher risk of hemorrhage and whose AVM cannot be removed completely or treated by radiosurgery because of its size, location, etc.

3. COMBINED MODALITIES

I have discussed the usefulness of preoperative embolization to facilitate the surgical excision and have warned against its abuse. It is also frequent practice to use embolization before radiosurgery. The rationale for this has to be questioned. Frequently, embolization is used in large AVMs that normally would not be amenable to radiosurgery in order to make them "smaller" and therefore amenable to radiosurgery. This rationale is based on the assumption that areas of the AVM that do not fill angiographically immediately after embolization are indeed permanently occluded. However, we know that many of these portions of the AVM that appear to be completely occluded after embolization recanalize with time [15]. In fact, preoperative embolization has been one of the most important factors correlated with failure of radiosurgery [15]. Additionally, as we discussed above, there is no evidence that partial embolization reduces the risk of bleeding and in fact there is some weak evidence that it increases it [1]. Nevertheless, we do recommend embolization prior to radiosurgery for the occasional AVM that cannot be excised surgically without high morbidity and where the angiographic appearance of the AVM presents what we would consider significant risk factors for hemorrhage as listed above. In our opinion, pre-radiosurgery embolization simply to reduce the flow to the AVM or even to reduce its size, if such can really be accomplished, is not indicated and in fact, we feel, is contraindicated given the additional morbidity of embolization.

SURGICAL TREATMENT

1. GENERAL COMMENTS

I have written extensively about surgical techniques for AVMs [1, 9, 10] but I will reiterate here some points that I feel are important. I will begin by saying that AVM surgery generally should be elective surgery. There is the occasional patient with a large intracerebral hemorrhage that requires surgical evacuation as a life saving operation. In these cases, I prefer to evacuate the hematoma very conservatively making every effort not to disturb the AVM which is left to be treated at a later time. Of course, there are those instances in which a very small superficial AVM is readily identifiable in relation to the hematoma and it can be removed safely but generally, we prefer to wait a few weeks, repeat the angiogram which sometimes would reveal a very different anatomy that what an emergency angiogram after the hemorrhage would indicate, and then operate electively.

For deep lesions, we have found frameless stereotactic guidance very helpful and tailor a relatively small craniotomy to get us to the lesion through the shortest trajectory through non-critical brain. For large superficial lesions, we use a larger-than-necessary craniotomy to be able to map the surface vascular anatomy including feeding arteries that sometimes can be identified on the surface before they plunge deeply into a sulcus as they approach the AVM. More importantly, the superficial draining venous anatomy sometime requires a large craniotomy to be able to be clearly understood. After the superficial anatomy is well defined, we proceed to systematically open under the microscope all the sulci around the AVM looking for superficial feeders which can be coagulated and divided as they approach the AVM. Sometimes, it is difficult to differentiate arterialized veins from feeding arteries and in these instances, if simple microsurgical observation under high power is not sufficient to differentiate them, we use a temporary clip which would show collapse of the vessel away from the AVM in the case of an arterialized vein. In critical areas of the brain, the surgeon must take feeding vessels only after he is absolutely sure the particular artery goes to the AVM and nowhere else. Arteries *en passage* that give small lateral branches to the AVM and go on to supply normal brain are a particular problem with AVMs in the Sylvian fissure and with pericallosal AVMs. In these cases, the artery needs to be meticulously "skeletonized" taking all the small side branches to the AVM and preserving the main trunk until the surgeon is sure that the artery goes on to normal brain without any further branches to the AVM. Of course, we try to preserve all arterialized veins but occasionally sacrifice one or more small superficial veins provided that there is ample venous drainage left intact. After we have identified all the superficial feeders to the AVM by opening all the adjacent sulci, we proceed with a circumferential corticectomy around the AVM. Empirically, we have found that if we carry that corticectomy to about 2.5–3 cm in depth, all the superficial arterial supply would be identified and occluded. After this is done, we proceed with a process of "spiraling" dissection around the AVM until we reach its deepest aspect. It is very important not to confuse loops of the AVM that project into normal brain with feeding arteries or draining veins. Coagulation and interruption of these loops could lead to significant bleeding from the AVM which is hard to control. As the deeper portion of the AVM is approached, frequently the surgeon encounters significant bleeding which of course is the Achilles tendon of AVM surgery. In the case of AVMs that reach the ventricle, frequently the bleeding will not stop until the ependyma of the ventricle has been reached and small ependymal feeders to the AVM are controlled. These deep vessels are extremely difficult to coagulate or clip and we have found that the small micro clips designed by the late Dr. Sundt specifically for this purpose, are extremely useful for these tiny fragile vessels. At times, in spite of meticulous technique, the surgeon encounters significant bleeding from the AVM and when this is the case, it is frequently possible to place a small cottonoid patty over the point of bleeding, against the AVM, and if necessary, place gentle traction with a retractor on that area and proceed with dissection elsewhere. It is of course essential never to pack bleeding away from the AVM since this can result in significant parenchymal or intraventricular hemorrhage.

Bipolar coagulation is the mainstay of AVM surgery. I teach my residents that they must learn how to use bipolar coagulation properly with simpler cases only to have perfected the technique by the time they are ready to operate on AVMs. I prefer steady bursts of coagulation lasting one or two seconds without bringing the tip of the forceps together and under constant irrigation. It is essential for the scrub nurse to have the bipolar tips perfectly clean before returning them to the surgeon. As soon as the surgeon observes any "dirt" at the tip of bipolar forceps, he should have the nurse clean them and use a new perfectly clean bipolar forceps. Having one of these fragile deep AVM vessels "stick" to the bipolar tips is simply intolerable and can lead to major problems with avulsion of the vessel and retraction of the proximal end into the parenchyma with significant hemorrhage. Frequently I use bipolar coagulation to stroke the loops of the AVM in an effort to shrink it away from normal brain when the lesion is located in critical areas. However, this maneuver is only safe when a substantial amount of the arterial input to the lesion has been controlled and the AVM has become relatively "soft".

2. SPECIFIC LOCATIONS

I will proceed to discuss my preferred surgical approach to cerebral AVMs that do not have a convexity surface representation.

2.1 Medial temporal AVMs

The more anteriorly located of these lesions, in the region of the uncus, amygdala and the anterior hippocampal complex are approached through the medial aspect of the Sylvian fissure using a pterional craniotomy. As the Sylvian fissure is opened and the temporal lobe is retracted laterally, the feeding vessels to the AVM come nicely into view and can easily be identified. From superficial to deep, these branches are usually anterior temporal branches of the middle cerebral artery (MCA), the anterior choroidal artery and its branches and branches of the posterior communicating artery as well as some early temporal branches of the posterior cerebral artery. All these feeders must be controlled and divided while preserving the draining veins which drain both anteriorly into the sphenoparietal sinus and medially into the basal vein. Once all the arterial supply is controlled, the lesion can be removed with little difficulty.

The more posteriorly located lesions of the medial temporal lobe involve the hippocampal and parahippocampal region as well as the fusiform gyrus and can extend back to the trigone. These lesions are approached through a temporal craniotomy working either subtemporally or through the inferior temporal gyrus as I described before [6]. The transtemporal approach has the advantage over a subtemporal approach of not stretching the vein of Labbe which may be arterialized. In either case, the direction is towards the temporal horn, which once identified, serves as a good anatomic landmark for orientation. The anterior choroidal artery, which invariably supplies these lesions, is identified at the choroidal fissure in the most anterior aspect of the temporal horn. A superior quadrantanopia has frequently resulted from using this approach, but this is well tolerated by most patients.

2.2 Insular AVMs

Those AVMs that involve the insula are approached through the Sylvian fissure with skeletonization of the MCA Sylvian branches to control the medially directed feeders to the AVM that sits just deep to the web of the Sylvian complex. Unfortunately, these lesions frequently have lenticular striate perforator supply which can be problematic at surgery (Fig. 2). If that supply is predominant, we may prefer to refer these lesions for radiosurgery if the size allows.

2.3 Trigonal AVMs

We use two different approaches for AVMs in this region. For those lesions located inferiorly involving the floor and lateral wall of the trigone, we prefer a transtemporal approach through the inferior temporal gyrus on the dominant side and either through the inferior temporal gyrus or the middle temporal gyrus on the non-dominant side. Again, a quadrantanopia may result from this approach. The lesions involving the medial aspect of the trigone and the parasplenial region which also frequently involve the roof of the trigone and at times even the dorsal surface of the pulvinar, are approached through a transcortical parieto-occipital approach that I have described before [7]. With this latter approach, which essentially is centered at a point 9 cm above the inion and 3.5–4 cm lateral to the midline, we are usually able to avoid significant motor sensory deficits as well as a significant visual field defect since the incision in the brain is between the parietal sensory association fibers and the occipital visual association fibers. Needless to say, frameless stereotaxis is extremely helpful to define the transcortical trajectory.

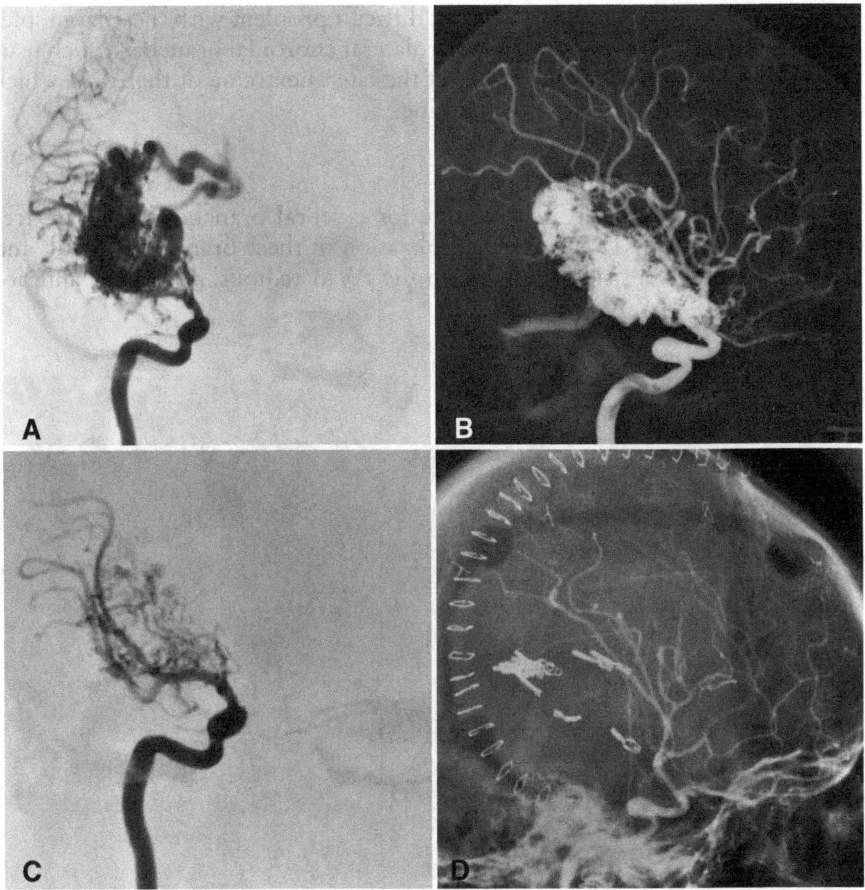

Fig. 2. Large left insular AVM. **A** A-P carotid injection. **B** Lateral carotid injection. **C** Early arterial phase of the A-P carotid injection demonstrating substantial lenticulostriate supply. **D** Postoperative lateral carotid injection. The lesion was successfully and completely removed by a trans-sylvian approach

2.4 Splenial-posterior third ventricular region

The difference between these AVMs and those that involve primarily the trigone is that the former are fed not only by posterolateral choroidal arteries coming from laterally into the trigone but also by posteromedial choroidal branches that come from medially. To control the latter, a parasagittal approach is preferable. For this approach, we prefer to use the lateral position with the ipsilateral side down and we have found that crossing veins are not a problem when a parieto-occipital trajectory is used. A lumbar drain is important in these cases to allow sufficient relaxation of the brain so as to not have to retract the brain forcibly. The most difficult problem with these large splenial AVMs is the control of the posterolateral choroidal branches which usually come along the choroid plexus at the lateral extreme of the AVM which may be as far as 3.5 cm from the midline.

2.5 Callosal AVMs

These lesions are usually fed by anterior cerebral branches which are frequently *en passage*. This makes embolization of these branches difficult and control of the small side branches to the AVM tedious. The more anterior

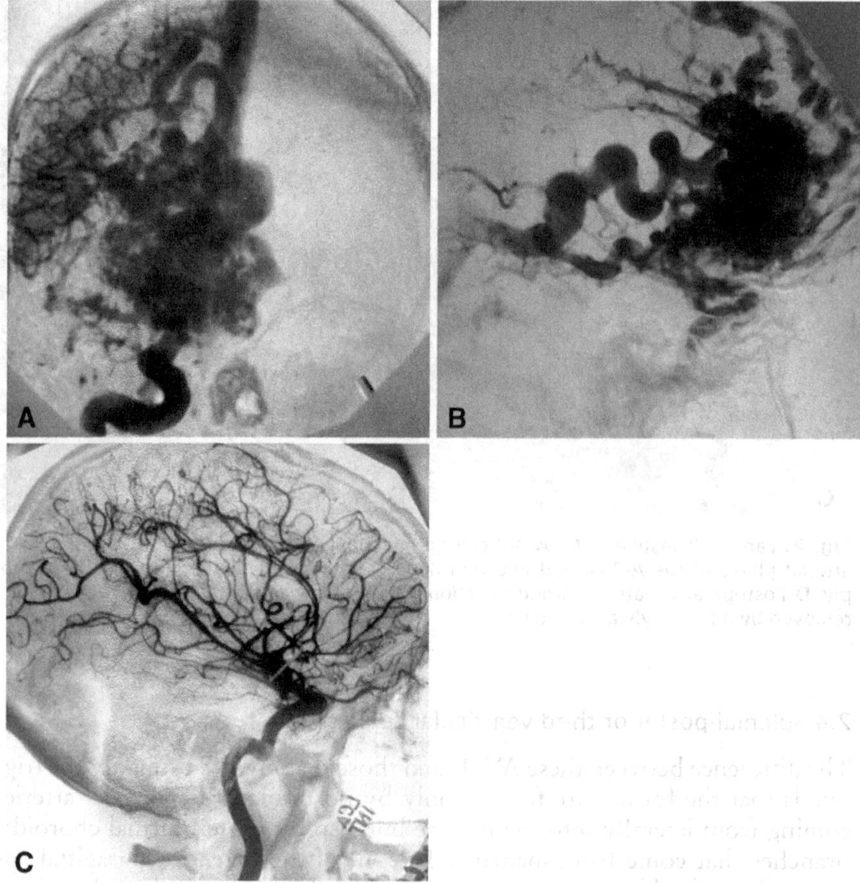

Fig. 3. Large anterior callosal and left deep frontal basal AVM. **A** A-P carotid injection. **B** Lateral carotid injection. **C** Postoperative carotid injection. The lesion was successfully and completely removed through a combined pterional and superior interhemispheric approach

large lesions frequently involve the head of the caudate nucleus and may extend to the anterior limb of the interior capsule which invariably implies arterial supply by deep perforators from the medial portion of the MCA and from the recurrent artery of Heubner. Some of these lesions can be very large and involve the basal-medial aspect of the frontal lobe. We have had a couple of these large AVMs that required the sequential use of a basal pterional approach and then a superior parasagittal approach through a large combined craniotomy and a change in the position of the head (Fig. 3). When these lesions are very large and have exuberant lenticulostriate supply, the surgical morbidity is likely to be high and conservative treatment may be an option.

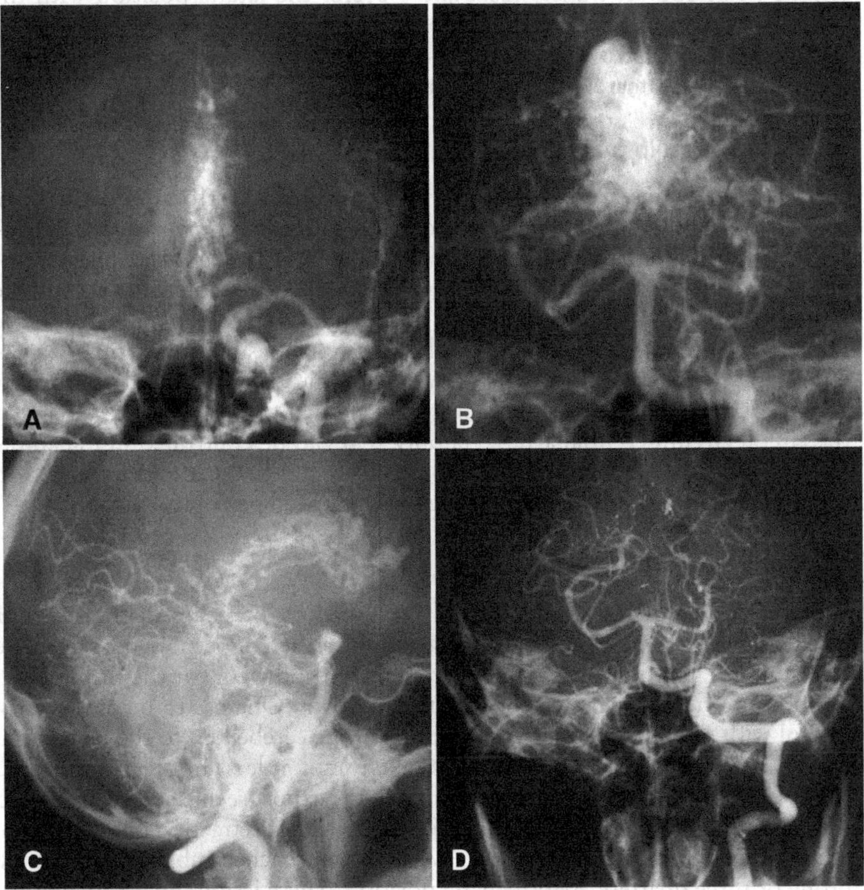

Fig. 4. Large intraventricular AVM occupying all the roof of the third ventricle. **A** A-P left carotid injection. **B** A-P vertebral injection. **C** Lateral vertebral injection; note predominant posteriomedial choroidal supply without any thalamoperforating supply. **D** Postoperative A-P vertebral injection. The lesion was successfully and completely removed through a transcallosal approach with the craniotomy centered at the coronal suture

2.6 Intraventricular AVMs

In my opinion, these lesions have a rather bad natural history with repeated hemorrhages and I tend to be aggressive with them. Resectability is determined by the predominance of choroidal supply as opposed to deep perforating supply. When the latter predominates, which of course means that the lesions involve the parenchyma of the thalamus, conservative therapy may be preferable unless the lesion is small enough to be treated with radiosurgery. When the supply is exclusively or predominantly choroidal, the latter can be controlled readily in the ventricle even when the lesion extends along the entire length of the roof of the third ventricle (Fig. 4). The approach to these lesions is, of course, transcallosal and I prefer the lateral position with the ipsilateral side down. Perhaps the most difficult aspect of operating on these intraventricular AVMs is the preservation of the internal cerebral veins which are frequently intimately related to the lesion.

2.7 Striato-capsulo-thalamic region

When these lesions are large and have predominant perforator supply, we prefer to leave them alone unless the entire lesion can be covered with radiosurgery. Lesions lateral to the internal capsule involving the lateral basal ganglia and insula, as indicated before, can be operated upon with acceptable morbidity, but the perforator supply is a significant problem that makes me reluctant to operate in many of these lesions. Small lesions involving the posterolateral inferior aspect of the thalamus or the anterio-medial ventricular surface of the thalamus can frequently be removed with safety, particularly if the lateral circumferential arterial supply that can be controlled in the ambient cistern in the former and the choroidal supply that can be controlled in the ventricle in the latter predominate over the deep perforator supply.

2.8 Cerebellar AVMs

Superior vermian AVMs are invariably supplied by branches of the superior cerebellar arteries, most frequently bilaterally. To reach these branches safely, we prefer an infratentorial supracerebellar approach and we favor the sitting position in order to allow the cerebellum to fall down. One has to be particularly careful with arterialized veins that drain from the cerebellum to the tentorium. These arterialized veins should not be taken until at least most of the arterial supply is controlled which sometimes makes the exposure difficult by having to work around these veins and with minimal downward retraction of the cerebellum. Posterior and inferior vermian AVMs are approached suboccipitally in the prone or three quarters "park bench" position. These lesions are supplied predominantly by posterior inferior cerebellar (PICA) branches but they frequently get deep arterial supply from the superior cerebellar arteries. Frequently they reach the fourth ventricle and here they get small transependymal supply which is difficult to control. The more lateral hemispheric AVMs, which frequently can be quite large, are generally approached on the lateral position through a retromastoid craniectomy which can be extended to the midline and supplemented by a far lateral suboccipital approach. In this fashion, the arterial supply from the PICA can be controlled infero-laterally, the anterior inferior cerebellar supply can be controlled at the cerebellopontine angle, and the superior cerebellar supply can be controlled superolaterally over the cerebellum.

2.9 Brainstem AVMs

I generally do not operate on AVMs located within the parenchyma of the brainstem. These lesions are generally fed by perforating arterial branches

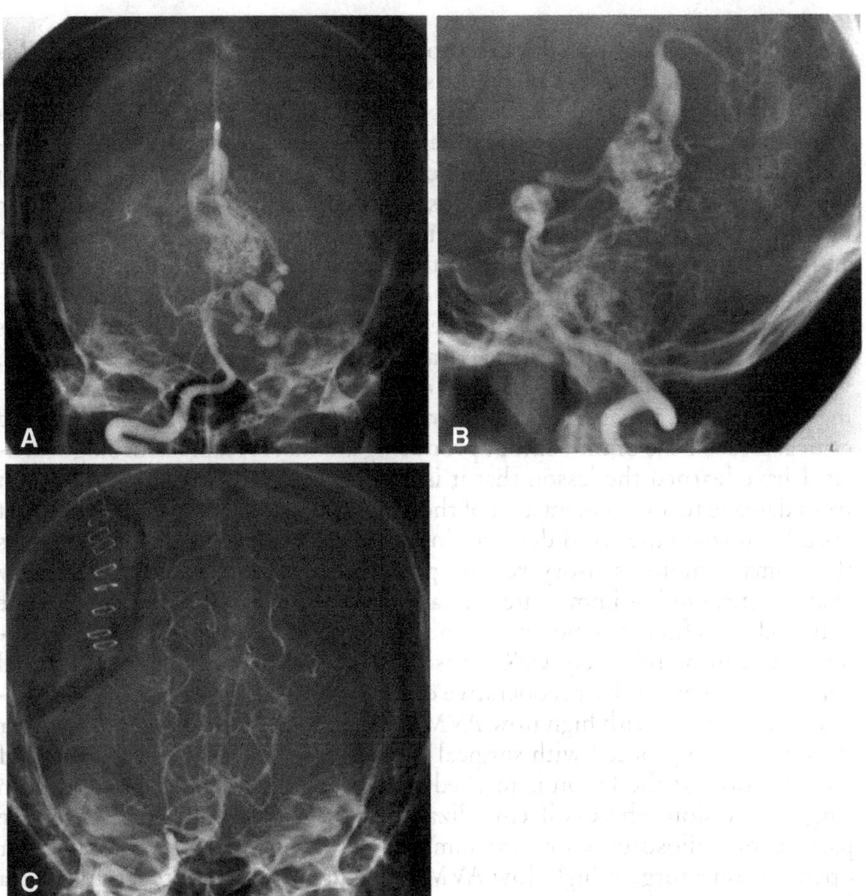

Fig. 5. Moderate sized tectal AVM. **A** A-P vertebral injection. **B** Lateral vertebral injection. **C** Postoperative A-P vertebral injection. The lesion was successfully and completely removed using a posterior temporal transtentorial approach to gain early access to the superior cerebellar supply, which in this case was unilateral

which cannot be controlled early in the dissection and surgical morbidity is forbidding. I am not sure of whether these lesions should be treated with radiosurgery given the high morbidity from radionecrosis in this location. I generally recommend a conservative approach to patients with these lesions unless they have bled more than once or have progressive symptomatology. The few lesions in the brainstem that I have operated are mostly pial lesions with primarily circumferential arterial supply that can be controlled in one of the surgical surfaces of the brainstem. Some tectal lesions are also amenable to surgery, particularly if the patient already has a Parinaud's syndrome (Fig. 5).

HOW TO AVOID COMPLICATIONS

We have categorized and discussed our complications with cerebral AVMs before [1, 9, 10]. Probably our most significant complications can be attributed to faulty surgical judgment; in other words, operating on patients that should not have been operated. This error was most commonly due to a misjudgment about the exact topographical localization of the AVM and the fact that it involved critical brain regions. These mistakes were more common before the days of MRI when we had to depend on a relatively crude CT scan and the angiographic anatomy to estimate whether a lesion, for example, was restricted to the cerebellar peduncle or it actually extended into the brainstem. With the advent of MRI and later functional MR, these mistakes are less common. Early in my experience, I adhered to the belief that there was no viable brain within the AVM and was overconfident in several cases in believing that I could resect a large or even a moderate sized AVM that involved critical areas of the brain without producing an unacceptable neurologic deficit. I have learned the lesson that it is best to expect the appropriate deficit from damage to an eloquent area of the brain when the AVM is located in that area. Even when the AVM does not involve a critical area of the brain such as the primary motor sensory region, primary speech areas and the primary visual cortex but it is immediately adjacent to these areas, the surgeon must be extremely careful in his judgment. I now prefer not to tackle these lesions unless they can be relatively well devascularized by early access to its arterial supply at surgery or by preoperative embolization. At times, I use preoperative embolization with high flow AVMs adjacent to a critical region and defer the decision to proceed with surgical excision until I can assess the result of embolization. If the lesion is markedly devascularized, I may proceed with surgical excision whereas if embolization was insufficient, I may refer the patient for radiosurgery or treat him conservatively. The reason that I fear operating on a turgent high flow AVM immediately adjacent to a critical area is that, in my opinion, the best way to remove these lesions is to gently stroke the loops of the AVM in the plane close to critical brain so as to shrink the AVM loops away from the brain and, as discussed earlier, it is too dangerous to do this when the lesion is still turgent and extensively arterialized.

Unnecessary parenchymal damage to normal brain can occur in a variety of ways. In my experience, this has occurred on a few occasions because I used an excessively generous margin of resection; in other words, as the AVM started bleeding, I moved the dissection to a "safer" plane around the AVM where there was no bleeding, thus injuring unnecessarily normal brain. Obviously, the way to avoid this is by staying right at the margin of the AVM and being patient with the bleeding which frequently can be controlled with relative ease by placing a patty and gentle retraction against the AVM. Another mistake that can result in unnecessary parenchymal damage is to take feeders at a distance from the AVM. Of course, there are areas where this can be done safely when the lesion is far away from critical areas, but generally it is best to follow each feeder until there is no question that the feeder goes exclusively to the AVM; most frequently this has to be done by a wide opening of the sulci around the AVM. Probably the most common cause of unnecessary parenchymal damage has been deep bleeding from the AVM and our efforts to control such bleeding by sometimes suctioning normal brain trying to get control of those feeders as they retract into normal brain parenchyma. As mentioned earlier, for the last several years I have depended very heavily on the Sundt AVM microclips to control these vessels as soon as they are identified rather than trying to follow them through normal white matter. I have commonly misjudged the significance of deep perforators which in the preoperative angiogram sometimes appear to be rather small and innocent. Deep bleeding from these perforators and the need to control them through important brain regions such as the brainstem, the basal ganglia and the thalamus has resulted in significant neurologic deficit. The lesson here is that when the AVM has significant deep perforating supply that is not amenable to preoperative embolization or to early surgical control, it may be best not to attempt surgical excision of the lesion. We commented before on vessels *en passage* which are a particular problem with Sylvian AVMs and with callosal AVMs and how their inadvertent occlusion can cause significant neurologic deficits.

Intraoperative hemorrhage into the brain parenchyma or the ventricle has resulted in several of the neurologic deficits that I have produced operating on some of the more difficult AVMs. I mentioned before the mistake of packing bleeding away from the AVM which should never be done. The surgeon should be doggedly persistent in stopping all bleeding from the "brain side" before moving to dissection in another plane. Intraventricular bleeding with lesions that reach the ventricle can be a significant problem because it is frequently not recognized immediately.

We have learned to minimize retraction damage by being more and more thoughtful about positioning the patient and using CSF drainage such as to insure that the brain "falls away", for example, in parasagittal and subtemporal approaches. Retraction can not only damage the brain directly, but also can result in damage to bridging veins. To avoid this, we sometimes resect a small portion of the brain in relatively silent areas such as the inferior temporal lobe to avoid injury to the vein of Labbe [7].

Even when the patient wakes up satisfactorily from surgery, there are a variety of causes of postoperative deterioration. The most dreadful, of course, is postoperative hemorrhage from retained AVM; with routine use of intraoperative angiography, this problem should not be seen. The problem of normal perfusion breakthrough which unquestionably was a significant one in the days before embolization, has practically been eliminated by preoperative embolization of the very high flow lesions that are likely to result in this problem.

Finally, there is of course, the problem of postoperative epilepsy. We have reviewed this topic in detail [13]. We observed new onset of seizures in 15% of the patients that did not have epilepsy before surgery. Most of these patients had only one or two seizures and only a handful had true epilepsy with repeated convulsions. We routinely use anti-convulsants after excision of supratentorial AVMs but generally discontinue these drugs after 3–6 months if the patients have had no seizures. Therefore, we do not know if the incidence of postoperative seizures would have been higher were it not for this policy.

SURGICAL RESULTS

Table 1 summarizes my personal results with surgical excision of cerebral AVMs since 1981. Four of these patients required re-operation for residual AVM which in two cases resulted in postoperative hemorrhage and in the other two, it was detected by postoperative angiography in the days before routine use of intraoperative angiography. Intraoperative or postoperative angiography was performed in all of my patients with exception of a handful that had a very small AVM in a non-eloquent area of the brain and I was sure that the AVM was completely excised. In all the others, intraoperative or postoperative angiography showed complete excision of the AVM with exception of the two patients that needed to be re-operated for residual AVM in whom angiography

Table 1. Early surgical results (1981–2008)

Grade (S & M)	No. of patients	Good	Fair*	Poor	Dead	Major M & M
I	101	97	4	0	0	0%
II	172	160	10	2	0	1.1%
III	186	139	31	15	1**	8.6%
IV	113	72	25	15	1**	14.1%
V	45	15	10	19	1	44.4%
Total	617	483	80	51	3	8.7%

*Minor or moderate neurologic deficit in immediate postop period not likely to result in permanent disability

**These two patients died from complications related to preoperative embolization

subsequent to the second operation demonstrated complete excision. To my knowledge, none of these patients has re-bled except for the notable exception of a 15 year old boy who had the AVM completely resected as demonstrated by postoperative angiography. Two years later he died of an intraventricular hemorrhage due to a recurrent AVM.

A brief perusal through Table 1 indicates that Grades I and II AVMs can be operated upon with minimal morbidity and essentially no mortality. This has been demonstrated repeatedly in almost all of the large AVM series by experienced surgeons. On the other hand, the morbidity with Grade IV and especially with Grade V AVMs, has been unacceptably high in my hands as it has been demonstrated in most other large series. Almost all of the patients with Grade V AVMs in my series and many of the patients with Grade IV AVMs were operated upon before we did an extensive review of my early experience which was reported in 1990 [12]. At that time, I reported that the permanent (all patients had at least a six month follow-up and the average follow-up was three years) serious morbidity when Grade IV and Grade V AVMs were considered together was 17.7% and the mortality was 3.2%. These numbers were sobering enough that since then I have been much more conservative with these high grade lesions. I believe it is fair to say that this change to a very conservative surgical attitude in patients with Grade IV and Grade V AVMs is currently shared by the majority of experienced neurovascular surgeons including Dr. Spetzler and his group [5]. On the other hand, the excellent results with Grade I and II AVMs and with the majority of Grade III AVMs in most series confirms my strong bias towards surgical excision of these lesions. Clearly, there are some Grade III lesions, for example, a moderate sized AVM involving the primary motor sensory region that should not be operated.

CONCLUSIONS

Cerebral AVMs are complicated neurovascular lesions that require decision making by a neurosurgeon with significant experience with these lesions. The natural history seems to be similar for AVMs that have bled as for unruptured AVMs with exception that the risk of hemorrhage is a bit higher during the first year after a hemorrhage. Thereafter, the annual rate of hemorrhage appears to be 3–4% annually with an approximate 30% morbidity and 10% mortality for both ruptured and unruptured AVMs. In my opinion, the neurosurgeon should recommend to the patient unambiguously what he feels is the best option for treatment of that particular patient with that particular AVM. Inferior options should not be presented as equivalent or alternatives to the "best option". Radiosurgery is a great advance in the treatment of AVMs and is usually the best treatment option for patients with small AVMs that because of their location would present unacceptable surgical risk. I feel strongly that radiosurgery should not be presented as an acceptable alternative to open surgical excision in relatively young patients in good health with Grade I and Grade II AVMs.

Preoperative embolization can greatly facilitate surgical excision, but it should be used only when the combined risk of embolization plus surgical excision is lower than the estimated risk of surgical excision alone. In general, embolization should not be presented to the patient as an acceptable alternative to surgical excision in patients with Grade I or II AVMs which can be surgically excised with less morbidity than the morbidity of embolization as demonstrated by most modern surgical and embolization series. The indications for palliative or pre-radiosurgery embolization are very limited and generally restricted to lesions that cannot be excised surgically with acceptable morbidity and that present clinical or angiographic features suggestive of a considerably higher than average risk of hemorrhage. Finally, most Grade V AVMs and many Grade IV AVMs should be treated conservatively since they are generally too large for radiosurgery, present unacceptable surgical morbidity, can only rarely be completely occluded by embolization and incomplete embolization, which is risky, does not improve and may worsen the natural history.

References

[1] Baskaya MK, Jea A, Heros RC, Javahery R, Sultan A (2006) Cerebral arteriovenous malformations. Clin Neurosurg 53: 114-144

[2] Brown RD Jr, Weiber DO, Torner JC, O'Fallon WM (1996) Incidence and prevalence or intracranial vascular malformations in Olmsted County, Minnesota, 1965–1992. Neurology 46: 949-952

[3] Crawford PM, West CR, Chadwick DW, Shaw MDM (1986) Arteriovenous malformations of the brain: the natural history in unoperated patients. J Neurol Neurosurg Psychiatry 49: 1-10

[4] Graf CJ, Perret GE, Torner JC (1983) Bleeding from cerebral arteriovenous malformations as part of their natural history. J Neurosurg 58: 331-337

[5] Han PP, Ponce F, Spetzler RF (2003) Intention to treat analysis of Spetzler-Martin Grades IV and V arteriovenous malformations: natural history and treatment paradigm. J Neurosurg 98: 3-7

[6] Heros RC (1982) Arteriovenous malformations of the medial temporal lobe: surgical approach and neuroradiological characterization. J Neurosurg 56: 44-52

[7] Heros RC (1990) Brain resection for exposure of deep extra-cerebral and paraventricular lesions. Surg Neurol 34: 188-195

[8] Heros RC (2005) Obliterated arteriovenous malformations. J Neurosurg 102: 829-831

[9] Heros RC (1993) Parenchymal cerebral arteriovenous malformations. In: Apuzzo MLJ (ed) Brain surgery – complication avoidance and management, vol 2 (Part 3). Churchill Livingstone, Los Angeles, pp 1175-1193

[10] Heros RC (1995) Surgery for arteriovenous malformations of the brain (Chapter 27). In: Ojemann RG, Ogilvy CS, Croswell RM, Heros RC (eds) Surgical management of neurovascular disease, 3rd edn. Williams & Wilkins, Baltimore, pp 420-475

[11] Heros RC, Korosue K (1990) Radiation treatment of cerebral arteriovenous malformations. N Engl J Med 323: 127-129

[12] Heros RC, Korosue K, Diebold PM (1990) Surgical excision of cerebral arteriovenous malformations: late results. Neurosurgery 26: 570-577

[13] Korosue K, Heros RC (1990) Complications of complete surgical resection of AVMs of the brain. In: Barrow DL (ed) Intracranial vascular malformations. Neurosurgical topics. American Association of Neurological Surgeons, Park Ridge, Ill, pp 157-168

[14] Ondra SL, Troupp H, George ED, Schwab K (1990) The natural history of symptomatic arteriovenous malformations of the brain: a 24 year follow-up assessment. J Neurosurg 73: 387-391

[15] Pollock BE, Kondzioka D, Lunsford LD, Bissonette D, Flickinger JC (1996) Repeat stereotactic radiosurgery of arteriovenous malformations: factors associated with incomplete obliteration. Neurosurgery 38: 318-324

[16] Taylor CL, Dutton K, Rappard G, Pride GL, Reploge R, Purdy PD, White J, Giller C, Kopitnik TA, Samson DS (2004) Complication of preoperative embolization of cerebral arteriovenous malformations. J Neurosurg 100: 810-812

[17] Valavanis A, Yaşargil MG (1998) The endovascular treatment of brain arteriovenous malformations. Adv Tech Stand Neurosurg 24: 131-214

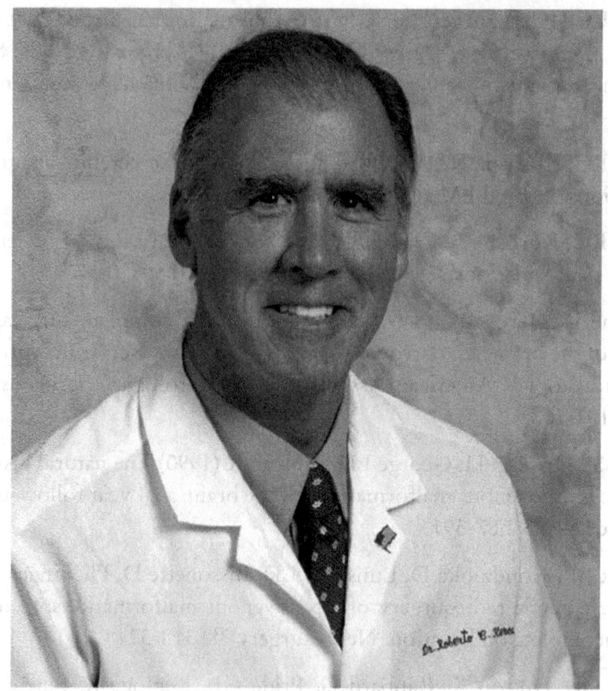

Roberto C. Heros

Roberto C. Heros is Professor, Co-Chairman and Program Director of the Department of Neurosurgery at the University of Miami. Formerly, he was the Lyle A. French Professor and Chairman of the Department of Neurosurgery at the University of Minnesota and before that he was Professor of Neurosurgery and Director of Cerebrovascular Surgery at the Massachusetts General Hospital/Harvard Medical School. Dr. Heros is the President of the XIV World Congress of Neurological Surgery and he has been President of the American Association of Neurological Surgery and the American Academy of Neurological Surgeons. He is widely recognized as an expert in the treatment of cerebral arteriovenous malformations and he has written over 30 original articles, editorials and book chapters on this topic.

Contact: Roberto C. Heros, Department of Neurosurgery, University of Miami School of Medicine, 1095 NW 14th Terrace, Miami, FL 33136, USA
E-mail: rheros@med.miami.edu

INTRACRANIAL CAVERNOMAS

H. BERTALANFFY

INTRODUCTION

Cavernous malformations form between 8 and 15% of all cerebral vascular malformations of the brain and constitute circumscribed benign vascular hamartomas. From the clinical point of view, these lesions show a great variability both morphologically and in terms of their behaviour. As the prevalence of cavernomas is rather low, it is sometimes quite challenging to decide whether an operation is indicated or not.

Many cavernomas are rather small in size (up to 20 mm) and may be well accessible even if they are not readily visible on the surface of the brain. Deep-seated cavernomas, such as those located in the subinsular area or the basal ganglia, within the thalamus and particularly within the brainstem, form a special subgroup. Apparently, these deep-seated lesions more frequently tend to bleed, and because of their highly eloquent location, severe neurological symptoms are more likely to occur than in other locations.

RATIONALE

When treating a cavernous malformation of the brain, a clear therapeutic goal has to be defined. Cavernomas may cause epilepsy in about 30% of cases, haemorrhage in about 15%, focal neurological deficit in 25%, headache in 6%. For clinicians it is important to know that cavernomas may appear as an asymptomatic (incidental) finding in up to 20% of cases. Treatment may either focus on avoiding or ameliorating epileptic fits in the future, on evacuating a large or compressing haematoma or, as a prophylactic measure, on avoiding future haemorrhages by completely eliminating the pathological lesion from the brain. The situation may be more complicated in the presence of multiple cavernous malformations within the brain, in lesions with high propensity for bleeding or in lesion that perhaps do not bleed but clearly increase in size over time. Estimating the risk of haemorrhage or re-haemorrhage in a certain specific case is one of the great challenges posed by these vascular malformations and needs many years of clinical experience. The coexistence of a venous and cavernous malformation may additionally complicate the clinical situation, particularly in the presence of a very large venous malformation. Moreover, these lesions may behave differently in the sporadic form of this disease where cavernomas

Keywords: brainstem, cavernoma, venous malformation, surgical technique

usually occur as a solitary lesion and in the hereditary form (found in up to 20% of cases) where multiple lesions and de novo formations may be observed more frequently than in the previous one. In such cases, several surgical procedures may be needed over time.

DECISION-MAKING

Due to their specific appearance on MRI, cavernous malformations of the brain can be diagnosed in the vast majority of cases with high accuracy. Most of the lesions, albeit not all, may show a more or less evident surrounding zone of hemosiderin-loaded gliosis that can best be detected on gradient echo sequences; frequently this marginal zone can also be observed on T2-weighted MR images. In most cases we can estimate the amount of intralesional hematoma within the entire pathological mass and this information may be quite helpful for the surgeon.

At present, the only efficient treatment modality for cerebral cavernous malformations is total microsurgical removal. Epilepsy caused by a cavernoma may be treated medically; however, this may not influence the risk of a new or recurrent haemorrhage. Gamma knife radiation treatment has been applied and reduction of bleeding risk has been claimed by several authors who applied this treatment. However, according to the available data, gamma knife surgery by no means does completely eliminate the risk of re-haemorrhage. Additionally this technique, has its own complication rate. As I have

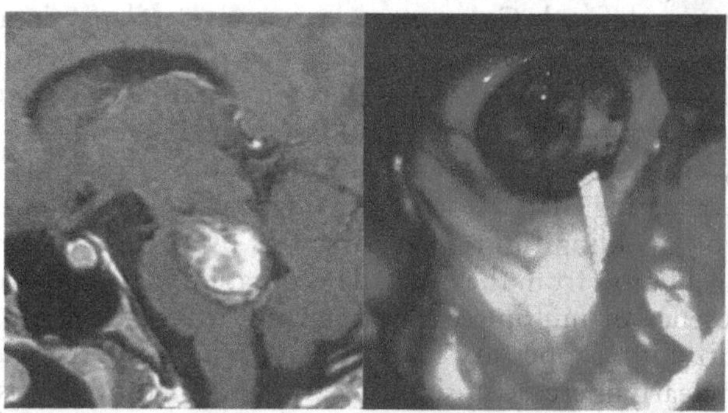

Fig. 1. Mid-sagittal T1-weighted contrast-enhanced MRI (*left*) showing a large dorsal pontine lesion composed to a great extent of intralesional hematoma. The cavernoma was located predominantly in the superior and anterior portion of the pathological mass. Part of the cavernoma is bulging dorsally towards the floor of the fourth ventricle. The lesion was excised through the rhomboid fossa using the supracolicular entry zone in the right paramedian region. The intraoperative photograph (*right*) shows the cavernoma cavity after complete removal and local haemostasis. During surgery the facial colliculus was identified and monitored by direct electrical stimulation. The location of the facial colliculus is inferior to the cavernoma cavity; the function of the nerve remained intact on both sides

observed in many cases, the pathological lesion may be formed of a high percentage of haematoma – sometimes over 90% – while the true cavernous malformation may be small and confined to a limited area of the lesion seen on MRI (Fig. 1). Applying radiation therapy to the entire pathological mass that is composed to a great extent by pure haematoma would require an inadequately high radiation dose that still may remain inefficient because the radiation may not be focused upon the malformation itself.

If the patient presents with acute neurological symptoms and in the early stage of bleeding, and if the images show a well-circumscribed and well-accessible lesion, surgery should be done in the acute stage because this will immediately eliminate the local pressure caused by the hematoma and allow for safe dissection of the malformation before significant scar formation has occurred. If the patient presents in the subacute or stable phase after a first haemorrhage, the size, location and particularly the morphologic aspect of the lesion are the most important criteria for decision making.

In some cases, an initial rather large haematoma may practically disappear by resorption without any treatment within two or three months, and MRI may only show residual hemosiderin or perhaps a small haemorrhage cavity but no more active cavernoma. In such cases surgical exploration is not indicated and a yearly MRI control is recommendable. I have observed many patients in whom one initial bleeding has not recurred over many years and the MRI aspect as described above has remained unchanged (Fig. 2).

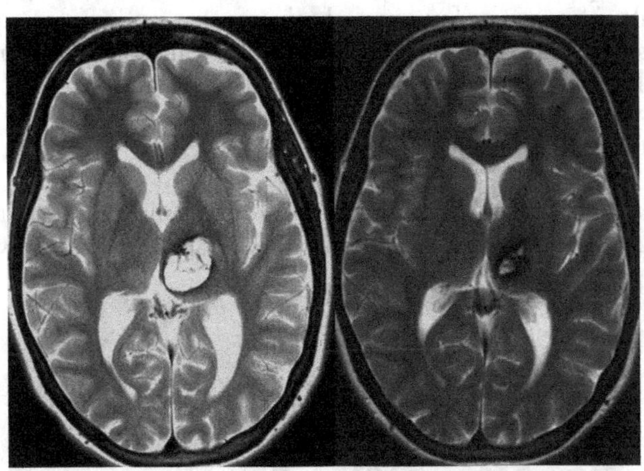

Fig. 2. T2-weighted axial MRI (*left*) showing a significant hemorrhagic lesion most likely caused by a cavernous malformation within the left posterior thalamus that has caused a contralateral sensory disturbance. Six months later the symptoms had disappeared and control MRI (*right*) demonstrates that the haematoma had been completely resorbed. Apart from residual haemosiderin deposits, no active cavernous malformation can be detected; there is no indication for surgical exploration in this case

SURGERY

1. CHOICE OF THE SURGICAL APPROACH, POSITIONING OF THE PATIENT AND CRANIOTOMY

In many cases of intracranial cavernoma the surgeon may have more than one option for the surgical approach. Great experience is required to choose the optimal approach particularly in deep-seated lesions. An optimal approach is one that gives a straight-line access to the lesion with the least impact on the surrounding brain and also allows for a certain manipulation around the lesion in order to be able to completely resect the vascular malformation.

As cavernomas may occur practically in all areas of the brain, they can be accessed in the same fashion as other lesions such as well-circumscribed tumors, etc. Neuronavigation and intraoperative ultrasound are of great help to precisely localize the lesion and adequately place the bone flap. We have previously described this technique for lesions located within the subinsular area or within the basal ganglia [1, 3]. Apart from the frontal, parietal, temporal or occipital access routes to various lesions of the hemispheres, the interhemispheric transcallosal approach was applied to expose intraventricular lesions, the pterional or, less frequently, the orbitozygomatic craniotomy have been used for hypothalamic or anterior midbrain lesions. Posterior thalamic and tectal cavernomas of the midbrain were accessed by the supracerebellar infratentorial approach. The patient was placed either in the sitting or in the lateral or prone (concorde) position. Lesions of the cerebellum, pons and medulla were frequently accessed by the midline or lateral suboccipital approach. Of particular importance for certain brainstem cavernomas were the subtemporal transtentorial and the suboccipital lateral transcondylar routes that give access to the lateral aspect of the brainstem (Figs. 3 and 4).

2. EXPOSURE OF THE LESION

Each of the mentioned approaches allows for visualizing a certain area of the brain including the brainstem. However, each specific surgical window ob-

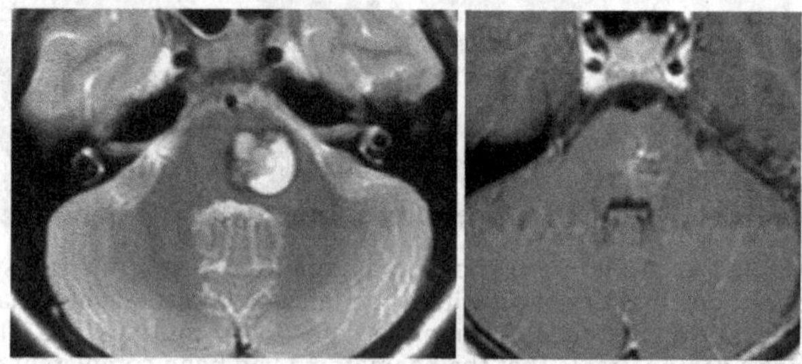

Fig. 3. Preoperative (*left*) and postoperative MRI (*right*) of a 13 years-old female patient who presented with a double vision and gait ataxia. The cavernous malformation was removed by microsurgical resection via a left-sided infratentorial far lateral approach as shown in Fig. 4

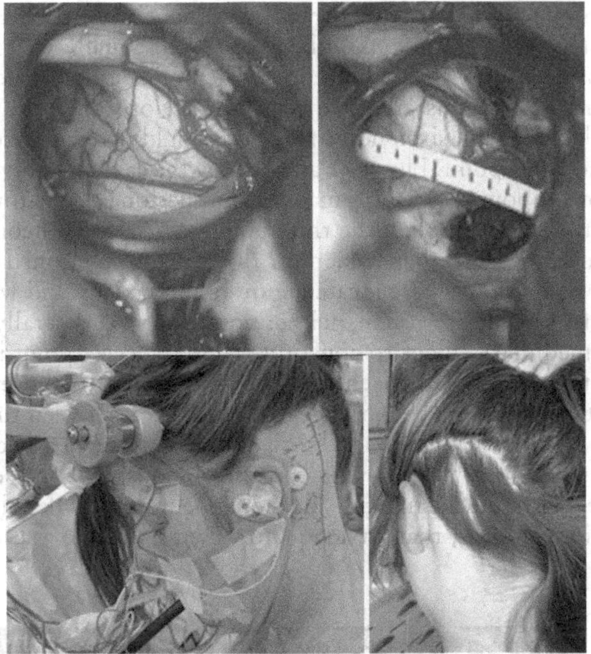

Fig. 4. Intraoperative images before (*upper left*) and during microsurgical resection (*upper right*) of the cavernous malformation located within the lower pons on the left side. Note that the malformation is not visible on the surface of the brainstem so that the exact entry point has to be defined by the surgeon. The region of the exit zones of cranial nerves seven, eight and nine was exposed from inferolaterally and the entry zone into the brainstem was chosen below the fibres of the facial nerve and superior to the exit zone of the ninth cranial nerve within the pontomedullary sulcus. Cavernous malformation and intralesional haematoma were removed through a small opening measuring not more than five millimetres in diameter. The patient was operated on in the sitting position (*lower left*); the postoperative course was uneventful with good cosmetic result (*lower right*) and without additional neurological deficits

tained with a certain approach has limits that should be well-known to the surgeon. Therefore, in case of a larger lesion, a combination of two different approaches can sometimes be useful as we have described at an earlier occasion [1]. Intraoperative guidance with navigation and ultrasound (or both in combination) may be most helpful. Nevertheless, these tools should never completely replace well-known anatomical landmarks, particularly when operating on a brainstem lesion. Such landmarks may be for instance the exit zones of various cranial nerves.

To access a cavernoma through the floor of the fourth ventricle requires bilateral sectioning of the tela choroidea and posterior medullary velum covering the inferior fourth ventricle. Sufficient exposure of the rhomboid fossa and visualization up to the aqueduct was always obtained with this technique. On the other hand, whenever possible, I avoided accessing the cavernoma via the rhomboid fossa because this area is more sensitive than the lateral part of the brainstem. If the lesion could be approached equally well from laterally, this approach was my first preference as the brainstem tolerates surgical manipulation better in this area than within the floor of the fourth ventricle. Particularly facial and sixth nerve functions could better be preserved by using a lateral entry point. Figures 3 and 4 show the case of a 13-year-old female with a lower pontine cavernoma and intralesional hematoma. Although accessing the lesion through the rhomboid fossa seemed theoretically possible, I choosed the lateral approach for the reasons mentioned above. Cavernoma and hematoma where located entirely intraaxially and were not visible on the surface of the brainstem, neither posteriorly nor laterally. I have found the pontomedullary sulcus to constitute an ideal access point into the brainstem, another "safe" lateral entry-zone in addition to those described by Recalde et al. [2]. In my experience, the small area between the exit zone of the facial glossopharyngeal nerves on the ventrolateral aspect of the pontomedullary region of the brainstem can obviously be incised over a few millimetres without causing any additional neurological deficits. One has to bear in mind, though, that an adequate viewing trajectory can only be ob-

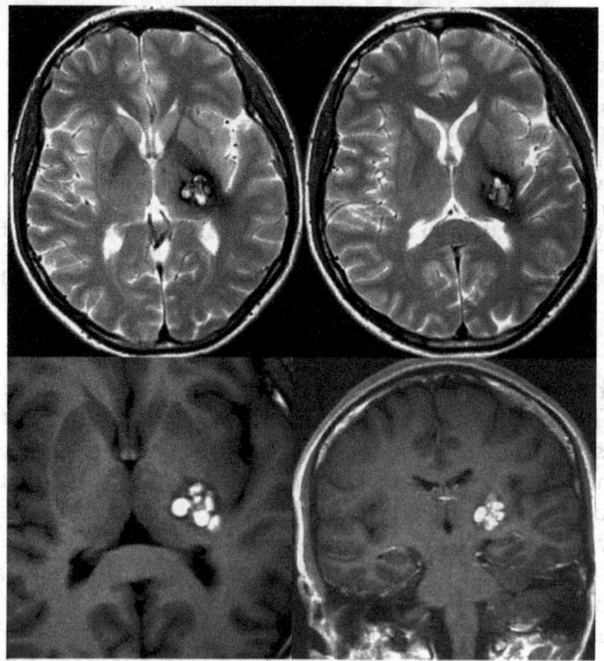

Fig. 5. Preoperative MRI of a 43-year-old female suffering from right-sided hemihypaesthesia. The lesion measuring 18 mm in diameter involved the posterior limb of the internal capsule and the left thalamus and did not reach the surface of the left insula

tained using the lateral suboccipital transcondylar approach. This special access route allows for sufficient manipulation in a lateral-to-medial and inferior-to-superior direction as shown in Figs. 4 and 5, so that the lesion can be

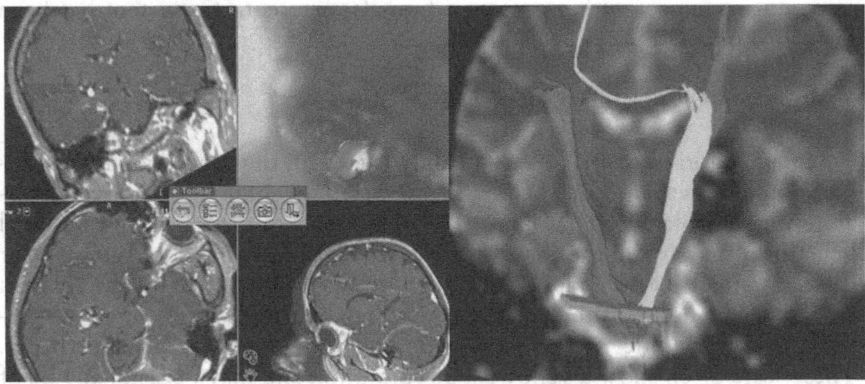

Fig. 6. Intraoperative screen shot from the neuronavigation monitor (*left*). Neuronavigation played an important role in determining the optimal trajectory through the posterior Sylvian fissure to reach the lesion in this specific case. The corticospinal tract is shown on preoperative MRI with fiber tracking to be located medial to the lesion with a slight lateral-to-medial shift

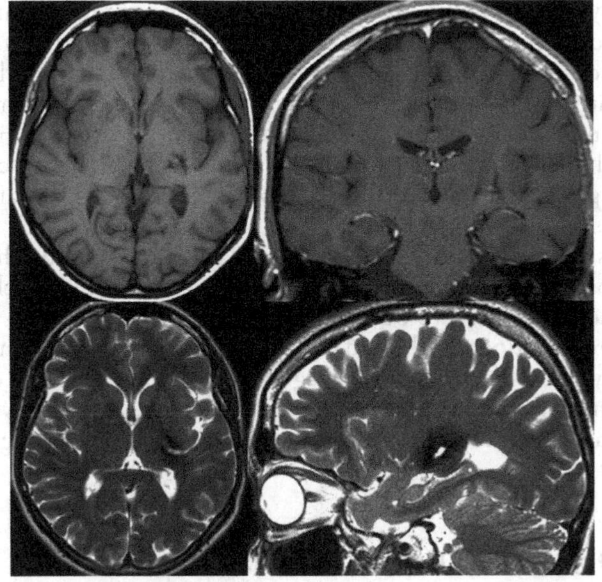

Fig. 7. Postoperative triplanar MRI of the same patient showing complete removal of the lesion. There is no reaction as consequence of microsurgical manipulation, neither by the transsylvian approach nor within the perilesional area. Accordingly, there were no additional neurological deficits, and particularly no speech disturbance occurred postoperatively

completely excised under good visualization. I have used this exposure and entry zone into the brainstem successfully in a number of similar cases.

The true value of neuronavigation becomes obvious in cavernous malformation of the subinsular region as shown in Figs. 5–7. Our technique of intraoperative image guidance using a frameless stereotactic system has been described in detail [3].

3. MICROSURGICAL DISSECTION TECHNIQUE

Once the lesion has been identified and visualized, the intralesional hematoma should be evacuated as the first surgical step. In some lesions, several separately encapsulated hematomas may be present; in others an intralesional hematoma may totally be absent. The next step should be identifying a clear dissection plane between lesion and surrounding brain parenchyma. This can sometimes be quite difficult as the lesion may be firmly adherent to the surrounding tissue due to scar formation following previous haemorrhages. These scars often show a yellowish discoloration and may occasionally be of extremely high consistency; in such cases precise severing with microscissors is required. The plane of dissection must be established in four directions; superior, inferior and bilateral. During the procedure, one must always be aware of and remain within this plane of dissection that can best be visualized with the aid of small cotton pledges. Tiny arteries supplying the malformation usually appear within this space; they must be coagulated and occasionally divided with microscissors. Tearing the lesion should be avoided as this manipulation may harm the surrounding tissue, particularly when working within a highly eloquent area. The surface of the dissected malformation should then gradually be coagulated and shrunk. Portions of the lesion that have already been separated from the surrounding parenchyma can be sharply excised; gradually, additional space is obtained allowing for safely continuing the dissection within a deeper area until the entire lesion is removed. In some cases the caverns of the lesion may lack a surrounding hemosiderin-loaded gliosis, and the caverns may be hidden within the parenchyma. These parts of the lesion deserve our particular attention in order to ensure their complete exstirpation. At the end of this surgical step, the lesion cavity must be precisely examined under high magnification to ascertain the complete removal of the cavernoma and to obtain meticulous hemostasis by using direct bipolar coagulation at a low current intensity alternated by slight irrigation with saline solution.

HOW TO AVOID COMPLICATIONS

Complications may be related either to the surgical approach, to the positioning of the patient, to anesthesia, to injury of surrounding vessels or brain tissue or to inadequate surgical technique. Thus, a great variety of complications may theoretically occur. However, in our series of over 300 procedures performed for cavernous angiomas in practically all areas of the brain, the complication rate remained in a low range (less than 3%) while the surgical mortality was 0.3%. Minor complications were local wound infections or wound hematomas. An early intraaxial rebleeding occurred in one patient harbouring a pontine cavernoma. The hematoma was evacuated on the same day and the patient eventually had an uneventful postoperative course without additional neurological deficits. One patient experienced a hemorrhage within the temporal lobe on the left side due to compression of the vein of Labbé while using the subtemporal approach. An initial speech disturbance completely resolved within the next 14 days.

Generally, an accentuation of pre-existing neurological deficits or new deficits may occur postoperatively that may not necessarily be considered a complication, particularly when such deficits rapidly recover.

In order to avoid complications after surgery of a cavernoma, I have learned over the years to pay attention to a number of aspects:

- Carefully selecting the optimal surgical approach
- Anticipating the surgical window and trajectory obtained with a specific surgical approach and verify whether this surgical window is sufficient in a specific case.
- Applying intraoperative image guidance for rapid and precise localization of a deep-seated lesion.
- Dissecting and separating the vein of Labbé from the temporal lobe so that the brain retractor can be placed below the vein while the patency and integrity of the vein can be preserved despite slightly elevating the temporal lobe; generally, however, brain retraction should be completely avoided or at least minimized.
- Paying attention to an associated venous malformation that must not be coagulated except for small tributaries that drain the vascular malformation itself.
- Using minimal manipulation of the surrounding brain tissue.
- Establishing a clear plane of dissection between lesion and brain parenchyma at the very beginning of dissection.
- Favouring the lateral aspect of the brainstem as preferred entry zone whenever possible.
- Working under continuous electrophyiological monitoring (SEP, MEP, AEBP, direct cranial nerve EMG).
- Avoiding a midline incision in the central area of the rhomboid fossa where the posterior longitudinal fascicles decussate.
- Performing a meticulous hemostasis within the lesion cavity at the end of dissection with low intensity bipolar coagulation.
- Using a watertight dural closure in order to avoid CSF leakage.

CONCLUSIONS

Complete microsurgical removal of a cerebral cavernoma presently constitutes the state-of-the art treatment of these heterogeneous vascular malformations. Generally, a symptomatic cavernoma should be treated surgically. Occasionally, small cavernous malformations can lead to a significant initial intracerebral haemorrhage with subsequent complete resorption of the hematoma. In such cases, the only finding on control MRI may be a hemosiderin spot without clear evidence of an active vascular malformation. Such lesions may remain silent over many years following the initial hemorrhage and do not require surgery or any other treatment.

Several relevant aspects of cavernoma treatment have been discussed in this chapter, emphasizing the importance of the surgical approach and microsurgical technique of cavernoma removal. Although modern technical tools such as navigation, ultrasound and electrophysiological monitoring play an important role in the management of these lesions, the surgeon's experience and anatomical knowledge remain important factors that influence the surgical result as well.

References

[1] Bertalanffy H, Benes L, Miyazawa T, Alberti O, Siegel AM, Sure U (2002) Cerebral cavernomas in the adult. Review of the literature and analysis of 72 surgically treated patients. Neurosurg Rev 25: 1-53

[2] Recalde RJ, Figueiredo EG, de Oliveira E (2008) Microsurgical anatomy of the safe entry zones on the anterolateral brainstem related to surgical approaches to cavernous malformations. Neurosurgery 62(3 Suppl 1): 9-15

[3] Tirakotai W, Sure U, Benes L, Aboul-Enein H, Schulte DM, Riegel T, Bertalanffy H (2003) Image guided transsylvian, transinsular approach for insular cavernous angiomas. Neurosurgery 53: 1299-1304

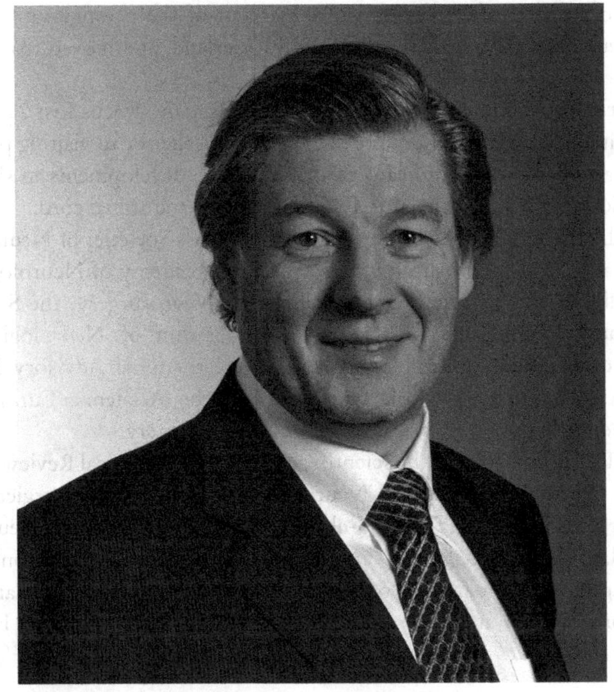

Helmut Bertalanffy

Helmut Bertalanffy is Professor of Neurological Surgery and Chairman of the Department of Neurosurgery of the University of Zurich, Switzerland. He received his neurosurgical training from the Albert Ludwigs University of Freiburg im Breisgau, Germany, where he completed with honors a Medical Doctorate in 1986 and obtained the qualification as board certified neurosurgeon in 1990.

Dr. Bertalanffy spent more than 2 years from 1990 to 1992 at the Department of Neurosurgery of the Keio University, Tokyo, Japan, as a scientific fellow of the prestigious Alexander von Humboldt Foundation, Bonn, Germany, and the Japan Society for the Promotion of Science, Tokyo, Japan, working in the fields of cerebral and spinal microcirculation and skull base surgery.

He served as vice chairman of the Department of Neurosurgery of the Technical University of Aachen, Germany from 1992 to 1997. The Friedrich Wilhelm Foundation of the Technical University of Aachen honoured Dr. Bertalanffy with the "Friedrich Wilhelm" Prize in 1994 given annually for outstanding scientific work.

In 1997 Dr. Bertalanffy was appointed to Professor on a permanent basis by the State of Hessen, Germany, and served as Professor and Chairman of the Department of Neurosurgery of the Philipps University of Marburg for 10 years. In July 2007 he accepted the position of Professor and Chairman of the prestigious Department of Neurosurgery of the University of Zurich, Switzerland, and moved from Marburg to Zurich.

He has been listed among the best doctors in Germany (Focus List 2001) and is frequently invited to meetings or congresses as guest speaker or to visiting professorships worldwide and has made significant contributions to developments in skull base surgery and microsurgery of vascular lesions of the brain and spinal cord.

Dr. Bertalanffy is a member of the German and Swiss Societies of Neurosurgery, the German Academy of Neurosurgery, the American Academy of Neurological Surgery (corresponding member), the World Academy of Neurosurgery, the Skull Base and the nominating committees of the World Federation of Neurological Surgeons (Chairman of the nominating committee), the International Advisory Board of the American Association of Neurological Surgeons, the Academia Eurasiana, and an honorary member of the Romanian Society of Neurosurgery.

He is the Editor-in-Chief of the scientific journal Neurosurgical Review and lends his expertise to the Editorial Boards of Neurosurgery, Acta Neurochirurgica, Techniques in Neurosurgery, Neurologia Medico-chirurgica and Zentralblatt für Neurochirurgie.

Dr. Bertalanffy has published 144 articles in peer reviewed journals, contributed over 50 book chapters or other articles to medical texts, and presented more than 300 lectures as visiting professor or at various congresses and symposia worldwide. He is married and has 2 daughters.

Contact: Helmut Bertalanffy, Professor and Chairman, Department of Neurosurgery, University Hospital of Zurich, Frauenklinikstrasse 10, 8091 Zurich, Switzerland
E-mail: helmut.bertalanffy@usz.ch

CAROTID ENDARTERECTOMY

V. BENEŠ

INTRODUCTION

Carotid endarterectomy (CEA) is a means for the secondary prevention of stroke that is caused by embolisation from carotid plaques. CEA is by far the most thoroughly studied surgical procedure as well as one of the most frequently used surgical techniques. Thrombendarterectomy was first performed by DeBakey in 1953. The number of surgeries increased steadily until the 1980s when, in the wake of extracranial-intracranial arterial bypass study, neurologists first questioned the rationale of CEA. The neurologists recognised that CEA was used to prevent stroke, but that stroke may happen during or after CEA as well. At that time the role of distal embolisation was not sufficiently understood and appreciated. The dangers of carotid stenosis were seen in terms of a reduction and interruption in blood flow. Only later was the embolic origin of the majority of strokes fully appreciated and antiaggregant treatment initiated. Such a treatment proved to be effective and thus the value of CEA was questioned even further.

Largely at the initiative of neurologists, randomised CEA versus the best medical treatment protocols were initiated. Altogether, four important studies (NASCET, ECST, ACAS, ACST [3–6]) led the American Heart Association (AHA) to postulate indication criteria for surgery. The latest guidelines were published in 2006 [11] and recent criteria for CEA are as follows: symptomatic stenosis >50%, provided the surgical morbidity/mortality (M/M) rate is <6% and in asymptomatic patients stenosis is >60%, provided M/M rate is <3%. Patient considered for CEA should have a 5-year life expectancy. This condition is difficult to establish precisely but should be kept in mind. Research indicates that the effect of CEA in women is lower than in men [2] and greater in older patients than in younger patients [1].

The trials proved CEA to be a very effective and safe procedure, which led to an increase in the number of procedures performed. In the USA, roughly 100,000 CEAs are performed each year, split nearly evenly between neuro- and vascular surgeons. In Europe, the majority of procedures are performed by vascular surgeons. It is my strong conviction that CEA could be useful to the neurosurgical armamentarium. The neurosurgeons are those with comprehensive experience and education in clinical neurology and neuroradiolo-

Keywords: brain, ischemia, endarterectomy, carotid artery, vertebro-basilar system

gy. Moreover, they possess the technical skills and necessary equipment. The target of CEA is the brain, not the vessel, and as such, the procedure is in the domain of neurosurgeons.

In general, the cerebral vasculature, including the magistral vessels, is very complex and the procedures to treat the lesions from aortic arch to distal branches of the middle cerebral artery are numerous. Another major impetus derives from the endovascular field and nowadays we hardly encounter stenotic lesions that are not amenable to some kind of correction. The description of various procedures is beyond the scope of this chapter. CEA is by far the most common vascular surgical procedure and the general rules of CEA are applicable to most of the other stenotic lesions. Neurosurgical involvement in the whole field of cerebral ischaemia is both exciting and rewarding.

CEA has not undergone so many technical changes: the basics involve longitudinal arteriotomy followed by plaque removal and vessel suture. Eversion endarterectomy technique was introduced, indwelling shunts and their use were discussed in the past and patching techniques are used by some surgeons on a regular basis. Numerous and long-lasting discussions exist between those advocating general anaesthesia and those operating in local and regional anaesthesia. Overall, it was demonstrated in several studies that the results of different anaesthesia techniques are not significantly different. Their use depends on institutional and individual experience and customs and is actually not that important.

The most important development came in the 1990s from the field of interventional neuroradiology, namely, the carotid stenting procedures (CAS), which are now being compared with CEA in several randomised studies. None of these randomised studies shows a superiority of CAS, some show non-inferiority of CAS as compared with CEA and the majority are not able to prove the non-inferiority of CAS. On the other hand, meta-analyses have indicated that CEA is superior to CAS in the majority of cases [7, 8].

RATIONALE

The goal of surgery is to eliminate the source of emboli. Carotid bifurcation is a predominant location for atherosclerotic plaque formation. Such a plaque may be fragile, where the intraplaque material sometimes has a mudlike consistency. As soon as the intimal layer is disrupted, the debris may embolise distally into the brain circulation. The tighter the stenosis, the thicker the plaque and the higher is the likelihood of embolisation. Clinically, the consequence of embolisations is transient ischaemic attacks (TIAs), both ocular and hemispheric, or completed stroke. Not an uncommon finding in stroke patients is carotid stenosis and embolic occlusion of the M1 segment.

Alternatively, the carotid artery may thrombose, which causes stroke. Once occluded, the internal carotid artery (ICA) is seldom the target of either emergency thrombendarterectomy or elective stumpectomy, which is to prevent embolisation via collaterals.

1. CLINICAL PRESENTATION

The patients considered for CEA are either asymptomatic or symptomatic. In asymptomatic patients the stenosis is diagnosed either accidentally or, more frequently, during the targeted evaluation of the patients at risk of atherosclerotic cerebral occlusive disease. Symptomatic patients present with the whole clinical spectrum, starting with TIAs, hemispheric or ocular, and ending with deep completed stroke. Patients with major ipsilateral completed stroke are considered for CEA with some reservations. The symptoms can be either relevant to the stenosis in question or relevant to a different territory (contralateral carotid, or vertebrobasilar territory). Clinical findings should always be evaluated carefully and individually.

2. RADIOLOGICAL WORK-UP

All patients must be subjected to basic radiological work-up, either brain CT or MR imaging. Any other than ischaemic lesion must be ruled out and the extent and "age" of eventual ischaemia must be clearly documented. In the past, digital subtraction angiography (DSA) was the most important and only reliable diagnostic procedure. Important randomised studies are based on DSA findings. However, DSA is an invasive mode of examination and the M/M rate of this procedure must be added to the surgical M/M. Recent M/M rates of diagnostic DSA do not exceed 1% (0.1% at the author's institution). In the past decade, non-invasive modalities have gradually taken over. Duplex ultrasonography (US) is an excellent tool provided the procedure is performed by an experienced professional. US is now preferable in screening and post-operative follow-ups. MR and CT angiography are now frequently used techniques in diagnosing and evaluating carotid stenosis. Both these techniques have the advantage of displaying the whole vasculature. Actually, the correlation of diagnostic methods and actual stenosis as measured on a removed plaque is not good. We have studied this problem for several years (supported by grants of the Czech Ministry of Health, IGA NR 9435-3). Our findings show that both DSA and US significantly underestimate the actual stenosis. CT and MR angiography are now under investigation.

DECISION-MAKING

The decision to treat carotid stenosis is based on AHA guidelines. AHA guidelines provide general recommendations based on firm scientific foundations. The presentation and discussion of AHA guidelines far exceeds the format of this chapter and the reader is therefore recommended to check the guidelines directly at http://stroke.ahajournals.org/cgi/content/full/37/2/577. However, some patients do not fit the criteria but still CEA can and, in some instances, should be indicated. The most typical example is a stenosis below the set value of 50% that is ulcerated and where US shows fragile material and the patient suffers repeated TIAs despite the best medical treatment. Another condition is a floating thrombus. In such a case the stenosis is negative according to NASCET measurements. All indications that do not fit AHA criteria should be strictly individual and based on individual and institutional experience.

1. TIMING

Timing depends on several factors. One factor is the patient's condition. In patients with recent major stroke the procedure should be postponed for an arbitrarily set interval of 6 weeks. Another factor is the CT finding. In patients with recent ischaemia on the basis of CT images the surgery should be postponed for the risk of haemorrhagic conversion of the infarcted region. Again, an interval of 6 weeks is recommended. However, it seems the risk of haemorrhagic conversion is not that high and thus the interval of 6 weeks has recently been questioned. In patients with TIAs, CEA should be performed as soon as possible. One study showed that 23% of major strokes were preceded by TIAs, and 43% of these strokes appeared within 1 week after the initial TIA [10]. Recently, CEA has been recommended within a week after TIA: ideally, TIA should be handled as an emergency and consequently treated by CEA. Unfortunately, this policy exceeds the efficiency of any recent medical system. In asymptomatic patients the timing does not apply.

1.1 CEA versus CAS

The interventional neuroradiologists simply took over the CEA indication criteria and applied them to CAS. CAS procedures, especially after the introduction of distal protection, seemed very attractive and promising for both patients and physicians. Actually, the general impression a few years ago was that these techniques would likely replace CEA. Thus far, this does not seem to be the case and, quite surprisingly, randomised trials comparing both techniques have shown either similar results for both techniques or CAS' inferiority. The last major trial (EVA-3S) was prematurely terminated because of CEA's superiority [9]. The SPACE study could not confirm the non-inferiority of CAS versus CEA [12]. Recently, the M/M rate of endovascular techniques exceeded the requirements of AHA, i.e. 6% of the M/M rate in symptomatic patients and 3% in asymptomatic patients. The value and possible indications for CAS should be solved by major ongoing randomised trials (ICSS, CREST, ACST-2). At our institution, after the first wave of enthusiasm, CAS is currently reserved for patients for whom the general anaesthesia is too risky from a medical point of view, for patients with carotid restenosis and carotid

Table 1. CEA and CAS results at the author's institution

	CEA	CAS
Number of procedures	1335	363
Mean age (years)	64	72
30-day morbidity/mortality	2.00%	4.68%
TIA within 30 days after procedure	1.49%	7.43%
Minor complications	10.07%	17.63%

dissections, for patients with tandem lesions and for post-irradiation stenosis. In unfavourable anatomical situations, CAS is also preferred: in extremely obese patients and patients with carotid bifurcation above the C2 level. CAS is also used in patients with a contralateral cranial nerve lesion (VIIth, Xth, XIIth). These guidelines were set at the present author's institution after the EVA-3S publication; earlier, the choice of treatment modality was more liberal. From 1982 to 2007, 1335 CEAs were performed. From 2001 to 2007, 363 CAS interventions were performed. In our material CEA proved to be safer (Table 1). Apart from carotid stenosis, of which CEA seems to be superior, in all other locations endovascular techniques are preferred (vertebral artery origin stenosis, intracranial stenosis, etc.).

SURGERY

1. SURGICAL PROCEDURES

1.1 Anaesthesia

All CEAs at the author's department are performed under general endotracheal anaesthesia with arterial line placement for continuous blood pressure monitoring. The controversy between general and local/regional anaesthesia is long-lasting and as of yet unresolved. The ongoing GALA trial, however, should shed some light on this issue. General anaesthesia has several advantages, including easier surgical manoeuvres, handling of complications and easier patient monitoring. On the other hand, clinical monitoring, which is allowed by local/regional anaesthesia, is unsurpassed by any other means. It seems that local/regional anaesthesia decreases the number of medical complications at the expense of neurological complications.

1.2 Patient positioning

The patient is positioned supine and the head is slightly turned to the opposite side and extended. A small pad is placed under the ipsilateral shoulder and the arm is extended downwards. The entire operating table is slightly (10%) elevated head-wise.

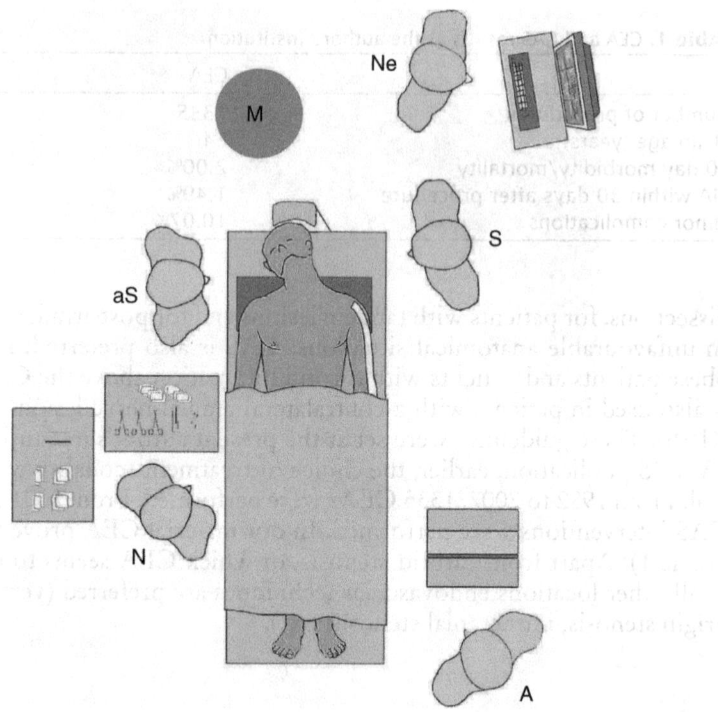

Fig. 1. Operation room team position during CEA. *S* Surgeon, *aS* assisting surgeon, *Ne* neurophysiologist, *A* anaesthesiologist, *N* nurse, *M* microscope

At this point, the transcranial Doppler (TCD) probes are fixed in place. Somatosensory evoked potential (SSEP) needles are introduced into the scalp and electroencephalography (EEG) electrodes are fixed. Figure 1 shows the operation room team position during CEA. The procedure starts once it is ascertained that the monitoring system is functioning properly.

1.3 Carotid dissection

The incision runs along the anterior border of the sternocleidomastoid muscle (SCM), never above the angle of the jaw. Skin and platysma are incised and along the anterior border of the SCM the dissection proceeds deeper. The only traversing structure is the facial vein in the upper third of the approach. The vein is ligated and divided. The jugular vein is not dissected free; it is merely identified and left untouched. The common carotid artery (CCA) is gently palpated at the lower aspect of the wound and the carotid sheath exposed. Longitudinally, along the CCA runs the hypoglossal ansa, which is mobilised and moved anteriorly. The carotid sheath is then incised and the CCA exposed. The dissection proceeds cranially up to the carotid bifurcation and external carotid (ECA) and the superior thyroid arteries are exposed to allow the application of the aneurysm clip. Only the self-retaining retractors are used throughout the procedure.

At this point, the microscope is introduced and the ICA is exposed as high up as needed using microsurgical techniques. Extreme care is taken not to harm the cranial nerves. The hypoglossal nerve is running immediately below the inferior head of the digastric muscle and its branch: the ansa cervicalis is running along the artery and at the level of the thyroid gland and curving anteriorly. The lower branch of the facial nerve runs transversally above the jaw angle in superficial layers. To protect this nerve in higher approaches the microscope is angled and higher up dissection runs only at and below the level of the digastric muscle. The lower head of this muscle may be transected, which would allow an even higher approach. The ICA is dissected well above the plaque, which is either seen at the vessel even from outside or can be gently palpated. The handheld retractors used by some surgeons to expose the distal ICA are never used for fear of injuring the peripheral nerves (VIIth and XIIth).

The ICA is usually positioned slightly lateral and posterior to the ECA. However, in some cases the ICA is hidden behind the ECA. The bifurcation complex is then dissected free from all the attachments and whole bifurcation is rotated using a sling around the ECA and eventual stitches in the adventitia are used to rotate the bifurcation.

Any manipulation of the vessels, especially at the level of stenosis, is strictly avoided. The arteries are not completely dissected from their attachment to the carotid sheath, i.e. they are dissected free only at points where clips are going to be placed. This procedure minimises the manipulation with the vessels and decreases the risk of embolisation.

If at this point in the procedure the SSEPs drop by 50% in three consecutive runs, the procedure is terminated. We have found this the hard way in the sense that neurological complications appeared always whenever the SSEPs dropped by more than 50% at the dissection phase. Such a decrease in SSEPs seems to indicate major distal embolisation. The significance of such an embolisation may not be sufficiently appreciated on TCD.

1.4 Cross-clamping and endarterectomy

Dose of 5000 units of heparin (protocol at the author's institution) is administered before the clip application, a solution of local anaesthetics is applied to the region of glomus caroticum locally to block the carotid reflexes. The first clip is applied to the ICA, then one each to the ECA and the superior thyroid artery and finally to the CCA. The regular carotid clamp is used only for the CCA: all other clips are Yasargil aneurysm clips (slightly curved in order not to obscure the surgical field). The surgeon now waits about 1 minute for the electrophysiologist who closely monitors the SSEPs. Only if the SSEPs drop by more than 50% is longitudinal arteriotomy performed and the intraluminal shunt inserted (less than 3% in the last 500

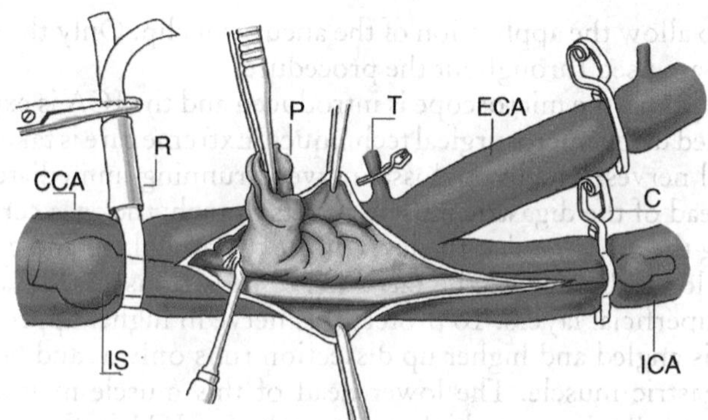

Fig. 2. CEA technique with intraluminal shunt. *IS* Intraluminal shunt, *R* rubber band around the CCA, *C* window aneurysm clip at the ICA, *P* plaque, *T* superior thyroid artery

surgeries at our institution). If the shunt is used, it is kept in place by a rubber band around the CCA and by the window aneurysm clip at the ICA (Fig. 2). The appropriate aperture of the clip is chosen to hold the shunt and block any back bleeding from the ICA. If the shunt is not needed, the CCA is incised some 2 cm caudally from the bifurcation and the proper plane of dissection is found (colour of the vessel wall slightly deeper than the colour of the plaque, smooth surface). The plaque is transversally cut in the most caudal aspect of the arteriotomy. The plaque is then separated without cutting it longitudinally and the arteriotomy proceeds cranially stepwise always after the segment of the plaque is dissected free. The arteriotomy is slightly lateral to the midline (from the surgeon's point of vision); especially at the bifurcation it runs some 3 mm lateral from the upper aspect of the bifurcation (Fig. 3). When the cranial end of the plaque is reached, it is sharply divided. Lastly, the plaque is dissected from the ECA. Extreme care

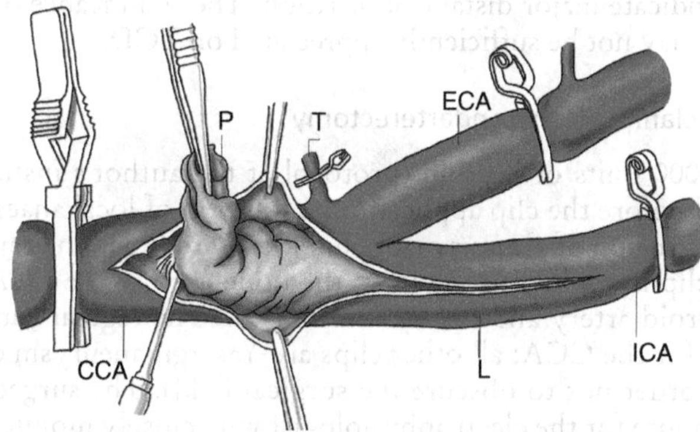

Fig. 3. Standard CEA technique. *P* Plaque, *T* superior thyroid artery, *L* longitudinal arteriotomy

is necessary when dissecting hard, calcified plaques. In these cases the risk of injuring the thinned vessel wall is high and the calcified plaque always has firmer attachments to the outer vessel layers. Somewhat more comfortable is to cut through the plaque to the lumen, cutting it longitudinally until the healthy ICA is reached. Dissection then starts on the lateral aspect of the incision at the ICA origin where the proper plane is most easily encountered. At the author's institution, the uncut plaque is removed because it is used in a research protocol to compare the morphological stenosis with radiological findings. The whole plaque is fixed and cut transversally, where the slice with maximum stenosis is found and used for further studies.

After plaque removal, the whole arteriotomised segment is closely inspected and any loose material removed. The vessel wall is repeatedly flushed with a heparin solution to disclose any remnants. Extreme care is given to the distal end of the plaque. All flaps that are best seen under the jet of heparin solution are removed. In case this is not possible, two to four 8/0 tacking sutures are used. The stitches are positioned at 6, 9 and 12 hours "looking into ICA lumen" (Fig. 4). The 4th firm point is the first stitch starting the closure (at 3 hours on Fig. 4). If only two stitches are used, these are positioned at 7 and 11 o'clock. The stitches are introduced from outside of the vessel into the lumen and back outside again.

Eversion endarterectomy represents another technique of CEA when the ICA is transversally cut, plaque is removed after eversion of the ICA wall and the ICA is finally sutured to the CCA (Fig. 5). This technique is not performed at the author's institution.

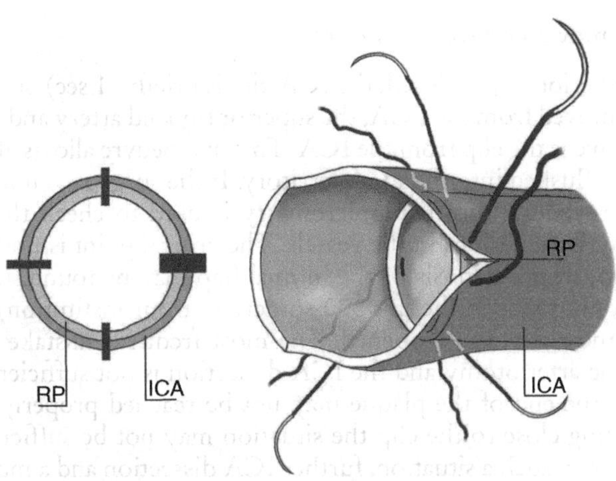

Fig. 4. Technique to secure the distal end of the plaque. In case it is not possible to remove all remnants of plaque in the distal end of ICA and the intima is loose, tacking sutures are used. The stitches are positioned at 6, 9 and 12 hours "looking into ICA lumen". The 4th firm point is the first stitch starting the closure (at 3 hours). *RP* Residual plaque

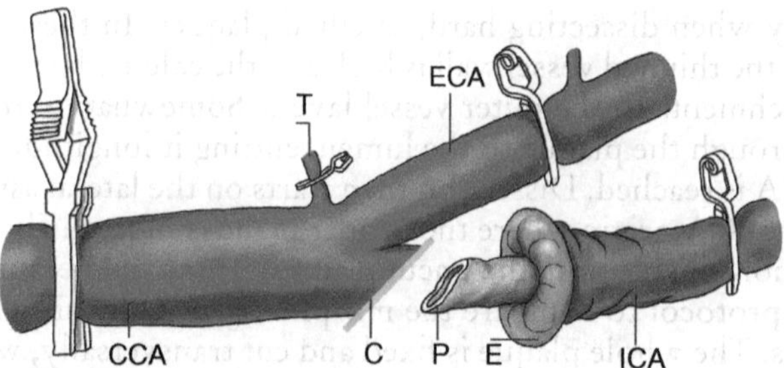

Fig. 5. Eversion CEA technique. *C* Point where ICA is cut, *E* eversed ICA wall, *T* superior thyroid artery

1.5 Arteriotomy suture

Arteriotomy is closed by the 6/0 running suture that starts at the cranial end. By using a microscope and microtechniques, we always have an abundance of the vessel wall, which obviates the need for patching. The first running suture is tight, short spaced. Before its completion, the ICA is shortly opened and flushed. Next, the artery is flushed with heparin solution. After completion of the first suture, the second suture, which is looser, is introduced, usually one stitch to each 2–3 of the first suture line. This is done because of the risk of suture material rupture. The second suture is for security. More knots are used – usually five – and the ends of the stitches are cut longer, some 5–6 mm from the knots. Again, this is for security purposes.

1.6 Clip removal and wound suture

After the arteriotomy is closed, the ICA clip is briefly (1 sec) opened. The clips are then removed from the ECA, the superior thyroid artery and the CCA. The last to remove is the clip from the ICA. This manoeuvre allows all the potential debris to be flushed into the ECA territory. If the surgeon is not fully satisfied with the procedure, direct dopplerometry is used to check the patency and disclose any irregularities in the vessels. The critical point is the cranial end of arteriotomy, where stenosis or the intimal flap may be found. In case of such an event (only twice in the last 500 surgeries at our institution), the clips are reapplied and the vessel reopened. The most frequent mistake is insufficient length of the arteriotomy and the ICA dissection is not sufficiently cranial, in which case the end of the plaque may not be reached properly and with the suture starting close to the clip the situation may not be sufficiently appreciated. To correct such a situation, further ICA dissection and a more cranial clip position are sufficient. The arteriotomy can then be sufficiently prolonged and any plaque remnants or intimal flaps can be handled.

In some cases, kink is appreciated at the end of the plaque and the ICA remains kinked even after the endarterectomy is completed. These kinks are not excessive and usually simple caudal displacement of the bifurcation area suffices to straighten the kinks. Desired position is secured by 6/0 stitches between the CCA adventitia and the muscles (omohyoid, sternocleidomastoid).

The heparin is not reversed. Haemostasis is meticulous and any tiny bleeding points are coagulated by bipolar coagulation. The arteriotomy usually leaks a small amount and sometimes even a small jet of blood may be encountered. However, this event is not a reason to add extra stitches. Leaking arteriotomy is covered for some 3–5 min by muslin soaked in warm Ringer solution. Bleeding usually stops spontaneously. Finally, the arteriotomy is covered by a small strip of oxycellulose. The suction drain is positioned along the vessels and the wound is closed in two layers (platysma, skin).

After dressing the wound, the anaesthesia is terminated and the patient is awakened in the OR suite. The patient is then transferred to a semi-intensive care unit. Usually, 24 hours later the arterial line is removed and the patient is allowed to ambulate. The patient is usually dismissed on the 3rd or 4th postoperative day.

2. RESULTS

From a technical point of view, the results of CEA are very satisfactory. In the long run, restenosis appears in less than 5% of the procedures. There are two types of restenosis. First, is the recurrent atherosclerotic process, and second, the myointimal hyperplasia. It seems that recurrent stenosis is a far more benign process than primary stenosis and it is questionable whether some active means should be taken at all. Ultimately, the vessel becomes occluded without causing symptoms. However, because the patients are followed and restenosis diagnosed in time, the restenosis is usually treated according to the same criteria as those applied to primary stenosis. In the present author's series over the past 10 years all restenoses are treated by endovascular means, either by stenting or by percutaneous transluminal angioplasty.

From a clinical perspective, the results, i.e. a serious M/M rate, must be compared with the natural course of patients who are treated properly with antiaggregants. AHA allows for a 6% M/M rate in symptomatic stenosis and a 3% M/M rate in asymptomatic stenosis.

The number of patients needed to treat to prevent one stroke differ according to the degree of stenosis and the patients' symptomatology (Table 2).

Table 2. The number of patients needed to treat to prevent one stroke

Symptomatic stenosis (NASCET)		Asymptomatic stenosis (ACAS)
>70%	50–69%	>60%
6	**15**	**67**

In our material of 1335 consecutive CEAs, the overall serious M/M rate (death and completed stroke within 30 days after the CEA) was 2.02%. Minor complications constitute another 10%. These minor complications included TIAs, various minor medical complications, cranial nerve palsies, hyperperfusion syndromes, wound swelling and wound haematomas, infections, etc. For various reasons, 3% of our patients underwent revision surgeries.

3. COMPLICATIONS

3.1 Medical

Medical complications depend on the patient population. We are treating seriously ill patients, usually in their 6th or 7th decennium. A typical patient is one that suffers from the combination of carotid occlusive disease (stenosis at relevant bifurcation only is very rare and other sclerotic findings are usually found elsewhere), ischaemic heart disease, arterial hypertension and diabetes mellitus. Consequently, the patients should be carefully selected and prepared for surgery. An experienced anaesthesiologist is far more important than the surgeon. He or she must collect all vital information about the patient, must be aware of all possible threats in the perioperative period and must be well prepared to deal with them effectively. The two possible serious complications likely to occur are myocardial infarction or cardiac failure during the perioperative period and a decrease in blood pressure during the perioperative period. A decrease in blood pressure, even a short and minor one (some 20 Torr), can cause stroke.

Another very dangerous condition in the immediate post-operative period is wound swelling and/or wound haematoma. Wound problems may cause breathing distress leading to myocardial infarction or failure with all possible consequences. As soon as the distress is noted after surgery, the patient should be taken back to the OR and the wound reopened, the haematoma removed and haemostasis achieved. If the haematoma is not present, the patient is intubated and ventilated for a few days. The sooner the action is taken, the better; in other words, the physician must "proact", not react.

3.2 Neurologic

The most frequent and unwelcome complication from surgery is exactly the disaster we want to prevent by surgery, namely, stroke. Stroke can be caused by a drop in blood pressure (see above), vessel thrombosis or by embolisation from the endarterectomised vessel. In case of stroke that is caused by thrombosis the patient must return to the OR and the vessel reopened. Any deep neurological deficit appearing in the immediate post-operative period is an indication for immediate investigation and revision in selected cases. This is an emergency and the success depends on timing. An immediate CT scan of the brain is indicated and CT angiography is very useful (if available).

TIAs, which appeared in 1.5% of our patients, should be treated as such (a single TIA can be considered inconsequential if CT and CT angiography is negative).

Hyperperfusion syndrome is characterised by unilateral headache and confusion. Close monitoring and maintaining the blood pressure within normal limits are manoeuvres to combat this condition.

In our series we have seen two typical hypertonic haematomas, both ipsilateral to the CEA and of grave consequences. To prevent intracerebral bleeding from reoccurring, close blood pressure monitoring and management are necessary.

3.3 Local complications

Cranial nerve injury. Nerve palsy appeared in 3.93% of our surgeries. The most frequently damaged nerve was the XIIth followed by the lower branch of the VIIth and recurrent nerve. In the majority of cases the palsy was caused by direct damage during surgery. Our experience shows that the function typically recovers within months. Inadvertent interruption of the nerve is a rare condition. If the surgeon is aware of the problem (in our material once in XIIth), the nerve should be sutured. We have encountered one permanent recurrent nerve palsy, two VIIth and four XIIth palsies.

Wound. As previously mentioned, wound haematoma and excessive wound swelling are potentially very dangerous. Haematoma should be removed and any swelling should be closely followed. Local infections are extremely rare (we encountered one early in the series).

HOW TO AVOID COMPLICATIONS

1. PATIENT SELECTION

Patients scheduled for CEA are usually generally quite ill, having a combination of atherosclerotic changes in more than one system. It is therefore mandatory to perform an exhaustive pre-operative assessment (e.g., functional cardiac tests and full laboratory battery). It is also necessary to evaluate the whole cerebral vasculature in order to determine whether there are any other pathological findings. An experienced anaesthesiologist is a conditio sine qua non. The anaesthesiologist should see and evaluate the patients well prior to the procedure. The final indication should be set by the vascular panel composed of all involved specialists. This scheme is the best prevention of post-operative medical complications. However, in very few patients surgery is declined. The patients should be prepared for surgery and active treatment of any concurrent disease before surgery is mandatory. Since 1999, all those patients found unsuitable for surgery were treated by CAS (based on SAPPHIRE study-13). In the past 2 years, CAS has been less frequently used, however, and the patients are very thoroughly prepared for surgery in general anaesthesia.

2. ANAESTHESIA

Very gentle and smooth anaesthesia is a must, where it is crucial that the anaesthesiologist keeps the patient's blood pressure some 20 Torr above his/her normal range. Any reduction in blood pressure is dangerous and hence should be strictly avoided. An arterial line for continuous blood pressure monitoring is mandatory throughout surgery and should continue another 24 hours post-surgery.

3. MONITORING

Monitoring is essential for selective intraluminal shunting. A decrease in SSEP during the dissection phase of surgery should lead to immediate abandonment of the procedure, which, however, could be repeated in a week or CAS may be a sensible alternative. If changes in SSEP appear later in surgery, the surgeon should work faster and the anaesthesiologist should increase blood pressure. TCD backup is helpful but we do not rely on it as the only monitoring technique. PostCEA direct dopplerometry is useful in checking the endarterectomised segment. Whenever reopening of the vessel is considered, it should be done as it could be too late later.

4. DISSECTION AND ENDARTERECTOMY

Sharp dissection with meticulous haemostasis throughout the whole procedure is required. Sufficient length of the vessels must be dissected free though the dissection should not reach caudally beyond the omohyoid muscle (recurrent nerve) and cranially above the angle of the jaw (facial nerve) above the lower head of the digastric muscle unless the hypoglossal nerve is dissected free. This strategy ensures good orientation within the surgical field and prevents peripheral nerve injury. After plaque removal, extreme care must be exercised on removal of all loose remnants. Otherwise, these loose remnants could embolise distally into the brain circulation after clip removal. The crucial point is the distal end of endarterectomy; the intima must be smooth and any flap either resected or fixed by stitch. This phase is the point where post-operative thrombosis can start. A meticulous surgical technique is the best prevention of post-operative thrombosis.

5. CROSS CLAMPING

Proper sequence of clip application and removal decreases the risk of perioperative embolisation.

6. HAEMOSTASIS

Step-by-step meticulous haemostasis provides the best prevention of post-operative haematoma and swelling with all the concomitant consequences.

7. HEPARIN NON-REVERSAL

Non-reversal or partial reversal of heparin only diminishes the risk of post-operative thrombi formation.

8. POST-OPERATIVE CARE

Some 24 hours of close monitoring after surgery ensures early detection and proper handling of any possible complication.

CONCLUSIONS

CEA is a rather safe and effective procedure. Its rationale has been proven by several major trials and its durability demonstrated over a long period. If indicated, and executed properly, it is a very effective method for the prevention of stroke. The risk of stroke, however, is not completely eliminated because only a tiny part of the vasculature is treated and the whole underlying process (atherosclerosis) remains unchanged. Thus, there is the need for lifelong medical treatment and regular exams.

CEAs should be performed only at institutions with a high volume of patients and a proven low M/M rate. Surgically, CEA in experienced hands is an easy and fast procedure. On the other hand, the patients are usually seriously ill with higher than usual surgical risks. Thus, to treat these patients effectively a dedicated team composed of neurologists, internists, anaesthesiologists, radiologists and neurosurgeons (vascular surgeons) is necessary.

The above described surgical techniques cannot be dogmatic. They work well at our institution, where they were developed and proven over the past 25 years (the author performed his first CEA in 1982). It has been shown that the same results were published with routine use of shunt, routine patching, eversion CEA, etc. Further, the monitoring system described here is not the only one providing the surgeon with relevant information. General versus local/regional anaesthesia is still under scrutiny. Concerning this matter, we are awaiting the GALA trial results. The important issues are not small differences in technique but final clinical results.

Acknowledgements

J. Kacvinsky (for preparation of figures) and D. Netuka (for help with text preparation) are to be acknowledged.

References

[1] Alamowitch S, Eliasziw M, Algra A, Meldrum H, Barnett HJ; North American Symptomatic Carotid Endarterectomy Trial (NASCET) Group (2001) Risk, causes, and prevention of ischaemic stroke in elderly patients with symptomatic internal-carotid-artery stenosis. Lancet 357: 1154-1160

[2] Alamowitch S, Eliasziw M, Barnett HJ; North American Symptomatic Carotid Endarterectomy Trial (NASCET); ASA Trial Group; Carotid Endarterectomy (ACE) Trial Group (2005) The risk and benefit of endarterectomy in women with symptomatic internal carotid artery disease. Stroke 36: 27-31

[3] Asymptomatic Carotid Surgery Trial (ACST) Collaborative Group (2004) Prevention of disabling and fatal strokes by successful carotid endarterectomy in patients without recent neurological symptoms: randomised controlled trial. Lancet 363: 1491-1502

[4] Barnett HJ, Taylor DW, Eliasziw M, Fox AJ, Ferguson GG, Haynes RB, Rankin RN, Clagett GP, Hachinski VC, Sackett DL, Thorpe KE, Meldrum HE, for the North American Symptomatic Carotid Endarterectomy Trial Collaborators (1998) Benefit of carotid endarterectomy in patients with symptomatic moderate or severe stenosis. N Engl J Med 339: 1415-1425

[5] European Carotid Surgery Trialists' Collaborative Group (1998) Randomised trial of endarterectomy for recently symptomatic carotid stenosis: final results of the MRC European Carotid Surgery Trial (ECST). Lancet 351: 1379-1387

[6] Executive Committee for the Asymptomatic Carotid Atherosclerosis Study (1995) Endarterectomy for asymptomatic carotid stenosis. JAMA 273: 1421-1428

[7] Kastrup A, Gröschel K (2007) Carotid endarterectomy versus carotid stenting: an updated review of randomized trials and subgroup analyses. Acta Chir Belg 107(2): 119-128

[8] Luebke T, Aleksic M, Brunkwall J (2007) Meta-analysis of randomized trials comparing carotid endarterectomy and endovascular treatment. Eur J Vasc Endovasc Surg 34: 470-479

[9] Mas JL, Chatellier G, Beyssen B, Branchereau A, Moulin T, Becquemin JP, Larrue V, Lièvre M, Leys D, Bonneville JF, Watelet J, Pruvo JP, Albucher JF, Viguier A, Piquet P, Garnier P, Viader F, Touzé E, Giroud M, Hosseini H, Pillet JC, Favrole P, Neau JP, Ducrocq X, EVA-3S Investigators (2006) Endarterectomy versus stenting in patients with symptomatic severe carotid stenosis. N Engl J Med 355: 1660-1671

[10] Rothwell PM, Warlow CP (2005) Timing of TIAs preceding stroke: time window for prevention is very short. Neurology 64: 817-820

[11] Sacco RL, Adams R, Albers G, Alberts MJ, Benavente O, Furie K, Goldstein LB, Gorelick P, Halperin J, Harbaugh R, Johnston SC, Katzan I, Kelly-Hayes M, Kenton EJ, Marks M, Schwamm LH, Tomsick T (2006) Guidelines for prevention of stroke in patients with ischemic stroke or transient ischemic attack: a statement for healthcare professionals from the American Heart Association/American Stroke Association Council on Stroke: co-sponsored by the Council on Cardiovascular Radiology and Intervention: the American Academy of Neurology affirms the value of this guideline. Stroke 37: 577-617

[12] SPACE Collaborative Group, Ringleb PA, Allenberg J, Brückmann H, Eckstein HH, Fraedrich G, Hartmann M, Hennerici M, Jansen O, Klein G, Kunze A, Marx P, Niederkorn K, Schmiedt W, Solymosi L, Stingele R, Zeumer H, Hacke W (2006) 30 day results from the SPACE trial of stent-protected angioplasty versus carotid endarterectomy in symptomatic patients: a randomised non-inferiority trial. Lancet 368: 1239-1247

[13] Yadav JS, Wholey MH, Kuntz RE, Fayad P, Katzen BT, Mishkel GJ, Bajwa TK, Whitlow P, Strickman NE, Jaff MR, Popma JJ, Snead DB, Cutlip DE, Firth BG, Ouriel K (2004) Stenting and Angioplasty with Protection in Patients at High Risk for Endarterectomy Investigators. Protected carotid-artery stenting versus endarterectomy in high-risk patients. N Engl J Med 351: 1493-1501

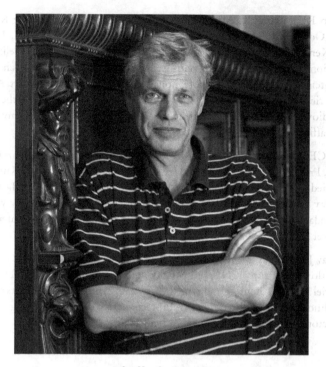

Vladimír Beneš

Vladimír Beneš is Professor of Neurosurgery and Chief of Neurosurgery at the 1st Faculty of Medicine, Charles University, Prague, Central Military Hospital and Postgraduate School of Medicine. Vice-President EANS 2003–2007, Chairman of the EANS Training Committee 2007–, President of the European Skull Base Society 2007–, President of the Czech Neurosurgical Society 2002–. Special interest in cerebrovascular surgery, cerebral ischaemia, intracranial aneurysms, AVMs, cavernomas. Research of correlation of diagnostic methods (digital subtraction angiography, Doppler ultrasonography, MR angiography, CT angiography) and morphological findings in carotid stenosis. Clinical research in psychological sequellae of aneurysm treatment (clipping and coiling), clinical management of arteriovenous malformations. Involvement in neurooncology, meningiomas, pituitary adenomas and sellar lesions in general. Local principal investigator and coordinator in international studies: ACST, ISAT, Glioma ARC Study, STICH. 200 publications, eight books and book chapters.

Contact: Vladimír Beneš, Department of Neurosurgery, Charles University, 1st Faculty of Medicine, Central Military Hospital, U nemocnice 1200, 16902 Prague 6, Czech Republic
E-mail: vladimir.benes@uvn.cz

BRAIN REVASCULARIZATION BY EXTRACRANIAL–INTRACRANIAL ARTERIAL BYPASSES

Y. YONEKAWA

INTRODUCTION

The therapeutic idea of anastomosis of the external carotid artery, or one of its branches, with the internal carotid artery above the area of narrowing was advocated by C. Miller Fisher in 1951. This was actually realized in another way than originally suggested at the cervical region, but in the form of superficial temporal artery–middle cerebral artery (STA-MCA) bypass using microsurgical technique by Donaghy and Yaşargil in 1967 [22]. Thereafter, applications of the revascularization technique have been reported for one cerebral vascular territory after the other. It was the international cooperative study of extracranial–intracranial (EC-IC) bypass, whose final results in 1985 called the role of the procedure in prevention of further recurrent stroke into question [5]. Most neurosurgeons were disappointed at the results then and apparently have lost interest in performing microvascular anastomosis. This tendency has been enhanced by the development of interventional neuroradiology represented by percutaneous an transluminal dilatation (PTA) pioneered by A. Grüntzig in 1979 and later with additional stenting procedure.

However, there are recently signs of a revival of interest in microsurgical revascularization, as some studies indicate the benefit of the bypass procedure in stroke prevention and also the limitation of the endovascular method has become gradually evident. In this chapter we present our method of revascularization, including indication, technique and results.

RATIONALE

Occlusion or hemodynamically significant stenosis of cerebral arteries mostly due to atherosclerotic process cause symptomatic cerebral ischemia of varying severity: transient ischemic attacks (TIAs) or strokes, depending on the degree of reduced regional cerebral blood flow (rCBF). Clinical manifestation and pathophysiological changes are dependent on inherent collateral

Keywords: brain revascularization, ischemia, brain revascularization, extra-intracranial arterial bypasses

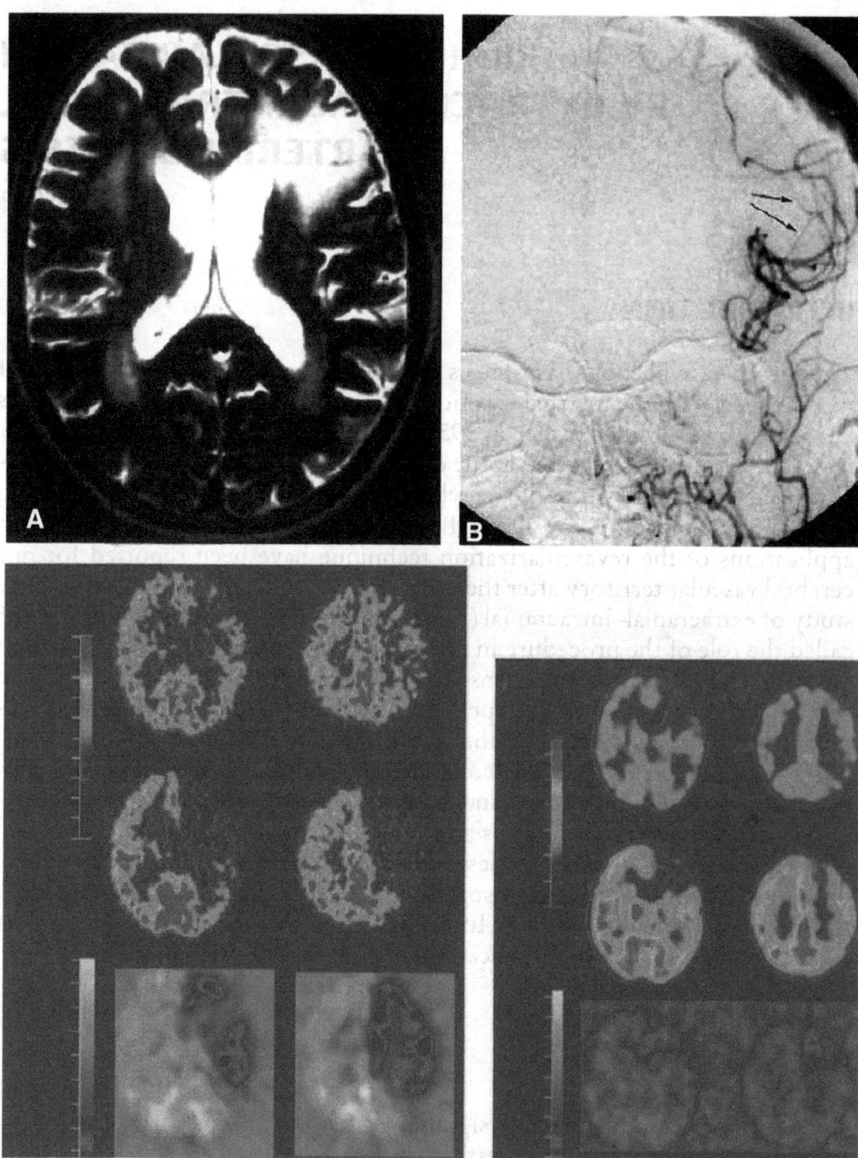

Fig. 1. 75-year-old female with completed stroke due to left ICA occlusion resulting in infarction in the frontal lobe (**A**). Despite antiplatelet therapy she had further TIAs presenting with aphasia and right hemiparesis. The preoperative PET scan revealed decrease of CBF in the left hemisphere along with decreased hemodynamic capacity on the Diamox test; there was even a steal phenomenon (**C**). Postoperative angiography showed an excellent filling of the MCA from the STA-MCA bypasss (**B**). The patient was asymptomatic and free of TIAs after the bypass procedure. The 3-month follow-up postoperative PET scan showed increased CBF and normalized hemodynamic capacity except for the infarcted area (**D**)

circulation which brings various hemodynamic, physiologic and metabolic situation (Fig. 1). Hemodynamic compromise or hemodynamic failure in cases with occluded cerebral arteries is represented on the PET (positron emission tomography) images with reduced CBF unaccompanied by proportional reduction in cerebral metabolic rate of oxygen and increase of oxygen extraction fraction, namely, misery perfusion [3], or accompanied by reduced cerebrovascular reactivity CVR on Diamox loading (Fig. 1). These can be detected more or less also by single-photon-emission computed tomography (SPECT) [15, 25].

Recurrence of cerebral ischemia has been reported to be around 30–40% (this rate has been reported to be approximately halved by the administration of Aspirin or anticoagulants) in five years and to be more frequent in cases with reduced CBF or/and reduced hemodynamic reserve. Klijn and coworkers reported in 1997, in review of literature, that patients with symptomatic carotid occlusion and hemodynamic compromise have a higher risk of strokes: 12.5%/year for all strokes and 9.5%/year for ipsilateral stroke, as compared with 5.5% and 2.1%, respectively, in cases without hemodynamic compromise [30].

Augmentation of CBF by around 10% obtainable by bypass surgery is considered to prevent recurrence of cerebral ischemia in cases with hemodynamic failure, which could not be selected out as a group for the international EC-IC bypass study in the 1980s. At that time a subgroup of the Japanese-Asian group under study which mainly consisted of MCA occlusive lesions did however show less incidence of stroke recurrence in the surgical group, though of no decisive statistical significance [25]. Recently, the newly organized Japanese EC-IC trial study (JET) showed the role of bypass in stroke prevention in cases with compromised cerebral hemodynamics with CBF of <80% and regional cerebrovascular reactivity of <10%, namely, stage 2 after Powers [15], as inclusion criteria [7]. Better perfusion of the ischemic penumbra (16–20 ml/100 g/min) around an infarcted area by bypass surgery has been considered to contribute also to functional recovery, although there are still objections to this view representing the penumbra allegorically as "sleeping beauty" [1, 25].

Moyamoya angiopathy (MMA), discovered in 1955, proved to occur not only in Japanese and Asian but also in Caucasian populations (USA, Europe) though with less incidence and is known to present mainly with ischemic cerebral symptomatologies in accordance with a varying degree of hemodynamic disturbances [10, 27]. The revascularization procedure has been reported to prevent recurrent cerebral ischemia and neurological deterioration due to hypoperfusion or hemodynamic failure and also to prevent intracerebral hemorrhage due to rupture of the Moyamoya vasculature or related microaneurysms in the basal ganglia, which is another manifestation of MMA [8, 27]. The role of bypass surgery in prevention of bleeding has still to be defined systematically [27]. Indirect revascularization method, using burr

Table 1. Representative type of extracranial–intracranial bypass procedure

1. Anterior circulation	STA-MCA bypass, OA-MCA bypass, STA-ACA bypass, STA-M2-3 bypass
2. Posterior circulation	STA-SCA bypass, OA-PICA bypass, OA-AICA bypass, OA-SCA bypass, OA-PCA bypass
Interposition graft bypass	Subclavia (CCA, EA, C4)-C2 or M2 bypass (high flow), Bonnet bypass (low flow)

holes, dural reflection, putting arteries or omentum on the brain surface, ideas related with the concept of Henschen's encephalomyosynangiosis described in 1950, are not discussed in this chapter in detail though they are rather in prevalent use as surgical treatment of MMA. For these, the various relevant articles should be referred to [13, 27, 28].

Reconstructive surgery of venous system including venous sinus is beyond the scope of this chapter and hence relevant articles should be referred to [17].

Revascularization using microvascular technique to be discussed in this chapter is represented with following bypasses (Table 1): the superficial temporal artery STA or the occipital artery OA of around 1 mm in diameter is dissected in situ and anastomosed with a cortical branch of the middle cerebral artery (STA-MCA bypass or OA-MCA bypass), with the superior cerebellar artery (STA-SCA bypass) or with the posterior inferior cerebellar artery (OA-PICA bypass) in accordance with the location of the territory of hemodynamic failure. The STA- or OA-MCA bypass are considered to deliver 10–20 ml/min flow at the beginning of bypass construction and to deliver as much as 100 ml/min flow after several weeks to months according to the need of the ischemic brain territory in question, so that hemodynamically compromised brain can obtain around 10% increase of CBF [16, 25].

Pressure difference between the extracranial artery and the cortical arteries has been reported to be around 20% at normal condition without any occlusive lesion and much more consequently in an ischemic brain, so that a flow reversal from intracranial to extracranial direction cannot take place through the newly constructed bypass route [29].

Combination of bypass surgery with therapeutic occlusion of parent artery of aneurysms is another indication of the revascularization procedure. A special type of revascularization high-flow bypass using saphenous vein graft or radial artery graft is also dealt with in this chapter.

DECISION-MAKING

Candidates for surgery for prevention of recurrent cerebral ischemia (transient ischemic attack TIA or/and stroke) *must fulfil all three criteria* as shown in Table 2. (1) Symptomatology and neurological signs should cor-

Table 2. Indication criteria of the STA-MCA bypass for the anterior circulation (modified inclusion criteria of the international cooperative study [5] and those of JET study [7])

1. Clinically: TIA or minor stroke with no or minor neurological deficits (Rankin 1, 2, 3)
2. Angiographically: a. MCA-M1 occlusion or stenosis (more than 50%)
   b. ICA occlusion
   c. ICA stenosis (more than 50%) above the mandibulomastoid line
3. Hemodynamic compromise (identified by PET scan or SPECT): CBF<80%, Acetazolamide loading <10%

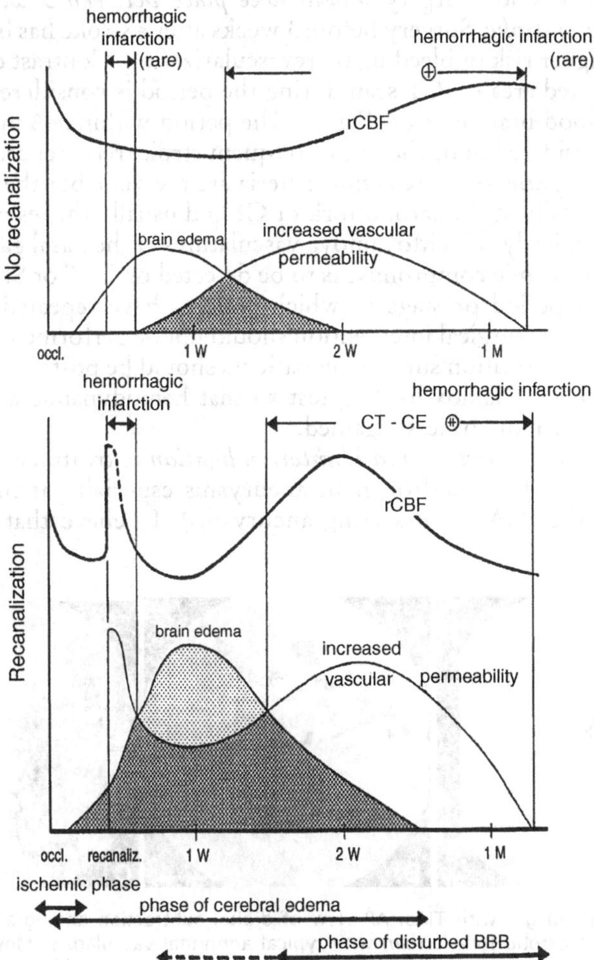

Fig. 2. Pathophysiological time course of an infracted area after Mizukami [14]. With this diagram one can understand the pathophysiological process of an infarction is very dynamic and complicated within three weeks after the onset, especially at the time of recanalization or revascularization

respond with the lesion but the patients should not have severe neurological deficits (up to moderate disability of Rankin scale 3) due to the above mentioned lesion. (2) Selection criteria of angiographically identified occlusive lesions responsible for the ischemia are the same as those for international cooperative study for the ICA territory and these can be extended to the vertebrobasilar artery territory. (3) Hemodynamic compromise should be detected either by $H_2{}^{15}O$ PET or SPECT (iodine-123-labeled amphetamine [IMP] or technetium-99m) with Diamox loading represented typically with decreased basal rCBF and reduced reactivity [7, 15, 25].

Revascularization surgery *should take place between 3 weeks and 3–6 months after a stroke*. Surgery before 3 weeks after a stroke has been reported to have a higher risk of bleeding on revascularization. Contrast enhancement of the infracted area on CT scan during the period is considered to indicate impaired blood brain barrier (Fig. 2). The period within 3–6 months after a stroke is considered to be the one of frequent stroke recurrence.

For MMA patients the selection criteria are the same but the occlusive lesion lies typically at the carotid fork or C1 and usually the lesion is bilateral combined typically with Moyamoya vasculatures at the basal ganglia (Fig. 3) [27]. Hemodynamic compromise is to be detected on PET or SPECT examination. At a period or stage in which patients have repeated or frequent ischemic attacks, surgical intervention should not be performed. In our experience, revascularization surgery on patients should be postponed more than 48 hours after a Diamox loading test so that hemodynamic and metabolic stability can be more or less regained.

Combination of bypass and Hunterian ligation as treatment for intractable aneurysms (large and/or giant aneurysms especially at the cavernous portion of the ICA or dissecting aneurysms). I believe that the ligation

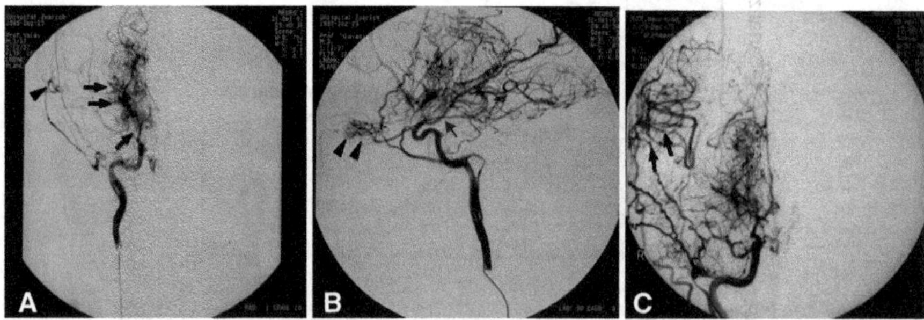

Fig. 3. 9-year-old girl with TIAs. AP view of digital subtraction angiography showing a stenosis at the carotid fork (arrow) with typical abnormal vasculature (Moyamoya) in the basal ganglia (double arrow). A vault Moyamoya (arrowhead) supplied by the middle meningeal artery is also seen (**A**). Lateral view showing typical stenosis at the carotid fork (arrow). Ethmoidal Moyamoya (double arrowhead) supplied by the ophthalmic artery is seen (**B**). AP view of the postoperative digital subtraction angiography showing a well functioning bypass supplying the MCA (double arrow) through the STA (**C**)

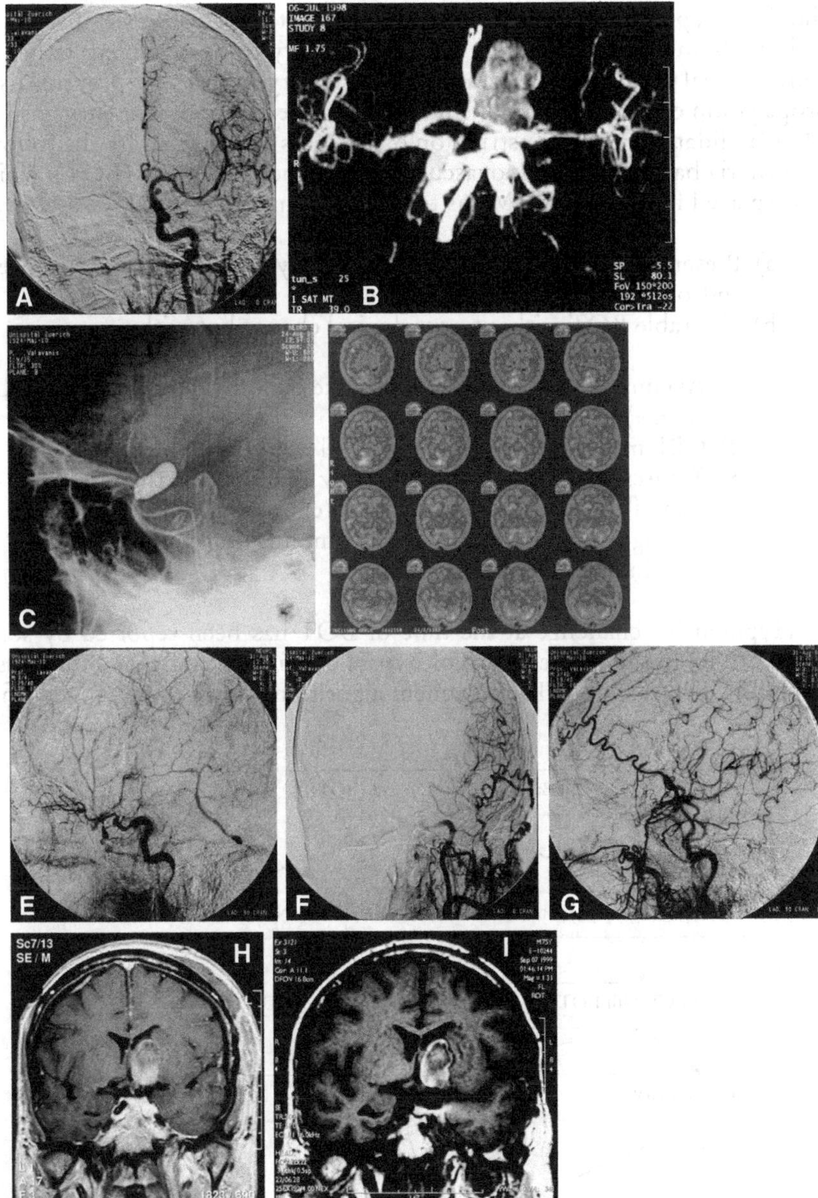

Fig. 4. 74-year-old male suffering from a growing mostly thrombosed giant aneurysm of the left ICA (**A**, **B**). He underwent the BOT (**C**), which was well tolerated but associated with asymmetry in SPECT (**D**). He underwent a standard STA-MCA bypass in combination with carotid occlusion just distal to the origin of the ophthalmic artery without any postoperative problems (**E**). The 3-month follow-up angiography showed an excellent filling of the MCA through the STA (**F**, **G**) and shrinkage of the thrombosed aneurysm (**H**, preoperative; **I**, one year postoperative)

should be replaced by a trapping procedure (distal occlusion site just proximal of a branching artery from the parent artery to be occluded) either by conventional surgery or by endovascular surgery in order to prevent distal propagation of thromboembolism or retrograde refilling of aneurysms [12, 32]. Candidates for the construction of a bypass are selected by the following criteria based on the endovascular balloon occlusion test (BOT), which has replaced formerly used Matas test and tournique test [30]:

a) Presentation of ischemic symptomatology such as hemiparesis, speech and/or consciousness disturbance
b) Tolerable BOT without neurological change but with
    1) Asymmetry of radionuclide uptake on SPECT study during BOT (Fig. 4)
    2) CBF measurement: less than 30 ml/100 g/min
    3) Transcranial Doppler sonography (TCD): less than 30% fall of mean flow velocity or less than 20 cm/s
    4) Changes of neurophysiological monitoring with EEG, SEP or near-infrared spectrophotometry

Hypotensive challenge at the time of BOT has been reported by some groups to be useful for selection of bypass candidates and type of bypasses (high flow or low flow). The treatment algorithm shown in Fig. 5, modified

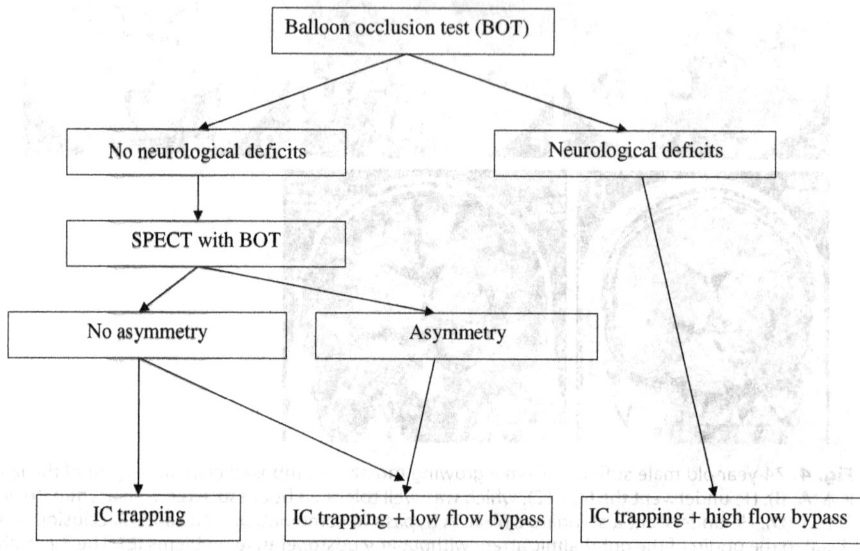

Fig. 5. Treatment algorithm with the use of balloon occlusion test (BOT) (modified from those suggested by Kawano et al. [4] and Date et al. [9])

Table 3. Contraindications and/or conditions in which bypass surgery should not be performed

a. cancer other than skin cancer (including lymphoma, leukemia)
b. renal failure (BUN > 50 mg%)
c. congestive heart failure (past or present)
d. severe hepatic or pulmonary disease constituting anesthetic risk
e. stroke acute stage less than 3 weeks after the onset.
Furthermore
f. blood sugar > 300 mg%
g. diastolic pressure >110 mmHg
These should be brought into the normal range and stabilized before surgery

from those proposed by Kawano et al. in 1991 and Date et al. in 2008, may also help to select patients and flow type of bypasses.

In bypass surgery for aneurysms indication has to be sometimes reviewed on individual basis in emergency settings of aneurysm surgery and in therapy-resistant vasospasm [12].

Contraindications. Most of the revascularization procedures are carried out for the prophylactic purpose, so that preoperative neurological and general physical status should not deteriorate after surgery. Items listed in Table 3 which were mostly exclusion critera of the international EC-IC bypass study can be considered as contraindication.

SURGERY

1. BYPASS SURGERY FOR ANTERIOR CIRCULATION

1.1 Operative technique of the standard the STA-MCA bypass (Fig. 6)

Under general anaesthesia, the head is fixed with a Mayfield apparatus in supine position with slight elevation of the shoulder on the side of surgery with insertion of a cushion underneath, so that the plane of the squama temporalis as horizontal plane comes at the top of the operative field. To be cared for are the turning and flexion-deflexion of the head with due regard to cervical spondylosis, venous return and endotracheal tube. Arm rest is indispensable for performance of microvascular surgery.

Dissection of the STA

After the scalp to be operated has been shaved, one assesses, guided by Doppler sonography, the course of the STA parietal branch and also the frontal branch if necessary. One may dissect the STA with a diameter of around 1 mm in the skin flap after reflection of a question mark incision as originally described. The STA can be dissected also under a linear incision for a length

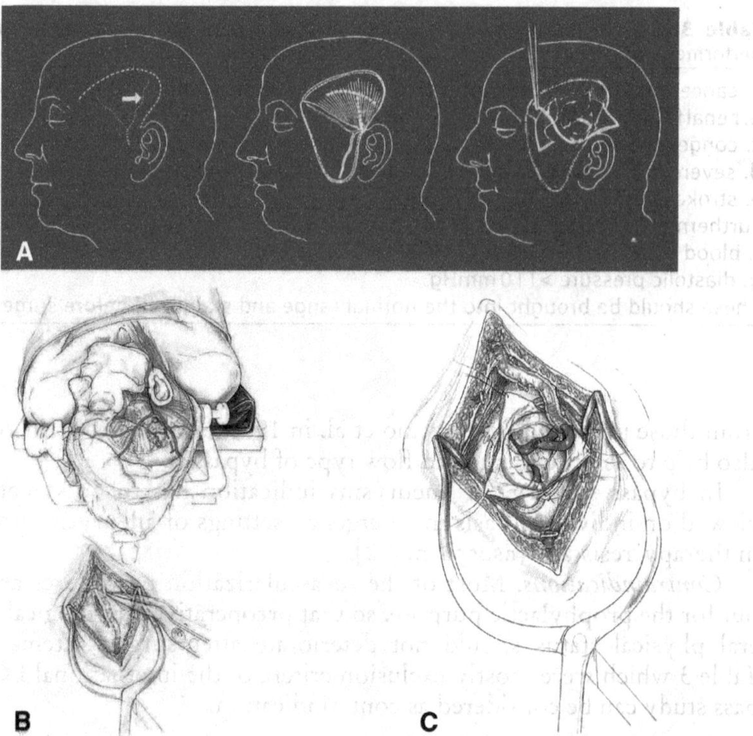

Fig. 6. Standard STA-MCA bypass. **A** Dissection of the STA from the skin flap. Frontal branch can be included also in the flap in case of necessity of its use [22, 29]. **B** Positioning of the head and dissection of the STA parietal branch by linear incision. **C** Completed STA-MCA bypass after a small craniotomy with its center placed 6 cm cranial to the external acoustic porus.

of 8–10 cm. The arterial dissection is done including periadventitial tissues so that it can be performed quickly and atraumatically protecting arterial walls within it. After having cut the temporal musculature along its fibre direction, the squama temporalis is exposed by spreading the cut muscular line.

Craniotomy
The center of the craniotomy is placed at a point about 6 cm cranial to the porus acusticus externus. This point is supposed to correspond with the end of the Sylvian fissure, from which branches of the MCA with a diameter of about 1 mm emerge onto the cortical surface. These arteries are the angular artery, posterior parietal artery or posterior temporal artery and suitable as recipient artery for end-to-side microvascular anastomosis with the dissected parietal branch of the STA as donor.

An alternative method is to use 3-D CT angiography or MR angiography for navigation to the location of the target cortical artery and perform a craniotomy accordingly [11]. One burr hole is placed just caudal to the sutura squamosa and from this hole a small bone flap of around 3 cm is sawed out towards cranially so that the above mentioned cortical arteries can be dissected after dural opening [25, 29].

End-to-side microvascular anastomosis
After having opened the arachnoidea, one of the cortical arteries of around 1 mm in diameter in the operating field is dissected in a length of 1 cm, with several tiny branches of the artery being coagulated and cut. A rubber dam is inserted between the cortical surface and the dissected segment of the cortical artery for the isolation of the latter. After the segment has been closed with temporary mini-clip at its proximal and distal ends, a longitudinal arteriotomy or an elliptical arteriotomy for a length of 1.0–1.5 mm is done on the superior surface of this recipient artery.

The cut end of the already dissected STA is brought over onto the recipient artery. The lengths should be optimally redundant to enable the whole anastomotic procedures and its torsion and strangulation should be avoided. After its temporary occlusion at the proximal part and irrigation of the lumen with heparin solution (1000–2500 IU/100 ml saline), the periadventitia is peeled off at its distal end and made ready for the anastomosing procedure. The end is cut so that the diagonal diameter corresponds with the opening of the recipient artery mentioned above. An end-to-side anastomosis is accomplished usually with 8 interrupted sutures with a 10-0 monofilament Nylon thread after the method described elsewhere for the laboratory training. This procedure needs around 20–30 minutes. This duration of blood flow interruption at the segment is considered acceptable and of no harm to the corresponding perfusion territory of the brain.

In MMA patients, especially in children, the cortical arteries are as small as 0.5 mm in diameter, so that around 6 sutures with a 11-0 monofilament are enough to complete an end-to-side bypass.

After the suture line has been checked, the temporary clips are transiently opened one by one, at first those applied to the cortical artery and then those at the STA. This procedure serves to check for the necessity of additional sutures around the anastomotic suture line and also to seal it. After completion of anastomosis by definite removal of the temporary clips and the rubber dam, the patency is checked representatively by micro-Doppler sonography or other methods such as fluorescence angiography, thermal clearance Peltier stack, or infrared probe, etc. We are using micro-Doppler sonography for its practical convenience and reliability.

Closure of the craniotomy
After oxycellulose has been applied around the suture line, the dura is approximated and closed not necessarily watertight but replacing the air with saline as much as possible. Strangulation of the donor STA is to be avoided at

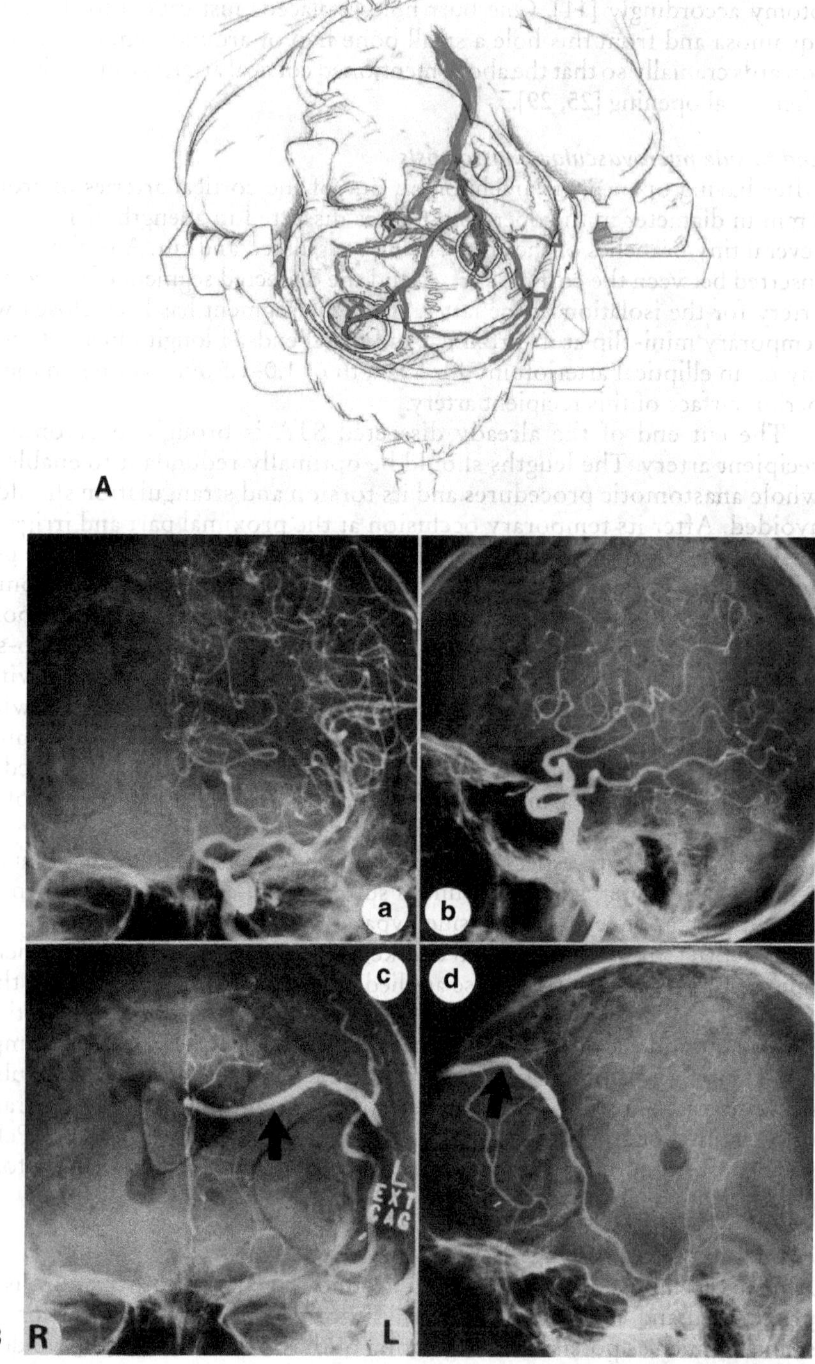
A
a
b
c
d
L
EXT
CAG
B
R
L

the time of bone replacement and muscle fascia and skin closure. Neither epidural nor subgaleal drainage is necessary.

As a modified method, the STA can be anastomosed with M2 or M3 by opening the Sylvian fissure, for example, at the time of aneurysm surgery, so that the frontal branch of the STA should always be included and kept intact in the skin flap [12].

Peri- and intraoperative management and follow-up

Anticoagulant therapy and or Aspirin therapy should be discontinued prior to surgery, mostly 3 days before. We are doing surgery rather under some influence of such therapy in order to prevent thromboembolism cerebral as well as cardiopulmonal. Appropriate hydration is necessary and dehydration is contraindicated. In MMA patients, CBF measurement examination with Diamox loading should have been completed more than 48 hours before surgery. Period of instable cerebral hemodynamics manifested with frequent TIAs especially in MMA patients should be passed over by administration of Dexamethasone and surgery shoud be carried out in stable situation.

Under general anaesthesia the patient is put on controlled respiration. pCO_2 is kept usually around 40 mmHg; both hypercapnea and hypocapnea should be avoided especially in MMA patients.

Postoperative blood pressure is kept in normal pressure range, especially systolic pressure is kept under 160 mmHg. Prophylactic antiepileptics is considered to be not necessary but prophylactic antibiotics is given intravenously only during surgery. Aspirin can be administered again after 24 hours postoperatively. Oral anticoagulant therapy can be resumed after a week. Patency of the bypass is followed up by Doppler sonography and whole postoperative follow-up hemodynamic check with angiography and water PET is done in 2–3 months postoperatively.

1.2 The STA-ACA bypass (Fig. 7)

As a special type of bypass procedure for the anterior circulation, the STA-ACA bypass is mentioned here. This bypass is indicated classically for MMA patients in which the ACA territory is hemodynamically compromised or for patients with large or giant aneurysms of the anterior communicating artery in which flow of the distal ACA is compromised by a clipping or coiling procedure. The frontal branch of the STA is anastomosed classically with the middle internal frontal artery (MIFA) at the medial corner of the frontal cortex located anterior to the coronal suture. Usually the end of the dissected frontal branch of the STA in its whole length at the frontal skin flap is long enough to reach the midline after stretching its curved and serpentine course

Fig. 7. STA-ACA bypass. **A** In MMA, the STA-ACA can be combined with STA-MCA bypass as illustrated. In this case, the interposition graft is taken from the distal STA (arrow). **Bc, Bd** Use of interposition saphenous vein graft in a patient with ACA occlusion (**Bab**)

and to anastomose with the MIFA. Otherwise, an interposition graft using a segment of the parietal branch of the STA, of the superficial temporal vein or of the distal saphenous vein is put between the MIFA and the end of the frontal branch [21].

1.3 Bypass surgery for posterior circulation

Bypass surgery for the posterior circulation is indicated as in the anterior circulation: prevention of recurrent stroke in the vertebrobasilar territory in cases with atherosclerotic occlusive lesion with hemodynamic failure or major arteries in the territory being compromised at the time of surgical or endovascular management of large or giant aneurysms.

The STA-SCA bypass (Fig. 8)
STA-SCA bypass surgery was initiated by Ausman in 1978 [2]. The technical outline is as follows [24]: After induction of general anesthesia and intubation, spinal drainage is put in order to reduce the temporal lobe retraction. The head and body position is the same as described above for the standard STA-MCA bypass. The STA parietal branch is dissected by linear skin incision up to the periphery for more than 10 cm to enable the end to reach the SCA in the depth for the performance of anastomotic procedure. The skin incision is extended curvilinear posterocaudally down to the posterior part of the mastoid process. The temporal craniotomy should be larger than 4 cm in diameter: anterior to the origin of the zygomatic arch, posterior to the sigmoid transverse sinus junction, caudal just above the porus acusticus externus. Then the temporal base including the outer portion of the pyramid is drilled away caudally down to the very basis in order to get a wide enough operative field. The mastoid cells may be partly opened inbetween and these should be closed meticulously with bone wax and fascia at the time of craniotomy closure. This procedure together with the above mentioned spinal drainage enables to perform the bypass procedure in the depth without excessive retraction of the temporal lobe and to minimize injury to the vein of Labbé. A small incision is made to the tentorium about 1 cm medially from the transverse sigmoid junction so that the superior surface of the cerebellum is exposed. The incision is extended toward the tentorial edge just 1 cm posterior from its attachment to the pyramid tip and the cut end of the tentorium is reflected. This procedure together with opening of the perimesencephalic cistern enables to expose the proximal part of the SCA

Fig. 8. STA-SCA bypass. **A** Illustration of the craniotomy and bypass procedure at the operating field by cutting the tentorium. **B** 56-year-old male underwent STA-SCA bypass due to basilar stenosis (**B1**) which turned out as occlusion on the 3-week follow-up angiography without any neurological deterioration. The bypass was patent (**B2**). The 3-month follow-up angiography on neurological deterioration showed patent bypass but propagation of thrombosis further distally up to the branching site of the anterior inferior cerebellar artery (**B4**). MRI showed pontine infarction (**B3**) but the patient could recover to Rankin 3

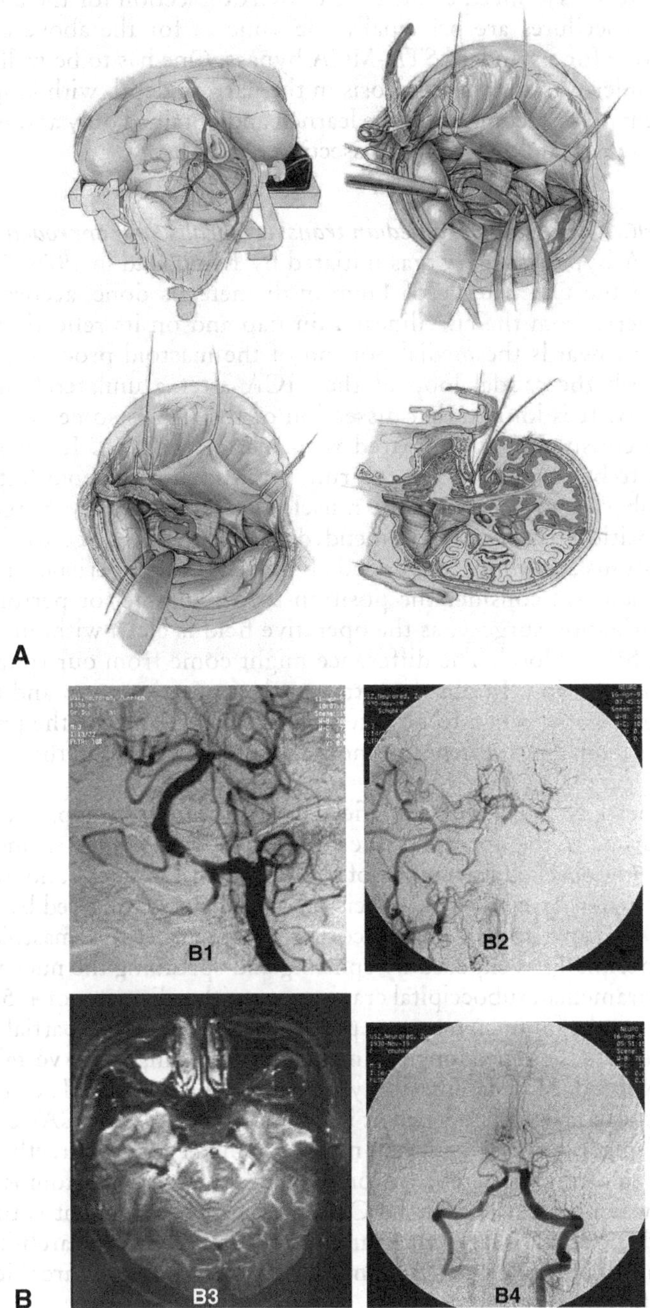
A
B1
B2
B
B3
B4

and its branches along with the trochlear nerve. There are practically no tiny branches to be sacrificed at the time of SCA dissection for the anastomosis. Further procedures are principally the same as for the above end-to-side anastomosis for a standard STA-MCA bypass. One has to be well trained to perform microvascular anastomosis in the narrow depth with longer micro-instruments. The technique can be learned and obtained only at the microsurgical laboratory and by cadaver dissection [23, 26].

The OA-PICA bypass by paramedian transvertebralis ring approach (Fig. 9)
OA-PICA bypass surgery was initiated by Khodadad in 1976 [2, 24]. Dissection of the OA usually of 1 mm in diameter is done, according to the early papers, from the curvilinear skin flap and on its reflection from the periphery towards the medial portion of the mastoid process and anastomosed with the caudal loop of the PICA after a unilateral suboccipital craniotomy. It is known that dissection of the OA is somewhat laborious and time consuming as compared with that of the STA. It has many tiny branches to be coagulated and cut, runs into the subcutaneous fatty tissue at the periphery and deep into the muscle layers proximally. Surgery in the sitting position has been recommended to be rather avoided for frequented complications according to Khodadad himself. Our experience, however, is different and we consider the position to be suitable for performing this revascularization surgery, as the operative field is clean without accumulation of CSF or blood. The difference might come from our routine use of the sitting position. In our department, the operating team and the anaesthesiologist know when to be careful and how to manage the problematic situations from an experience of more than 200 surgeries in the sitting position per year.

The head is fixed with Mayfield's three-point pin apparatus rotating ca. 30° turned to the operating side and flexed ca. 20° in the sitting position. After having checked the course of the OA with Doppler sonography, surgery is initiated by a linear skin incision over the OA followed by dissection of the OA down to the medial corner of the processus mastoideus. The squama occipitalis is exposed by splitting and spreading the nuchal muscles. After a paramedian suboccipital craniotomy with a diameter of 4–5 cm reaching down to the foramen magnum preferably followed by a partial condylectomy, the dura is opened longitudinally. The dural ring of the vertebral artery is thus exposed. Hemilaminectomy of C1 is not necessary. The arachnoidea of the cisterna magna is opened at its lateral corner. The PICA's caudal loop or lateral medullary segment of 1 mm in diameter comes directly into view after just elevating the cerebellar tonsil. The subsequent anastomosing procedure between the cut end of the OA and the PICA segment is the same as described above. Closure of the craniotomy should be done carefully to avoid strangulation of the donor OA, as muscle layers to be closed are thick to close after the bone replacement.

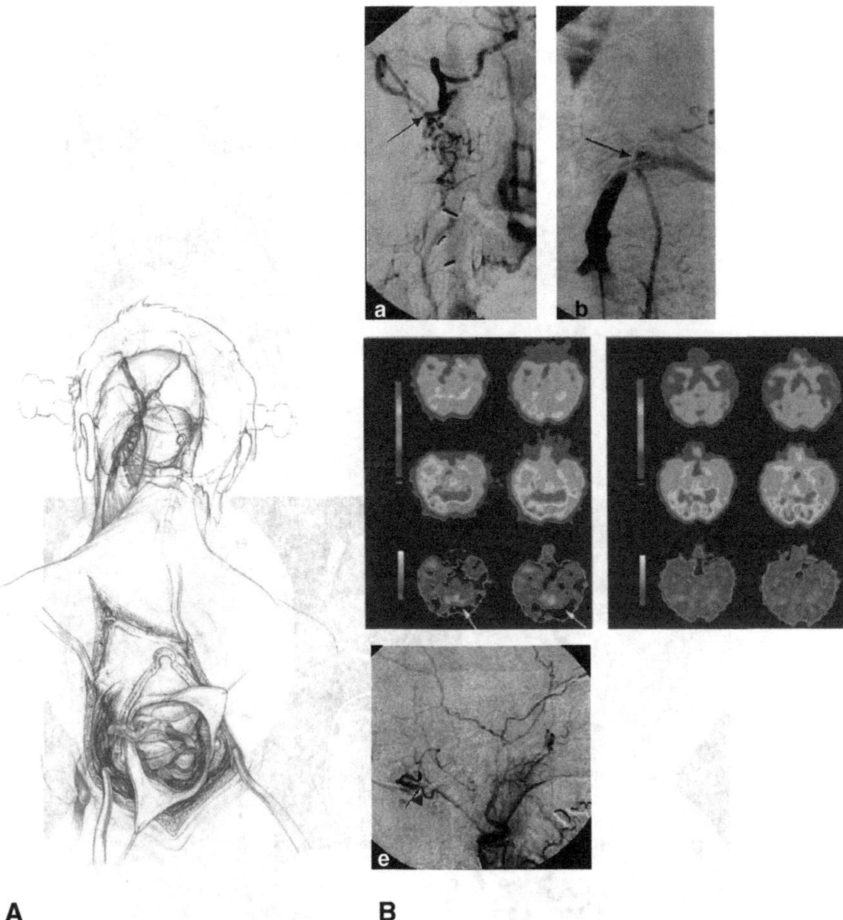

Fig. 9. OA-PICA bypass. **A** Illustration of the bypass by linear incision along the dotted line (see text). **B** 50-year-old male with both vertebral artery (VA) occlusion (**a** and **b**, arrow) and with hemodynamic compromise at the left PICA territory (**c**, arrows) underwent left OA-PICA bypass. The 3-month follow-up examination displayed a patent OA-PICA bypass (**e**, arrow) with improved hemodynamic capacity on the left cerebellar hemisphere (**d**)

The OA-SCA and OA-PCA bypass by supracerebellar transtentorial approach (Fig. 9)

The supracerebellar transtentorial approach in the sitting position has been reported by us in 2001 [31]. The OA is anastomosed either with the SCA or with the posterior temporal artery of the PCA. Dissection of the OA as long as possible is performed by linear incision in the same manner as described above. After a paramedian craniotomy, space between the tentorium and the cranial surface of the cerebellum is obtained by sacrificing one or two bridg-

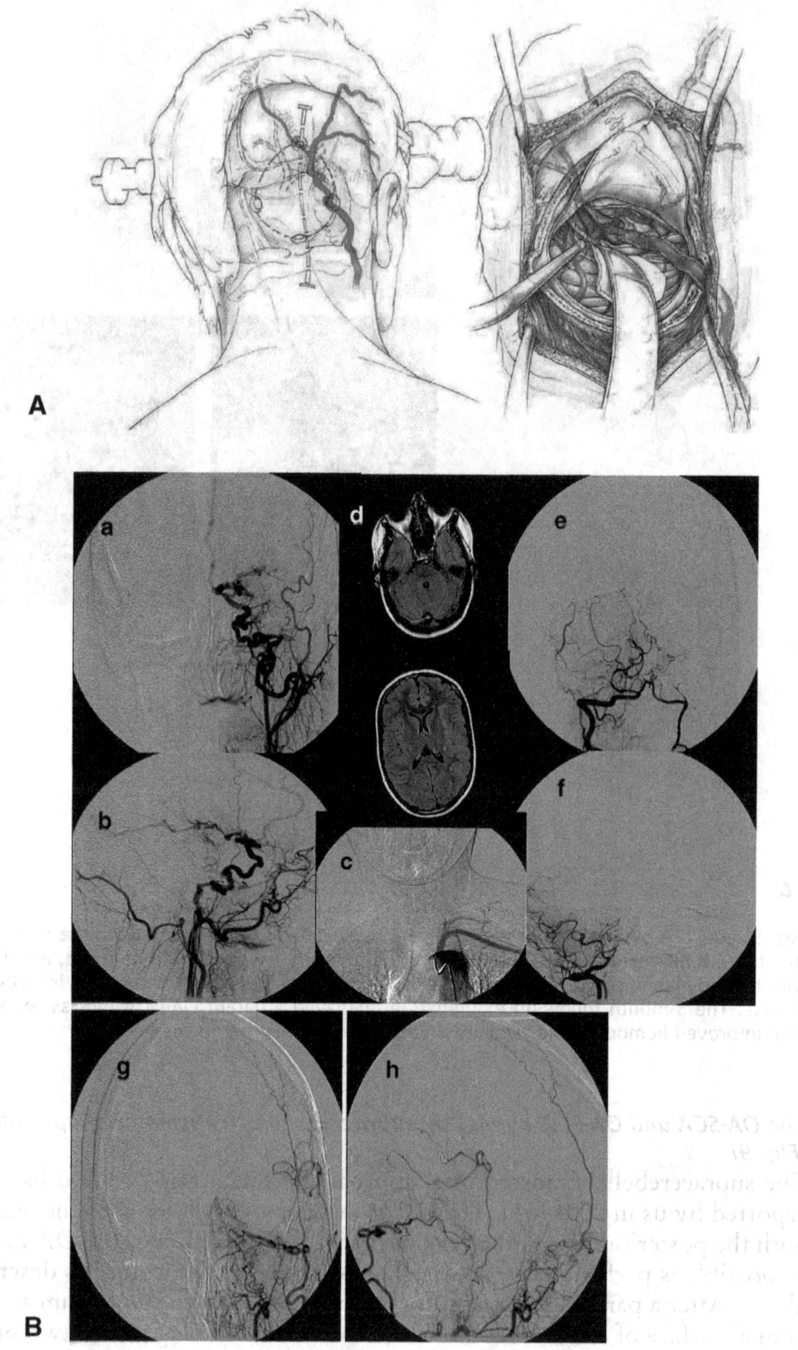
A
a
b
c
d
e
f
g
h
B

ing veins between them. The arachnoid of the cisterna magna is opened at its lateral corner for the purpose of CSF drainage beforehand, so that the mentioned space can increase. The tentorium is incised from the midway towards the tentorial notch. This procedure enables to obtain a spacious operative field and to obtain a cortical branch of the PCA as recipient artery around the corner of the parahippocampal gyrus and the lingual gyrus. The SCA marginal branch can be found together with the trochlear nerve at the cranio-anterior margin of the lobulus quadrangularis. The tentorial incision is done also for the OA-SCA bypass as this procedure brings about a more spacious and better illuminated operative field.

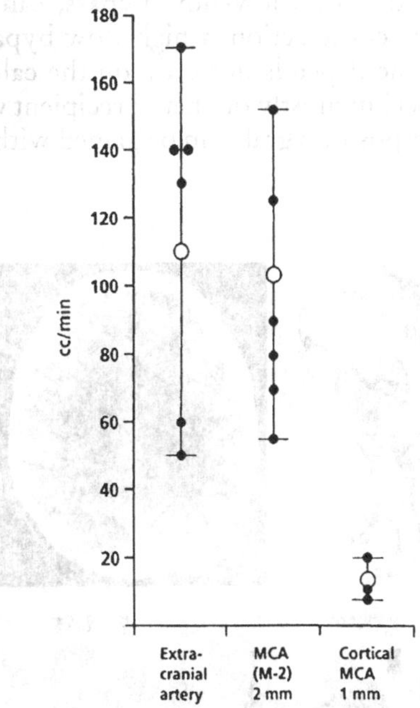

Fig. 11. Bypass flow vs. recipient diameter [30]

Fig. 10. OA-SCA and OA-PCA bypass. **A** Illustration of the bypass procedures via paramedian suboccipital craniotomy by linear incision. Note the tentorium is incised in both bypass procedures. The SCA and its branches are found just at the anterosuperior corner of the lobulus quadrangularis. The posterior temporal artery and its branches are found at the junction of the parahippocampal gyrus and lingual gyrus on the tentorial incision. **B** 21-year-old female with dysplastic ICA plus MCA occlusion on the left side (**a**, **b**) combined with aplasia of the left VA (**c**). The basilar artery was not opacified via the right VA. MRI did not show any abnormal findings. On the basis of PET findings the patient underwent STA-MCA and OA-SCA bypass. The 3-month follow-up examination demonstrated patency of both bypasses (**g**, **h**) with clinical improvement of cessation of vertigo attacks and hemodynamic improvement on PET scan

This type of bypass to the PCA does not need the use of the PCA trunk itself as in the STA-PCA interposition graft bypass [20], so that the possible complication of hemianopsia or hemiparesis can be avoided.

The end-to-side microvascular anastomosis is done in a similar fashion with long microinstruments as described above. The advantage of this procedure is again a clean operative field. The disadvantage of the sitting position, mainly the risk of air embolism, can be managed and overcome through experience of the anesthesiology team and operating team as mentioned above.

1.4 High-flow bypasses

While a usual bypass, that is, a low-flow bypass, can carry 10–20 ml/min blood flow just after its construction, a high-flow bypass can carry around 100 ml/min. This volume depends not only on the calibre of the donor or interposition graft vessel but mostly on that of recipient vessel (Fig. 11). Large calibre of donor or interposition graft can be gained with a saphenous vein or

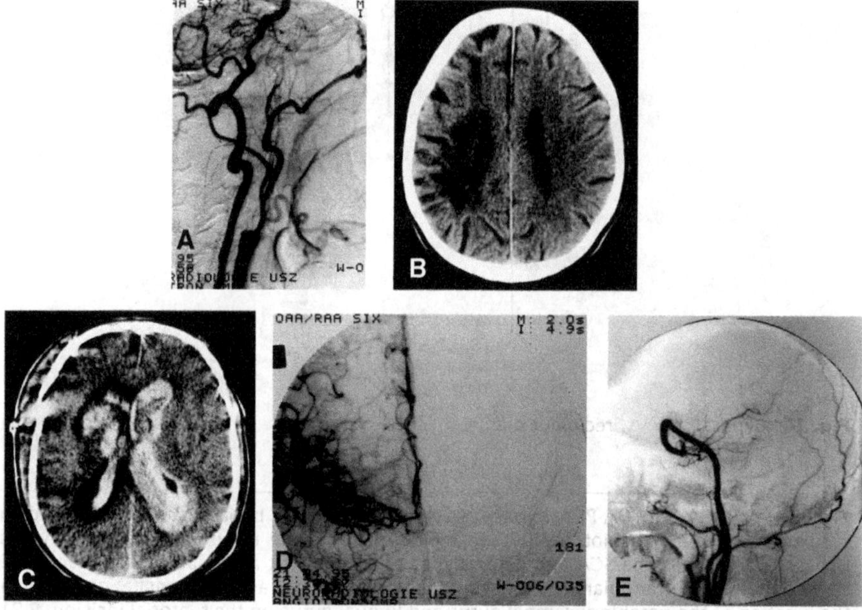

Fig. 12. High-flow venous graft bypass between the right common carotid artery and the MCA (M2). 58-year-old male with right ICA occlusion (**A**) with an extensive infarction on the right hemisphere (**B**) underwent this bypass surgery, as the STA as donor artery was not available. After an uneventful postoperative course, sudden neurological deterioration occurred on the 3rd postoperative day. The CT scan displayed bleeding into the infarcted area along with hematocephalus (**C**); and digital subtraction angiography, a patent high-flow bypass (**D**, **E**)

radial artery graft. One has to know that the length of a graft with blood flow would expand by around one-third as compared with an empty graft without blood flow.

Saphenous vein graft and radial artery graft (Fig. 12)
The saphenous vein is usually dissected at the medial side of the lower leg, beginning at the level of the maleolus medialis towards cranially up to the medial corner of the knee joint through a linear incision. We prefer harvesting this distal part of the saphenous vein to the proximal one of the upper thigh, as the calibre of the former is more suitable for anastomosis with intracranial arteries. For its dissection at a sufficient length, small tiny branches are coagulated and cut meticulously and the larger branches are closed with thread ligation or with metal clips. After blood remaining in the lumen of the harvested vein has been flushed, the segment is filled with heparin solution and preserved until its use slightly distended with temporary clips at both ends. Skin is closed in layers and then bandaged with slight compression. The graft may contain some venous valves which do not need to be removed as the graft is put according to the direction of the flow at the time of interposition. The proximal vessel to be anastomosed could be the subclavian artery, common carotid artery, proximal external carotid artery or C5 (after anterior perosectomy) and the distal one C2 (after selective anterior clinoidectomy), M2 or M3 portion of the MCA by opening the Sylvian fissure. This venous graft is used also as low-flow bypass to cortical arteries with diameters of 1 mm in which some technical difficulties of microvascular anastomosis due to a difference in graft and recipient artery calibre have to be overcome.

The radial arterial graft has been used also for the purpose of high-flow graft. The size of the cut end is just that of the M2 portion (2–2.5 mm in diameter). After tolerated Allen test, a graft as long as 20 cm can be harvested without compromise of blood supply to the forearm and volar portion of the hand. In comparison with the saphenous vein graft, the following advantages and disadvantages can be pointed out for the radial artery graft.

1. Microvascular anastomosis on artery is easier to perform due to less distensibility and to more rigidity of the arterial wall than that of venous wall.
2. Torsion and kinking of the graft can easily be prevented.
3. Graft dissection is easier.
4. Length of the graft is rather limited.
5. Because of the graft's arterial nature, problem of atherosclerotic change is possible.

In spite of the advantages of the arterial graft over the venous graft, I prefer to use the venous graft from the practical point view of easier availability.

Use of high-flow graft in various bypass procedures
A high-flow graft is used for the following bypasses:

1. Between extracranial supraaortic arteries such as common carotid and subclavian artery as in the subclavian steal syndrome
2. C5 to C2 bypass as in large and giant aneurysms in the ICA cavernous portion [6].
3. Subclavian artery, common carotid artery or external carotid artery to C2 or M2 as in intractable large or giant aneurysms in the ICA or MCA.

Although innovative techniques such as the use of excimer laser-assisted nonocclusive anastomosis for the construction of a high-flow bypass have been reported, in which no temporary occlusion of the recipient artery is necessary [19], the standard method with the use of microsutures of 8-0 to 10-0 monofilament under temporary occlusion of the recipient artery for around less than 30 min is still in wide practical use. Temporary occlusion of such duration is considered to be acceptable under general anesthesia with controlled hemodynamics and administration of neuroprotective drugs such as mannitol and barbiturate, and also with the use of mild hypothermia in extreme cases.

LONG-TERM RESULTS AND COMPLICATIONS

Microsurgical revascularization procedures was performed as follows during the period from 1993 through 2007 at the department of neurosurgery, University Hospital Zürich: 203 patients underwent 277 microvascular revascularization procedures: atherosclerosis 93 cases, MMA 47 cases, aneurysms 57 cases (50% intractable large or giant aneurysms, 40% emergengy bypass and 10% intractable vasospasm) and skull base tumors 6 cases. Most cases underwent revascularization to the territory of the MCA, 34 cases to the territory of the ACA and 13 cases to the territory of the posterior circulation. Multiple bypass procedures were necessary in most of the MMA patients followed by patients with atherosclerosis.

Bypass patency rate examined by follow-up angiography was 87%. Although the stroke recurrence rate in our recent series is still under investigation, the annual recurrence rate is expected to be around 2% (vs. 5% in conservative treatment) from our previous experience [25].

Major complications are listed in Table 4 and direct postoperative mortality was in 3 cases. Two cases of extensive ischemic swelling are cases of aneurysms: one is with symptomatic giant ICA aneurysm. ICA occlusion was interpreted as tolerable on BOT but with some asymmetry on SPECT, so that normal STA-MCA bypass was combined with therapeutic ICA occlusion.

Table 4. Complications[a]

Major complications (overlapped):
Extensive infarction – insufficient flow 2 cases*
Infarction – hemodynamic instability in 3 MMA cases
Infarction – conversion from stenosis to occlusion 1 case
Intracerebral hemorrhage into infarcted area 1 case
Epidural subdural, intracerebral hematoma 3 cases
Subdural hematoma-effusion 2 cases
Cardiopulmonary insufficiency 1 case*

[a]Asterisk indicates mortal cases (total, 3)

The patient died of extensive infarction in spite of subsequent decompressive craniotomy. The other patient was with ruptured giant anterior communicating aneurysm presenting with grade IV. One ACA had to be occluded at the time of radical clipping so that STA-ACA bypass was combined. The patient died of infarction and diffuse swelling due to SAH. The third case was a case of bonnet bypass [18] with the use of the brachio-cephalic vein as interposition graft. The patient expired 3 weeks after surgery due to cardiopulmonary failure. Postoperative ischemic complication in MMA patients was encountered in three cases. In another case of MCA stenosis of atherosclerosis, new ischemia was encountered at the basal ganglia originating in compromise of a lateral lenticulostriate artery due to conversion of MCA stenosis to occlusion after bypass procedure. Such conversion of stenosis into occlusion after bypass surgery with or without neurological deterioraton has been infrequently reported also in the vertebrobasilar territory. These should be kept in mind. Other complications were related to hemorrhage. One was a case of infarction which changed into hemorrhage three days after the construction of a common carotid–M3 high-flow bypass using a long saphenous vein graft (Fig. 12). The other cases are more or less related with antiplatelet or anticoagulant therapy: epidural and subdural hematomas.

HOW TO AVOID COMPLICATIONS

Complications can be classified into four groups:

1. ischemic complication
2. hemorrhagic complication
3. cardiopulmonary complication
4. minor complication such as wound healing problems, infection, CSF rhinorrhea, epileptic seizures, etc.

Strict attention should be paid to the following important items at perioperative care and management.

Good hydration. One of the most important things in the perioperative care is considered to be appropriate hydration. It is easy to understand that combination of hemoconcentration plus low perfusion can enhance the risk of rheological deterioration of the hemodynamic situation easily resulting in ischemia. This might be one of the reasons that cases with misery perfusion have also an elevated risk of ischemia.

Normotension. Excessive postoperative hypertension or hypotension should be avoided. We had some cases in the past in whom cerebellar hemorrhage complicated due to postoperative hypertension [25]. Hypotension would induce rheological deterioration and hence ischemic complication.

Normocapnea. Hypercapnea or hypocapnea must be avoided especially in MMA patients. Intraoperative regulation of pCO_2 around 40 mmHg is considered to be optimal in MMA patients and cases with atherosclerotic lesion. Diamox loading test is a good and simple procedure to find out hemodynamic failures but may induce metabolic acidosis and hypovolemia. Aggressive intervention of bypass surgery should be postponed until 48 hours after the test.

Complication of *subdural hematoma* has been observed in cases with infarction of considerable size and postoperative subdural air accumulation would turn to subdural effusion and then to hematoma under the necessary medication of antiplatelet agent [25]. Therefore, we are recommending to drive out subdural air by replacing it with saline as much as possible at the time of dural closure and bone replacement. Use of a linear incision for donor artery dissection instead of that in the skin flap seems to reduce the problem of *wound healing* and the method would reduce duration of surgery.

CONCLUSIONS

State-of-the-art of microvascular intracranial revascularization procedures for both the anterior and the posterior circulation, indication, technique and results have been outlined. Negative results of international cooperative study of the procedure in stroke prevention would not justify to abandon the technique. We now are relatively sure that the procedure is effective in stroke recurrence prevention in the group of *hemodynamic compromise*. This procedure can be extended for the *treatment of MMA, aneurysms* and some *skull base tumors* in combination with other surgical or endovascular treatment.

Technique of revascularization microsurgery can be obtained only by microsurgical training in the laboratory [22, 23, 26]. Prerequisite for its clinical use is a 100% patency rate obtained at any performance of an end-to-end or end-to-side anastomosis of vessels with a diameter of 1 mm in the laboratory.

Acknowledgement

I am indebted to P. Roth for the artist drawings.

References

[1] Astrup J, Siesjö BK, Symon L (1981) Threshols in cerebral ischemia – the ischemic penumbra. Stroke 12: 723-725

[2] Ausman JL, Diaz FG, De Los Reyez RA, Pearce JE, Schronitz CE, Pak H (1985) Microsurgery for atherosclerosis in the distal vertebral and basilar arteries. In: Rand RW (ed) Microneurosurgery. CV Mosby, St Louis, Mo, pp 497-510

[3] Baron JC, Bousser MG, Rey A, et al. (1981) Reversal of focal "misery-perfusion syndrome" by extra-intracranial arterial bypass in hemodynamic cerebral ischemia: a case study with ^{15}O positron tomography. Stroke 12: 454-459

[4] Date I, Tokunaga K, Sugiu K (2008) Multimodality therapy for large and giant intracavernous internal carotid artery aneurysms. Surg Cereb Str (Jpn) 36: 12-18

[5] The EC/IC Bypass Study Group (1985) Failure of extracranial-intracranial arterial bypass to reduce the risk of ischemic stroke. Results of an international randomized trial. N Engl J Med 313: 1191-1200

[6] Fukushima T (1992) Operative technique of the skull base bypass. Jpn J Neurosurg 1: 41-47

[7] JET Study Group (2002) Japanese EC-IC Bypass Trial (JET Study): the second interim analysis. Surg Cerbr Stroke (Jpn) 30: 434-437

[8] Karasawa J, Kikuchi H, Furuse S, Kanamura J, Sakaki T (1978) Treatment of Moyamoya disease with STA-MCA anastomosis. J Neurosurg 49: 679-688

[9] Kawano T, Yonekawa Y, Miyake H, et al. (1991) Balloon occlusion test and Matas test – clinical efficacy, indication and practice. Neurosurgeons (Jpn) 10: 42-56

[10] Khan N, Schuknecht B, Boltshauser E, Capone A, Buck A, Imhof HG, Yonekawa Y (2003) Moyamoya disease and Moyamoya syndrome: experience in Europe; choice of revascularisation procedures. Acta Neurochir (Wien) 145: 1061-1071

[11] Kikuta K, Takagi Y, Fushimi Y, Ishizu K, Okada T, Hanakawa T, Miki Y, Fukuyama H, Nozaki K, Hashimoto N (2006) "Target bypass": a method for preoperative targeting of a recipient artery in superficial temporal artery-to-middle cerebral artery anastomoses. Neurosurgery 59(4) (Suppl 2): ONS320-ONS327

[12] Krayenbühl N, Khan N, Cesnulis E, Imhof HG, Yonekawa Y (2008) Emergency extra-intracranial bypass surgery in the treatment of cerebral aneurysms. Acta Neurochir Suppl 103: 93-101

[13] Matsushima Y, Fukai N, Tanaka K, et al. (1981) A new surgical treatment of moyamoya disease in children: a preliminary report. Surg Neurol 15: 313-320

[14] Mizukami K (1985) cited from Yonekawa Y: Cerebrovascular disease. In: Takakura K, Abe H (eds) (1996) Neurosurgery. Nankodo, Tokyo (Jpn), pp 239-291

[15] Powers WJ (1991) Cerebral hemodynamics in ischemic cerebrovascular disease. Ann Neurol 29: 231-240

[16] Schmiedek P, Piepgras A, Leinsinger G, Kirsch CM, Einhäupl K (1994) Improvement of cerebrovascular reserve capacity by EC-IC arterial bypass surgery in patients with ICA occlusion and hemodynamic cerebral ischemia. J Neurosurg 81: 236-244

[17] Sindou M, Daher A (1987) Autogenous vein grafts for arterial and venous brain vascularization. Neurosurgeons (Jpn) 6: 231-239

[18] Spetzler RF, Roski RA, Rhodes RS, Modic MT (1980) The "bonnet bypass". Case report. J Neurosurg 53: 707-709

[19] Streefkerk HJ, Bremmer JP, Tulleken CA (2005) The ELANA technique: high flow revascularization of the brain. Acta Neurochir (Suppl 94): 143-148

[20] Sundt TM, Piepgras DG, Houser OW, Campbell JK (1982) Interposition saphenous vein grafts for advanced occlusive disease and large aneurysms in the posterior circulation. J Neurosurg 56: 205-215

[21] Tanaka K, Yonekawa Y, Satou K, Katagiri K, Kouno H (1992) STA-ACA anastomosis with interposed vein graft. A case report. No Shinkei Geka 20: 171-176

[22] Yaşargil MG (1969) Microsurgery: applied to neurosurgery. Thieme, Stuttgart

[23] Yaşargil MG (1967) Experimental small vascular surgery in the dog including patching and grafting of cerebral vessels and the formation of functional extra-intracranial shunts. In: Donaghy RMP, Yaşargil MG (eds) Microvascular surgery. Thieme, Stuttgart, pp 87-126

[24] Yonekawa Y (1988) Posterior fossa revascularization – indication, technique and results. The Mt. Fuji Workshop on CVD 6: 71-76

[25] Yonekawa Y (1988) Prevention of relapsing cerebral ischemia by the EC–IC bypass – Reevaluation of results of the EC–IC bypass international cooperative study and those of our cases. Shinkei Shinpo (Jpn) 32: 320-327

[26] Yonekawa Y, Frick R, Roth P, Taub E, Imhof HG (1999) Laboratory training in microsurgical techniques and microvascular anastomosis. Oper Tech Neurosurg 2: 149-158

[27] Yonekawa Y, Khan N (2003) Moyamoya disease. In: Barnett HJM, Bogousslavsky J, Meldrum H (eds) Ischemic stroke. Advances in neurology, vol 92. Lippincott Williams & Wilkins, Philadelphia, pp 113-118

[28] Yonekawa Y, Yaşargil MG (1977) Brain vascularization by transplanted omentum. A possible treatment of cerebral ischemia. Neurosurgery 1: 256-259

[29] Yonekawa Y, Yaşargil MG (1976) Extra-intracranial arterial anastomosis. Clinical and technical aspects. Results. Adv Tech Stand Neurosurg 3: 47-78

[30] Yonekawa Y, Fandino J, Taub E (2001) Surgical therapy. In: Fisher M, Bogousslavsky J (eds) Current review of cerebrovascular disease. 4th edn. Current Medicine, Philadelphia, pp 219-232

[31] Yonekawa Y, Imhof HG, Taub E, Curcic M, Kaku Y, Roth P, Wieser HG, Groscurth P (2001) Supracerebellar transtentorial approach to posterior temporomedial structures. J Neurosurg 94: 339-345

[32] Yonekawa Y, Zumofen D, Imhof HG, Roth P, Khan N (2008) Hemorrhagic cerebral dissecting aneurysms: surgical treatment and results. Acta Neurochir Suppl 103: 61-69

Contact: Yasuhiro Yonekawa, University of Zurich, Haldenbachstrasse 18, 8091 Zurich, Switzerland
E-mail: yasuhiro.yonekawa@usz.ch

MANAGEMENT OF INTRACRANIAL VENOUS PATHOLOGIES – POTENTIAL ROLE OF VENOUS STENTING

J. D. PICKARD

INTRODUCTION

The anatomy and physiology of the cerebral venous system has received much attention. Through trial and error, the rules for safely dealing with the local venous drainage in various surgical approaches are well established. Many pathologies affect the cerebral venous system including

- Traumatic injury to the major dural sinuses
- Carotico-cavernous fistulae
- Dural arteriovenous fistulae
- Developmental venous anomalies
- Arterial venous malformations
- Meningiomas involving the dural sinuses
- Pineal and glomus tumors
- Cerebral venous thrombosis
- Pseudotumor cerebri syndrome (PTCS, benign intracranial hypertension (BIH), idiopathic intracranial hypertension (IIH))
- Giant arachnoid granulations.

Through study of PTCS, it is now becoming recognised that some patients have venous sinuses that reversibly collapse in the face of raised cerebrospinal fluid pressure. Venous stenting was recently developed by Higgins et al. in Cambridge to help some of these patients and has subsequently proven to be of value in managing challenging lesions within the venous sinuses presenting with raised CSF pressure such as meningiomas and giant arachnoid granulations.

This chapter will focus, firstly, on the general principles of protection of venous drainage during surgery for many different conditions and, secondly, on the potential of the recent advance of venous sinus stenting.

RATIONALE

Careful consideration needs to be given to the local venous drainage when planning and executing most microsurgical approaches to the brain and base

Keywords: intracranial venous pathologies, benign intracranial hypertension, venous shunting

of skull. Comprehensive accounts of the relevant anatomy and congenital variations are widely available. Sindou and Auque have provided a helpful account of which venous structures are "dangerous" to sacrifice including the mid third and posterior third of the superior sagittal sinus (SSS), the lateral sinus where it is dominant, the large calibre midline afferent veins to the SSS (including Trolard), interior cerebral veins (including Labbe), the large calibre superficial Sylvian veins and the deep cerebral veins including the vein of Galen, the thalamo-striate vein and the superior petrosal vein.

The experimental consequences of venous occlusion depend upon the species, acuity and method of occlusion presumably reflecting the ability of the venous collateral capacity to cope. In some studies, but not all, dural sinus occlusion leads to increased cerebral blood volume and cerebral water content resulting in raised intracranial pressure and reduced cerebral blood flow. Intraparenchymal haemorrhage and blood brain barrier disruption reflect the additional occlusion of cortical veins. Experimentally, chronic elevation of venous sinus pressure may induce either hydrocephalus or PTCS depending in part on whether the cranial sutures are open or closed. Venous sinuses that are compressed by raised CSF pressure may compound the increase in intracranial pressure (Figs. 1 and 2) [7].

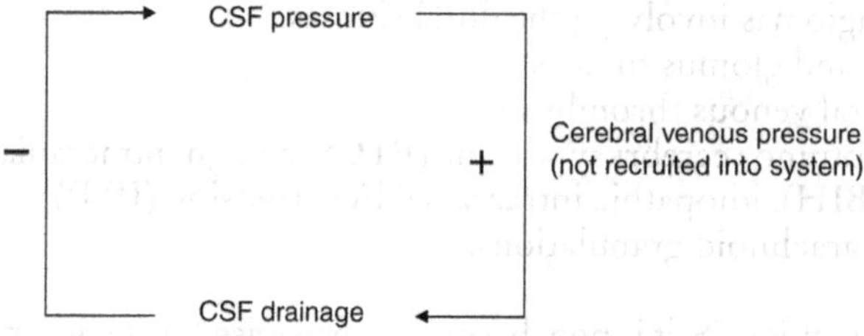

Fig. 1. Normal negative feedback – Increases in CSF pressure are controlled by an increase in the rate of CSF absorption as it is a pressure dependent process

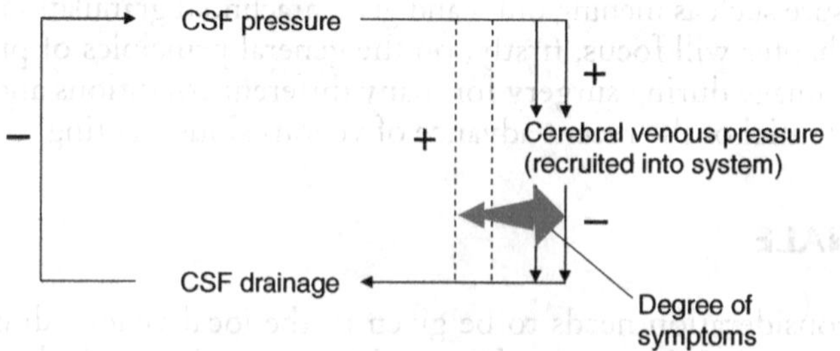

Fig. 2. Disordered positive feedback – Recruitment of the cerebral venous sinuses into the feedback loop due to venous sinus collapse, secondary to increased CSF pressure, causes venous sinus pressure (particularly SSS pressure) to increase. This inhibits CSF drainage and results in further increases in CSF pressure and so on

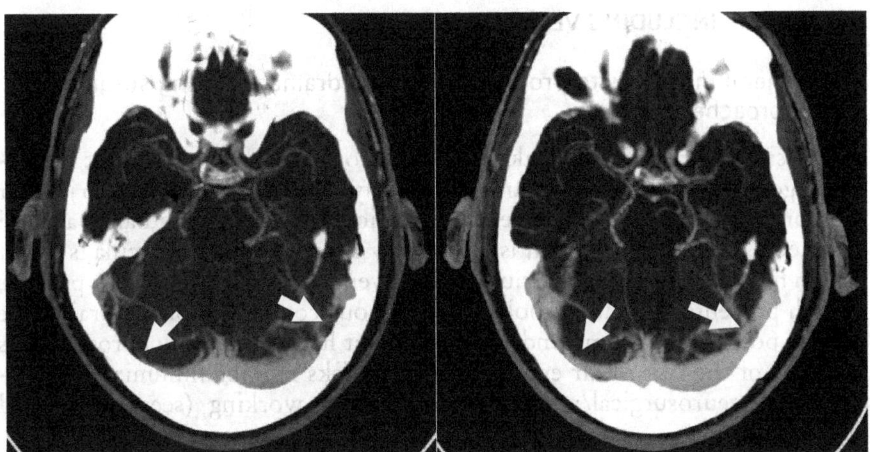

Fig. 3. CT venogram in a case of PTCS with compressible veins: immediate effects on the transverse sinuses of CSF withdrawal by lumbar puncture. Courtesy of Dr. N. Higgins

It is now clear that many sinus narrowings are not fixed obstructions but are reversible by lowering CSF pressure (Fig. 3).

DECISION-MAKING

Magnetic resonance (MR), computerized tomography (CT), digital subtraction angiography (DSA) and direct retrograde cerebral venography (DRCV) all have their part to play in investigating the cerebral venous circulation. MR venography in its various forms including phase contrast or time of flight supplemented where appropriate with intravenous Gadolinium injection provides a comprehensive view of the intracranial venous circulation. CT venography with contrast is useful for examining the transverse sinuses. Conventional and digital subtraction angiography are useful particularly where there is a suspicion of a dural arteriovenous fistula.

Direct retrograde cerebral venography (DRCV) combined with manometry is the investigation of choice for venous sinus obstruction. It provides the most accurate information including the functional significance of any obstruction in terms of pressure gradient and clarification of whether MR appearances of sinus narrowing are genuine or the result of so-called "contrast streaming". DRCV is invasive and carries a small risk of perforation of a vein or sinus by the guidewire and of thrombosis around the catheter. Temporary balloon occlusion of a sinus is occasionally used to assess whether it would be safe to sacrifice a lateral sinus during surgery.

1. SURGERY INCLUDING VENOUS STENTING

1.1 General measures to protect the venous drainage during surgical approaches

Obsessional care should be taken with the positioning of any patient in neurosurgery to minimize intracranial venous hypertension secondary to jugular compression caused by extreme neck positions or constricting bands around the neck. Modest head-up tilt is commonly used – when the torcula is about 15 cm higher than the right atrium, cranial venous pressure is slightly positive which prevents both air embolism and venous congestion of the brain. The sitting position is recommended by some but hated by other neurosurgeons because of the risk of air embolism. These risks may be minimized by obsessional neurosurgical/neuroanaesthetic team working (see Sindou and Auque).

As always, excessive brain retraction must be avoided or venous drainage will be endangered. Unlike arterial bleeding, venous bleeding usually responds to gentle measures including gentle pressure and onlay of Surgicel or Spongistan, bone wax and disciplined use of bipolar diathermy. Small holes in veins including bridging veins may be controlled simply by wrapping with Surgicel or Spongistan. Veins that obstruct the surgical approach or are at risk during retraction should be sacrificed as little as possible. Sugita's technique for the dissection of bridging veins is helpful.

If a vein has to be sacrificed, it should be temporally occluded for a few minutes to see if the brain swells. Sindou's technique for dividing a bridging vein distal to its last bridging point is useful.

Various techniques have been described for the reconstruction of bridging veins by silicone tubes and vein grafts. Such techniques are not in common use and there is always the risk of unduly extending the duration of the operation.

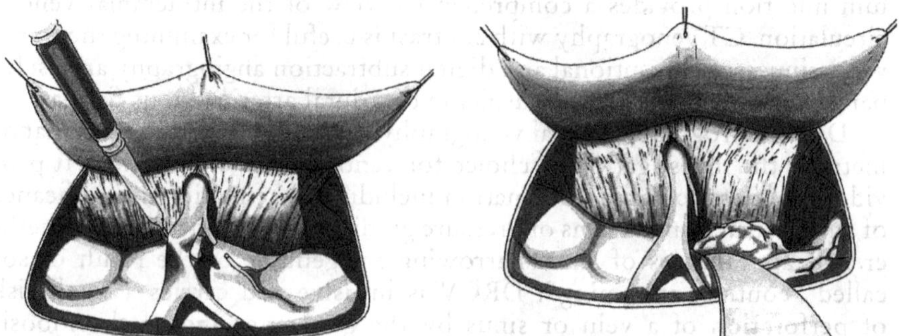

Fig. 4. Sugita technique for dissection of bridging veins (Source: Sindou M and Auque J (2000) The intracranial venous system as a neurosurgeon's perspective. Adv Techn Stand Neurosurg 26, p 169, Fig. 22)

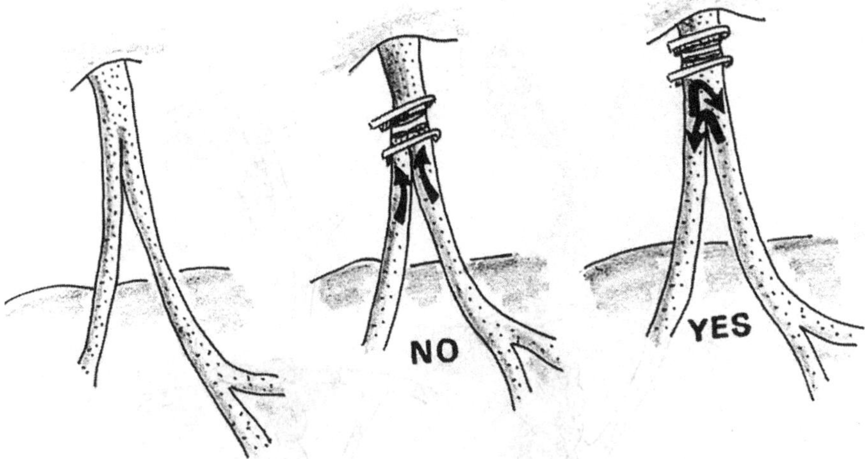

Fig. 5. The best way to *divide a bridging vein* (if necessary), according to the authors (Source: Sindou M and Auque J (2000) The intracranial venous system as a neurosurgeon's perspective. Adv Techn Stand Neurosurg 26, p 170, Fig. 23)

During closure, some surgeons wash the operative catheter with 10% papaverine in saline combined with Jugular compression to check that complete haemostasis has been secured.

Inadvertent tear of a dural sinus is best controlled by a skilled assistant gently applying a flat retractor whilst the surgeon stitches in a flap of dura or peracranium.

Where a meningioma involves the wall of a sinus, a similar technique may be used depending on the degree of invasion (see chapter by Sindou):

Type I: Excision of the outer layer, leaving a clean and glistening dural surface and coagulation of the dural attachment;

Type II: Removal of the intraluminal fragment through the recess and repair of the dural defect by re-suturing the recess or by closing it with a patch or sealing up the opening with aneurysm clips provided this does not cause stenosis;

Type III: Resection of the sinus wall and repair with a patch;

Type IV: Resection of both invaded walls and reconstruction of the two resected walls by patches;

Type V: This type can be distinguished from type VI only by direct surgical exploration of the sinus lumen. Where the opposite wall to the tumor side is free of tumor, Sindou prefers to reconstruct the invaded wall with a patch after resection rather than perform a bypass;

Type VI: Removal of the involved part of the sinus and restoration by venous bypass.

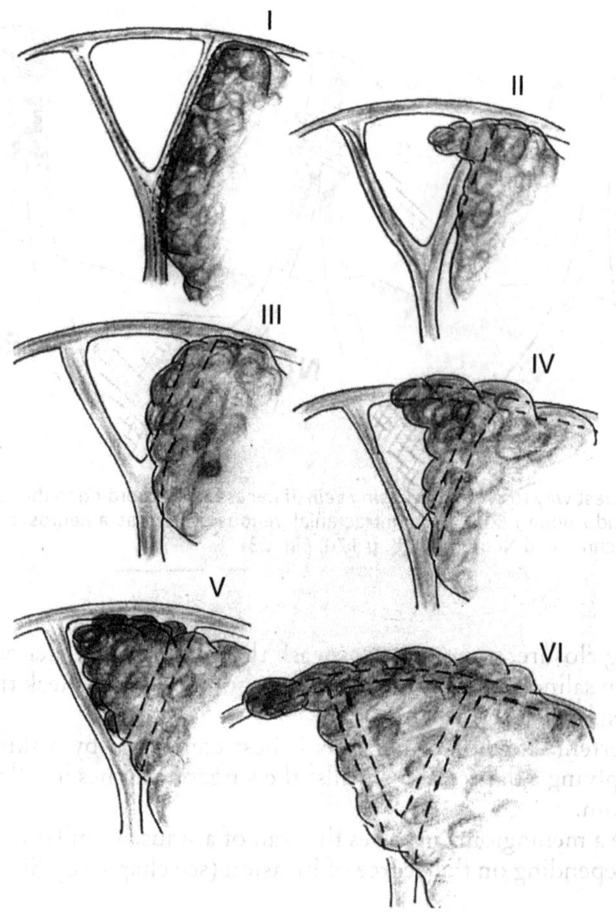

Fig. 6. Classification of meningiomas according to the degree of dural venous sinus involvement. *Type I*: meningioma attached to outer surface of the sinus wall; *Type II:* lateral recess invaded; *Type III*: lateral wall invaded; *Type IV*: entire lateral wall and roof of the sinus both invaded; *Types V and VI*: sinus totally occluded, one wall being free of tumor in type V. This classification is a simplified one from Krause F (1926) Operative Freilegung der Vierhuegel, nebst Beobachtungen über Hirndruck and Dekompression. Zentralbl Chir 53: 2812-2819; Merrem G (1970) Die parasagittalen meningeome. Fedor Krause-Gedächtnivorlesung. Acta Neurochir (Wien) 23: 203-216 and Bonnal J, Brotchi J, Stevenaert A, Petrov VT, Mouchette R (1971) Excision of the intrasinusal portion of rolandic parasagittal meningiomas, followed by plastic surgery of the superior longitudinal sinus. Neurochirurgie 17: 341-354 (Source: Sindou M and Auque J (2000) The intracranial venous system as a neurosurgeon's perspective. Adv Techn Stand Neurosurg 26, p 186, Fig. 29)

1.2 Venous bypass grafts

Sindou has pioneered the use of venous bypass autologous vein grafts for cases completely occluded by a tumor, venous thrombosis and jugular steno-

Table 1. Current published experience of stenting for PTCS ('IIH')

Higgins JN, Owler BK, Cousins C, Pickard JD (Cambridge; Lancet. 2002;359:228-230)	First case-report
Higgins JN, et al. (Cambridge; J Neurol Neurosurg Psychiatry 2003;74:1662-1666)	12 patients: 5 asymptomatic 2 improved 5 unchanged
Owler BK, et al. (Sydney; J Neurosurg 2003;98:1045-1055)	4 patients: headaches improved in all vision improved CSF leak resolved in one case
Ogunbo B, et al. (Newcastle; Br J Neurosurg 2003;17:565-568)	1 patient became asymptomatic
Rajpal S, et al. (Wisconsin, USA; J Neurosurg 2005; 102(3 Suppl): 342-346)	15 yr old boy; headache and papilloedema resolved
Donnet A, et al. (2008) (Marseille; Neurology 2008;70:641-647)	10 patients: papilloedema resolved in all; headache: 6 asymptomatic; 2 less; 2 no change
Thurtell M, et al. (2008)	27 patients – presented at INOS 2008

sis and bony obstruction of the venous system (Achondroplasia, complex craniostenoses). Long term patency is difficult to achieve but Sindou argues that even short term patency allows venous collaterals to develop. In contrast, some neurosurgeons prefer subtotal section of a sinus meningioma followed by radiotherapy or a staged approach. Intra-operative sinus pressure monitoring has been used to select those patients who really need sinus reconstruction with a bypass.

1.3 Venous stenting

A new approach to such a conundrum may be venous stenting. Venous stenting was introduced recently for venous thrombosis (2001) and by Higgins and colleagues for sinus stenosis causing or exacerbating PTCS (2002). The technique has now been extended by Higgins and colleagues for patients where raised intracranial pressure has been caused by sinus meningiomas (Fig. 7).

Raised intracranial pressure and vasogenic oedema have been successfully managed by stenting followed as appropriate by radiotherapy and/or surgery.

Venous sinus stenting is performed under general anaesthesia. The guide catheter is directed into the lateral sinus, usually from a percutaneous jugular puncture, and the stent deployed across the stenosis supported by a guidewire. In some patients overlapping stents have been deployed because of the length

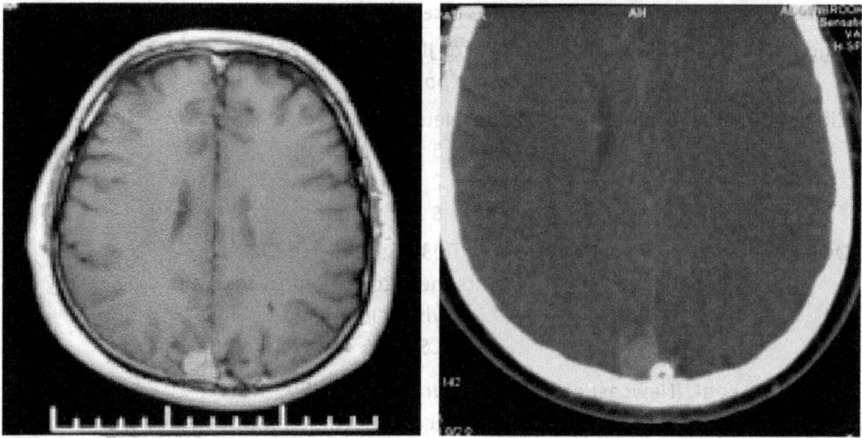

Fig. 7. Tumor in sagittal sinus on axial T1 weighted MR after Gadolinium and the stent in the right side image

of the stenosis and development of "floppiness" either side of the initial stent. In the minority of patients, bilateral stents have been used for PTCS. Patients are heparinized during the procedure, subsequently converted to warfarin and then to low dose aspirin or clopidogrel after eight weeks. Follow upon venography and manometry is usually undertaken once anticoagulation has been discontinued.

RESULTS

1. COMPLICATIONS OF VENOUS STENTING FOR PTCS

Probable intra-luminal thrombosis was observed in two patients which was successfully treated with thrombolytic therapy with resolution of symptoms. Ipsilateral headache over the side of the stent occurs in the minority of patients and resolves with time. Transient hearing loss ipsilateral to the side of stenting occurs in the minority but resolves within a few days as did unsteadiness in one patient. Anecdotally, acute subdural haematomas have been seen but not in the Cambridge series of over 50 cases.

CONCLUSIONS

The rules for preserving the integrity of the venous circulation during surgical approaches to the brain skull base are well described. Considerable surgical ingenuity has been displayed in developing techniques to preserve bridging veins and for reconstructing sinus obstruction caused by tumor, bony narrowing and thrombosis. Venous stenting has recently been introduced and has considerable potential as a way of re-establishing venous outflow in the face of thrombosis and intrasinus obstructing lesions.

References

[1] Auer LM, Loew F (eds) (1984) The cerebral veins. Springer, Wien New York

[2] Ganesan D, Higgins JN, Harrower T, Burnet NG, Sarkies NJC, Manford M, Pickard JD (2008) Stent placement for management of a small parasagittal meningioma. J Neurosurg 108: 377-381

[3] Higgins JN, Owler BK, Cousins C, Pickard JD (2002) Venous sinus stenting for refractory benign intracranial hypertension. Lancet 359: 228-230

[4] Higgins JN, Burnet NG, Schwindack CF, Waters A (2008) Severe brain edema caused by a meningioma obstructing cerebral venous outflow and treated with venous sinus stenting. Case report. J Neurosurg 108: 372-376

[5] Johnston I, Owler B, Pickard J (2007) The pseudotumor cerebri syndrome. Cambridge University Press, Cambridge

[6] Kapp JP, Schmiedek HH (eds) (1984) The cerebral venous system and its disorders. Grune and Stratton, New York

[7] Owler BK, Parker G, Halmagyi GM, Johnston I, Besser M, Pickard JD, Higgins JN (2005) Cranial venous outflow obstruction and pseudotumor cerebri syndrome. Adv Tech Stand Neurosurg 30: 107-174

[8] Sindou M, Auque J (2000) The intracranial venous system as a neurosurgeon's perspective. Adv Tech Stand Neurosurg 26: 131-216

[9] Sugita K, Kobayashi S, Yokoh A (1982) Preservation of large bridging veins during brain retraction. Technical note. J Neurosurg 57: 856-858

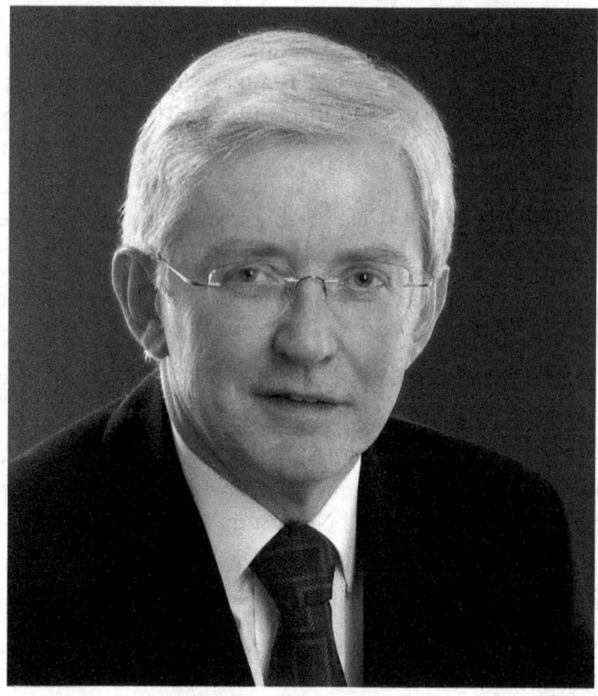

John D. Pickard

John D. Pickard is Professor of Neurosurgery in the University of Cambridge at Addenbrookes Hospital and Chairman of the Wolfson Brain Imaging Centre. He trained in Cambridge, London, Glasgow and Philadelphia and was Consultant Neurosurgeon (from 1979) and latterly Professor of Clinical Neurological Sciences in Southampton before moving in 1991 to the newly established Chair of Neurosurgery in Cambridge. His research interests include the pathophysiology and management of brain injury and disorders of the CSF circulation and impaired consciousness. He is the Immediate Past-President of the Society of British Neurological Surgeons.

Contact: John D. Pickard, Academic Neurosurgery Division, Box 167, Level A4, Addenbrooke's Hospital, Cambridge CB2 0QQ, UK
E-mail: prof.jdp@medschl.cam.ac.uk

TRAUMAS, CEREBROSPINAL FLUID, INFECTIONS

THE GLASGOW COMA AND OUTCOME SCALES: PRACTICAL QUESTIONS AND ANSWERS

G. M. TEASDALE

INTRODUCTION

Since they were described, the Glasgow Coma Scale [6] and Outcome Scale [1] have gained wide acceptance and are now in use throughout the world. Nevertheless, such commonplace use can engender a feeling of familiarity that can lead to them being used less effectively than ideal. Usually this is the result of some of the factors that were crucial in their development, and remain important in their day to day application, being overlooked. It is therefore appropriate to re-visit some of the features that are the basis of reliable, robust use of the scales and in the interpretation of their findings.

The reader of this handbook will already have, at the very least, an elementary knowledge of the make up and application of the scales. The approach adopted in this review is based around a series of questions that are often posed to the author by colleagues seeking guidance about aspects of practical use. An awareness of the answers to these queries ensures that the scales will continue to play their maximum part in benefiting the treatment of patients with acute brain damage.

Why were the scales developed? Assessment of the initial severity and late outcome play a key role in the management and understanding of a wide range of acute injuries and insults to the brain. Although their consequences can include focal neurological impairments, relating to the particular location of damage, the severity of the more generalised effects on the brain are usually much more important in acute management and ultimate outcome. Such effects are expressed in the acute stage as the depth and duration of impaired consciousness and at a later stage in impairments of lifestyle.

Since the scales were developed, the methodology of development of clinical assessments has advanced considerably and expanded into the science of 'clinimetrics'.

THE GLASGOW COMA SCALE

What were the main factors in the design of the scale? We considered it to be important that the approach should be simple and practicable, useable

Keywords: comatous states, consciousness disorders, Glasgow Coma Scale

in a wide range of hospitals by staff without special training, reflecting the ubiquitous dispersion of head injured victims.

It is fundamentally unsound to expect clear watersheds in the continuous spectrum of states within the range of impaired consciousness and coma. We, therefore, did not seek to establish an overall classification with a series of arbitrary levels or steps. It is also important not to depend on only one type of response because this may, for various reason, becomes untestable and because different aspects of 'consciousness' such as arousal and awareness have different clinical expressions.

Eye opening was considered useful as a reflection of the intensity of impairment of activating functions. Verbal responses offer an index of higher cortical function. Motor responses are a way of investigating the integrity of the nervous system in patients who are not speaking. Subdivisions within the components reflected increasing degrees of impairment (Table 1).

How are the responses assessed and interpreted? The assessment had to have a high degree of consistency and be widely acceptable. The findings at any one point are less important than changes in the pattern over time and consistent communication about a patient is essential as responsibility for care is passed on between the staff of a unit or between units.

1. EYE OPENING

• *Spontaneous eye opening*, with sleep wake rhythms is the highest level. Although it indicates arousal mechanisms brain stems are active it should not be

Table 1. The Glasgow Coma Scale and Scores

Eye opening			
Spontaneous	4		
To pain	3		
To sound	2		
Absent	1		
Verbal response			
Orientated	5		
Confused	4		
Inappropriate	3		
Incomprehensible	2		
Absent	1		
Best motor response			
Original scale		*Expanded scale*	
Obey commands	5	Obey commands	6
Localise pain	4	Localise pain	5
Flexion	3	Normal flexion	4
Extension	2	Abnormal flexion	3
None	1	Extension	2
		None	1
Total Coma Score	14	Total Coma Score	15

taken to imply awareness. Indeed in the persistent vegetative or minimally conscious state, eye opening is characteristically dissociated from evidence of intellectual function.

• *Eye opening in response to speech* is sought by speaking or shouting at the patient. Any sufficiently loud sound can be used, not necessarily a command to open the eyes. This should be assessed before the patient is physically stimulated.

• *Eye opening response to pain* is assessed if the person is not opening their eyes to sound. It is essential that assessment is carried out using a consistent approach to stimulation, which does not give rise to ambiguous responses nor causes unnecessary injury to the patient. After extensive testing of various approaches, we recommended that the stimulus should be pressure on the bed of a fingernail. This gives a reproducible stimulation and also avoids the difficulty in interpretation that can arise if the person grimaces in response to a stimulus on the face. Options such as rubbing the sternum or pinching the chest or arm do not offer advantages.

• *An absence of eye opening* implies substantial impairment of brain stem arousal mechanisms. Before assigning this level of response, substantial effort should be made to ensure that this is not due to an inadequate stimulation. The key is that the examiner should be sure that if the patient would be examined subsequently by someone else, a higher level of response will not be elicited. It is also important to identify if a lack of eye opening is a consequence of local injury, for example fronto-basal fractures, or sedative and paralysing medication.

2. VERBAL RESPONSE

• *Orientation* is the highest level of response and implies awareness of self and environment. The person should be able to provide answers to at least three questions, who they are, where they are and the date – at least in terms of the year the month and day of the week. A person who can answer some but not all these questions can be subcategorised as partially orientated, either specifying what information that they are able to give or how many out of the three components they can provide.

• *Confused conversation* is recorded if the patient engages in conversation but is unable to provide any of the foregoing three points of information. The key factor is that the person can produce appropriate phrases or sentences.

• *Inappropriate speech* is assigned if the person produces only one or two words, in an exclamatory way, often swearing. It is commonly produced by stimulation and does not result in sustained conversation exchange.

• *Incomprehensible sounds* consist of moaning and groaning but without any recognisable words.

The verbal responses may be affected as a result of focal brain damage rather than a general impairment of function. For example, an impaired verbal response in an otherwise apparently alert person should raise the suspicion of dysphasia. The use of endotrachial intubation clearly precludes a verbal response.

3. MOTOR RESPONSES

The assessment of motor responsiveness becomes important in a person not conversing to at least a confused level.

• *Obeying commands* is the best response possible. It is important to be aware that motor responses can occur as a primitive grasp reflex or a startle response or a even simple posture adjustment and these should not be interpreted as a high level response. If in doubt, confirmation of the specificity of the response should be sought, for example by squeezing and releasing the fingers or holding up the arms or other movement elicited by verbal command.

If someone is not obeying commands, the pattern of motor responses to physical stimulation provides a very valuable method of assessing dysfunction. Stimulation should be applied in a standardised way and maintained until maximum response is obtained.

• Although stimulation of the fingernail will usually already have been applied to assess the level of eye opening, assessment for *localisation* should start with the application of pressure to a point in the head and neck – the supraorbital notch or styloid process behind the mandible. In order to be sure that the response is a specific motor response to a specific site of stimulation, localising should be recorded only if the person's hand reaches above the clavicle in an attempt to remove the stimulus. Stimulus to the trunk may result in the arms moving across the chest in a way that does not represent a specific localised response. If in doubt, stimulation can be applied to more than one site to ensure that the hand attempts to remove it.

• *A flexion response* is recorded if the elbow bends but the movement is not sufficient to achieve localisation whereas in *extension* the elbow only straightens. Before recording that someone has no motor response, vigorous and varied efforts should be made.

What kind of flexion movements can be recognised? A range of movements may be seen in patients with marked impairment of consciousness who do not localise painful stimulation. At one end it is often possible to recognise a relatively *normal flexion* movement characterised by rapid withdrawal, abduction of the shoulder, and external rotation which varies from stimulation to stimulation. At the other end, *abnormal flexion* is clearly present when the response is slow, stereotyped – that is repeated time after time – and results in the arm moving to an adducted internally rotated position, characteristic of the hemiplegic or so called decorticate posture. Nevertheless, between these two clear patterns, varied patterns can be seen and some patients showing both types of movement at the same examination.

Experienced observers, particularly after careful training and discussion, can distinguish the two kinds of flexion response with an adequate degree of reliability. However, inexperienced staff, particularly working outside neurosurgical centres, find the distinction very difficult to make with consistency. For this reason, in the acute stage, it is sufficient in monitoring most patients to record simply that flexion is present.

The distinction is not crucial in the acute phase when deciding the need for action such as intubation to protect the airway or the performance of a CT scan – these will be indicated in any person not localising to a painful stimulus. Furthermore, transition between a normal and an abnormal flexion response is rarely sufficiently clear to signal deterioration or improvement in a way requiring alteration of management.

The distinction is useful prognostically and it is in this context that it is most relevant, for example when considering a likely outcome or in comparing series of patients.

Why is it the best motor response? The scale is based upon taking account of the best response of the better limb. Thus, during examination, a patient may show varying patterns with better responses occurring as the patient is more aroused. The highest level of response achieved provides the most consistent assessment of the patient's state and the best guide to the integrity of brain function remaining. A difference between the two sides may indicate focal brain damage. The worst or most abnormal response also should be noted in order to identify the site of focal damage, for the purpose of assessing the degree of impaired consciousness, it is the best response from the better limb that is relevant.

• *Absence of motor response.*

What needs to be checked if there is apparently no response? An absence of motor response clearly equates to a severe depression of function. Before ascribing this to structural damage it is important to exclude other causes – for example the effects of systemic insults such as hypoxia, hypotension or the use of drugs. Also, comparison should be made of the responses in the legs and arms with those in head and neck in order to alert the examiner to the possibility of spinal cord or brain stem injury. It is also important to ensure a stimulus of adequate intensity has been applied.

DISCUSSION

How consistent is the use of the scale? The initial development of the scale was strongly influenced by the findings of studies in the Glasgow unit in which several observers were asked to examine patients and compare their findings [8]. These guided the way that the scale could be used with equal consistency by nurses and non-specialist doctors, as well as by experienced neurosurgeons. Since these original studies, inter-observer consistency has been examined by many investigators and has been shown to be robust in a wide, relevant range of circumstances including emergency departments, intensive care units and in pre-hospital care. However, consistency cannot be assumed and should be confirmed and enhanced by training and communication between staff.

How soon and how often should a patient be assessed? Although these questions are frequent, common sense dictates that there are not simple single answers. The issue of when to commence observations reflects the need to distinguish between the use of the scale as a measure of early progress and as a predictor of ultimate outcome. Thus, when tracking the condition of a patient in the acute stage, the sooner an observation is made, the more useful it is as a guide to interpretation of later findings. Conversely, it is the very lability in the acute state that can make prognosis difficult so that most estimates of prognosis have been based upon an assessment after sufficient time has passed in order to ensure that the patient's state is not influenced by remedial disorders – for example hypoxia or hypotension or a developing intracranial haematoma. Later observations are often characterised as 'post resuscitation GCS' but it can sometimes be difficult to determine precisely when this is. Sometimes the 'time after injury' has been used, for example 6 hours, but this implies the time of injury is known, which is not always the case, and that emergency measures have been applied effectively.

Questions about the frequency of observations can likewise usually be resolved by common sense in relation to the likelihood that an influential change may take place. The shorter the time between an injury or other event and the assessment, the more the security about the stability of a patient's condition so that observations at frequent intervals are appropriate for example every few minutes and at least several times within an hour. As time passes the frequency can be reduced, and related to whether or not there are reasons for considering the patient needs continuing observation and care.

How much change matters? Questions are asked about the extent of change that should take place in order to trigger action. This may be simply to request assessment by another colleague or consultation with a more senior medical colleague. It may determine transfer to another unit e.g. from a general to a specialist neurosurgical department. Again, hard and fast rules are not appropriate.

The general guidance is that it depends upon where the patient is showing change from and the extent of the change. Thus, in a patient with no or mild impairment of responsiveness the certainty about a change may be less and the consequences of a small change also less so that a further period of observation and repeat assessments perhaps by a second colleague, can be appropriate. Conversely, the worse the patient's initial state, the more adverse the effect of a further deterioration and the greater the need for to avoid this. It is also the case that there is a greater degree of consistency in the assessment of the motor component of the scale than the verbal and eye features [8].

When in doubt, the safe thing is to consult and discuss, based upon a full description of all three aspects of the patient's condition and their changes over time and the time over which change has been taking place.

What is the relationship between the scale and the score? Our aim was for the approach to be useful both in practical day to day monitoring of patients with acute brain damage and in studies of prognosis, management and outcome. To enable the computerised analysis essential for such scientific studies, we assigned numbers to each response so that clinical recordings could be entered into a coding proforma [7].

For each of the three components of the scale, an absence of response was assigned the number 1 in order to make it clear that this was a positive identification of unresponsiveness. Increasingly high numbers were assigned to successively better responses and the three results entered separately. Inevitably, the temptation to sum together the three numbers into a total score became irresistible!

The total or sum score was initially used as a way of summarising information, in order to make it easier to present group data. However, the resulting score proved a useful and powerful summary of the extent of brain dysfunction and showed a strong relationship with prognosis [7]. The coma score has been the measure reported in most scientific papers and as a consequence as least as popular as the scale. It is, however, important to be aware of the pros and cons of the two approaches, how they are complementary and the circumstances in which one or other is more appropriate.

What are the roles of the scale and the score? When describing an individual patient, especially when communicating with colleagues, it is always preferable to refer to the responses observed and not to rely upon communication through the intermediary of numbers or a total score.

A major limitation of the total score is that it can be made up of a number of combinations of performance on the different components of the scale. This makes it difficult to translate the score into a clear picture of the patient's actual condition. This is particularly a risk in telephone exchanges.

Another problem with the total score is that if one component of the scale is untestable, this precludes allocation of a total score. Extrapolating and assigning an estimated score on the basis of the findings of only two components of the scale cannot be done reliably between the eye opening and the verbal responses nor between either the eye or verbal responses and the upper ranges of a motor response. Reporting what can be observed according to the framework of the subscales will convey whatever information can be reliably obtained.

Is the total score 14 or 15? Systems of numbering resulting in total scores of either 14 or 15 came about as a result of the differences in the approaches to assessment of flexion motor responses. In the simpler system, recommended for routine use in patient monitoring, no attempt is made to distinguish between normal and abnormal flexion. This results in a system summing to a total of 14. On the other hand, if the distinction between normal and abnormal flexion is considered to be reliable and to be useful, the total score possible becomes 15.

The approach giving a score of 15 has become most widely used, reflecting the way that the score was popularised through research papers. It is now not realistic to seek to establish one or other approach as the 'official' method. In order to avoid confusion if a patient is described by the total coma score, it should be made clear which system is being used by reporting the relevant total, i.e. a score out of 14 or 15.

Does an early assessment of Coma Scale and Score relate to later events and outcome? There are now many studies relating both the components of the scale [3] and the total score [7] to the occurrence of complications such as an intracranial haematoma in the acute stage and to late outcome after acute brain injuries. These provide a picture of a strong, close association. Moreover, where sufficient numbers have been studied, the relationship is both continuous (that is with each 'step' in the total score there is a change in outcome distribution) and almost quantitative (the extent of difference is similar across all steps). Although the way that the score came about was accidental, by good fortune it does provide a useful number!

THE GLASGOW OUTCOME SCALE

Why was an Outcome Scale needed? An understanding of how outcome can be described after acute brain insult is as important as early assessment. Anxiety about the ultimate outcome is often foremost in the minds of patients and their families from the very moments after an acute insult. They need to be given a realistic and understandable account of the range of possibilities and kept informed as the prospects evolve as time passes and advised how to plan for the likely outcome.

Many decisions in the acute management of the patient depend crucially upon the outcome that it is expected will likely follow. Balancing the consequences of one option versus another, and how this is informed by the previous experience of the unit or in the literature, requires a succinct, relevant and readily comprehensible method of describing the different forms of outcome. There are, however, a number of challenges in assigning outcome to a brain damaged patient.

One challenge is that the consequences of brain injury can be expressed in such a wide variety of ways through disturbances in mental function, over and above any physical neurological defects or deficits. A thorough assess-

Table 2. Original and extended Glasgow Outcome Scale

Original	Symbol	Extended
Good recovery	GR	Upper good recovery Lower good recovery
Moderate disability	MD	Upper moderate disability Lower moderate disability
Severe disability	SD	Upper severe disability Lower severe disability
Vegetative state	PVS	
Dead	D	

ment from a multitude of perspectives may be necessary to fully understand the detailed picture in an individual but this does not yield the overall summation that can be used to encapsulate the extent of the impact on a patient's lifestyle. Moreover, the impact upon a person's lifestyle is often more determined by changes in emotional, behaviour and personality than in more specific aspects of neurological and neuropsychological function.

Another challenge is that the approach must be capable of integrating the perspectives of patient and family as well as clinicians. Finally, in view of the large number of patients with acute brain damage that need follow up, the approach must be capable of application without the need to spend time and resources on extensive testing.

What factors influenced the design of the Glasgow Outcome Scale? Unlike the Coma Scale, the Outcome Scale [1] was based upon an approach in which a number of features were integrated into a hierarchy of states, ranging from death to good recovery (Table 2). Assignment depended upon comparison between information about a patient and a description of the characteristics of each of the four categories of survival.

How are the outcomes defined and assigned?

1) Good recovery is assigned if the patient is able to return to their previous level of lifestyle, including social and family activity as well as return to work – indeed it is the capacity to return to work rather than actually having done so that is relevant. Many people who otherwise clearly have made a good recovery do not return to work for a variety of reasons. Conversely, neurological, mild neuropsychological limitations or other deficits may be present without impairing the person's lifestyle.

2) Mild disability (also referred to as independent but disabled), refers to a patient who is able to look after themselves but has not regained their previous lifestyle in some significant way. If working, as some do, they have not attained their previous level, and there is substantial limitation of lifestyle and other social functions. Personality changes and memory and other cognitive problems are common but in some the restriction appears to reflect a failure to cope with residual deficits. The crucial factor is the person is able to care for themselves for at least 24-hours in society, including an ability to shop and, if applicable, travel reliably by public transport.

3) In *severe disability* (also referred to as conscious but dependent) the person requires the support of some other person for some activities at least within every 24-hours. The worst affected have a combination of severe mental and physical disability but some are so seriously affected only mentally that they require support and supervision on a daily basis either by family or in residential care. This categorisation of severe disability is much broader than used for example by geriatricians or physicians in regard to aspects of daily living. For the latter, independence may indicate someone having no more than the ability to attend to their basic personal needs at home but be unable to be mobile outside their home or organise their living without assistance. Failure on either of these criteria would result in assignment to severe disability on the Glasgow Scale.

4) The *vegetative state* was defined by Jennett and Plum in 1972 as being survival with no evidence of psychologically meaningful activity as judged behaviourally. Their criteria included cycles of spontaneous eye closure and opening but a strict absence of obeying simple commands, expression of any words or evidence of appropriate responsiveness to the environment.

How long the vegetative state should be present before being referred to as *persistent* has usually been taken as at least 3 months but improvement can occur after this. For many purposes at least a year should elapse before it is considered *permanent*. Definition of this state has become more difficult leading to the additional concept of the minimally responsive state.

Why is there an extended Glasgow Outcome Scale? The categories in the original scale were considered by some to be too broad to be able to affect important differences between patients or in the evolution of the same patient with recovery over time. In 1981, the scale was extended by sub-division of the categories of conscious survival (severe and moderate disability and good recovery) into upper and lower bands. This produced an eight-point version (Table 2). Although this allowed greater discrimination, this was off-set by a much lesser degree of consistency of allocation.

How was inconsistency dealt with? The problem of variable assessment led to the development of a structured approach to the assignment of outcome on both the original and extended scales [11]. The questions reflected an emphasis on social disability and the multiple aspects of outcome in the original approach. Areas covered include consciousness, independence in the home and outside, work status, social and leisure activities, relationships with family and friends and a return to the lifestyle normal for that individual, always considering potential rather than actual achievement. No weighting is put on the different aspects but the relevance of the components varies across the spectrum of outcome.

The questionnaire also includes specific guidance about the outcome to which the patient would be allocated, depending upon the response obtained. The structured approach also made it possible to take into account previous disabilities, which are found in a sizeable minority of patients with head injury and other intracranial insults.

The inter-observer reliability of the structured approach has been studied extensively. It shows a high degree of consistency when applied by the same observer on different occasions, by two observers on the same occasion, by comparison between face to face and telephone interview and also between assessments using self completed a postal questionnaire. Nevertheless, discrepancies are not entirely eliminated and can occur either in relation to the detailed information that is obtained or how this is translated into the overall score. Improvement can be obtained by training and by the use of a single central reviewer to allocate the scale on the basis of the detailed information.

What are the relationships between the Glasgow Outcome Scale and other indicators of outcome?

Jennett and Bond's work [1] preceded many of the other approaches to assessing aspects of outcome after brain injury have been made, these support its validity and utility [9].

1) The *World Health Organisation* described a classification of impairments, disabilities and handicaps some years after the Glasgow Outcome Scale. It is important to appreciate that the term disability is used very differently in the two approaches. In the WHO system it rates much more closely to a specific deficit in functional activity whereas in the Glasgow system disability refers to the net effects, and corresponds more to the concept of handicap in the WHO system. Direct comparison is therefore not possible.

2) The relationships between *neuropsychological measures* of intellectual impairment and the Glasgow Outcome Scale have been extensively studied. Highly significant associations exist between the categories of both the original five point scale and the extended 8 point scale and a wide range of assessments. Nevertheless, these associations in group findings go along with substantial variability of performance among patients in a particular outcome category. It is difficult to predict from any one specific assessment how a person will be in terms of overall lifestyle and social reintegration.

3) The *Disability Rating Scale* is widely used in rehabilitation after brain damage. Although there are overall correlations between the two scales there are important differences. The disability rating scale has an emphasis on neurological limitations and activities of daily living and systematically underreflects the disability or handicap shown in the Glasgow Outcome Scale. It was originally proposed as a method for tracking individuals through rehabilitation. In contrast, it is important to be aware that the degrees of disability on the Glasgow Outcome Scale cannot be assigned to a patient while they are still undergoing in patient care.

4) A number of *'quality of life'* assessments have been described, based upon summation of multi-item variables. One of the most widely advocated is the SF36. Comparison of assignments on the Glasgow Outcome Scale with

findings on each of the components of the SF36 showed a very significant relationship in each area with, reassuringly, with the greatest separation in the area of social handicap [9].

What are the roles of the original and extended scales? The two approaches to assignment of outcome have merits in different circumstances. In clinical care in the acute stage what is valuable is the predictability of outcome for an individual patient. Although there are clearly established correlations between initial clinical state as assessed by the coma scale and later outcome these correlations apply most clearly to the extremes of outcome, i.e. death or good recovery, and the extent of disability is very difficult to predict. For this reason, even the simpler original scale categories are often reduced to three: death or vegetative state versus severe disability, versus moderate disability or good recovery. There is little evidence of ability to discriminate between categories in the extended scale.

The value of the extended approach lies in the later stages after injury. It can be useful for tracking the progress of an individual patient and detect changes not evident in the original scale. It can also be useful in making more sensitive comparisons between groups of head injured patients. The distinction between upper and lower levels of severe disability is considered to have particular importance from an economic perspective – reflecting the much greater cost of care of the very severely disabled person. Conversely, the original scale performs well across the spectrum of head injuries and is sufficiently sensitive to detect the disability that commonly follows so-called mild injury [10].

What is the utility of "dichotomous" division of outcome and how should it be done? Division of outcome into only two options (dichotomisation) is common in research studies. The alternatives are referred to as favourable or unfavourable, worthwhile or not worthwhile, acceptable or unacceptable. Although these terms imply some value judgement, the approach initially was based more on the statistical merits in research of compressing even the five point scale into two different options. This maximises the numbers of people in the two categories rather than having them spread across five. This increases the statistical precision or confidence in the quoting of a percentage for either group and hence the greater reliability in comparing findings with another group. The division after a severe head injury is usually made between severe and moderate disability but other points can be appropriate, for example after less severe injury.

HOW SHOULD THE RESULTS OF THE GLASGOW COMA SCALE AND OUTCOME SCALE BE PRESENTED IN SCIENTIFIC REPORTS

The use of the Coma Score is firmly established as a valid measure in the description of early severity. The issue is how the distribution of severity in a group of patients should be summarised. It is essential not to treat the findings as if the score provided 'real' numbers – they are derived from rankings and the lowest score is not 0, nor even, 1 but 3! It is therefore completely invalid to summarise findings in a mean or average GCS – and even more to calculate this to a decimal point. Although quoting a median is more reasonable, the proper method is to present the distribution of the numbers of patients across the range of scores of interest. This may be by each step in the scale or in certain constellations, e.g. scores between 3 and 8 out of 15 are equated with a severe head injury, between 9 and 11 with a moderate injury and 12 to 15 as a mild injury. However, variations exist and the method used should always be specified.

In reporting outcome, there is no basis for referring to a Glasgow Outcome Score. It must be emphasised that the outcome assessment depends upon assignment to a scale. This simply presumes a hierarchy, with good recovery better than moderate disability, than severe disability, than vegetative state, than death. Numbers, or letters can be used only to indicate the rank order. What cannot be done is to assign a 'real' or cardinal value to any point. There is, therefore, no sensible way in which a numerical value can be assigned to any survival state as against another and even less sense in trying to decide how many times better than death is survival!

Recurring questions such as if death or good recovery should be given a score of one make no sense. It also is completely invalid to use summary statistics such as a mean or median to describe the findings of any numbers assigned to indicate order. Reports of outcome distribution should therefore provide the numbers of patients in each reported category, summarised if necessary in terms of proportion of the whole cohort studied.

CONCLUSIONS: DO THE GLASGOW SCALES REMAIN USEFUL TODAY

Although initially described three decades ago, the Glasgow approaches to assessment of initial severity and outcome of brain damage have weathered the test of time.

The *Coma Scale* is widely employed throughout the world in its own right and also through incorporation into recommendations for clinical care. These include the Advanced, Trauma and Life Support system and guidelines for head injury management from organisations such as the National Institute for Clinical Excellence in the UK, the Brain Trauma Foundation and the World Federation of Neurosurgical Societies. It remains the standard for acute assessment [5] .

The *Outcome Scale* is the most widely used approach in papers describing outcome after acute brain damage and its value is being enhanced by the increasing utilisation of the structured approach.

Alternatives to and adaptations of the Glasgow Scales have been described. Some of these have clear advantages, for example in relation to children.

Others find relevance to only very restricted groups of patients or in a particular clinical unit and have not been found to be useful replacements for the Glasgow Scales across the world.

It is, nevertheless, important to guard against this familiarity resulting in the scales being applied less rigorously and effectively than needed to ensure their value is used to the utmost. If issues arise about their application, relevance, reliability, interpretation or other aspects of their use and utility, these should be readily resolved by reference to the essential features of each of the two scales, to the factors underlying their application and the adoption of a common sense, flexible approach as set out in this account.

References

[1] Jennett B, Bond M (1975) Assessment of outcome after severe brain damage: a practical scale. Lancet 1: 480-484

[2] Jennett B, Plum F (1972) Persistent vegetative state after brain damage: a syndrome in search of a name. Lancet 1: 480-484

[3] Marmarou A, Lu J, Butcher I, Mc Hugh G, Murray GD, Steyerberg EW, Shkudiani NA, Choi S, Maas A (2007) Prognostic value of the Glasgow Coma Scale and pupil reactivity in traumatic brain injury assessed pre-hospital and on enrollment: an IMPACT analysis. J Neurotrauma 24: 270-280

[4] Reilly PL, Simpson DA, Sprod R, Thomas L (1988) Assessing the conscious level in infants and children: a paediatric version of the Glasgow Coma Scale. Child's Nerv Syst 4: 30-33

[5] Servadei F (2006) Coma Scales. Lancet 367: 548-549

[6] Teasdale G, Jennett B (1974) Assessment of coma and impaired consciousness: a practical scale. Lancet 2: 81-84

[7] Teasdale G, Jennett BJ (1976) Assessment and prognosis of coma after head injury. Acta Neurochir 34: 45-55

[8] Teasdale G, Knill-Jones R, Van der Sande J (1978) Observer variability in assessing impaired consciousness and coma. J Neurol Neurosurg Psychiatry 41: 603-610

[9] Teasdale GM, Pettigrew LEL, Wilson JTL, Murray G, Jennett B (1998) Analysing outcome of treatment of severe haed injury: a review and update on advancing the use of the Glasgow Outcome Scale. J Neurotrauma 15: 587-597

[10] Thornhill S, Teasdale G, Murray GM (2000) Disability in young people and adults one year after head injury. Br Med J 320: 1631-1635

[11] Wilson JTL, Pettigrew LEL, Teasdale G (1998) Structured interviews for the Glasgow Outcome Scale and Extended Outcome Scale: guidelines for their use. J Neurotrauma 15: 573-585

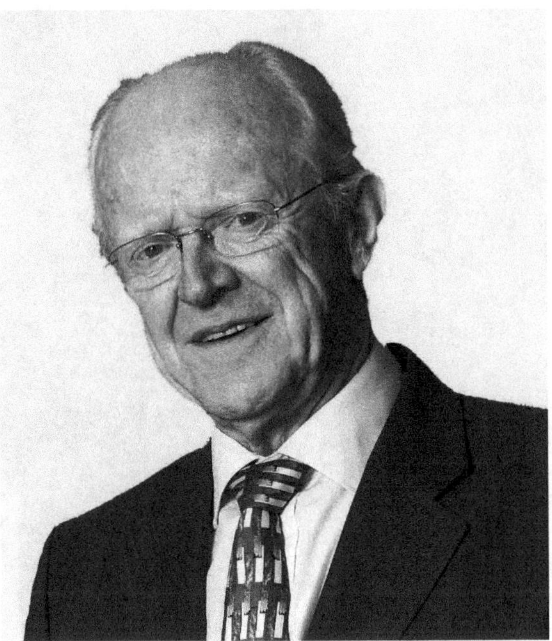

Graham M. Teasdale

Graham M. Teasdale was Professor and Head of the Department of Neurosurgery, University of Glasgow (1981 to 2003). He qualified in medicine at the University of Durham. His career has been dedicated to improving the assessment, management and outcome of people suffering from acute brain damage from head injury and other causes. He is the author of more than 300 publications on topics including the Glasgow Coma Scale and the management of head injury. He was President of the Royal College of Physicians and Surgeons of Glasgow, Chairman of the European Brain Injury Consortium and of the International Neurotrauma Society. He is currently Editor in Chief of Acta Neurochirurgica, the European Journal of Neurosurgery, and Chairman of NHS Quality Improvement Scotland. He has received many awards and distinctions including the Medal of Honour of the World Federation of Neurosurgical Societies in 2005 and was made a Knight Bachelor in the 2006 New Year Honours list for services to Neurosurgery and victims of head injuries. He is FRCS Edinburgh; FRCPS Glasgow; FRCP London; FRCP Edinburgh; Honorary FRCS England, Ireland; MD Hon Causae Athens; Honorary International Fellow, American College of Surgeons; Fellow of the Academy of Medical Sciences; Fellow of the Royal Society of Edinburgh.

Contact: Graham M. Teasdale, The Royal College of Physicians and Surgeons Glasgow, 232-242 St. Vincent Street, Glasgow G25RJ, UK
E-mail: graham.teasdale@hotmail.co.uk

CRANIAL TRAUMA IN ADULTS

P. J. A. HUTCHINSON

Dr. Mathew R. Guilfoyle, Academic Clinical Fellow, University of Cambridge, is co-author of this chapter.

INTRODUCTION

Cranial trauma and its sequelae present one of the most challenging areas of any healthcare system. Around 1% of all adult deaths annually result from head injury, with all age groups affected; in the young it accounts for up to a third of fatalities. Patients suffering trauma to multiple organ systems are up to ten times more likely to die if they have a concomitant brain injury. Moreover, those surviving severe brain injury have significant morbidity and disability with often devastating physical and psychological implications for the individual and, major economic burdens to society [4].

RATIONALE

1. SKULL FRACTURE

Direct blows to the head can result in a variety of fractures to the cranial vault and skull base. Linear fractures of the vault usually result from diffuse low-energy trauma and, other than serving as a pointer to mechanism and severity of injury, are not of clinical significance unless associated with suture diastasis or an underlying extradural haematoma. Depressed fractures are caused by focal high-energy impacts, typically over the fronto-parietal convexities and vertex, which result in comminuted fragments of bone being displaced inwardly. Fragments that are significantly displaced – defined by depression equal or greater than the thickness of the vault – are elevated to help minimise complications such as post-traumatic epilepsy, and restore the normal contour of the head. Patients with scalp lacerations and compound vault fractures are at risk of developing infection involving the soft tissues, bone, meninges, CSF, or cerebrum, particularly if heavily contaminated (e.g. farmyard injuries). Similarly to other open fractures, early (<6 hours) debridement reduces this likelihood.

Linear fractures of the skull base are associated with a number of complications including cerebrospinal fluid fistula, cranial nerve palsies, and vascular

Keywords: cranial traumas, adults brain injury, cerebral oedema, intracranial pressure

injury. Fractures through the anterior fossa floor involving the orbital plate of the frontal bone present with "raccoon eyes" and with extension into the ethmoid bones there is often a dural tear causing CSF rhinorrhoea together with shearing of the olfactory nerves as they pass through their foramina in the cribriform plate resulting in anosmia.

Temporal bone fractures are classified into three types: (I) longitudinal fractures directed along the axis parallel to the petrous ridge, (II) transverse fractures oriented between foramen magnum and middle fossa, and (III) a mixed or oblique fracture pattern. Fractures that run through the mastoid typically manifest with mastoid ecchymosis (Battle's sign) and CSF otorrhoea. The seventh nerve is vulnerable in its course through the temporal bone and is most often injured in transverse fractures. Complete facial palsy at presentation suggests nerve transection and has a poor prognosis whereas immediate but partial palsy may be recoverable with timely decompression of the nerve. Delayed facial palsy is caused by swelling around the fracture and in most cases resolves completely with conservative management. Hearing loss is a frequent complication of temporal bone fracture with a variable prognosis depending on whether there is a conductive deficit from disruption of the ossicular chain, which is potentially repairable with surgery, or a sensorineural deficit due to cochlear injury, which is less likely to recover. Fractures involving the foramen lacerum should raise the suspicion of carotid artery injury.

Linear fractures of the occipital bone can be associated with tears to the venous sinuses and posterior fossa extradural haematomas. Fractures running into the jugular foramen, hypoglossal canal, and occipital condyles can present with constellations of lower cranial nerve palsies. Three types of occipital condyle fractures are described: (I) impaction from axial loading, (II) extension of a linear fracture from the occipital bone, and (III) avulsion as a consequence of high velocity rotation. Only type III fractures result in potential instability of the cranio-cervical junction.

2. TRAUMATIC BRAIN INJURY

The primary brain injury sustained at the time of trauma remains the principal determinant of neurological outcome [7]. Severity is classified clinically on the basis of a patient's initial (post-resuscitation) neurological status defined by the Glasgow Coma Scale (GCS; Table 1) and further by the appearance of computed-tomography imaging [3] (Table 2).

Table 1. Severity of traumatic brain injury

Minimal	GCS 15, no LOC or PTA
Mild	GCS 14–15 with brief LOC and PTA
Moderate	GCS 9–13 or LOC > 5 min or focal deficit
Severe	GCS 3–8
Critical	GCS 3–4

Table 2. CT classification

Diffuse I	No visible pathology on CT
Diffuse II	Basal cisterns present with MLS 0–5 mm and/or high or mixed density lesion density present <25 ml
Diffuse III	Basal cisterns compressed or absent with MLS 0–5 mm with no high or mixed density lesion density present>25 m l
Diffuse IV	MLS >5 mm high or mixed density lesion density present>25 m l
Evacuated mass lesion	Any lesions evacuated
Non-evacuated mass lesion	Any lesions of high or mixed density lesion density present >25 ml not evacuated

Epidural haematomas are caused by tearing of dural vessels, typically branches of the middle meningeal artery, and are associated with skull fracture in most cases. Subdural haematomas usually arise from disruption of bridging veins between cortex and the venous sinuses but can occasionally be due to arterial bleeding.

Injury to the brain parenchyma is classified as focal or diffuse. Cerebral contusions and haematomas characteristically occur in the frontal and temporal lobes as these are susceptible to impacting the skull following trauma. Diffuse axonal injury results from shearing of neurons at the neocortical-white matter junction during rapid deceleration. In high-energy trauma there is typically a combination of focal and diffuse parenchymal injury and, importantly, both are associated with delayed cerebral oedema and intracranial hypertension. Traumatic subarachnoid and intraventricular haemorrhage are both indicators of severe injury and poor prognosis.

Approximately 5% of traumatic intracranial haematomas occur in the posterior fossa with similar aetiologies as in the supratentorial compartment. Neurological impairment associated with posterior fossa lesions is due to a combination of direct pressure on the brainstem and obstructive hydrocephalus.

The degree of primary brain injury cannot be improved by current treatment modalities. Instead, the focus of management is averting secondary insults in the minutes, hours, and days following trauma that promote further derangement of glioneuronal metabolism and, ultimately, cell death. Fundamentally the aim is to prevent and aggressively treat cerebral ischaemia. Autoregulation of cerebral blood flow (CBF) is complex, but the principal modifiable factors are intracranial pressure (ICP), mean arterial pressure (MAP), arterial carbon dioxide tension, temperature, and serum osmolality. CBF is critically dependent on cerebral perfusion pressure CPP = MAP – ICP) and is therefore reciprocally related to ICP. In addition, raised ICP causes secondary brain displacement and herniation through the fixed openings in the dura and skull resulting in brainstem ischaemia.

In the context of trauma, a rise in ICP is most often due to evolution of intra- or extra-axial haematomas, hydrocephalus, or cytotoxic/vasogenic oedema. Left untreated, as ICP escalates and cerebral ischaemia ensues, energy failure results in cell breakdown and loss of blood–brain-barrier integrity with consequent increase in cytotoxic oedema. Compensatory mechanisms including cerebral vasodilatation further compound the cycle of worsening intracranial hypertension.

Medical control of ICP aims to lower cerebral metabolic demand with anaesthesia and hypothermia, counter oedema with administration of hypertonic solutions, and reduces cerebral blood volume by cautious application of moderate hyperventilation to induce controlled cerebral vasoconstriction whilst avoiding ischaemia. Ventriculostomy for external drainage of CSF can further significantly improve compliance. If ICP remains intractable despite these interventions then the only remaining option is to effectively increase the size of the cranial vault by decompressive craniectomy.

DECISION-MAKING

1. DIAGNOSIS AND IMMEDIATE MANAGEMENT

Improving neurological outcomes from TBI is critically dependent on instituting secondary prevention as early as possible. Detailed protocols exist for the prehospital and emergency department management of patients with (suspected) head injury with which all neurosurgeons should be familiar, particularly when advising referring physicians and transfer teams [1]. In short, patients should be managed in accordance with general advanced trauma and life support principles, and in particular resuscitated to a MAP of >90 mmHg, normoxia, normoglycaemia, and if signs of neurological deterioration (>2 GCS points) or herniation develop (uni- or bilateral pupillary dilatation) then hyperosmolar therapy with mannitol or hypertonic saline should be considered. A clear record of GCS at scene and initial hospital is invaluable in assessing severity of injury, prognosis, and making management decisions once the patient has been transferred to the neurosurgical centre.

Computed tomography (CT) is the investigation of choice to assess cranial trauma. Opinions on which patients should undergo CT vary widely; recent guidelines from the UK National Institute of Clinical Excellence are very helpful in this respect. In most circumstances a standard non-contrast scan with brain and bone windows is sufficient. Consideration should be given to performing any necessary spinal CT at the same time and if there is suspicion of vascular injury then a CT angiogram or venogram may be useful.

On the basis of the patient's neurological condition and CT findings a decision is made whether immediate surgery is necessary, guided by evidence-based criteria set out by the Brain Trauma Foundation [2] (Table 3). If a mass lesion requires evacuation this should be performed promptly – delays in surgery are well proven to have a major negative impact on outcome [11].

Table 3. Criteria for emergency surgery

Extradural haematoma				
Volume ≥ 30 cm³	or	Volume ≤ 30 cm³	and	• Thickness ≥ 15 m • MLS ≥ 5 mm • GCS ≤ 8 • Focal deficit
Subdural haematoma				
Thickness ≥ 10 mm MLS ≥ 5 mm	or	Thickness ≤ 10 mm MLS ≤ 5 mm	and	• Deterioration to G CS ≤ 8 since time of injury • Unequal pupils • Fixed and dilated pupil(s)
Parenchymal contusion/haematoma				
Volume ≥ 50 cm³	or	Volume ≥ 20 cm³	and	• GCS ≤ 8 • MLS ≥ 5 mm • Cisternal effacement
Posterior fossa				
Any lesion causing mass effect (distortion or obliteration of fourth ventricle, effacement of basal cisterns, or obstructive hydrocephalus) or neurological impairment/deterioration				

If operation is not initially indicated the surgeon needs then to judge whether invasive ICP monitoring is required. Patients with post-resuscitation GCS of < 9 without mass lesion needing evacuation should have an ICP monitor. Patients with a GCS of 8–14 present a difficult decision as often they are agitated and combative necessitating sedation, or require intubation for management of concomitant systemic injuries. Some have suggested that serial CT and assessment of basal cistern effacement is sufficient to monitoring in patients under 40 years, however given the low risk associated with modern ICP monitoring and the potentially devastating and irretrievable effect on outcome of undiagnosed intracranial hypertension we recommend that any patient with TBI who cannot be assessed neurologically at regular intervals with sedation breaks should have ICP monitoring. Adjunct multimodality monitoring varies between centres and includes microdialysis, brain tissue oxygen sensor, and thermodilution blood flow probes.

2. ICP CONTROL

Once invasive monitoring is instituted ICP should be managed aggressively with a standardised escalating protocol aimed at maintaining a target ICP of less than 25 mmHg and CPP of 60–70 mmHg [3]. An example from our Neurosciences Critical Care Unit is set out in Fig. 1. If medical therapy (including

Addenbrooke's NCCU: ICP/CPP management algorithm

All patients with or at risk of intracranial hypertension *must* have invasive arterial monitoring, CVP line, ICP monitor and Rt $SjvO_2$ catheter at admission to NCCU.

- This algorithm should be used in conjunction with the full protocols for patient management.
- Aim to establish multimodality monitoring within the first six hours of NCCU stay.
- Interventions in stage III to be targeted to clinical picture and multimodality monitoring.
- CPP 70 mmHg set as initial target, but CPP>> 60 mmHg is acceptable in most patients.
- If brain chemistry monitored, PtO_2 >1 kPa & LPR < 25 are 2° targets (see full protocol)

Evacuate significant SOLs & drain CSF before escalating medical Rx.
Rx in italics and Grades IV and V only after approval by NCCU Consultant.

I

- **10-15° head up, no venous obstruction**
- **CPP ≥ 70 (CVP 6-10; ± PAC); *2° targets: PtO2 >1 kPa; LPR < 25***
- **SpO_2 ≥ 97%; PaO_2 ≥ 11 kPa, $PaCO_2$ 4.5-5.0 kPa**
- **Temp ≤ 37°C; SjO_2 > 55%; blood sugar 4-7 mmol/l**
- **Propofol 2-5 mg/kg/h; Fentanyl 1-2 μg/kg/h; atracurium 0.5 mg/kg/h (consider indications for midazolam, remifentanil)**
- **Ranitidine 50mg 8° iv (or sucralfate 1g 6° NG if enteral access)**
- **Phenytoin 15 mg/kg if indicated (fits, depressed # etc)**

ICP < 20 CPP >> 60 → **yes** (return to I) / **no** (to II)

II **Drain CSF via EVD if possible and evacuate significant SOLs**

-Recent CT? -Low risk of new SOL? → **yes** (to III) / **no** → **CT** → **SOL?** → **No** (to III) / **Yes - Evacuate**

III

- **5% NaCl 2ml/kg (repeat if Na < 155 mmol/l, Posm < 320)**
- **20% mannitol 2ml/kg X 3 or till plasma 320 mosm/l**
- **PAC, volume ,vasoactives: trial of ↑↑CPP (>>70 mmHg)**
- **Temp ~ 35°C, Daily lipid screen if still on propofol**
- **EEG: ? fits -> Institute or escalate antiepileptic therapy**
- ***Reduce $PaCO_2$ to ~ 4.0 kPa providing SjO_2 stays >> 55%***
- ***Consider 0.3M THAM 1-2 ml/kg if chronically ↓ $PaCO_2$***

CPP < 60; ICP > 25 (Check probe, ? re-CT)

IV

Temp 33°C (discontinue propofol)

CPP < 60; ICP > 25 (Check probe, ? re-CT)

V

Try iv anaesthetic (e.g.Propofol 1mg/kg), maintain CPP (fluids & vasoactives). If ICP and CPP improve start thio (250 mg boluses up to 3-5 g, then 3-8 mg/kg/hr to maintain burst suppression). Monitor EEG if available.

Consider decompressive craniectomy as an alternative to medical therapy for uncontrolled intracranial hypertension

Menon. Version 12. August 2004

Fig. 1. Intracranial pressure management protocol

ventriculostomy and drainage of CSF) has been exhausted and refractory intracranial hypertension persists then craniectomy should be considered. The role of decompressive surgery is currently being evaluated in the RESCUEicp randomised controlled trial (www.rescueicp.com).

3. DEPRESSED SKULL FRACTURES

For closed injuries elevation is indicated if the fracture is depressed by more than the width of the skull. The same rule is applied to compound fractures but debridement, washout and closure of wounds may be necessary even if the fracture itself does not require elevating.

4. BASILAR SKULL FRACTURES

Management is directed at preventing and treating complications. As a rule, traumatic CSF fistulae usually settle without intervention. Ongoing leak after seven days should prompt insertion of a lumbar drain to promote sealing off of the dural tear. Only a small minority of patients fail these measures and require operative repair either via sinus endoscopy or craniotomy. There is no evidence that antimicrobial prophylaxis reduces the risk of meningitis and such treatment should be reserved until there is indication of infection.

Temporal bone fractures with early facial palsy should be discussed with the ENT surgeons who may wish to undertake decompression of the nerve. Delayed palsy is managed expectantly. Steroid treatment remains controversial and of uncertain value in both settings. Hearing loss does not benefit from emergent investigation or intervention and should be assessed following the acute episode. If a fracture involves the carotid canal then angiography must be considered, particularly if there is atypical distribution of subarachnoid haemorrhage in the basal cisterns and sylvian fissue, or if there is otherwise unexplained poor GCS or lateralising neurological signs.

Potentially unstable occipital condyle fractures necessitate the hard cervical collar to be kept on and consideration of either internal fixation or conservative management with definitive immobilization in a halo vest.

5. SURGICAL APPROACH

For the majority of lateralised supratentorial injuries the standard frontotemporoparietal flap is the approach of choice. This craniotomy affords sufficient access to the structures most commonly injured in trauma – middle meningeal vessels, temporal and frontal poles, bridging veins to the sagittal sinus – and allows the surgeon to comfortably evacuate clot and obtain haemostasis. Furthermore, if at the end of surgery the brain is oedematous leaving the bone flap out provides a suitable decompressive craniectomy.

The craniectomy performed for decompression of predominantly diffuse injury is dictated by any signs suggesting more severe oedema in one hemisphere (e.g. midline shift, unilateral cisternal effacement) in which case a frontotemporoparietal flap is suitable. In generalised oedema a bifrontal craniectomy is the procedure of choice.

SURGERY

1. OPERATIVE TECHNIQUES

1.1 General considerations

Most procedures for trauma affecting the supratentorial compartment are performed with the patient supine and the head turned to the side contralateral to the lesion, with the exception of the bifrontal craniotomy which is performed with the head in a neutral position. A horseshoe headrest is sufficient for closing scalp lacerations and elevating uncomplicated depressed skull fractures, however procedures potentially involving craniotomy should be performed with the head secured in the three-pin Mayfield clamp. Jugular venous obstruction from excessive neck rotation is avoided by elevating the shoulder and hip ipsilateral to the operative side. If there is potential cervical spine instability instead of rotating the neck the patient is placed in the lateral position. If the thoracolumbar spine is not cleared then the procedure can still be carried out in the supine position but the whole spine should be maintained in neutral alignment by extensively padding the shoulders, back, hips, and knees.

For posterior fossa craniectomy the patient is turned prone with the head secured in the Mayfield clamp. Great care should be taken during positioning of a patient with cervical spine injury in a prone postion as the immobilizing collar will need to be removed to allow for the approach.

Trauma procedures are often performed in patients who have multiple injuries, physiological derangements (including coagulopathy), and potential haemodynamic instability. Precautions such as large-bore venous access and readily available blood cross-matched products are mandatory. Close communication with the anaesthetist and theatre staff is essential in maintaining optimal cerebral physiology during surgery and in making procedures as uncomplicated as possible.

1.2 Depressed skull fracture

In a compound injury it is usually possible to incorporate the laceration in a linear or lazy-S incision to provide adequate exposure of the fracture. A caveat to this is in a fracture involving the frontal air sinus where, rather than extend lacerations on the forehead it is preferable to perform a bicoronal incision.

The bone fragments are often impacted. Elevation can be performed either via a burrhole sited alongside the fracture or by using a high-speed burr on the fragments to free them. Each piece of bone is removed, avoiding downward pressure, to reveal the dura and, following thorough inspection, any tears are washed out and closed in a watertight fashion. If the bone fragments are large enough they should be reconstructed using bioplates and replaced to fill the defect. Otherwise, and only if there is no evidence of infection, a titanium mesh cranioplasty should be fashioned and the scalp closed in layers. If there is gross contamination of the wound the bone defect should be left and the scalp closed in a single layer with monofilament suture.

Fractures involving only the anterior wall of the frontal sinus may be fixed as described above or if the depression is not cosmetically significant then closure of any forehead lacerations is sufficient. When both the anterior and posterior walls are fractured the risk of infection and CSF leak is much higher and it is necessary to perform a bifrontal craniotomy (see below) to allow full inspection for dural tears and to repair the fracture. The pericranium is developed in a separate layer whilst reflecting the myocutaneous flap. Depressed fragments of the anterior wall are reconstructed and fragments of the posterior wall are removed – however, it is usually not necessary to formally remove the entire posterior wall ("cranialising" the sinus). The mucosa of the sinus is stripped and pushed down to occlude communication with the ethmoidal and nasal cavities and may be sealed with fibrin glue. Once any dural tears have been addressed the pericranial flap is laid over the frontal sinus. If there are associated fractures of the ethmoids or anterior cranial fossa floor these can be repaired with more fibrin glue or fascia lata graft if the pericranium is insufficient. A layered repair can be secured over the fracture with a small titanium mesh if necessary. The bone flap is replaced with four craniofix and the galea and skin are closed in the usual fashion over a suction drain. If the patient had a pre-operative CSF leak or is at high risk then a lumbar drain for 3–5 days post-operatively is prudent.

Elevation of fractures involving a venous sinus should be planned on the assumption of a bone fragment having perforated the sinus wall. Preparations for rapid haemorrhage should be in place and an assistant should be ready to manoeuvre the operating table at a moments notice. At surgery, decompression of the fragments may release any tamponade resulting in profuse bleeding and risk of air embolism. Continuous generous irrigation over the sinus during elevation reduces the chance of embolism and wet swabs should be at hand to immediately cover the sinus. Small holes or tears can be managed with surgicel or gelfoam and gentle pressure. Direct closure of tears can be performed if it does not result in sinus stenosis. For larger ruptures a patch repair using pericranium or fascia lata is required.

1.3 Frontotemporoparietal craniotomy

The "question-mark" incision begins 1cm anterior to the tragus and is first curved superioposteriorly over the ear, then superiomedially to reach within 1 cm of the midline and continued anteriorly ending just before the hairline, or, optionally, curved 2–3 cm across the midline. Below the superior temporal line (STL) the incision is to the galea, above the incision is made directly on to bone. At 10 cm intervals bleeding from larger scalp vessels is controlled with bipolar diathermy and Raney clips are applied to the skin edges, and then the incision is continued. Once the incision is complete, temporalis fascia and muscle is divided in line with its fibers down to bone with cutting monopolar diathermy, half a centimetre from the skin margin. The myocutaneous flap is then reflected inferiorly elevating the periosteum from the frontal and parietal bones and temporalis off the temporal bone with a combination of sharp dissection and diathermy until the keyhole is exposed and the orbital rim palpable. The flap is retained by placing three or four sutures as low as possible in the undersurface of temporalis and securing these under tension to the drapes with artery or towel clips. It is important to control any bleeding from branches of the superior temporal artery now to avoid problematic haemostasis later in the operation.

Burrholes are placed at the inferior point of the temporal bone, the most anteromedial point of the frontal bone, the most posteromedial point on the parietal bone, the keyhole, and midway between temporal and parietal burrholes along the wound margin (Fig. 2). A free bone flap is completed with the craniotome extending medially to within 1–2 cm from the sagittal sinus cutting the section parallel to the sinus last. In patients precipitously deteriorating prior to induction or with escalating ICP the temporal burrhole should be made first and quickly extended circumferentially with Kerrison's rongeurs, (and the dura incised in cruciate fashion in the case of SDH) and clot suctioned as a temporising measure whilst the remainder of the craniotomy is completed. The sphenoid wing should then be nibbled down, any bleeding bone edges controlled with wax, and the edge of the craniotomy lined with surgicel.

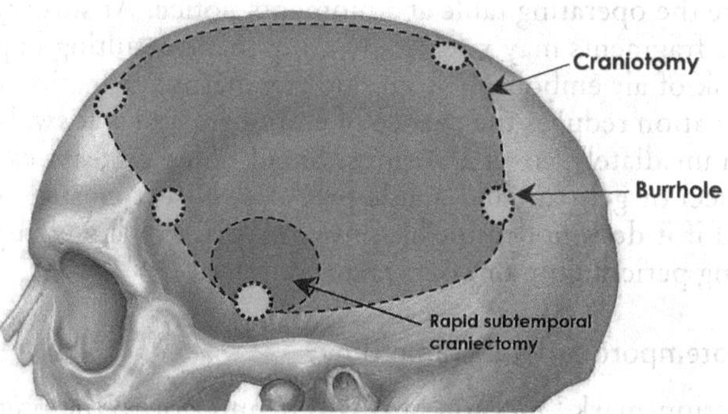

Fig. 2. Frontotemporoparietal craniotomy

1.4 Evacuation of extradural haematoma

Extradural haematoma is removed using suction and generous warm irrigation; clot can be gently stripped off the dura with forceps if necessary. As the evacuation proceeds bleeding points (usually from middle meningeal branches) should be controlled with bipolar diathermy. If bleeding continues despite cauterizing the visible branches of the middle meningeal then, with an assistant providing suction and irrigation, the temporal lobe is retracted to reveal the foramen spinosum and this is packed with a combination of bonewax and surgicel or gelfoam. Once any brisk haemorrhage has been stopped further haemostasis is best achieved by placing hitch stitches at 1–2 cm intervals along the dural margin to tamponade residual venous ooze and prevent recollection. These may be tethered to the periosteum and subgaleal tissue or oblique holes can be drilled in the bone edge. If there is suspicion of a concomitant subdural haematoma (either from preoperative imaging or at operation) a 5–10 mm incision can be made in the dura for inspection and closed if negative. To close, a sheet of surgical is laid on the dura and the bone flap is replaced with three craniofix. The central dura is hitched via two holes drilled in the centre of the bone flap. Galea and skin are closed over a suction drain.

1.5 Evacuation of subdural haematoma

A frontotemporoparietal craniotomy is performed as described above. To access the subdural space a wide dural incision is made based on the sagittal sinus or inferior extent of the craniectomy. Subdural haematoma is removed with suction and warm irrigation, with particular care taken to not to unduly disrupt the arachnoid and pia. Bleeding points on the cortical surface are controlled as the evacuation progresses toward the part of the haematoma nearest the sagittal sinus. Great care is taken not to tear bridging veins whilst suctioning the haematoma, however, if one of the veins is bleeding or avulsed then it should be controlled with bipolar diathermy. A very proximal tear to a bridging vein or one that involves the sinus wall is better controlled with surgicel applied with gentle pressure using a patty, which is then left to tamponade whilst evacuation and haemostasis in other areas is attended to. Using a broad spatula the frontal, temporal, and parietal lobes are gently retracted in turn and the subdural space inspected for residual haematoma. Hitch stitches place at 2–3 cm intervals are useful again as epidural oozing often begins following decompression of the SDH.

If the brain is slack following evacuation of the haematoma and the dura is easily approximated then it is closed in a watertight fashion with running 3-0 Vicryl. The bone flap is replaced with three craniofix and the frontal burrhole filled with bone dust.

If there is any concern regarding intracranial pressure from residual mass lesions such as parenchymal contusions (which may potentially evolve) or from brain oedema then further releasing incisions are made in the dural edges and the dural flap is laid on the brain surface but not closed. A large sheet of surgicel is laid over the brain and dura, the bone flap is not replaced and the galea and skin are closed meticulously to avoid CSF leak.

1.6 Evacuation of intracerebral haematoma and contusions

Following craniotomy, evacuation of an intracerebral haematoma proceeds as for spontaneous or aneurysmal haemorrhage. If the clot points to the cortical surface then it is entered through this point, otherwise a small corticotomy over the haematoma is made. The central bulk of the haematoma is removed with suction and irrigation and the cavity is then thoroughly inspected using the operating microscope. Once there has been satisfactory decompression haemostasis is achieved by lining the cavity with surgicel. As for SDH, a decision then has to be made whether to replace the bone flap.

Adequate surgical decompression in patients with diffuse injury and contusions depends on craniectomy. Contusions may be evacuated in the process of obtaining haemostasis and this is particularly true at the temporal tip where contusions frequently evolve and haemorrhage further. However, other than for these reasons, the additional benefits of debriding contusions is questionable as potentially eloquent or salvageable brain is removed together with haematoma and may negatively impact on outcome.

1.7 Bifrontal decompressive craniectomy

The patient is positioned as above with the head positioned neutrally and the neck slightly flexed. A bicoronal incision connecting the two points 1cm in front of the tragi is made behind the hairline. The scalp is reflected forward in the aponeurotic layer until the orbital rim is palpable. The temporalis muscle

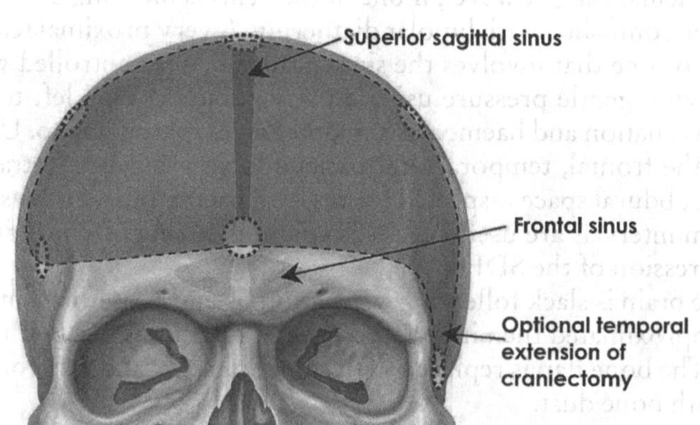

Fig. 3. Bifrontal decompressive craniectomy

is divided along its fibers half a centimetre in front of the incision and reflected anterioinferiorly. Depending on the degree of injury to the temporal lobes the craniotomy can be taken to just below the superior temporal line or more inferiorly. Burrholes are placed in the temporal area and keyhole point bilaterally (Fig. 3). Two further burrholes are placed on the midline over the sagittal sinus at the anterior and posterior extents of the intended craniotomy, with the option for intermediate burrholes to free the dura from the bone. Anteriorly it is preferable to avoid entering the frontal sinus and the distance above the orbital rim at which the sinus ends should be gauged from the CT scan. Lateral to the frontal sinus the craniectomy is taken as close to the orbital rim as possible. Posteriorly the burrhole should be placed 1cm in front of the skin incision to facilitate future cranioplasty. Particular attention should be paid to stripping the dura around the midline burrholes and it is helpful to begin a channel for the craniotome with Kerrison's rongeurs to minimise the chance of injury to the sagittal sinus. The craniectomy is then completed on both sides cutting away from the sinus. Raising the bone flap presents the greatest risk of tearing the sinus and should be performed with great care. If there is a sinus injury then prevention of air embolism and repair are performed as described above. If the frontal air sinus has inadvertently been entered then it should be occluded as detailed above. Strips of surgicel are placed along the sinus and around the margins of the craniotomy and bonewax applied liberally to the bone edges. Symmetrical U-shaped dural flaps are cut based on the sagittal sinus and further releasing cuts in the dural edges can be made if the brain is very tense. Lastly, the sagittal sinus is ligated no more than 1 cm from its most anterior point and then the frontal lobes are gently retracted to allow division of the insertion of the falx into the anterior fossa floor with scissors. The dural flaps are laid over the cortical surface and two large squares of surgicel are placed over each hemisphere. The galea and skin are closed in the normal fashion.

1.8 Posterior fossa craniectomy

Post-traumatic haematomas in the posterior fossa are evacuated via bilateral suboccipital craniectomy. A linear midline incision is made from 1 to 2 cm superior to the external occipital protruberance to the level of C2–3. The paraspinal muscles are dissected in the avascular median raphe which is continued superiorly in a Y-shape parallel to the superior nuchal line to leave a cuff of tissue for closure. The muscles are dissected from the skull base with monopolar diathermy. For rapid decompression multiple burrholes can be made and the craniectomy completed with Kerrison's rongeurs. Alternatively burrholes are placed laterally over the transverse sinus and a bone flap can be completed using the craniotome. As in the supratentorial compartment extradural haematomas are removed with irrigation and suction with meticulous control of bleeding points with bipolar diathermy. Bleeding from the transverse sinus or, less commonly, the sigmoid sinus should be stopped with surgicel applied with gentle pressure using a cottonoid patty. Larger tears should be managed similarly to the sagittal sinus (above). Hitch stitches should be placed circumferentially before closing.

The durotomy to evacuate subdural haematoma is performed in a Y-shaped fashion taking care to ligate the occipital sinus if patent. Clot is then gently suctioned and a thorough inspection is undertaken to identify any bleeding from bridging veins or the sinuses. The dura is not closed primarily and is either left open or an expanding duraplasty can be performed with a suitable synthetic dural graft. Hitch sutures should be placed around the dural edges.

Traumatic cerebellar haematomas are evacuated via a small corticotomy made with the bipolar diathermy and using the operating microscop0065. Once the bulk of haematoma is removed the cavity is lined with surgicel to obtain haemostasis. When substantial swelling is anticipated the posterior arch of the atlas can also be removed to make further room.

In all posterior fossa procedures meticulous closure of the fascia, subcutaneous layer and skin are paramount to prevent post-operative cerebrospinal fluid fistula.

2. PROGNOSIS AND OUTCOME

The standard assessment of outcome following TBI is the Glasgow Outcome Score at six months post-injury. In clinical trials, the GOS is often dichotomised into favourable (GOS 4–5) and poor (GOS 1–3) outcomes. Recent studies have shown that TBI management in neurosurgical centres significantly improves outcome compared with non-specialist centres [10]. Implementing standardised ICP protocols and surgical interventions has significantly improved outcome compared to historical controls with yearly reductions in mortality. Despite this progress, mortality at 6 months in severe TBI remains approximately 30% [8]. A further 20% of patients are in the vegetative state or severely disabled leaving 50% with favourable outcome. Several models have been developed to help predict outcome for individual patients and in general concur that the principal factors are age, motor component of the initial GCS, and pupil reaction [6, 7, 9].

Data on long-term outcomes are lacking, particularly with respect to patient reported measures of quality of life. Nevertheless, it is clear that many survivors of TBI have problems with cognition, emotional difficulties, dependence for activities of daily living, and few return to their previous level of employment [12].

HOW TO AVOID COMPLICATIONS

1. INEFFECTIVE OPERATION

Management of raised ICP is inherently time critical, and inadequate decompression, whether evacuation of haematoma or craniectomy may drastically change outcome for a patient. In contrast to current trends toward minimally invasive surgery, trauma procedures necessitate large craniotomies for evacuation of haematoma, thorough inspection, and haemostasis. Moreover when decompression is required if the craniectomy is too small the pressure against the brain at the bone edges may cause venous infarction and further oedema. Generally, in supratentorial compressive craniectomy a minimum bone flap size of 12 cm diameter is recommended.

2. RECOLLECTION OF HAEMATOMAS

Meticulous haemostasis is imperative intra-operatively and both anaesthetic and critical care teams should aggressively correct coagulopathy. Avoiding venous obstruction and dural hitch sutures are important in stopping ooze which develops when venous tamponade is released during haematoma evacuation and decompression. The operating microscope is invaluable to assist in obtaining haemostasis within haematoma cavities.

CONCLUSIONS

Operative intervention in cranial trauma has an ancient history but until relatively recently a pessimistic view prevailed on the supposition that the severity of injury was the only real determinant of outcome, and subsequent treatment beyond supportive care did not change prognosis. However, in the latter half of the 20th century parallel advances in neuroimaging, anaesthesia, intracranial monitoring, and our knowledge of the basic pathophysiology underlying brain injury prompted a reappraisal of TBI management. There is now ample evidence to demonstrate that significant improvements in outcome can be gained by prompt institution of standardised care. Perhaps more than in any other aspect of neurosurgery a good working understanding of both medical and surgical treatment modalities is necessary to manage the individual patient and optimise their recovery.

Acknowledgement

Original images were produced by Patrick J. Lynch.

References

[1] Badjatia N, Carney N, Crocco TJ, et al. (2008) Guidelines for prehospital management of traumatic brain injury, 2nd edn. Prehosp Emerg Care 12 Suppl 1: S1-S52

[2] Brain Trauma Foundation (2006) Guidelines for the surgical management of traumatic brain injury. Neurosurgery 58: S1-S62

[3] Brain Trauma Foundation (2007) Guidelines for the management of traumatic brain injury. J Neurotrauma 24: vii-viii

[4] Maas A, Stocchetti N, Bullock R (2008) Moderate and severe traumatic brain injury in adults. Lancet Neurol 7: 728-741

[5] Marshall L, Marshall S, Klauber M (1991) A new classification of head injury based on computerized tomography. J Neurosurg 75: S14-S20

[6] MRC CRASH Trial Collaborators (2008) Predicting outcome after traumatic brain injury: practical prognostic models based on large cohort of international patients. BMJ 336: 425-429

[7] Murray G, Butcher I, McHugh G, et al. (2007) Multivariable prognostic analysis in traumatic brain injury: results from the IMPACT study. J Neurotrauma 24: 329-337

[8] Murray G, Teasdale G, Braakman R, et al. (1999) The European brain injury consortium survey of head injuries. Acta Neurochir (Wien) 141: 223-236

[9] Mushkudiani N, Hukkelhoven C, Hernandez A, et al. (2008) A systematic review finds methodological improvements necessary for prognostic models in determining traumatic brain injury outcomes. J Clin Epidemiol 61: 331-343

[10] Patel H, Bouamra O, Woodford M, et al. (2005) Trends in head injury outcome from 1989 to 2003 and the effect of neurosurgical care: an observational study. Lancet 366: 1538-1544

[11] Seelig J, Becker D, Miller J, et al. (1981) Traumatic acute subdural hematoma: major mortality reduction in comatose patients treated within four hours. N Engl J Med 304: 1511-1518

[12] Willemse-van Son AHP, Ribbers GM, Verhagen AP, et al. (2007) Prognostic factors of long-term functioning and productivity after traumatic brain injury: a systematic review of prospective cohort studies. Clin Rehabil 21: 1024-1037

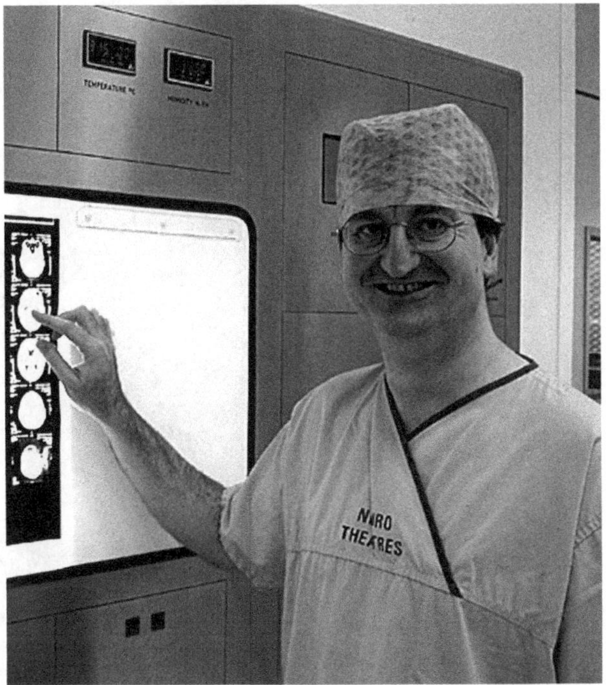

Peter J. A. Hutchinson

Peter Hutchinson holds an Academy of Medical Sciences/Health Foundation Senior Surgical Scientist Fellowship within the Department of Clinical Neurosciences, University of Cambridge and Honorary Consultant Neurosurgeon post at Addenbrooke's Hospital. He has a general neurosurgical practice with subspecialist interest in the management of neurotrauma. He has a research interest in traumatic brain injury, multimodality monitoring in neuro-critical care and functional imaging. He is running the MRC funded RESCUEicp decompressive craniectomy study, www.RESCUEicp.com, and is chairman of the EANS Research Committee.

Contact: Peter J. A. Hutchinson, Department of Clinical Neurosciences,
Neurosurgery Unit, University of Cambridge, Cambridge CB2 3EB, UK
E-mail: pjah2@cam.ac.uk

HYDROCEPHALUS IN ADULTS (INCLUDING NORMAL PRESSURE HYDROCEPHALUS SYNDROME)

T. TROJANOWSKI

INTRODUCTION

Hydrocephalus is defined as an increase of the amount of cerebrospinal fluid (CSF) within the cerebral ventricles and/or subarachnoid spaces of the brain which equals an enlargement of the intracranial spaces containing CSF.

It can result from loss of equilibrium between production (overproduction) and elimination (impaired absorption) of the CSF or an obstruction in its circulation.

Hydrocephalus was first described and named by Hippocrates (466-377 BC). Andreas Vesalius (1514–1564) presented the concept of hydrocephalus as accumulation of water inside the ventricles. In 1701 Pacchioni discovered arachnoid granulations but wrongly associated them with secretion of CSF. In the beginning of 20th century Walter Dandy and Kenneth Blackfan studied hydrocephalus in an animal model and showed that removal of the choroid plexus, before occlusion of aqueduct or of the foramina, prevented development of hydrocephalus. This showed that plexus is generating much of the CSF. It was only in the second half of the century when extensive research on hydrocephalus provided understanding of its pathophysiology and provided concepts for treatment. Removal of the choroid plexus proposed by Dandy was replaced by open third ventriculostomy performed in 1940 by White and Michelsen, Dandy and Stookey and an endoscopic method described by Mixter.

A major progress in the management of hydrocephalus came with introduction of a variety of shunting procedures, diverting excess of CSF into various body cavities or vessels.

In the recent years multiple studies searched for methods of selecting patients with NPH who would benefit from treatment by shunting. Progress in imaging and improvements in shunt technology, particularly introduction of an anti-siphon device, flow controlled valves and those with externally

Keywords: hydrocephalus, idiopathic normal pressure, shunt adjustable opening pressure enhanced understanding and management of the condition.

RATIONALE

Overproduction of CSF in excess of its absorption is rare and may occur in neoplasms of the choroid plexus: papillomas and choroid plexus carcinomas. Reduced absorption capacity of the CSF follows in some patients subarachnoid or ventricular haemorrhage, meningitis, or accompanies increased venous pressure in the superior saggital sinus occurring in superior vena cava syndrome and in sinus thrombosis. Disturbed CSF circulation results from obstruction of the CSF pathways. This may occur in the ventricles, but can also take place in the subarachnoid space at the base of the brain or over the convexity. Tumors, haemorrhages, congenital malformations and infections can cause obstruction at any point in the pathways [7].

The intracranial pressure may increase under the influence of the mechanisms leading to hydrocephalus but it may also remain at the normal level.

Different forms of hydrocephalus are given specific names indicating basic differences between them.

Communicating hydrocephalus occurs when a patent communication between the ventricles is maintained and the flow is disturbed after CSF exits the ventricles into the subarachnoid space.

Non-communicating or *obstructive*, *occlusive* hydrocephalus develops when CSF flow is obstructed within the ventricular system leading to enlargement of the isolated parts of the ventricular system. *Normal pressure hydrocephalus* is recognized when cerebral ventricles are enlarged without increase in intracranial pressure and a characteristic set of neurological symptoms is presented. *Hydrocephalus ex vacuo* is a form of cerebrospinal spaces enlargement resulting from reduction of the volume of the brain damaged by ischemia, injury or degeneration. Intracranial pressure in those cases is normal. Enlargement of the cerebral ventricles is merely a replacement of lost cerebral tissue with CSF and no imbalance in fluid production and absorption exists. Some authors hesitate to diagnose this condition a hydrocephalus. *Arrested hydrocephalus* is a stable enlargement of the ventricles in patients whose neurological status do not change. It represents a condition persisting after a temporary enlargement of the ventricles triggered by a transitory cause.

Development of a hydrocephalus may be rapid in *acute hydrocephalus* or may take weeks to years in *chronic hydrocephalus*.

Paediatric hydrocephalus has its specific causes, course, pathology and treatment and is presented in another chapter. *Adult hydrocephalus* is of an acquired type, communicating or non-communicating. The main form is normal pressure hydrocephalus (NPH) which needs to be differentiated from hydrocephalus ex-vacuo.

DECISION-MAKING

1. SYMPTOMS OF ADULT-ONSET HYDROCEPHALUS

Symptoms of adult-onset hydrocephalus vary depending on the ICP level associated with the condition.

In *occlusive hydrocephalus* with elevated ICP symptoms may include headache, nausea, vomiting and, sometimes, blurred vision. There may be problems with balance, walking and poor motor coordination. Irritability, fatigue, seizures, and personality changes, difficulties in concentration or memory deterioration may also develop. Drowsiness and double vision occur with higher ICP levels.

Normal pressure hydrocephalus (NPH) also called Hakim-Adams syndrome after the first authors who described it in 1965 presents in adults and is of a chronic, communicating type. A decrease in absorptive capacity of the arachnoid villi in the subachnoid space leads to increase of the CSF outflow pressure. This may result from a subarachnoid hemorrhage, head trauma, infection, neoplasm or complications of surgery. However, in many patients NPH occurs even when none of these conditions is present. It can occur at any age, but it is most common over the age of 50 with the mean age at onset close to 70. In cases with unknown aetiology it is called *idiopathic normal pressure hydrocephalus* (INPH). It has been shown, that in NPH and INPH there are periodical fluctuations of intracranial pressure with high level intervals, at least in the early stages of the disease. Therefore the name normal pressure may be misleading. Presence of intermittent elevation of ICP provides also a rationale for treatment by shunting, which cuts off the peaks of ICP waves, damaging the brain. NPH is caused by a blockage of the CSF draining pathways in the brain with increasing outflow or absorption pressure. Although the ventricles enlarge, the pressure of the CSF remains within normal range. The syndrome is important because it accounts for 5 to 6 percent of all cases of dementia, and occurs in 0.4% of the population [7].

NPH has a very distinct symptomatology. It is a triad of progressing symptoms consisting of gait disturbances, incontinence and cognitive decline eventually leading to dementia.

Walking disturbances are characterised by general slowing of movements. Gait is wide-based, steps are short, and shuffling. There are difficulties in going up and down stairs and over the curbs which may result in frequent falls. These disturbances range in severity from mild imbalance to the inability to stand or walk at all. Patients may have difficulty turning around. They turn very slowly with multiple steps. Gait disturbances are usually the first, most consistent and most pronounced symptom.

Impairment in bladder control in mild cases consists of urinary frequency and urgency whereas in more severe cases a urinary incontinence occurs.

Mental impairment and dementia presents as a loss of interest in daily activities, gradual loss of short-term memory, leading to difficulties in carrying routine tasks. In NPH those symptoms are often overlooked for years or accepted as an inevitable consequence of aging. The patients themselves may be less aware of their deficits because of the cognitive impairment. The symptoms get worse over time. Neuropsychological testing plays an important role in identifying intensity of mental impairment.

Because NPH symptoms may also be present in other disorders such as Alzheimer's disease, Parkinson's disease and Creutzfeldt-Jakob disease, correct diagnosis requires additional tests, including CT and MR brain scans, CSF dynamics, intracranial pressure monitoring and neuropsychological testing. Using MR it has been established that mean intracranial CSF volume in INPH is 280 ml compared to 195 ml in controls [9].

Differentiating NPH from ventricular enlargement in the course of brain atrophy and ageing is still difficult, despite a great variety of tests used to evaluate CSF flow dynamics, isotopic cisternography, MR flow studies, ICP monitoring, infusion test, CSF evacuation and neuropsychology [7].

Syndrome of hydrocephalus in young and middle-aged adults (SHYMA) is a recently described form of hydrocephalus. It is different from hydrocephalus diagnosed in infancy and early childhood as well as from adult-onset NPH. The syndrome name proposed by Dr. Michael Williams is described in the literature under a variety of self-explanatory terms like: late-onset idiopathic aqueductal stenosis, long-standing overt ventriculomegaly of the adult, and late-onset acqueductal stenosis. The cause of SHYMA may be congenital with a few or no symptoms in childhood, acquired after head injury, following meningitis or in the course of a brain tumor. It is idiopathic when no cause can be identified.

SHYMA is characterized by headache, subtle gait disturbance, urinary frequency, visual disturbances and some level of impaired cognitive skills. The job performance and personal relations of those patients can be affected at various degree. Early diagnosis is an important factor in obtaining resolution of symptoms.

In patients with disturbed gait, bladder control and mild dementia, SHYMA is diagnosed using a combination of CT and MR brain scans, intracranial pressure monitoring, lumbar puncture, ICP monitoring, measurement of CSF outflow resistance, isotopic cisternography and neuropsychological tests.

In properly diagnosed cases, treatment with shunting can reverse many of the symptoms, restoring much cognitive and physical functioning. In untreated patients symptoms can become disabling, leading to severe cognitive and physical decline [3].

2. ADULT HYDROCEPHALUS

Adult hydrocephalus is treated in the ways appropriate to the type of hydrocephalus and its mechanism.

In occlusive hydrocephalus the cause of CSF pathways obstruction, usually a tumor, should be removed. If this is not possible a diversion of the fluid with endoscopic third ventriculostomy or a shunt is an option. Endoscopic third ventriculostomy is applicable when cerebrospinal pathways are obstructed beyond the third ventricle and absorptive capacity of the arachnoid remains adequate [4].

In most cases symptomatic non-communicating hydrocephalus needs to be treated before permanent neurologic deficits develop or neurologic deficits progress.

In urgent situation of rapid development of acute hydrocephalus it can be treated with temporary measures using ventricular drainage before the underlying condition, for example a posterior fossa tumor is removed, or intraventricular blood absorbed.

CT and MR scan delineates the degree of ventricular enlargement and in many cases discloses the causal aetiology. The degree of the ventricular enlargement can be evaluated by an Evan's index, which is a ratio of greatest width of the frontal horns of the lateral ventricles to the maximal internal diameter of the skull. An index exceeding 0.3 is indicative of a hydrocephalus. T2-weighted MR images can show transependymal flow of CSF and subependymal white matter damage. Widened temporal horns and flattened cortical sulci at the top of the brain are also found in NPH [2].

Differential diagnosis is based on a combination of clinical symptoms, imaging and tests predicting likelihood of improvement after shunting. All types of hydrocephalus may present with disturbed balance and gait, as well as cognition. It is important to identify patients with dementia in the course of subcortical or vascular dementia in Binswanger's or Alzheimer's disease and in Parkinson's disease in whom treatment with shunting is ineffective. Extensive leukoaraiosis is more common in vascular dementia then in ventricular dilation in INHP.

Predictive tests either measure CSF flow dynamics or simulate shunting by removal of the CSF.

Isotopic cisternography monitors absorption of CSF by tracing with gamma-camera a radioactive isotope injected into the lumbar subarachnoid space. Accumulation of isotope over the cortical surface indicates normal flow distribution. In NPH isotope enters the ventricular system. This method has not been proven to be reliable and was generally abandoned after 1992.

Infusion tests are based on recording of ICP during infusion of artificial CSF into the lumbar subarachoid space or into the lateral ventricle. It allows calculation of CSF outflow resistance, compliance, CSF formation rate and dural venous pressure. Despite variations in the conduction and interpretation of the test the outflow resistance is regarded to be the most reliable predictor of effectiveness of shunting. Patients correctly selected for shunting based on elevated outflow resistance may not improve if the disease has reached an irreversible stage [8].

The flow within the CSF spaces can be studied non-invasively with MR. Increased velocity or volume of natural pulsatile flow in the aqueduct following blood pulsations predict favourable outcome of shunting.

Draining of 40–50 ml of CSF by lumbar puncture or continuous drainage of 150–250 ml a day in 2–4 days should temporarily relive NPH symptoms, but not those related with other forms of dementia. The method has not proved to be particularly reliable with false positive and false negative results. Lumbar puncture can be simultaneously used to measure intracranial pressure, and provide samples of CSF for analysis. It should only be performed after imaging studies rule out an obstruction of the ventricular system and increased ICP [8].

ICP monitoring over a period of at least 24 hours with a pressure transducer inserted into the brain or cerebral ventricle permits detection of pressure waves that speaks for presence of NPH and indicates choice of treatment. Slow, rhythmic oscillations in pressure described as B-waves are regarded to be a good indicator of NPH likely to benefit from shunting, however evidence exists that only a week correlation between ICP and surgical outcome exists [10].

Biomarkers offer some hope in enhancing diagnosis. Patterns of the concentration of neurofilament protein light (NFL), hyperphosphorylated tau (P-tau) and beta-amyloid (Aβ42) may help in differentiation of INPH from subcortical atherosclerotic encephalopathy [1].

Those supplemental tests can improve the accuracy of predicting a response to surgical treatment. CSF shunting provides significant symptom improvement in the majority of appropriately evaluated patients.

Patients with NPH who are considered for shunting should have gait disturbances and at least one of the two other elements of the triad: disturbances of urination and cognition. They should have dilatation of ventricles confirmed by imaging and an obstruction of the ventricular system excluded. Neuropsychological testing together with imaging help to exclude vascular dementia in Alzheimer's disease. At least one of the CSF dynamics tests should be indicative of a reduced compliance of the CSF flow. In our institution a lumbar infusion test with lumbar pressure measurement followed by evacuation of 50 ml of CSF and neurological and neuropsychological evaluation are done before decision making. In rare case ICP monitoring over 2 days is performed [6].

SURGERY

1. OPERATION

In the majority of NPH patients fulfilling above described criteria a ventriculo-peritoneal shunt is implanted.

Out of the great variety of shunting devices a variable opening pressure valves with an antisyphon are mostly used. It enables adjustment of opening pressure of the valve without operation. The initial opening pressure of the valve is set at the mean ICP level of the patient. This pressure is measured during pre-operative CSF-dynamic studies. The opening pressure is adjusted as necessary to counteract over- or under-drainage and resulting complications.

Shunt implantations are done in an operating theatre as the first procedure of the day, with additional restrictions in personnel circulation during the procedure to maintain highest level of asepsis. A single dose of prophylactic antibiotic approved for the whole hospital is used. The patient in general anaesthesia is placed supine on the operating table with the head resting on a horse-shoe support to allow repositioning during surgery, important at the stage of passing under the skin a guide from head to chest. The head is rotated to the left, hair shaved in the right frontal, temporal and retroauricular area. Upper part of the chest is elevated with a support across the shoulder blades to reduce curvature between the head, neck and chest to facilitate passage of the shunt passer without additional skin incisions between the head and abdomen. Incisions on the head and abdomen are marked and the skin in the area of shaved head, neck, chest and upper abdomen scrubbed with an antiseptic solution, covered with adhesive plastic and draped. A semicircular skin and periosteal incision is made immediately in front of the coronal suture and 2–3 cm to the right of the midline. It is slightly larger then the planned size of the burr hole. The skin flap with galea and pericranium is separated from the bone and retracted with a small self-retaining retractor. A burr hole is made with an electric drill. The diameter of the hole should be sufficient to accommodate the valve or a reservoir or provide space for the ventricular drain, depending on the construction of the shunt. The wound is temporarily covered with saline soaked gauze. A 4 cm long linear horizontal skin incision is made in the right upper quadrant of the abdomen. Appropriately moulded short passer is pushed under the skin from the frontal incision to the retroauricular area, where a secondary small straight skin incision is made. A long passer is guided under the skin between the abdominal and retroauricular incisions. Depending on the construction of the shunt modifications of this stage of operation may be necessary. We try to make as few secondary incisions as possible. In most cases one behind the earlobe is sufficient. Space in the subcutaneous tissue is prepared to accommodate valve and/or reservoir depending on the shunt type. In shunts without a tube shape passer pulling of the abdominal drain with a thread passed through the subcutaneous tunnel may facilitate the process. The peritoneal drain is passed from the frontal to the abdominal skin incisions. The dura and cortical arachnoidea are incised with No 11 blade and coagulated with a bipolar cautery. Making an incision prior to coagulation gives better control of the size of the dural opening and secure haemostasis. The size of the incision should be just large enough to allow passage of the ventricular drain. Larger opening increases the risk of

CSF subcutaneous leak along the drain. The ventricular drain of the length determined preoperatively on the MR is inserted perpendicularly to the bone into the lateral ventricle, anterior to the foramen of Monroe using a stylet. It is rarely necessary to use a ventriculoscope to confirm correct placement of the tip of the catheter, away from the choroid plexus. Proximity of ventricular catheter tip to the choroid plexus increases the risk of drain occlusion by adhesions with plexus. The usual length of the catheter is 5–6 cm. If shunt construction requires connecting ventricular and peritoneal catheters it is done at this stage. Drains are secured on the connector with a non-absorbable thread. Making a knot connecting both ligatures decreases the risk of disconnection. Free flow of the CSF from the peritoneal end of the shunt confirms patency of the system. Now abdominal straight muscle is split along its fibre lines, peritoneum elevated, opened with scissors and secured with clamps. The distal catheter of the shunt is introduced through the opening into the peritoneal cavity. It is suggested that a single-end hole catheters are more resistant to occlusion then those with multiple side holes or slits. A length of around 40 cm of catheter is left in the peritoneal cavity with a purse-string suture of the peritoneun tied around the entry point. Placing the drain over the liver is believed to reduce the risk of occlusion by peritoneal adhesions. Skin wounds are sutured in layers and dressing applied.

A lumboperitoneal shunt may be used as an alternative to the commonly used ventriculoperitoneal shunt. They are used if ventricles are small, like in pseudotumor cerebri. They tend to overdrain and cause headache, therefore a positional valve turning off the flow of CSF when the patient is upright is recommended.

Other types of shunts, like ventriculo-atrial or ventriculopleural are used very rarely in NPH and usually in special circumstances. Ventriculoatrial shunting is used in patients with contraindications for insertion of an abdominal catheter, which occurs after multiple abdominal operations, in extensive peritoneal adhesions, malabsorptive peritoneal cavity. Complications of the ventriculoatrial shunt include renal failure, great vein thrombosis, catheter thrombosis or cardiac arrhythmias. They are more common and severe then complications in ventriculoperitoneal shunts [5].

Shunting should not be performed in infected patients or those with high CSF protein level of >150 mg/dL.

2. POSTOPERATIVE CARE

Wounds are kept dry under sterile dressings. Skin sutures on the head are removed on the 5th postoperative day and those on the abdomen on the 7th day.

Plain radiographs of the implanted shunt provides control of the position of the shunt and connections as well as a good baseline for the future. In patients with variable pressure valve it confirms the setting of the opening pressure.

Postoperative CT scan is used to document ventricular size, although a scan performed shortly before the operation may suffice.

Patients with high brain compliance should be mobilized and brought to the upright position gradually to reduce the incidence of overdrainage and subdural haematoma formation.

3. COMPLICATIONS

Shunts are prone to complications. They include mechanical failure, infections and obstructions.

If the volume of drained CSF is inadequate the problem of overdraining or underdraining occurs. It results from an inappropriate opening pressure of the shunt system for the individual patient.

A shunt malfunction may be indicated by headaches, vision problems, irritability, fatigue, personality change, loss of coordination, difficulty in waking up or staying awake, a return of walking difficulties, mild dementia or incontinence.

Overdraining may lead to collapse of the ventricles and development of slit ventricle syndrome or to tearing of blood vessels resulting in formation of a subdural hematoma. The risk can be reduced by using antisiphon devices and avoiding selection of too low opening pressure of the valve. In adjustable pressure valves overdrainage can be overcome by increasing opening pressure.

Underdraining occurs when the volume of drained CSF is too low. In those cases the symptoms of hydrocephalus do not retreat or recur. It is managed by increasing opening pressure of the valve, but sometimes requires occlusion of the shunt system.

Collapse of the ventricular walls and occlusion of the ventricles lead to slit ventricle syndrome. It is rare condition occurring after ventriculitis or shunt infection. Usually high ICP develops. The slit ventricle syndrome does not imply overdrainage. It manifests with symptoms high intracranial pressure. Collapsed ventricle tends to block ventricular catheter, which may be resolved by a subtemporal decompression creating a pressure reservoir allowing expansion of the ventricle.

Infections of the shunt system are a serious and common complications of shunting. It is estimated that between 5 and 15% of the devices become infected, of which more then a half within the first month after surgery [5].

Eradication of the bacteria, commonly staphylococci, from the foreign body of the shunt is extremely difficult and usually is achieved only after removal of the system. Infection causes fever, symptoms of meningitis or encephalitis, swelling and tenderness along the shunt drains. Infection is usually combined with dysfunction of the valve and sometimes recurrence of the hydrocephalus symptoms.

Prognosis of the treatment of INPH with shunting is uncertain. It depends on the stage of the NPH and the level of brain damage before treatment. Complications of shunts and their dysfunction further increase the failure rate. While the success of treatment with shunts varies, many patients, close to 80% of cases diagnosed early, treated in time with proper indications, recover almost completely and have a good quality of life.

HOW TO AVOID COMPLICATIONS

Complications are unavoidable but we can reduce their frequency. To achieve this goal reliable diagnosis of NPH should be made, appropriate selection of patients with high likelihood of effectiveness of shunting. Meticulous execution of implantation plays an important role in complication avoidance. Too long or too short ventricular catheter, placed sub optimally in the ventricular system, mechanical damage of the shunt system by inadequate handling or bad instruments, too long operation time, violation of strictly aseptic technique increase the risk of shunt dysfunction or infection.

CONCLUSIONS

Hydrocephalus in adults is different from that occurring in childhood. The most common and typical is normal pressure hydrocephalus, presenting a typical triad of symptoms. Treatment is basically implantation of a ventriculo-peritonael shunt. Success of the treatment depends on the proper selection of candidates for shunting and exclusion of those with dementia in other brain conditions. Treatment is safe but not free of complications. Most of them can be avoided by using good clinical judgement and meticulous surgical technique. Bolus resistance testing and gait improvement immediately following shunting are the best prognostic indicators of a favourable outcome. It is common that gait and incontinence respond to shunting, but dementia responds less frequently.

References

[1] Ågren-Wilsson A, Lekman A, Sjöberg W, Rosengren L, Blennow K, Bergenheim AT, Malm A (2007) CSF biomarkers in the evaluation of idiopatic normal pressure hydrocephalus. Acta Neurol Scand 116: 333-339

[2] Boon AJ, Tans JT, Delwel EJ, Egeler-Peerdeman SM, Hanlo PW, Wurzer HA, Hermans J (2000) The Dutch normal-pressure hydrocephalus study. How to select patients for shunting? An analysis of four diagnostic criteria. Surg Neurol 53: 201-207

[3] Cowan JA, McGirt MJ, Woodworth G, Rigamonti D, Williams MA (2005) The syndrome of hydrocephalus in young and middle-aged adults (SHYMA). Neurol Res 27: 540-547

[4] Dusick JR, McArthur DL, Bergsneider M (2008) Success and complication rates of endoscopic third ventriculostomy for adult hydrocephalus: a series of 108 patients. Surg Neurol 69: 5-15

[5] Epstein MH, Duncan JA III (2000) Surgical management of hydrocephalus in adults. In: Schmidek HH, Sweet WH (eds) Operative neurosurgical techniques. Indications, methods, and results. W. B. Saunders, Philadelphia

[6] Gallia GL, Rigamonti D, Williams MA (2006) The diagnosis and treatment of normal pressure hydrocephalus. Nat Clin Pract Neurol 2: 375-381

[7] Malm J, Eklund A (2006) Idiopatic normal pressure hydrocephalus. Pract Neurol 6: 14-27

[8] Marmarou A, Young HF, Aygok GA, Sawauchi S, Tsuji O, Yamamoto T, Dunbar J (2005) Diagnosis and management of idiopathic normal-pressure hydrocephalus: a prospective study in 151 patients. J Neurosurg 102: 987-997

[9] Tsunoda A, Mitsuoka H, Bandai H, Endo T, Arai H, Sato K (2002) Intracranial cerebrospinal fluid measurement studies in suspected idiopathic normal pressure hydrocephalus, secondary normal pressure hydrocephalus, and brain atrophy. J Neurol Neurosurg Psychiatry 73: 552-555

[10] Vanneste J, van Ecker R (1990) Normal pressure hydrocephalus: did publications alter management? J Neurol Neurosurg Psychiatry 53: 564-568

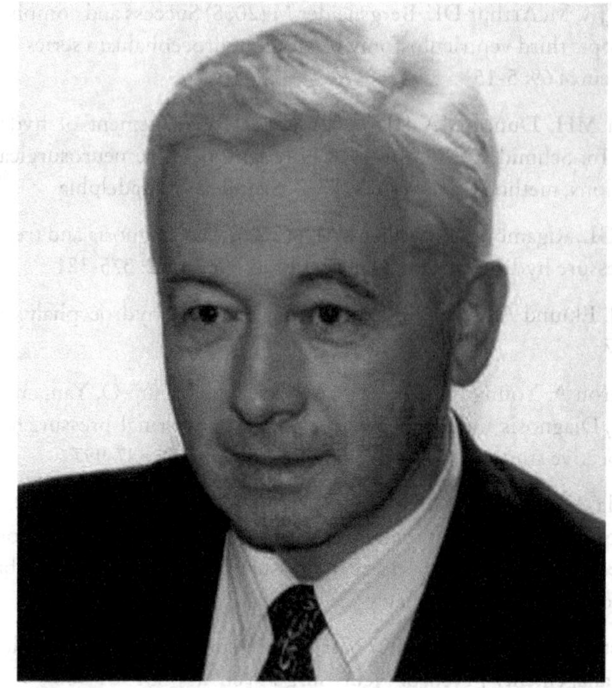

Tomasz Trojanowski

Tomasz Trojanowski is Chairman of the Department of Neurosurgery and Paediatric Neurosurgery at the Medical University in Lublin, Poland. Member of the Polish Academy of Sciences and of the Polish Academy of Arts and Sciences, born in 1947 in Lublin, Poland. Vice-President of the WFNS and of the EANS. Member of the Eurasian Academy of Neurosurgery, World Academy of Neurosurgery, German Academy of Neurosurgery, Turkish Academy of Neurological Surgery. Chairman of the JRAAC, Ethico-Legal Committee of EANS. President of the Section of Neurosurgery of UEMS. Honorary President of the Polish Society of Neurosurgeons, Honorary Member of the Polish Surgical Society, British Neurosurgical Society, Corresponding Member of the German Neurosurgical Society. Chairman of the Neuroscience Committee of the Polish Academy of Sciences. Main scientific interests: neurodiagnostics, vascular brain diseases, neurooncology, radiosurgery, neurosurgical technique, neuro-pathophysiology. Author of over 130 published papers, 180 congress presentations and chapters in 6 monographs.

Contact: Tomasz Trojanowski, Department of Neurosurgery and Paediatric Neurosurgery, Medical University in Lublin, Jaczewskiego 8, 20950 Lublin, Poland
E-mail: t.trojanowski@am.lublin.pl

ARACHNOID CYSTS

H. W. S. SCHROEDER

INTRODUCTION

Arachnoid cysts are congenital cerebrospinal fluid-filled lesions probably arising from anomalous splitting of the arachnoid during prenatal development [16]. In some cysts, a valve mechanism seems to play a major role in cyst enlargement [12, 13]. During life, these cysts may expand and cause symptoms by compressing the neighbouring brain structures or causing occlusive hydrocephalus. Therefore, they usually become symptomatic with signs of increased intracranial pressure. Furthermore, depending on their location, arachnoid cysts may cause seizures, hemisyndromes, increased head growth, ocular symptoms, cerebellar symptoms, endocrinological abnormalities, etc. Arachnoid cysts can be found anywhere in the brain, but are predominantly located in the Sylvian fissure [7]. With the increasing use of magnetic resonance (MR) imaging, arachnoid cysts are frequently discovered as an incidental finding. True congenital arachnoid cysts should be distinguished from acquired cysts which may occur after trauma, bleeding, or infection.

RATIONALE

The goal of surgery in arachnoid cysts is simply the creation of a communication between the cyst and the normal cerebrospinal fluid (CSF) spaces, i.e. the ventricles and/or the cisterns (Fig. 1). This communication should be large to avoid reclosure of the opening by scarring [2, 14]. When a large opening cannot be performed for anatomical reasons, a silicon catheter can be placed between cyst and CSF space. However, foreign material should be avoided whenever possible. When all fenestration attempts fail, a cystoperitoneal shunt has to be inserted as the final treatment option (Fig. 2).

DECISION-MAKING

1. DIAGNOSTIC CRITERIA

1.1 Imaging

MR imaging is the imaging modality of choice. Our standard protocol for arachnoid cysts includes T1- and T2-weighted sequences in axial, coronar,

Keywords: arachnoid cyst, endoscopy, endoscopic fenestration

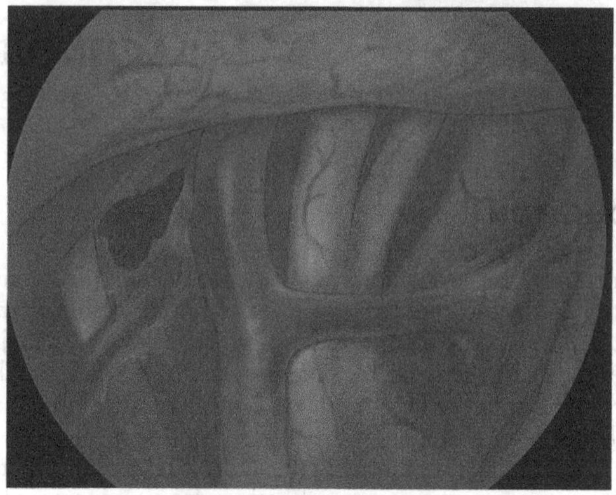

Fig. 1. Schematic drawing of a Sylvian arachnoid cyst showing the fenestration between carotid artery and oculomotor nerve which creates a communication to the prepontine cistern

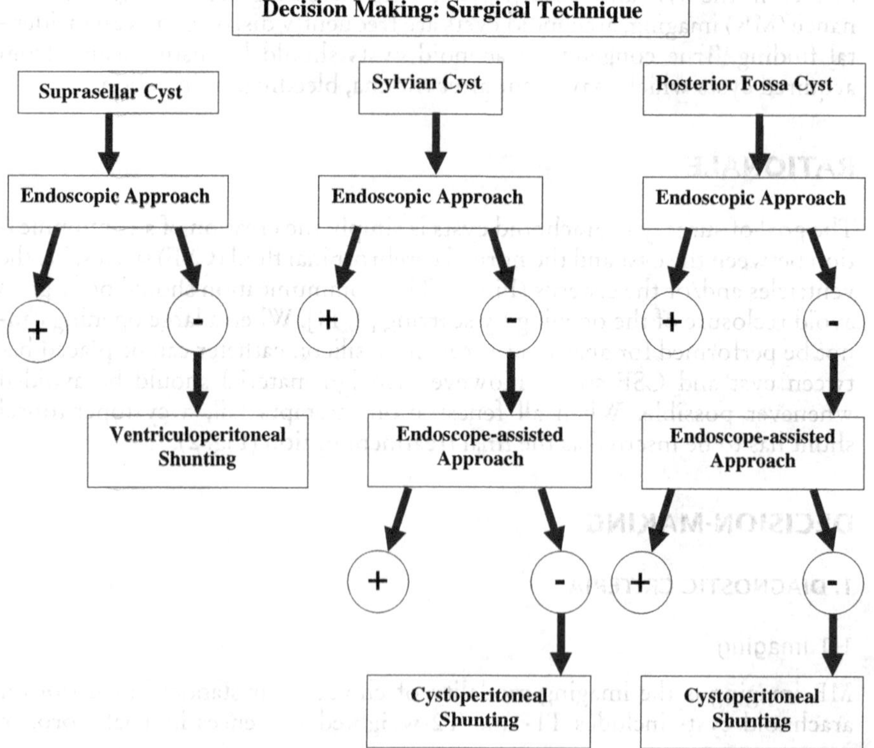

Fig. 2. Decision making for surgical technique

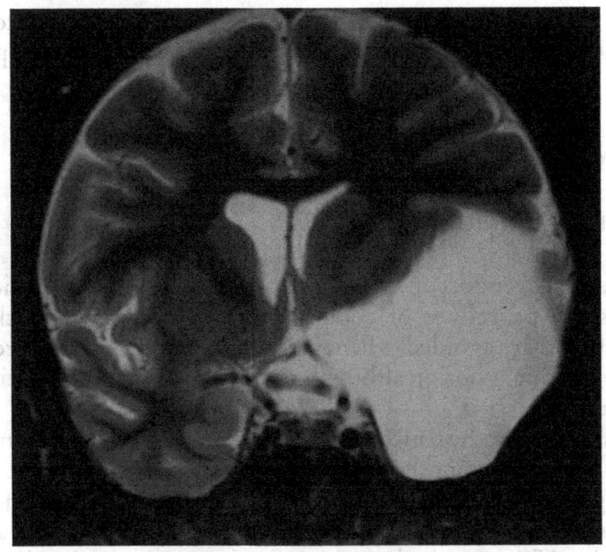

Fig. 3. Coronal T2-weighted MR image showing a Sylvian arachnoid cyst with midline shift and ventricular compression

and sagittal plane, as well as high resolution CISS (constructive interference in steady state) und IRTSE (inversion recovery turbo spin echo) sequences (plane depending from the location of the cyst). Size, configuration, mass effect and width of the ventricles were evaluated (Fig. 3).

1.2 Clinical symptoms

Headaches are the most common complaint. Other symptoms depend from the location of the cyst. Sylvian cysts may cause seizures and hemi-syndromes. Suprasellar cysts usually lead to obstruction of the aqueduct resulting in occlusive hydrocephalus. Therefore, signs of acute or chronic hydrocephalus may occur. Sometimes endocrine dysfunction, such as precocious puberty, is the initial symptom. Arachnoid cysts in the pineal region may cause Parinaud syndrome or diplopia. Infratentorial cyst often present with dizziness, balance problems, or cranial nerve dysfunction.

2. INDICATIONS

Symptomatic arachnoid cysts are an indication for surgery if no contraindications exist. Symptomatic cysts usually show a mass effect on MR imaging with flattening of cerebral gyri, midline shift, and/or ventricular compression. The surgical indication for asymptomatic arachnoid cysts remains controversial [1, 3, 10]. In my opinion, surgery for asymptomatic arachnoid cysts in adults is not justified although the vulnerability of arachnoid cysts in minor head trauma is well known. In children however, asymptomatic cysts with a significant mass effect that may hinder the normal development of the adjacent brain tissue should be treated surgically [1, 4, 11].

SURGERY

1. OPERATIVE TECHNIQUE

In my experience, endoscopic or endoscope-assisted microsurgical cyst fenestration is the procedure of choice in most intracranial arachnoid cysts. Shunting should be avoided whenever possible and is considered to be the last-in-line treatment option although some reports favour shunting over cyst fenestration [1, 4].

The positioning of the patient on the operating table depends on the location of the cyst. The entry point should be the highest point to prevent excessive CSF loss. After general anesthesia has been induced, the head is placed in three-pin fixation. Single shot antibiotic prophylaxis (1.5 g cefuroxime) is administered intravenously. When required, computerized neuronavigation is installed and referenced. Neuronavigation is helpful in selecting the ideal entry point and the best trajectory [15]. In cystic cavities, lacking anatomical landmarks, neuronavigation is sometimes mandatory to stay oriented. When neuronavigation is not used, the entry point is determined according to the best trajectory obtained from MR imaging. Then the operating field is prepared and draped.

If an endoscopic procedure is performed, a 10-mm burr hole is made at the entry point. The endoscopic sheath with trocar inside is inserted free-hand or under navigational guidance into the cyst or ventricle and fixed with a self-retaining holding device. Care is taken to avoid significant CSF loss when directly approaching the cyst cavity. Therefore, the endoscopic sheath is inserted immediately after incising the cyst membrane and cottonoids are densely packed around the sheath at the level of the burr hole. Then the trocar is removed and the endoscope is inserted to inspect the cyst. We use a recently developed rigid multipurpose ventriculoscope which has a 6° Hopkins II rod lens optic, a 2.9 mm working channel, and two 1.6 mm irrigation channels (Karl Storz GmbH & Co. KG, Tuttlingen, Germany). The operations are performed under continuous irrigation with Ringer's solution at 36°C. Depending on the cyst location, cystocisternostomies, ventriculocystostomies, or ventriculocystocisternostomies are made. Once the endoscopic fenestration is accomplished, the cyst is inspected to make sure that a sufficient communication between cyst and cistern or ventricle has been created. Then the operating sheath is withdrawn with the endoscope inside to look for active bleeding in the puncture canal. Since suture of the dura in adults is not feasible, we pack the burr hole with a gelatin sponge and tightly suture the galea to prevent subgaleal CSF accumulation and fistula formation. In infants, we suture dura, periost (if possible), temporal fascia, and galea. The skin is closed with a running atraumatic suture.

For endoscope-assisted microsurgical procedures, a mini-craniotomy (approx. 2 by 2 cm) is made and a fenestration or partial cyst resection performed under microscopic and endoscopic view. For endoscopic visualization, 2.7 mm Hopkins II rod lens optics (Karl Storz) with angulated eye piece and different angles of view are used. These endoscopes have no working channel. The instruments are guided around the endoscope. Because the endoscope is fixed with a self-retaining holding device, the surgeon has both hands free for bimanual dissection as he is used to do under the microscope.

2. SUPRASELLAR ARACHNOID CYSTS

Suprasellar arachnoid cysts are an ideal indication for an endoscopic approach. Usually large suprasellar arachnoid cyst cause occlusive hydrocephalus due to aqueductal obstruction (Fig. 4A and B). The ventricular dilation provides plenty of space for insertion of an endoscope. Because of their characteristic appearance on axial MR images these cysts are also referred to as Mickey Mouse cysts (Fig. 4C). The patient is placed supine with the head slightly anteflexed. A precoronal burr hole is made 2 cm paramedian on the right side. Thereafter, the endoscope is introduced into the right lateral ventricle (Fig. 4D). Usually the foramen of Monro is enlarged by the cyst (Fig. 4E). A large fenestration into the lateral ventricle (approx. 1 by 1 cm) is created in the cyst wall with the aid of bipolar coagulation and scissors (Fig. 4F and G). In cysts with a very thin cyst membrane, a bimanual technique is used to prevent collapse of the cyst. Via one irrigation channel a flexible forceps is introduced to hold the cyst membrane while scissors are used via the working channel to make the fenestration. Then the cyst membrane in front of the aqueduct is coagulated with a bipolar diathermy probe to shrink the collapsed cyst and restore CSF flow through the aqueduct. Once the fenestration has been accomplished (Fig. 4H), the inside of the cyst is inspected. The cranial nerves III to VII/VIII, basilar and vertebral arteries as well as pituitary gland can often be seen (Fig. 4I and J). If a valve mechanism is found around the basilar artery, this valve should be destroyed because a major pathogenic factor may be eliminated. If anatomically possible, a communication between the cyst and the basal cisterns is performed additionally to create a ventriculocystocisternostomy [5]. However, this step of the procedure seems to be not mandatory to be successful.

3. SYLVIAN ARACHNOID CYSTS

The optimal treatment for Sylvian arachnoid cysts is still under discussion. We prefer an endoscopic burr hole approach. However, when the cyst membrane turns out to be very tough or the windows between carotid artery, optic and oculomotor nerve are very narrow, we do not hesitate to switch to an endoscope-assisted microsurgical technique. Then, the burr hole is en-

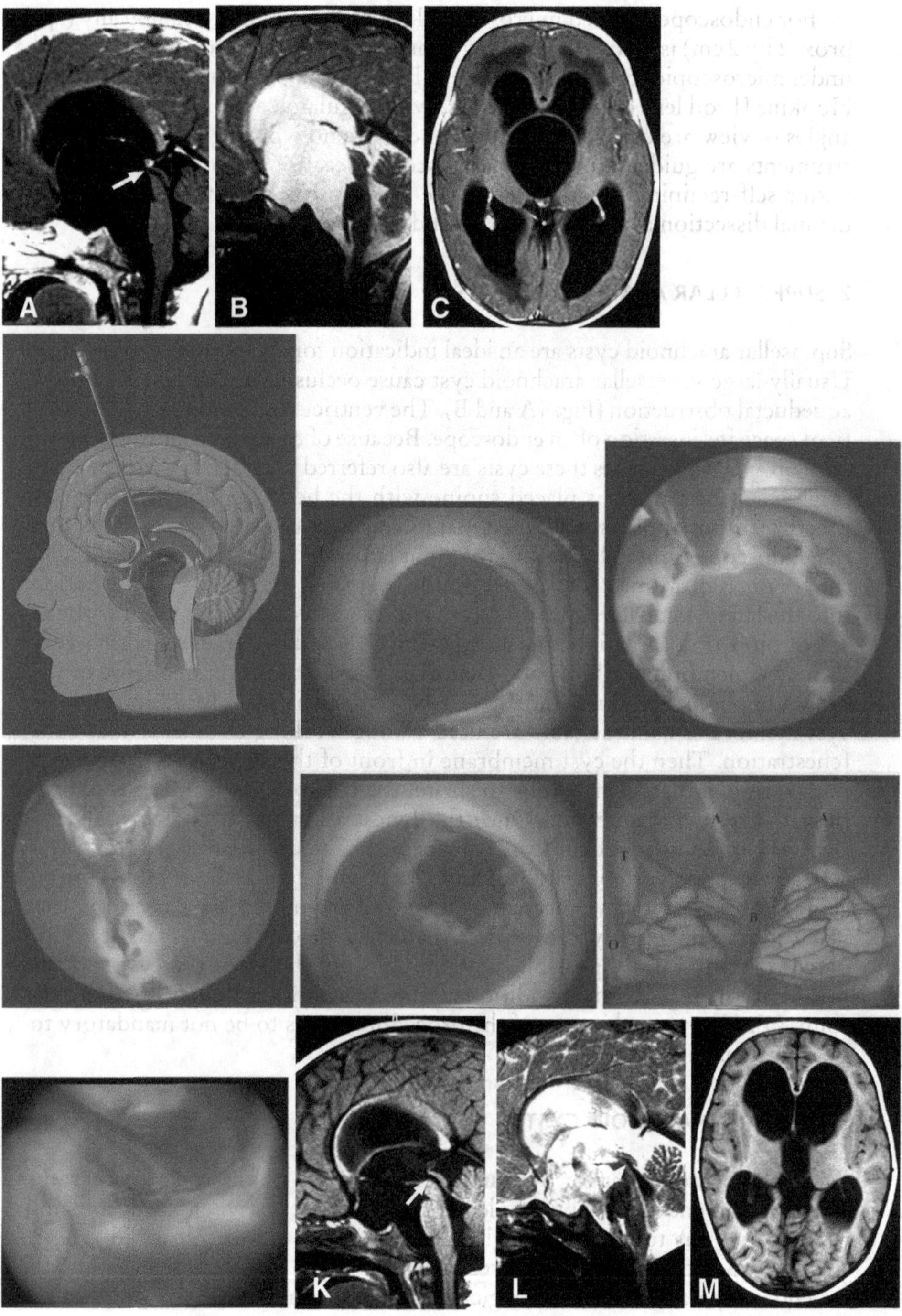
A
B
C
K
L
M

larged to a small craniotomy (2 by 2 cm), the CSF is sucked off, and the fenestration is performed under microscopic and/or endoscopic view. Since the approach goes through the cyst lumen, no higher rate of injury to brain tissue is caused with this approach compared with the pure endoscopic approach. However, the disadvantage of this technique is that the CSF has to be removed. That may result in cyst collapse and subdural effusions. Therefore, we start with the endoscopic inspection via a burr hole.

The patient is placed supine with the head turned to the contralateral side. Depending from the cyst size, the skin incision is placed more or less above the level of the zygomatic arch anterior to the ear. Neuronavigation is helpful to find the ideal entry point and the best trajectory to the basal cisterns without touching the brain. Care should be taken to spare the frontotemporal branch of the facial nerve. The temporal fascia and muscle are incised and the temporal muscle is dissected from the skull. A burr hole is made and a cross-shaped dura incision is performed. Then, the underlying cyst membrane is incised. It is of utmost importance to cauterize the fragile arachnoidal blood vessels in the entry zone to avoid bleeding induced by moving the endoscope. Outflow of CSF should be minimized and care has to be taken to prevent detaching the outer cyst membrane from the dura when inserting the operating sheath, which may result in cyst collapse and accumulation of CSF between the cyst membrane and dura which later may lead to subdural hematomas.

After insertion of the endoscope, the cyst is inspected (Fig. 5B). Usually orientation is easy because of the well known anatomical landmarks, such as the carotid and middle cerebral artery, optic nerves, and oculomotor nerve (Fig. 5C). In large cysts, even the frontal skullbase and olfactory tracts may be seen. In general, there is only a limited space for the fenestration of the cyst between carotid artery and oculomotor nerve or carotid artery and optic nerve. Rarely, the fenestration is performed lateral to the oculomotor nerve. Since blunt perforation of the cyst membrane is usually impossible, the membrane has to be cut with scissors. Sometimes parts of the cyst membrane can be removed with grasping forceps (Fig. 5D). After incision of the cyst wall, Liliequist's membrane comes into view (Fig. 5E). This membrane has to be incised too to create a communication to the prepontine cistern. Thereafter, the opening is enlarged by inflating the balloon of a No. 3 French Fogarty

Fig. 4. Suprasellar cyst in a 1-year-old girl presenting with head growth and vomiting. **A** T1-weighted sagittal MR image showing a large suprasellar cyst with occlusion of the aqueduct (arrow). **B** T2-weighted MR image revealing no CSF flow through the aqueduct. **C** T1-weighted axial MR image showing the typical Mickey Mouse cyst. **D** Schematic drawing showing the approach trajectory. **E** Enlarged foramen of Monro. **F** Circular coagulation of the cyst wall. **G** Cutting of the cyst wall with scissors. **H** Collapse of the cyst after fenestration. **I** View into the prepontine cistern showing basilar artery (*B*), oculomotor (*O*), trigeminal (*T*), and abducens (*A*) nerve. **J** View to the sella with pituitary gland. **K** T1-weighted sagittal MR image obtained 3 months after surgery showing the collapse of the cyst with patent aqueduct (arrow). **L** T2-weighted MR image obtained 3 months after surgery demonstrating vigorous CSF flow through the aqueduct (arrow). **M** T1-weighted axial MR image obtained 3 months after surgery showing a marked decrease in cyst size

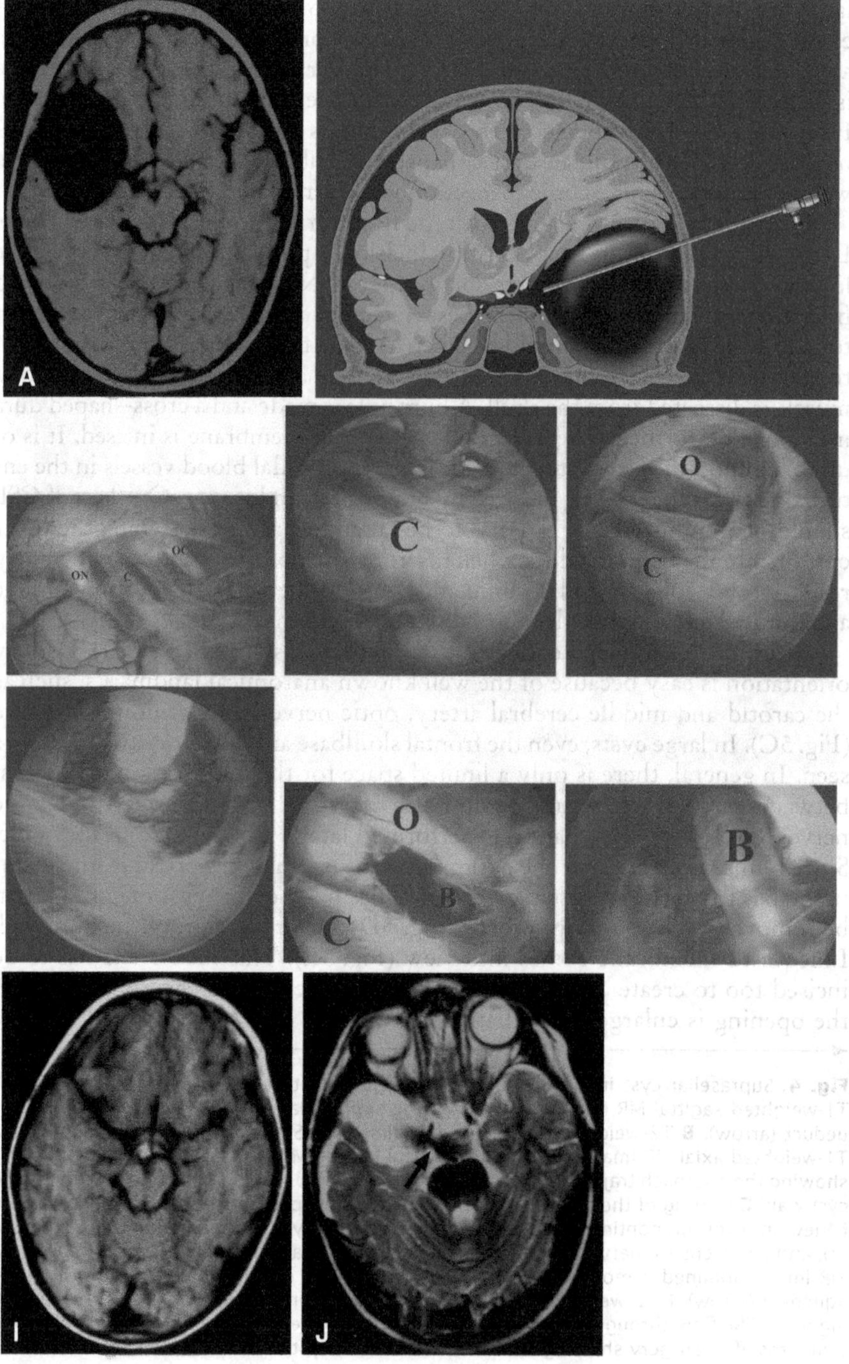
A
ON
C
OC
C
O
C
O
B
C
B
I
J

catheter (Fig. 5F) or with the aid of scissors and grasping forceps. Once the fenestration has been accomplished (Fig. 5G), the prepontine cistern with the basilar artery (Fig. 5H) has to be seen to make sure that a wide communication with the cistern has been created. Coagulation of the membrane should be avoided since the shrinking often leads to an even thougher membrane. If the created opening is too narrow and the risk of later occlusion by scarring is high, a fimbrial ventricular catheter may be inserted into the adjacent basal cisterns. Care must be taken not to injure the oculomotor nerve or branches of the carotid artery when advancing the catheter into the cistern.

When the endoscopic technique is not efficient because of anatomical conditions or a firm arachnoid membrane, we switch to an endoscope-assisted microsurgical technique [8].

4. ARACHNOID CYSTS OF THE POSTERIOR CRANIAL FOSSA

For small arachnoid cysts which are covered by cerebellar tissue, an endoscope-assisted microsurgical approach is used. For large cysts reaching the dura in the area of a potential approach, an endoscopic approach is preferable.

Patients with cysts of the cerebellopontine angle are positioned supine with the head turned to the contralateral side. A retrosigmoid suboccipital craniotomy is performed or a burr hole is placed just over the cyst. After incision of the outer cyst membrane, a fenestration to the prepontine cistern is created between the cranial nerves. Care must be taken to avoid injury to the adjacent cranial nerves and vessels.

Patients with midline cysts are placed prone with the head anteflexed (Concorde position). If possible, the location of the burr hole should allow a straight approach to the cyst and adjacent cisterns. With the aid of scissors and grasping forceps, a large fenestration connecting cyst and cisterns is created.

5. LONG-TERM RESULTS

According to the literature and my own experience the success rate of endoscopic cyst fenestration in suprasellar cysts is very high (90–100%) [2, 6, 10]. Only a few patients need to be shunted because of persistent or recurrent hy-

Fig. 5. Sylvian cyst in a 3-year-old boy presenting after a minor head injury. The cyst was an incidental finding. **A** T1-weighted axial MR image showing a large space-occupying Sylvian cyst. **B** Schematic drawing showing the trajectory of the approach. **C** Endoscopic view to the anterior clinoid with optic (*ON*) and oculomotor (*OC*) nerve as well as carotid artery (*C*). **D** Grasping of the thin arachnoid membrane between carotid artery (*C*) and oculomotor nerve. **E** After cyst fenestration, Liliequist's membrane comes into view below the carotid artery (*C*) and oculomotor nerve (*O*). **F** Enlarging the fenestration with a Fogarty balloon catheter. **G** After completed fenestration the basilar artery (*B*) is visible below the carotid artery (*C*) and oculomotor nerve (*O*). **H** View into prepontine cistern showing the basilar artery (*B*). **I** T1-weighted axial MR image obtained 1 year after surgery showing a marked decrease in cyst size. **J** T2-weighted MR image shows a strong flow void signal at the site of the fenestration indicating its patency (arrow)

drocephalus although the cyst fenestration has been successful. The same is true for arachnoid cysts of the posterior fossa. The majority of patients (80–100%) improve after fenestration [8–10]. In Sylvian arachnoid cysts, the success rate seems to be less good (approx. 60–90%) [8, 10]. In my own series of 22 arachnoid cysts including 12 Sylvian, 5 suprasellar, 2 posterior fossa, 2 intraventricular, and 1 intrameatal cyst the overall success rate of endoscopic fenestration was 81% with a mean follow-up period of 6.3 years, ranging from 1.1 to 11.4 years. In children, the decrease in cyst size was more striking than in the adult patients.

6. COMPLICATIONS

Severe complications resulting in mortality and permanent morbidity are fortunately very rare (0% in most reports in the literature). Subdural hematomas (10%), CSF leaks (5%), and meningitis (5%) were the most frequently reported complications [8, 10]. No permanent morbidity and mortality occurred in my own series. In one patient with a Sylvian cyst, a transient oculomotor palsy was observed which resolved completely within 2 months. In one boy, a subgaleal CSF accumulation occurred, but resolved spontaneously after 3 weeks. One patient had meningitis which responded quickly to antibiotic treatment. However, finally this patient needed to be shunted. Two patients presented with subdural collections on the routine postoperative imaging which did not require further surgical intervention.

HOW TO AVOID COMPLICATIONS

1. HEMORRHAGE

Before incising the arachnoid cyst membrane, care must be taken to coagulate all tiny arachnoidal vessels in the area of the approach. Oozing from these blood vessels may significantly blurr the endoscopic view. Furthermore, one must take care when incising and removing parts of the arachnoid membrane covering nerves and arteries when creating the fenestration to the cisterns.

2. SUBDURAL HYGROMA OR HEMATOMA

It is of utmost importance to avoid detaching the arachnoid membrane from the dura when inserting the endoscopic sheath into the cyst. Sometimes it is advisable to suture the arachnoid to the dura to prevent detaching and collapse of the cyst. Furthermore, one should make sure that excessive loss of CSF is avoided which contributes to subdural collections.

3. NERVE INJURIES

Since the space between nerves and arteries in Sylvian cysts is mostly narrow, care must be taken to avoid injury to these structures. Sharp dissection is recommended when the arachnoid membrane is tough to prevent traction injury to the nerves.

4. CSF FISTULA

In adults, CSF leaks are usually not a problem although water-tight dural suturing is not performed. However, in children water-tight closure of the dura should be achieved. Because of the thin scalp, the risk of subgaleal CSF accumulations or fistulas is high.

CONCLUSIONS

Endoscopic techniques are safe and effective options in the treatment of arachnoid cysts and should seriously be considered as the initial therapy. Should the endoscopic procedure fail, an endoscope-assisted microsurgical fenestration is the second line treatment. Shunting should be avoided whenever possible.

References

[1] Arai H, Sato K, Wachi A, Okuda O, Takeda N (1996) Arachnoid cysts of the middle cranial fossa: experience with 77 patients who were treated with cystoperitoneal shunting. Neurosurgery 39: 1108-1113

[2] Caemaert J, Abdullah J, Calliauw L, Carton D, Dhooge C, van Coster R (1992) Endoscopic treatment of suprasellar arachnoid cysts. Acta Neurochir (Wien) 119: 68-73

[3] Cincu R, Agrawal A, Eiras J (2007) Intracranial arachnoid cysts: current concepts and treatment alternatives. Clin Neurol Neurosurg 109: 837-843

[4] Ciricillo SF, Cogen PH, Harsh GR, Edwards MSB (1991) Intracranial arachnoid cysts in children. A comparison of the effects of fenestration and shunting. J Neurosurg 74: 230-235

[5] Decq P, Brugières P, Le Guerinel C, Djindjian M, Kéravel Y, Nguyen JP (1996) Percutaneous endoscopic treatment of suprasellar arachnoid cysts: ventriculocystostomy or ventriculocystocisternostomy? Technical note. J Neurosurg 84: 696-701

[6] Gangemi M, Colella G, Magro F, Maiuri F (2007) Suprasellar arachnoid cysts: endoscopy versus microsurgical cyst excision and shunting. Br J Neurosurg 21: 276-280

[7] Harsh GR IV, Edwards MSB, Wilson CB (1986) Intracranial arachnoid cysts in children. J Neurosurg 64: 835-842

[8] Hopf NJ, Perneczky A (1998) Endoscopic neurosurgery and endoscope-assisted microneurosurgery for the treatment of intracranial cysts. Neurosurgery 43: 1330-1336

[9] Jallo GI, Woo HH, Meshki C, Epstein FJ, Wisoff JH (1997) Arachnoid cysts of the cerebellopontine angle: diagnosis and surgery. Neurosurgery 40: 31-38

[10] Karabatsou K, Hayhurst C, Buxton N, O'Brien DF, Mallucci CL (2007) Endoscopic management of arachnoid cysts: an advancing technique. J Neurosurg 106: 455-462

[11] Okumura Y, Sakaki T, Hirabayashi H (1995) Middle cranial fossa arachnoid cyst developing in infancy: case report. J Neurosurg 82: 1075-1077

[12] Santamarta D, Aguas J, Ferrer E (1995) The natural history of arachnoid cysts: endoscopic and cine-mode MRI evidence of a slit-valve mechanism. Minim Invasive Neurosurg 38: 133-137

[13] Schroeder HWS, Gaab MR (1997) Endoscopic observation of a slit-valve mechanism in a suprasellar prepontine arachnoid cyst: case report. Neurosurgery 40: 198-200

[14] Schroeder HWS, Gaab MR, Niendorf W-R (1996) Neuroendoscopic approach to arachnoid cysts. J Neurosurg 85: 293-298

[15] Schroeder HWS, Wagner W, Tschiltschke W, Gaab MR (2001) Frameless neuronavigation in intracranial endoscopic neurosurgery. J Neurosurg 94: 72-79

[16] Starkman SP, Brown TC, Linell EA (1958) Cerebral arachnoid cysts. J Neuropathol Exp Neurol 17: 484-500

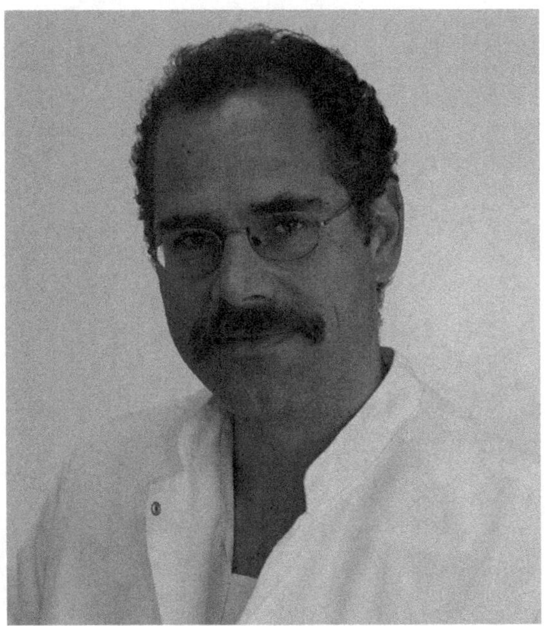

Henry W. S. Schroeder

Henry W. S. Schroeder is Professor of Neurosurgery and Chairman of the Department of Neurosurgery at Greifswald University. He was born in 1963 in Prenzlau, Germany. He studied medicine at the Ernst Moritz Arndt University at Greifswald, where he was a resident at the Department of Neurosurgery, 1989–1996. 1990, M.D. graduation; 1996, board certification as neurosurgeon; 2001, Ph.D. graduation, associate professor of neurosurgery; 2003–2004, acting chairman of the Department of Neurosurgery at Greifswald University. He is a member of the German Society of Neurosurgery, Congress of Neurological Surgeons, and American Association of Neurological Surgeons. His main interests are in endoscopic neurosurgery and endoscope-assisted skull base surgery.

Contact: Henry W. S. Schroeder, Department of Neurosurgery, University of Greifswald, Ferdinand-Sauerbruch-Strasse, 17475 Greifswald, Germany
E-mail: henry.schroeder@uni-greifswald.de

BRAIN INFECTIONS

R. D. LOBATO

INTRODUCTION

Brain infections can affect both its coverings and the brain parenchyma in either a diffuse or focal manner. Diffuse infections as meningitis and encephalitis are rarely subsidiary of surgical treatment. In contrast, intracranial focal purulent conditions are severe threatening pathologies in which surgery plays a keystone role. This chapter will focus on the latter i.e., brain abscess, subdural empyema and epidural abscess.

Before the 19th century, intracranial pyogenic infection was an almost uniformly fatal condition, rarely diagnosed before autopsy. The first surgical attempts to treat intracranial purulent collections are attributed to Galen, who as early as in the 2nd century used trepanation and trephination to drain pus underneath the skull. These procedures were also performed during the 17th and 18th centuries, and Morand is recognized to be the first in operating successfully an intracranial abscess of otic origin in 1752. In 1872 Weeds reported the successful drainage of a posttraumatic brain abscess. A few years later, Macewen published his monograph "Pyogenic infective diseases of the brain and spinal cord", an unique text systematically describing "Surgical anatomy", "Pathology of cerebral abscesses and meningitis", "Symptoms of abscess of brain and meningitis", "Thrombosis of intracranial sinuses", "Treatment" and "Results". He reported 25 brain abscesses 19 of which were operated on, with recovery in 18 cases [1]. Later on several techniques have been described to drain intracerebral abscess, including tube drainage, marsupialization, excision and tapping with aspiration. This last procedure was advocated by Dandy as a minimally invasive procedure, and has been refined in the modern era by using stereotactic techniques.

The other fundamental step in the treatment of intracranial pyogenic conditions was the development of antibiotic treatment introduced in the mid 20th century, with drugs such as penicillin or chloramphenicol. Currently new antimicrobials allow the treatment of almost every pathogen with reasonable risk of toxicity [4].

Finally, the development of neuroimaging techniques, namely the CT scan and MRI studies, have enormously improved not only initial diagnosis of these lesions by readily showing their number and location, but also the monitoring of treatment results.

Keywords: infectious diseases, brain infections, neurosurgery, antibiotics

RATIONALE

Brain abscesses are focal intraparenchymal infections that cause neural tissue damage through inflammation, oedema and compression. Infective pathogens can reach brain parenchyma by one of the following mechanisms [2, 4, 7]:

- *Extension in contiguity*: Direct extension from infections affecting the paracranial sinuses or ear remains the main pathophysiologic mechanism in the formation of brain abscess. This occurs through the invasion and destruction of the skull and cerebral envelopes by pathogens, although it can also proceed through septic thrombophlebitis of intra-extracranial venous channels. These infections are frequently polymicrobial.
- *Hematogenous spread*: It is the result of bacteriemic episodes secondary to infectious pathologies in other organs (endocarditis), or breaches (i.e. dental extractions, or invasive diagnostic studies) bringing micro-organisms into the blood stream, and is favoured by underlying conditions shunting the pulmonary filter such as arteriovenous fistulas or persistent foramen ovale. This is a frequent source of brain abscesses that tend to be monomicrobial and multiple.
- *Direct inoculation by means of trauma or surgery*: The increment of neurosurgical procedures added to the relative decrease in other sources of infection resulting from improvement in their medical management (mainly of otic infections), has increased the relative incidence of this mechanism that nowadays equals that of contiguous extension in some series. Infections following open traumatic injuries are infrequent.
- Still, the origin of brain abscesses remains unknown in 20–30% of the cases ("cryptic" abscess without obvious source).

The above classification, based on the origin of the infection, correlates with its intracranial location, and helps to predicting the most frequent etiology and directing empirical treatment (Table 1). However, in some cases the source of infection is unknown, or no micro-organism has been isolated, precluding an optimal medical management. The absence of a microbiological specimen has been related to the need for broad-spectrum antibiotherapy which carries a higher risk of toxicity, higher costs, greater number of follow up studies and more prolonged treatment [4]. In these cases a surgical procedure can be indicated to obtain tissue sampling for microbiological study, whereas antibiotic treatment is readily instituted when the causative microorganism is identified. However, it should be noted that antibiotics alone can fail to cure the infection because the extent to which they cross the blood–brain barrier, permeate the abscess capsule and diffuse into devitalized purulent tissue is usually restricted, so they can be eventually unable to eradicate the infectious reservoir. Independently

Table 1. Characteristics of intracranial infections regarding location, the most common causative organism and the recommended empirical treatment. Most of the data can be applied to brain abscess, subdural empyema and epidural abscess

Source	Abscess location	Frequent organisms	Empiric treatment
Paranasal sinuses	Frontal	Streptococci (aerobic and anaerobic) *Haemophilus* sp. *Bacteroides* sp. *Fusobacterium* sp.	Ceftriaxone 3–4 g/d + Metronidazole 500 mg/8 h
Otic infections	Temporal Lobe Cerebellum	*Streptococcus* sp. *Enterobacteriaceae* *Bacteroides* sp. *Pseudomonasa eruginosa*	Ampicillin 2 g /8 h+ Metronidazole 500 mg/8 h+ Ceftazidime 2 g /8 h
Hematogenous spread/ cryptogenic	Mainly middle cerebrala rtery territory, but any region can be involved Multiple abscesses	▪ Endocarditis *Staphylococcus aureus* *Streptococcus viridans* ▪ Urinary tract *Enterobacteriacea* *pseudomonas* ▪ Intra-abdominal *Enterobacteriacea* *Streptococcus* sp. *Anaerobes* ▪ Pulmonary abscess *Streptococcus* sp. *Actinomices* sp. *Fusobacterium* sp.	Endocarditis: Benzolpenicillin 1.8–2.4 g/6 h Ceftriaxone 3–4 g/24 h + Metronidazole 500 mg/8 h
Trauma	Depends on site wound	*Staphylococcus aureus* Clostridium Enterobacteriaceae	Cloxacillin 2 g /4 h or Ceftriaxone 3–4/g/24 h
Neurosurgery	Depends on operateda rea	*Staphylococcus aureus* *Staphylococcus epidermidis* Enterobacteriaceae Pseudomonas	Vancomicyn 1g/12 h+ Ceftazidime 1 g /8 h

of bacterial enzymes that can inactivate antibiotics, these drugs can be also neutralized by their binding to proteins present in pus fluid, or the pH of this material [6].

It has been found that patients with brain abscesses lesser than 2 cm in diameter have good outcomes with medical treatment alone, while sizes over this threshold increase the risk of treatment failure usually requiring surgical evacuation as an adjunctive therapy. It should be emphasized that in some instances the risk of neurological deterioration is very high with antibiotic treatment alone. Abscesses can reach a great volume causing significant mass effect and brain herniation prompting urgent surgical evacuation. In addition, the periventricular location carries the risk of intraventricular rupture and ventriculitis, due to the relatively poorer vascularization and capsule development from the ependymal side. This event can precipitate abrupt neurological deterioration and carry a very poor prognosis, mortality rate reaching 80% of the cases. Thus, surgical evacuation of these abscesses and of those other unresponsive to antibiotherapy is strongly recommended.

Subdural empyema is a loculated collection of pus in the subdural space causing inflammation and oedema of the underlying brain, septic thrombophlebitis and venous infarction, which can rapidly extend along the subdural space because of the absence of tissue barriers. Most subdural empyemas (between 41 and 67%) develop as a complication of cranial sinus infection, and the second most common cause is infection following intracranial surgery. Hematogenous spreading from a distant infective focus occurs in some cases, and infection of subdural effusions in children with meningitis may also cause subdural empyema. In any case, subdural empyema is a condition that carries a very high risk of clinical deterioration and rapid surgical evacuation is mandatory to avoid death or irreversible neurological complications [5].

Epidural abscesses are pyogenic collections developing in the virtual space between the cranial dura and bone. The occurrence of osteomyelitis and bone erosion is usually required to strip the dura mater off the bone to which it is tightly adherent, a characteristic that usually contains the extension of these lesions. Direct extension from paracranial sites, or postoperative intracranial infection is the main cause of this condition. Due to the relative isolation of brain tissue and the insidious progression of this process, epidural abscess tend to reach a significant size at diagnosis. This fact, along with the usual involvement of the bone resulting in osteomyelitis and devitalized bone fragments, favours the indication of surgery to facilitate antibiotic activity and diminish the risk for intracranial complications.

DECISION-MAKING

1. CLINICAL DIAGNOSIS

Clinical presentation of a brain abscess depends on its size and location. Nonspecific neurological manifestations such as headache, nausea, or vomiting depend on the presence of intracranial hypertension. Headache is the single most frequent symptom (49% of the cases), and alterations of the level of consciousness are present in many patients (51%). Focal neurological signs and symptoms depend on the involvement of eloquent areas by the lesion itself or surrounding oedema, and can occur in 25–50% of the patients. Meningeal symptoms or signs are present in about 25% of the cases, mainly when the lesion reaches the pial surface. However, the triad of headache, fever and focal neurological symptoms is rare. In fact, fever is not a constant sign, and is present in less than half of the patients (43%). Seizures may occur in 25–50% of the cases. Infections of the craniofacial area can be a clue to diagnosis, and should be investigated in every patient with suspected or demonstrated pyogenic intracranial infection. The non-specific presentation and rarity of this pathology accounts for the frequent delays in diagnosis, so a high index of suspicion is necessary [2, 4].

Subdural empyema is usually a fulminant disease with a rapidly progressive clinic of headache, fever, meningismus, seizures and focal neurological deficit and this type of progression is a hallmark of this condition [6]. In contrast with brain abscesses, local signs reflecting the origin of the infection are present in 60–90% of patients in the form of an infective focus in the ENT field, or inflammatory changes over the skull.

Epidural abscesses tend to present in a more indolent fashion due to the relative isolation of the brain. Symptoms include fever, headache and findings referred to the primary source of infection.

Postoperative purulent intracranial complications tend to manifest by the development of new focal deficits or worsening of pre-existing ones, and are usually associated with inflammatory signs over the surgical wound.

2. LABORATORY TEST AND IMAGING STUDIES

Blood test can sometimes show leucocytosis and abnormalities in certain inflammatory parameters (ESR, RCP). Blood cultures, which may be particularly useful when there is no available material from the pyogenic collection, are mandatory as they can identify the pathogen, orient to the systemic origin of infection, and initiate the most appropriate antibiotic therapy.

Lumbar puncture should be avoided in this clinical setting until the presence of intracranial mass effect has been ruled out, because the risk of brain herniation is very high (occurs in 15–33% of the cases).

Its widespread availability renders the CT scan the technique of choice for providing a rapid and precise diagnosis in patients with urgent pathologies such

Table 2. Stages of brain abscess formation and correlative imaging features

Stage	Days	Histology	CT picture
	1–3	Early infection and inflammation, poorly demarcated from surrounding brain	Focal hypodense area with/ without enhancement after contrast
Late cerebritis	4–9	Reticular matrix and developing necrotic center	Wider hypodense region with ringe nhancement
Early capsule	10–14	Neovascularity, necrotic center, reticular network surrounds	Ring enhancing lesion
Late capsule	>14	Collagen capsule, necrotic center, gliosis around capsule	Ring enhancing lesion

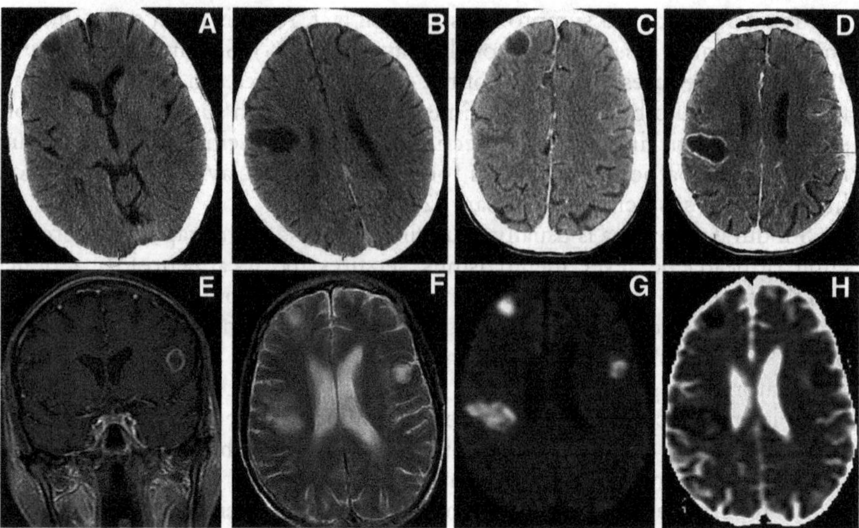

Fig. 1. CT and MRI findings in a patient with multiple brain abscesses caused by hematogenous spread after superior digestive tract endoscopy (*Streptococcus milleri*). CT scan images (**A–D**) show hypodense lesions with fine ring enhancement. MRI shows them as hypointense lesions with peripheral enhancement on contrast-enhanced T1 weighted images (**E**). On T2 weighted images the lesions appear hyperintense with a hypointense halo (**F**). On diffusion weighted images the abscesses displayed a marked restricted diffusion (**G**) with very low ADC (**H**)

as purulent intracranial infections. The CT scan not only shows the location, size and number of lesions, but facilitates urgent treatment planning when necessary. MRI, which is better in terms of sensitivity and specificity, is not always available in emergency conditions. The appearance of a brain abscess in the CT scan correlates with its pathological stage (Table 2). The typical picture of a brain abscess is that of a hypodense ring enhancing lesion with extensive perifocal oedema (Fig. 1). On MRI abscesses are usually seen as hypointense lesions on T1 weighted images which enhance following intravenous contrast injection in the same way as they do in the CT scan study. On T2 sequences they are seen as hyperintense lesions, and a hypointense rim may be seen when a fibrous capsule is already formed. FLAIR images help to better delineate those lesions in the vicinity of CSF containing spaces, as it suppress the CSF hyperintense signal. The differential diagnosis with other ring enhancing lesions such as glioblastoma, lymphoma, or metastases, which may share a similar appearance, has been greatly improved with the introduction of more specific MRI sequences such as the diffusion ones as purulent collections typically show a restricted diffusion and a diminished ADC, in contrast with the above mentioned conditions. Diffusion studies also help in the evaluation of treatment response of brain abscesses, as low signal intensity at diffusion weighted imaging with high ADC correlates with a good therapeutic response.

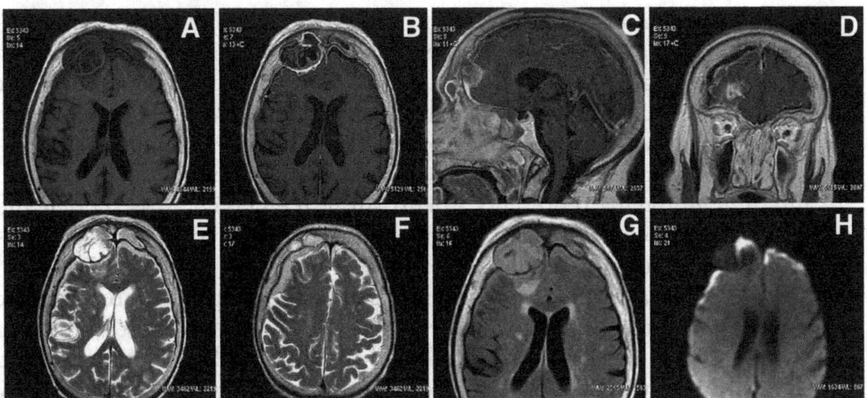

Fig. 2. MRI study of a patient with frontal mucopyocele complicated with intracranial infection. T1 (**A**) and contrast-enhanced T1 weighted images (**B–D**) demonstrate a small subdural hypointense collection surrounded by fine contrast enhancement. This collection appears hyperintense on T2 weighted (**E**, **F**) and FLAIR images (**G**) and shows restricted diffusion (**H**). These findings were diagnostic of subdural empyema that was operated on with positive cultures for *Streptococcus milleri*

In the case of subdural empyema CT scan shows an extra-axial collection with variable degrees of accompanying brain oedema and mass effect. A fine enhancement can be seen in the pial side following intravenous contrast injection. However, a subdural empyema can be missed by the CT scan, and MRI has become the best technique to find and delineate the extension of the pathology (Fig. 2). Again, diffusion MRI sequences may result definitive for distinguishing this condition from other types of fluid collections. However, it should be noted that some infectious collections fail to show a restriction in MR diffusion sequences, a finding observed at our clinic and also reported by other authors. Sensitivity exceeds 95% in spontaneously developing (non postsurgical or posttraumatic) pyogenic collections, but false positive and false negative results are seen in up to 37% of postoperative infections [3].

Epidural abscesses tend to offer less diagnostic difficulties due to their usual biconvex appearance and bigger volume once they become clinically expressive, as well as for the frequently associated lesions involving the overlying bone or the paranasal sinuses. Attention should be paid to the possible imaging abnormalities in neighbouring structures such as the ear and the frontal sinuses, as well as to the presence of osteomyelitis or foreign bodies.

Once a cerebral abscess has been diagnosed the main question arising is whether surgery is indicated or not. The following are classical surgical indications: (a) abscess diameter of >2 cm; (b) intracranial hypertension; (c) risk of intraventricular rupture; (d) absence of response to medical treatment; and (e) mycotic infections.

In our opinion, only those lesions less than 2 cm in diameter occurring in clinically stable patients can be managed non-surgically. If they are diagnosed in patients with a demonstrated infectious process and an identified causative organism, antibiotic treatment should be instituted or a microbiologic specimen taken from the original source. If no other infectious process is identified, basic investigation including urine analysis, body CT scan and an ENT examination should be performed, and when an etiologic diagnosis is not established following MRI and systemic studies, surgical aspiration and sampling is indicated.

Subdural empyema represents a neurosurgical emergency, as sudden and catastrophic neurological deterioration may occur, and once it has been diagnosed urgent evacuation should be performed.

Because of the anatomical peculiarities stated above epidural abscesses are less risky than their subdural counterparts. In fact the resistant duramater tightly adhered to inner table of the skull difficult spreading of infection and consequently decreases the risk for sudden neurological deterioration. In any case, the usually large volume of the collection along with the presence of bone erosion and fragments and the possibility of treating the underlying paracranial infection render surgery the most appropriate treatment.

SURGERY

The need for interdisciplinary and cooperative management of patients with pyogenic intracranial infections by neurosurgeons, neurologists, neuroradiologists and infectious diseases specialists has been progressively recognized. While the main tool in the treatment of brain abscesses are antibiotics, their correct choice and dosage, the indication for adjunctive surgical treatment, and the radiological follow-up monitoring may exceed the scope of a single specialist.

Although open surgical evacuation was the main treatment used for many years, needle aspiration has progressively substituted this technique, diminishing the aggressiveness of surgical approaches. This improved management has been possible thanks to the marriage of neuroradiological and stereotactic techniques which allow the precise puncture of these lesions through burr holes with minimal brain damage. Although it might be argued that there is a higher risk of recurrence with tapping and aspiration as compared to abscess removal, similar results have been reported with both techniques. In any case, repeated aspiration still represents a low risk procedure with the higher probability of success. Although free hand puncture and aspiration has been used, it is based on surface anatomy references, and thus subjected to spatial imprecision and higher risk of complications (multiple tracks, non rigid needle handling). In contrast, stereotactic approaches optimize the choice of the trajectory and needle positioning for pus aspiration.

Frame based stereotaxy has been the traditional method used for tapping intracranial pyogenic collections. In this case the patient is taken to the operating room where the stereotactic frame is placed with the aid of mild sedation end local anesthesia; blockade of supraorbital and occipital nerves can be performed 5 min before fixing the frame. Then the patient is moved to the CT scan/MR room for taking the integrated images showing both the lesion and frame marks. The coordinates of the target are calculated while the patient is returned to the operating room where puncture is planned through a safe trajectory avoiding eloquent areas, the ventricles and vessels. The patient is positioned either supine with the trunk slightly elevated and mild head flexion or semisitting. The frame is fixed to the operating table, the scalp is scrubbed, and the planned burr hole position marked over the skin. The coordinates are fixed in the frame and checked independently by the surgeon and an assistant. Draping the surgical field needs to allow the assemblage of the frame arch. A small longitudinal incision is made to the depth of the skull, a mastoid retractor is positioned and a burr hole is performed with an air driven craniotome. The dura is coagulated in a cross shape and then incised and coagulated to retract the small dural flaps. The arachnoid is open with diathermy coagulation and the needle is slowly advanced until reaching the target. Although the capsule can offer slight resistance in abscesses evolved to the late capsule stages, we have never found this to impede tapping. Then aspiration with a syringe is made without excessive suction until pus egress stops; thereafter slight irrigation of the abscess cavity can be performed. There is no scientific rationale for the instillation of antibiotics into the abscess cavity [7].

The introduction and development of frameless stereotactic systems has partly simplified this procedure, so we prefer to use neuronavigation. After initial diagnosis a contrast enhanced CT scan or MR is performed in adequate conditions for neuronavigation and the study is imported to the planning station where both the target and needle trajectory are calculated. In most patients we use general anesthesia for the sake of patient and surgeon comfort, although mild sedation and local anesthesia is preferably used in medically ill patients. In either case the patient's head is fixed in a Mayfield clamp, the neuronavigation system is prepared and the registration is performed. Patient's positioning is easier without the presence of the stereotactic frame, so lateral decubitus can also be used when dealing with temporal lesions. Registration is greatly aided with systems that allow face surface matching, although fiducial registration does not add significant difficulty. The rest of the procedure using a biopsy system adapted to the neuronavigation apparatus is identical to that explained above. When intraventricular rupture of the abscess does occur an external ventricular drainage can be inserted for the instillation of antibiotics.

There is still some controversy as to whether it is preferable to perform craniotomy or one/several burr-holes to drain a subdural empyema. Although good results have been reported using burr hole drainage, we prefer to perform a generous craniotomy covering as much as the affected brain surface as possible, crossing the midline when interhemispheric collections are present. Wide dural opening allows material sampling followed by drainage, debridement, and irrigation. The dura is closed when possible, without using allografts or any other foreign bodies. In cases without bone involvement this should be replaced, but craniectomy and delayed cranioplasty is preferred when bone infection is present or suspected.

In the case of epidural abscess the frequent bone involvement makes craniectomy mandatory to eliminating any osteomyelitic component. The abscess is drained and infectious debris over the dura are carefully curetted. Given that paracranial sinuses are often affected cranealization and sealing with a pericranial flap is also mandatory.

In patients with postoperative infectious complications we usually try antibiotic treatment when there are signs of cerebritis or surgical wound infection, but no collections are identified by MRI. When abscess or empyema are encountered surgical evacuation is indicated and allografts used to repair the dura or in cranioplasty, together with any devitalized tissue (bone flap, necrotic brain, etc.) should be removed because they act as a reservoir for infective organisms preventing antibiotic efficacy.

While antibiotic treatment can be directed in those cases with identified causative organisms, empirical treatment has to be instituted until cultures are available and when no germen is identified. The initial choice of antibiotics can be facilitated by patient premorbid conditions, the location of the abscess, the precipitating source of the infection (when identified) and Gram staining. Although available information is limited, Table 2 gives general treatment recommendations for covering a wide range of bacteria. The antibiotic treatment of postoperative infections should be tailored according to the pathogenic flora at each center. A high incidence in oxacillin resistant staphylococcus led us turn to vancomicyn and ceftazidine (vancomycin + meropenem for patients with long stay in the ICU because of resitant acinetobacter).

Intravenous antibiotics should be administered for 2 weeks, and then they can be switched to an oral route if a good clinico-radiological evolution has been observed and the therapy regimen allows this change. Oral antibiotics will be taken during 4 additional weeks, although longer courses are sometimes necessary (it occurs in 50% of the patients in some series) as judged depending on the evolution [2].

The use of steroids is controversial, because they can diminish bacterial clearance, antibiotic diffusion into the abscess and delay capsule formation. However, they can be beneficial in patients with marked secondary brain oedema causing intracranial hypertension or focal neurological deficits. We recommend the use of dexamethasone up to 10 mg/6 h in these instances, dosage being tapered once the patient reaches clinical stability thus avoiding the long term use of these drugs.

Seizures can present in the acute stage and occur in up to 70% of the cases when long term course of the disease is considered [5]. In light of these data some authors recommend antiepileptic prophylaxis, which we consider indicated in patients with lesions close to the cortical surface. Seizures are even more frequent in patients with subdural empyema (25–80%), in whom prophylactic treatment is mandatory [5].

HOW TO AVOID COMPLICATIONS

As the surgical technique does not carry great technical difficulty, the main way to achieve good results relays upon an appropriate overall management. Macewen stated that "One might almost conclude that in uncomplicated abscesses of the brain operated on at a fairly early period, recovery ought to be the rule" [1]. Certainly, and apart from the baseline patient characteristics, a good neurological status is the main prognostic factor and surgery, when indicated, should not be deferred based solely on clinical stability.

Although mortality rate in patients with intracranial pyogenic collections was reported to be as high as 50–70% in the past, it ranges from 2 to 10% in recent series [2].

CONCLUSIONS

Purulent intracranial infections can pose an important diagnostic problem when signs and symptoms are non specific, so a high index of suspicion needs to be kept in mind, mainly in patients with immunodepression, a past history of otic, dental or nasosinusal pathologies, bacteriemic conditions or surgical or traumatic antecedents.

Surgical treatment is a fundamental tool in the management of brain abscesses as it permits to identify the microoganism, relieve mass effect, decrease the risk of complications and fasten clinico-radiological improvement. Surgical treatment of the primary focus (e.g. an otic infection) when present is essential. Some small abscesses with known causative organisms can be managed with antibiotics alone.

Surgical empyema represents a surgical emergency, so craniotomy and evacuation are mandatory as soon as it is diagnosed.

Epidural abscesses need to be evacuated to eradicate the infection. Treatment of the primary infection can also be performed in the same intervention in most cases.

Pyogenic infections following neurosurgical procedures need surgery when there exits a purulent collection. In these cases surgical removal of foreign bodies and wound debridement offers a faster and safer recovery.

References

[1] Canale DJ (1996) William Macewen and the treatment of brain abscesses: revisited after one hundred years. J Neurosurg 84: 133-142

[2] Carpenter J, Stapleton S, Holliman R (2007) Retrospective analysis of 49 cases of brain abscess and review of the literature. Eur J Clin Microbiol Infect Dis 26: 1-11

[3] Farrell CJ, Hoh BL, Pisculli ML, Henson JW, Barker FG, Curry WT Jr (2008) Limitations of diffusion-weighted imaging in the diagnosis of postoperative infections. Neurosurgery 62: 577-583

[4] Mathisen GE, Johnson JP (1997) Brain abscess. Clin Infect Dis 25: 763-779

[5] Osborn MK, Steinberg JP (2007) Subdural empyema and other suppurative complications of paranasal sinusitis. Lancet Infect Dis 7: 62-67

[6] Wagner C, Sauermann R, Joukhadar C (2006) Principles of antibiotic penetration into abscess fluid. Pharmacology 78: 1-10

[7] Working Party of the British Society for Antimicrobial Chemotherapy (2000) The rational use of antibiotics in the treatment of brain abscess. Br J Neurosurg 14: 525-530

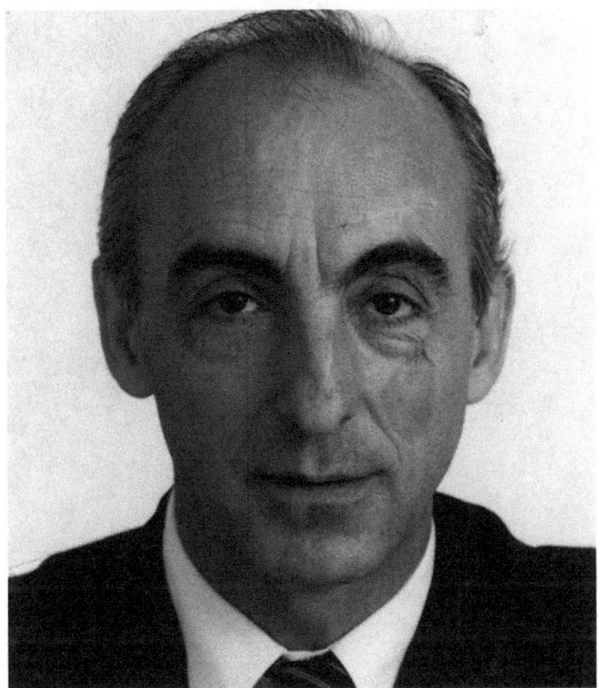

Ramiro D. Lobato

Ramiro D. Lobato is Chief of the Neurosurgical Service at Hospital "12 de Octubre" and Professor of Neurosurgery and Vicedean of the Faculty of Medicine at the Universidad Complutense, Madrid. The areas of special interest in his neurosurgical work have been craniocerebral trauma, primary intracranial hemorrhage (vascular malformations and vasospasm following aneurismal SAH) and hydrocephalus. Currently his main interest is focussed on cranial base surgery. He has ruled the Editorial Committee of the Spanish neurosurgical journal Neurocirugia and has published over 300 papers in national and international journals.

At the present time he is involved in academic activity at both undergraduate and postgraduate levels paying especial attention to the reform of undergraduate curriculum at the Universidad Complutense in Madrid.

Contact: Ramiro D. Lobato, Service of Neurosurgery, Hospital "12 de Octubre",
Avda Cordoba Km 6, 28041 Madrid, Spain
E-mail: rdiez.hdoc@salud.madrid.org

PARASITOSES OF THE CENTRAL NERVOUS SYSTEM: HYDATIDOSIS

B. ABDENNEBI

INTRODUCTION

Parasitic zoonoses, transmittable from animals to humans, remain a serious and significant public health problem in developing countries [1, 13]. Twenty-five percent of the world's population could be suffering parasitic infestation. Among these parasitoses, neurocysticercosis, infection of the central nervous system by Taenia solium metacestodes, is the commonest encountered cerebral parasitic infection in the world. It is the first cause of epileptic seizures in developing countries. The other zoonosis with a world-wide distribution is the hydatid disease which will be the topic of this chapter.

Hydatid is a word derived from the Greek "ydatos" which means water. Hydatid disease is a parasitic infestation caused by a dog tapeworm larvae of Echinococcus granulosus, a helminth belonging to the cestod group.

It is common in sheep farming in underdeveloped countries such as those located in Asia, Africa, South and Central America or in the mediterranean area. "It follows the sheep as his shadow". On the opposite, it is unusual in developed countries. Nevertheless, this notion should be attenuated by the movements of humans, especially migratory flows. Liver and lung, as big filters of the portal system, are the most infested organs, whereas involvement of brain, 2–3% of all body localisations, and spine, less than 1%, are rare. However, these spinal hydatid cysts (SHC) represent around 50% of the bone localisations.

Indeed, in Antiquity, according to Galen, Hippocrates (4th century AD) has evoked the disease and taught his students: "when liver is distended with water, it breaks in the epiploon, so the abdomen is full of water and the sick dies". Arateus, Galen (first and 2nd century AD, respectively), Al Rhazes (860–932 AD) and Avicenna (980–1037) reported also on human involvement by hydatidosis. John Hunter in 1773 described the morphological picture and Goeze in 1782 the microscopic picture of the cyst. The first description of vertebral echinococcosis was by Chaussier in 1807 [5]. Reydellet is believed to have performed the first surgical intervention for spinal hydatidosis in 1819. Virchow, for the first time in 1855, established the helminthic nature of alveolar cysts. The life cycle of the parasite was first described in 1862. In 1890, Graham and Clubb were the first neurosurgeons to perform removal of a brain hydatid cyst. Since the last century, it is usual to associate the following names with improvement of the surgical procedures of brain hydatid cyst:

Keywords: parasitoses, hydatidosis, hydatid cyst, brain, spine

Dowling [7], Da Gamma Imaginario and Goinard, Descuns [9]. More recently Arana-Iniguez [2] perfected the procedure giving birth to an unbroken cyst by irrigating saline isotonic solution between cyst wall and brain.

RATIONALE

The Echinococcus granulosus cycle requires two hosts: one intermediate, usually sheep, camel or swine, and the other final hosts represented by dog or fox. Dogs are infected by ingesting faeces or butchering infected animals containing cysts which develop into cestode, an adult tapeworm in their small intestine. Eggs included in some parts of the bowels pass out through faeces and contaminate pasture. When ingested by the sheep, the scolex or eggs become immediately infective by releasing larvae which cross the intestine wall. Then they are carried through the portal system to liver, where they develop into hydatid cysts. Occasionally humans can take the place of sheep as accidental intermediate hosts through contact with infected dogs or by oral ingestion of garden vegetables infected by the eggs of the parasite.

If the daughter cyst crosses the hepatic filter; then it is spread through the bloodstream to other organs, i.e. lungs, and less frequently to brain. Usually, the infestation goes up the systemic circulation to the parietal lobe via the middle cerebral artery as in all embolic diseases. Brain hydatid cysts (BHC) are spherical, or balloon-shaped, and are characterized by slow growth. At diagnosis, their size varies from few centimetres to huge volume of 15 cm or more (Fig. 1). Ventricles, brainstem and orbit are other exceptional localisations. The solitary aspect of the BHC is the most observed (85%), remaining cases are multilocular or multiple. Growth rate is slow and controversial, ranging between 1 and 10 cm per year. Rarely, BHC can be calcified, expression of their degeneration and death.

On the other hand, spinal involvement is possible, owing to direct portovertebral venous shunts. SHC is smaller either due to its growth inside the vertebra body or inside the spinal canal, being wedged by ligaments and disc. The thoracic spine is the most affected followed by the lumbar spine. Braithwaite and Lees [4] classified this spinal cord compression into five types: (1) primary intramedullary hydatid cyst; (2) intradural extramedullary hydatid cyst; (3) extradural intraspinal hydatid cyst; (4) hydatid disease of the vertebrae and (5) paravertebral hydatid disease. Involvement of the vertebra and extradural localisations are common. Although the supply is more favorable anteriorly, posterior arch involvement is most frequent. Contrary to the involvement of the spine, the skull is exceptionally affected, whereas the infection of the brain parenchyma is more frequent. Calcified SHC has never been reported.

Histologically, three membranes constitute the cyst wall (Fig. 1). From the outside:

- The external membrane or host derived adventitia is not easily defined in all cases.

- A thick acellular laminated layer, rich in amino carbohydrates, explains the Periodic Acid Schiff positivity. This nonnucleated membrane of parasitic origin surrounds also the daughter cysts.
- The inner germinal layer, composed of an alignment of nuclei which are cells of the parasite.

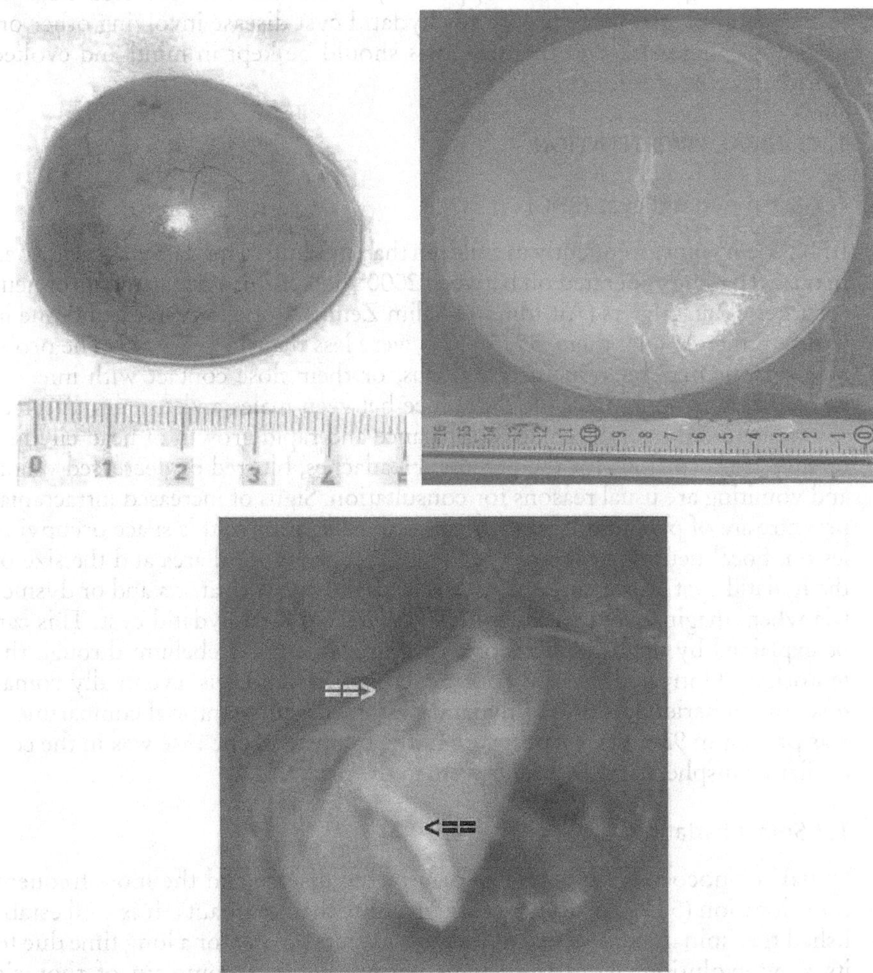

Fig. 1. *Top left*: Overall view showing the macroscopic aspect of the hydatid cyst covered with the host derived adventitia. *Top right*: Translucent cyst of 15 cm in diameter. We can distinguish many scolices and daughter vesicles arranged in bunch of grapes inside the cyst. *Bottom*: Gross pathology of the membranes of the open cyst demonstrating the adventitia externally (white arrow) and the thick acellular laminated layer intimately adherent to the inner germinal layer (black arrow)

The lumens of the cysts are filled with fluid, hydatid sand, daughter vesicles arranged in bunch of grapes, and protoscolices that have the capability to grow into adult worms if consumed by a definitive host.

DECISION-MAKING

Patients living in endemic areas, possibly in contact with infected dogs or those who had previous surgery for hydatid cyst disease involving other organs are at high risk and the diagnosis should be kept in mind and evoked before imaging studies.

1. CLINICAL PRESENTATION

1.1 Brain hydatid cyst (BHC)

BHC occurs more frequently in children than in adults. This data was confirmed in our 99 patients operated on between 2000 and 2007 in 4 departments of neurosurgery: 2 in Algiers (Ait Idir and Salim Zemirli), one in Annaba and one in Constantine. Among them, 59 (59.5%) were less than 15 years old. The probable reasons may be a ductus arteriosus, or their close contact with infected dogs. There is no appreciable difference between males and females affected: sex-ratio 46/53. In children, loss of balance and rapid growth of head circumference are suspicious for the parents. Headaches, blurred or decreased vision and vomiting are usual reasons for consultation. Signs of increased intracranial pressure are of paramount importance in the diagnosis of this space occupying lesion. Focal neurological deficit depends on the involved area and the size of the hydatid cyst. Nevertheless, some infants present with ataxia and or dysmetria when imaging features show huge parieto occipital hydatid cyst. This can be explained by the hypothesis of a pressure cone on cerebellum through the tentorium. Untreated, patient become lethargic, stuporous, eventually comatose. In our series, location of hydatid cyst in the supratentorial compartment was present in 92 cases, 4 cases were in the brainstem, one case was in the cerebellar hemisphere and two cases were in the orbit.

1.2 Spinal hydatid cyst (SHC)

Spinal echinococcosis is a severe form of the disease and the most frequent bone location (50%). It occurs more in adults than in infants. It is well established that spinal echinococcosis remains asymptomatic for a long time due to its slow evolution. After this latent period, patients complain of thoracic radicular pain symptoms. These symptoms are tolerable and not sufficient for the patient to seek medical attention. As the pain increases, it becomes resistant to medication. Compression leads to other symptoms, i.e., sensory and motor signs, in particular, hypoesthesia of the lower limbs, weakness and sphincter disturbances. The initial nerve root or spinal cord injury rapidly increases to paraplegia in few days to a few weeks. Paraplegia can sometimes occur acutely. Spinal cord compression is an emergency since it can lead to permanent paraplegia. Patient with physical examination of spinal cord compression, should undergo an adequate imaging check up and consequently an appropriate decompressive surgery as soon as possible.

2. DIAGNOSIS

2.1 BHC

Children treated for head injury may sometimes show split sutures indicative of increased intracranial pressure, leading to the incidental discovery of intracranial mass lesion. Skull X-rays can be useful, showing signs of raised intracranial pressure as suture diastasis, unilateral enlargement or erosion of the inner table of the skull, or decalcification of the posterior clinoid process in older patients. CT scan demonstrates non contrast enhancing circular hypodense lesion [8, 12]; ipsilateral ventricles can be compressed, effaced with midline shift to the controlateral hemisphere (Fig. 2). Sometimes one large cystic lesion with internal septations evocative of daughter cysts can be seen. Absence of surrounding oedema is usual. In our series, a diameter of 5–10 cm was the most frequent and was encountered in 56% of cases. In 51

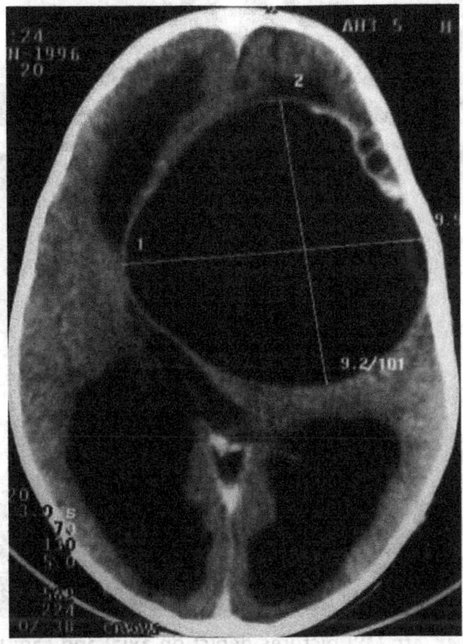

Fig. 2. CT scan reveals giant fronto temporal cystic lesion with two daughter vesicles. Note the important midline shift, the effacement of the ipsilateral frontal horn and the massive hydrocephalus

cases (51%), BHC was single and multiple in 49 patients. Due to increased intracranial pressure and worsening of the patient condition, MRI was not performed on many patients and the decision was to operate as soon as possible. MRI, axial, sagittal and coronal views, reveal spherical or egg-shaped lesions with CSF-like signal intensity both in T1 and T2 sequences: hypointense in T1 and hyperintense in T2 (Fig. 3). On T1 weighted images, the thin capsule is iso- or slightly more hypointense than the fluid content; enhancing ring lesion is observed in case of infected cyst. T2W images show a low inten-

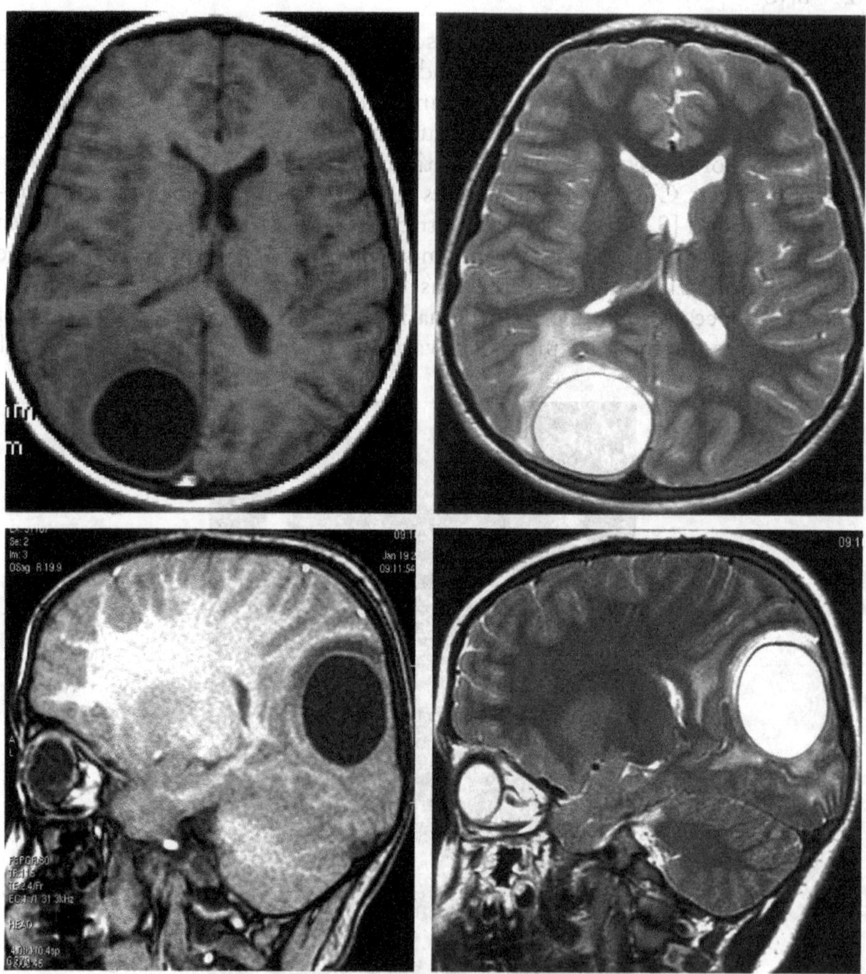

Fig. 3. *Upper and lower left*: MRI pictures depict on axial and sagittal T1-weighted images a hypointense occipital mass with no shift. *Upper and lower right*: Slices on T2-weighted images show a hyperintense occipital mass with hypointense capsule with slight surrounding oedema

sity rim which correlates to the external layer composed of fibrosis of surrounding brain tissue [11]. On the whole, image of BHC is a well recognized entity on CT scan, which is superior to MRI in depicting rare calcifications. On the other hand, MR imaging is more accurate in demonstrating the pericyst layer, which appears as a ring.

2.2 SHC

1. Antero posterior and lateral spine X-rays show multiple lytic lesions involving vertebral bodies and pedicles. It seems obvious that in the initial phase of the disease, especially in type 3, 4, and 5, the disc is spared which is explained by resistance of the anterior and posterior longitudinal ligaments.
2. Owing to its high bone resolution, CT scan demonstrates erosions of the posterior arch but also of the body of the vertebra in map shape configuration [4].
3. MRI is the best tool to illustrate spinal hydatid cysts: These lesions have a CSF-like intensity, i.e., isointense on T1 and hyperintense on T2 weighted images (Fig. 4). In intradural location SHC appears like a sausage, a date and in vertebral body as a green peas or grape bunch.

The growth of these cysts is surely limited by the osseous and ligamentous structures of the spine. Magnetic resonance imaging of the lumbar spine revealed: (a) one or numerous multiseptated cystic lesions inside the spinal canal, (b) cord compression, (c) possible intramedullary signal hyperintensity due to the pressure effect observed in case of chronic and severe compression, (d) contrast enhanced T1-weighted MR image shows thin walled cyst. Involvement of the vertebral bodies may not be obvious.

2.3 Serologic tests

The Casoni skin or intradermal test used to be the only test has now been replaced by hydatid serology which detects hydatid antibodies: hydatid immunoelectrophoresis, enzyme-linked immunosorbent assay (ELISA), latex agglutination (LA) and indirect haemagglutination (IHA) test. False results are possible. Tests can remain positive for a long time after surgery. Sensitivity varies with 4 parameters: the involved organ, intact or broken cyst, solitary or multiple cyst, and also the nature of test.

2.4 Differential diagnosis

a) BHC: it shoud be anticipated with the following, slow-growing space occupying lesion, in particular arachnoid cyst, epidermoid cyst and cystic astrocytoma. But in case of ring enhancement and perilesional oedema one should suspect brain abscess.
b) SHC: Pott disease and metastasis should be excluded.

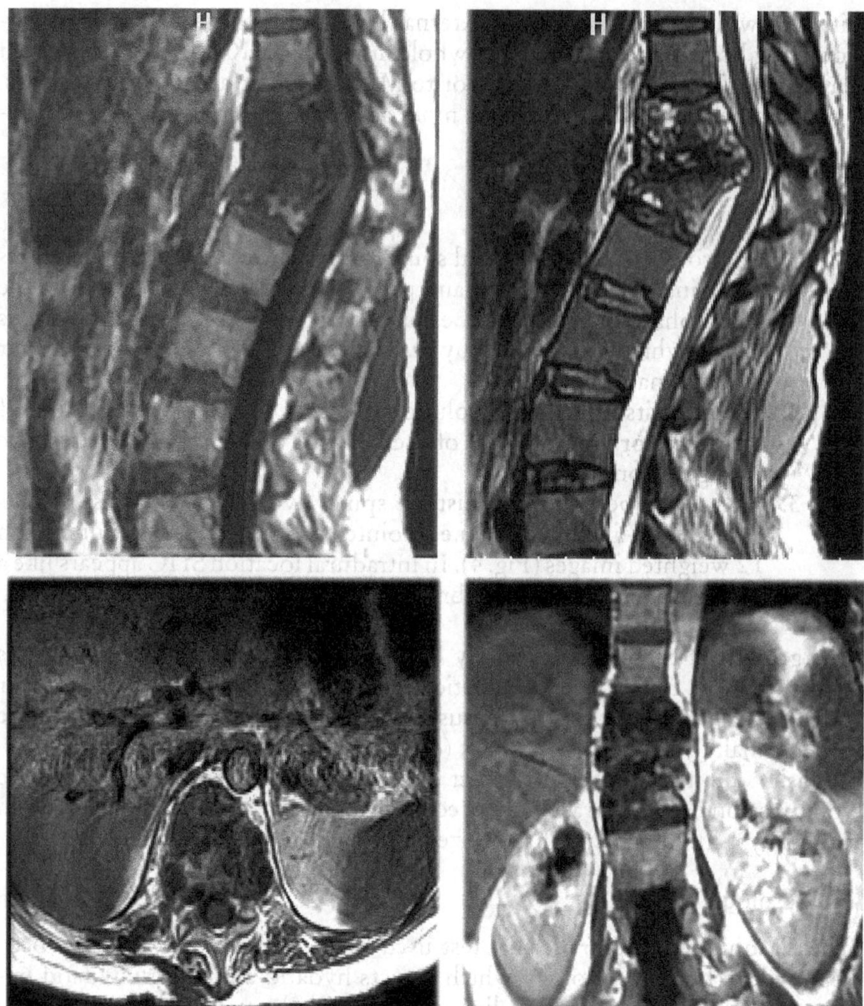

Fig. 4. *Top*: Sagittal T1 and T2 weighted images of the thoracic spine demonstrating multilocular vertebral body lesions involving T9 and T10 with CSF-like signal intensities and mass effect on the spinal cord. The CSF spaces are totally obliterated. *Bottom*: Axial T1 and coronal T2 weighted images of the same pathology described above

SURGERY

1. OPERATIVE TREATMENT

Multiple BHC is most likely secondary to locations in other organs. Hence, it is mandatory to look for the source in either the liver, lung or kidney. This will prevent unexpected complications like bronchial cyst rupture which can happen during intubation leading to hydatid vomit and spillage into the airway. Usually, this type of surgery does not require intraoperative blood transfusion.

1.1 BHC

As for most of the space occupying lesions, total surgical excision remains the only treatment. Complete removal of an unruptured cyst with preservation of adjacent brain parenchyma leads to cure. It is absolutely contraindicated to place a ventricle-peritoneal shunt prior to the removal of the unruptured cyst. The use of monopolar cautery is dangerous and has to be avoided. Operative microscope is not necessary for intracranial localisations which are removed with protective eye shield. The microscope can be used with SHC.

Surgery is performed under general anesthesia, in the supine position except when dealing with posterior fossa or occipital lesions. The head is secured in a Mayfield head rest, slightly elevated and rotated to the controlateral side of the lesion. Scalp is shaved around the involved area.

The following principles should be respected:

1. The size of the bone flap is key to a successful extirpation. This should allow maximum space for maneuvering the cyst expulsion (Fig. 5).
2. The greatest care must be taken in performing this flap. The inner table of the skull may be eroded and thin in close proximity of the cyst. The surgeon should be extremely careful when performing the burr holes. Hand drill and Gigli saw are more advisable than pneumatic drill. The free bone flap is removed.
3. Dura is tense. Meningeal vessels must be coagulated. Dural opening is meticulous, since it may be in close proximity or adherent to the cyst. This dural flap is reflected and held by sutures.
4. The brain surface, under pressure, has lost its gyri and sulci (Fig. 5). The cyst may be visible. Usually a limited corticectomy is sufficient and performed precisely above the lesion. Finding the cyst wall is crucial. Gentle dissection of the cyst from the surrounding brain tissue is performed by spatula, cottonoid and saline irrigation. Soaked cotton patties are placed in the dissected plane between the brain surface and the cyst wall in leafs of daisy (Fig. 5). The brain parenchyma should be respected. For other locations, the approach will be similar to that practised in case of tumor.
5. Huge cysts are more translucent than smaller ones. Attention is focused on preserving the integrity of the cyst. Its intra-operative accidental rupture is devastating and leads first to dissemination and consequently to recurrences because each protoscolex released may grow and become a new cyst, second, anaphylactic shock may occur.

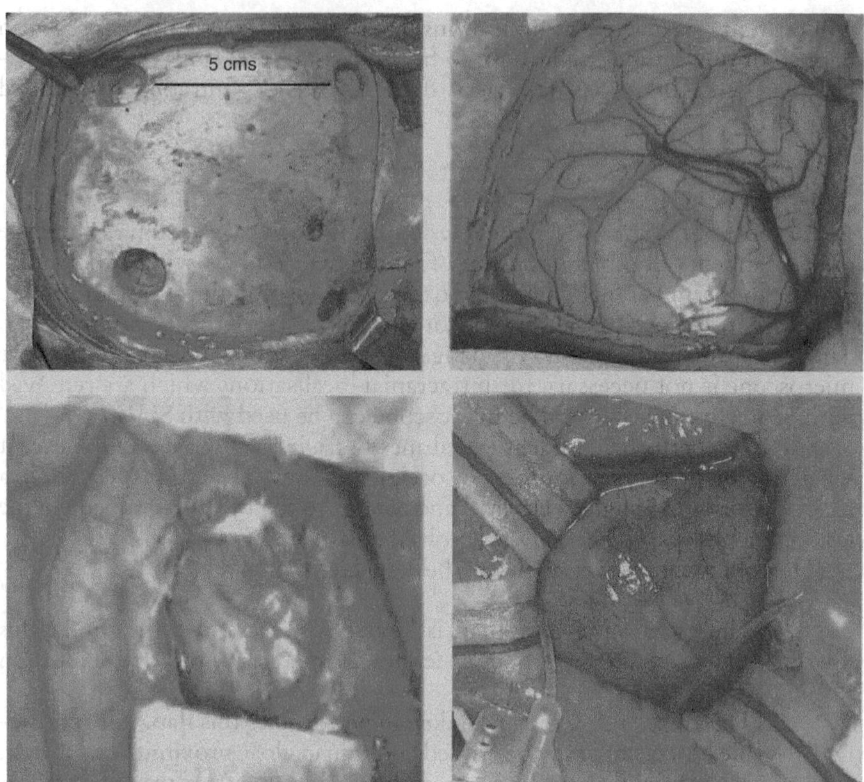

Fig. 5. Intraoperative photographs of the occipital hydatid cyst. *Upper left*: Position of burr holes: The bone flap is cut reaching the margins of sagittal and transverse sinuses. *Upper right*: In the lower right corner, the brain appears yellowish and less vascularized. *Lower left*: Corticectomy shows the cyst. *Lower right*: Dissection and hydropulsion of the hydatid cyst underway

6. Expulsion of the cyst is practised according to Dowling–Orlando technique [7] described in 1924, improved by Arana-Iniguez [2] based on water dissection. This technique is facilitated by the rarity of adherences between the cyst wall and the brain surface. It is necessary to pass two catheters laterally and then under the cyst. This step must be undertaken with extreme care. Then, isotonic solution is injected under pressure by two syringes, to facilitate the cyst expulsion without rupture outside the operative field. The cyst can break and rupture. Its content should be immediately sucked and the cyst wall removed.
7. Hydrogen peroxide soaked cottonoids are placed inside the operative field for two minutes. Then, we irrigate with hypertonic saline solution for five minutes to kill any remaining eggs or larvae before

closing. Some authors advocate the use of 10% formaldehyde solution or cetrimide. Some deep seated cysts can be unrecognized and lead to recurrences.

8. At the end, inspect the cavity looking for small cysts, fill the cavity with isotonic saline solution in order to prevent pneumatocele or translation of the brain. Complete haemostasis is ensured.
9. Ensure watertight dural closure. The bone flap is repositioned. The wound is closed in the usual multilayered fashion
10. Atypical aspects according to:

    a) Clinical status: In case of intracranial high pressure and eventually loss of consciousness, puncture aspiration of the cyst, easy to perform, is the adequate procedure realized in 16 patients (16%) of our series.
    b) Numerous cysts:

        - In the same hemisphere: Extirpation through one approach of all cysts whenever possible
        - In both hemispheres: a staged removal is considered. The procedure is first performed on the most symptomatic cyst.

1.2 SHC

The goal of surgery is to decompress the spinal cord and nerve roots by removing hydatid cysts. To avoid mistakes, particularly in dorsal spine, the affected vertebra level is marked on the skin over the spinous process with metallic marker for preoperative X-rays. The procedure is performed under general anesthesia, in prone position with the head lower than the lower limbs so that the cerebrospinal fluid (CSF) loss from the intracranial compartment is minimized.

Laminectomy is the most appropriate approach. However, through this route, it is impossible to reach the vertebral body without cervical or thoracic spinal cord injury. Hence, it is necessary at times to perform a posterolateral approach, i.e., a costo-transversectomy at the thoracic level.

A single level laminectomy provides sufficient exposure in case of one intradural cyst. In most instances, a multilevel laminectomy is necessary. After a midline longitudinal skin and aponeurosis incision centered over the targeted spinal level, bilateral subperiosteal dissection and retraction of paraspinal muscles is realized. Spinous process and interspinous ligaments are undercut and the laminae are exposed.

Two possibilities:

1. *Vertebral body or spinal extradural HC*: Using Kerrison rongeurs, ligamentum flavum is removed piecemeal and the affected lamina is taken. Involved bone is of poor quality, usually friable. This laminectomy is started at the lower level in a rostro-caudal direction. The extension of surgery may

need to include posterior structures, i.e., lateral masses, facets or extend as lateral as the transverse processes. To disturb the adjacent facet joints in the thoracic spine is without consequences for spine stability. Contrarily, stabilization may be required for cervical or lumbar spine lesions.

Devices such as curettes and suction are indispensable for removing intraosseous cysts. Multiple pearly and translucent cysts of different size are observed. Operative microscope is useful. The real difficulty is how to totally extirpate the cysts, which may count in tens or more with a size of pin-head to chick-pea. Unfortunately, some cysts are ruptured by the suction tip or other tools. Severe spinal cord compression may be observed. It is well understood that complete removal of all cysts is illusive and their dissemination possible. For this, hydrogen peroxide sopped cottons are placed in the operative field for 2 minutes, after which the surgical area is irrigated with hypertonic saline solution.

Accidental durotomy in case of extradural compression is a serious complication and should be avoided.

Wide laminectomy with removal of the posterior or anterior parts of the vertebra can destabilize the spine and lead to kyphosis and or scoliosis. To preserve spinal stability, bone fusion with posterior or anterior instrumentation is useful and could be performed on the same day [3]. Fascia and skin are closed in layers.

Despite immediate and significant postoperative improvement of the neurological symptoms, surgery of spinal echinococcosis is deceptive. Recurrences remain the major worry of the neurosurgeon due to small daughter cysts that are left behind, despite microsurgical technique.

2. *Intradural localisation.* Here, the lamina is healthy, bone resection should be carefully adapted to size of the intradural cyst. Dura is opened and held to paravertebral muscles. Once the dural edges are retracted, hydatid cysts of different sizes are seen. Spinal cord compression and distortion may be visible. Cotton strips are rostrally and caudally slipped in subarachnoid spaces delineating the pathology. The cyst walls are dissected away from the spinal cord. Contrary to BHC, there is no adventitia around the cyst. Posteriorly located lesions are easier to remove than those anteriorly placed. If needed, division of the dentate ligament or posterior root is justified.

Following decompression, the spinal cord is now free of any tension.

In case of intradural location with normal vertebra, complete removal of cysts is feasible. The operative bed is filled with hydrogen peroxide soaked patties for a few minutes and then washed with hypertonic saline solution.

Closure is carried out in multiple layers.

2. MEDICAL TREATMENT

1. Is there a successful antiparasitic chemotherapy for hydatidosis of the central nervous system? The answer remains controversial. Neurosur-

geons agree on the possible benefit of albendazole, a broad-spectrum oral antihelminthic drug, used in cases of multiple BHC or SHC. For the majority of cases, a postoperative course is sufficient, whereas in others pre- and postoperative albendazole may be considered. The dosage is 400 mg twice a day for 4 weeks in 4 cycles separated by 2 weeks free of drugs.

2. Patients with preoperative seizures require long-term antiepileptic therapy.
3. Last but not least is an adequate rehabilitation, crucial for a successful management.

3. LONG-TERM RESULTS

According to our series and current literature [1, 6, 10], patients who undergo BHC or SHC surgery show immediate resolution of their symptoms in the postoperative follow-up. This affirmation excludes blindness, seizures or flaccid paraplegia. This appreciable improvement of neurological signs is detected in 80% of patients. Reexpansion of the brain is usually complete within few days. Sometimes it is difficult to distinguish on postoperative MRI or CT scan residual cyst from postoperative changes, hence the need to base evaluation and outcome on the clinical presentation rather than the imaging findings.

In BHC, long-term recurrences occur in 10–20% of cases, 12% in our series, and are more observed when cyst is multiple or ruptured preoperatively. In SHC, earlier clinical deterioration and recurrence within 2 years are the rule and happen in 40–100% of cases, particularly in the types 4 and 5 of Braithwaite and Lees classification.

HOW TO AVOID COMPLICATIONS

Cyst rupture during dural opening or cyst dissection is redoubtable, providing ground for surinfection and what is more for recurrences. Hydrogen peroxide and hypertonic saline solution should be within hand-reach and used immediately. Anaphylactic shock can be observed when intraoperative spillage occurs. Antihistamines, hydrocortisone, crystalloids, adrenalin and high flow oxygen are administered according to the importance of the allergic reaction. Early postoperative complications include hematomas of the operative bed as well as epidural hematomas. Some of these may require repeated surgery if indicated by the neurological deterioration and the imaging findings.

This is avoided by ensuring of a perfect arterial and venous haemostasis of the operative field. Other complications are subcutaneous CSF collections, or leak which may be treated by repeated punctures or lumbar drainage.

In case of SHC, deep venous thrombosis are avoided with preventive measures such as intermittent calf pressure devices and if needed mild anticoagulation therapy.

Meningitis or abscess can occur. Postoperative spondilodiscitis can be observed in spinal surgery.

Kyphosis and other spinal deformities may be prevented by bone fusion. We deplore 5 deaths (5%). This concords with current literature.

CONCLUSIONS

In summary, the most important requirement for a successful surgery is the extirpation of an intact cyst which remains technically feasible. Nevertheless, this lesion may recur, even after this meticulous surgery. Total recovery in case of BHC is possible and should be the rule. Concerning SHC, prognosis is bleak, better in intradural involvement where cure is possible. In case of vertebral body involvement, poor results are observed despite aggressive therapy. This is due to the difficulty to remove all the cysts without rupture, which explains the high rate of recurrences recquiring several operations. This has been called "cancer blanc" or white malignancy by Dévé in 1948. Death may happen in a paraplegic patient due to complications of decubitus, mentioned above.

Like other parasitoses, regression of the disease is based on prophylaxis which includes improvement of sanitary services, elimination of carriers, i.e. dog, fox, and forbidding clandestine slaughtering of sheeps. This needs the collaboration between physicians, veterinarians and in particular full cooperation of the appropriate authorities. Public education includes preventive measures that break the infestation cycle and the hand–mouth contamination with the Echinococcus granulosus: meticulous hand washing before meals; fruits, vegetables and in particular salad cleaning prior to their consumption.

Due to globalisation, it is well understood that parasitoses of CNS are not a disease of the south hemisphere only but became a world-wide illness.

References

[1] Abada M, Galli L, Bousallah A, Lehmann G (1977) Kyste hydatique du cerveau, à propos de 100 cas. Neurochirurgie 23: 195-204

[2] Arana-Iniguez R (1978) Echinococcus. Infection of the nervous system. In: Vinken PJ, Bruy GW (eds) Infections of the nervous system, part III. Handbook of clinical neurology, vol 35. Elsevier/North Holland Biomedical Press, Amsterdam, pp 175-208

[3] Bozbuga M, Celikoglu E, Boran B (2005) Hydatid cyst of the craniocervical junction: case report. Neurosurgery 57(1): 193

[4] Braithwaite PA, Lees RF (1981) Vertebral hydatid disease. Radiological assessment. Radiology 140: 763-766

[5] Chaussier (1807) Un cas de paralysie des membres inferieurs. J Med Chir Pharmacol 14: 231-237

[6] Ciurea AV, Fountas KN, Coman TC, et al. (2006) Long-term surgical outcome in patients with intracranial hydatid cyst. Acta Neurochir (Wien) 148: 421-426

[7] Dowling E, Orlando R (1929) Quist hidatico del lobulo frontal derecho. Rev Espec Assoc Med Argent 4: 209-217

[8] Draouat S, Filali N, Abdenabi B, et al. (1986) Apport de la scanographie dans la pathologie hydatique cérébrale de l'enfant. J Radiol 67: 179-184

[9] Goinard P, Descuns P (1952) Les kystes hydatiques du nevraxe. Rev Neurol 86: 369-415

[10] Onal C, Unal F, Barlas O, et al. (2001) Long-term follow-up and results of thirty pediatric intracranial hydatid cysts: half a century of experience in the Department of Neurosurgery of the School of Medicine at the University of Istanbul (1952–2001). Pediatr Neurosurg 35: 72-81

[11] Ravalji M, Kumar S, Shah AK, et al. (2006) CT and MRI features of the typical and atypical intracranial hydatid cysts: report of five cases. Neuroradiology 16(4): 727-732

[12] Rudwan MA, Khaffaji S (1988) CT of cerebral hydatid disease. Neuroradiology 30: 496-499

[13] Vuitton DA (1997) The WHO Informal Working Group on Echinococcosis. Coordinating Board of the WHO-IWGE. Parassitologia 39: 349-353

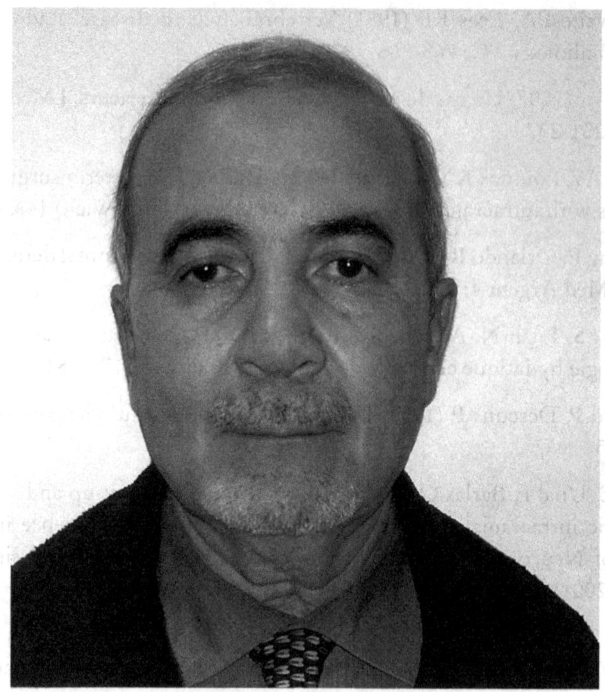

Benaissa Abdennebi

Benaissa Abdennebi is head of the Department of Neurosurgery at Salim Zemirli Hospital in Algiers. Medical degree: University of Algiers, 1975. Neurosurgical residency: University of Algiers Medical Centers, 1975–1979. Fellowships: Hopital Neurologique de Lyon (France) – Prof. M. Sindou, 1983–1984; Kantonspital Zurich (Switzerland) – Prof. J. Siegfried, 1984–1985. President of the Algerian Training Committee of Neurosurgery, 1989–1994. Member of the Editorial Board of the Panarab Journal of Neurosurgery and the African Journal of Neurosciences. Reviewer: Acta Neurochirurgica, Journal of Pediatric Neurology. Member of the French Speaking Society of Neurosurgery (SNCLF), 1986–present; president elect of the Panarab Neurosurgical Society in 2008; member of the Panarab Society of Neurosurgery (PAANS), 1997–present; member of the Stereotactic and Functional Neurosurgical Committee of the WFNS, 1999–2002 and 2005–present.

Contact: Benaissa Abdennebi, Department of Neurosurgery, Salim Zemirli Hospital, University of Algiers, Route de Baraki, Algiers, Algeria
E-mail: babdennebi@yahoo.fr

PARASITOSES OF THE CENTRAL NERVOUS SYSTEM: CYSTICERCOSIS

P. P. DIAZ VASQUEZ

INTRODUCTION

Cysticercosis is a parasitic infection that results from ingestion of eggs from the adult tapeworm, *Taenia solium*. When cysticercosis involves the central nervous system, it is called neurocysticercosis (NCC). Historically, neurocysticercosis was endemic to only Latin America, Asia, and Africa, although it has become increasingly frequent in the United States since the 1980s. It is the most common parasitic infection of the central nervous system (CNS) [7].

RATIONALE

1. LIFE CYCLE

Taenia solium, also called the pork tapeworm, is a cyclophyllid cestode in the family Taeniidae. It lives in the small intestine, adhered by the scolex (head). The scolex is provided with a rostellum, four suckers and a double-crown with 30 hooks. It can reach up to 5 m in length, and its scolex is followed by a neck and proglotids that content a ramified uterus filled with ova.

Humans are the only natural definitive hosts for the *Taenia solium*, which are aquired by the ingestion of undercooked or raw meat (most commonly pork) infested by larvae [9]. These larvae or cysticerci evaginate their scolex which adheres to the intestine and form proglotids, that develop into the adult form of the tapeworm. The proglotids eliminated along with feces free their eggs on the ground where they are ingested by the animals that will become the intermediate hosts. Humans may become accidental intermediate hosts by the ingestion of the parasite's ova, with development of cysticerci within organs. Cysticerci may be found in almost any tissue (Fig. 1). The most frequently reported locations are skin, skeletal muscle, heart, eye, and most importantly, the CNS.

2. PATHOLOGY

Cysticerci are vesicles consisting of two main parts, the vesicular wall and the scolex. The scolex has a similar structure to the adult *T. solium*, including a

Keywords: parasitoses, cysticercosis, brain, spine

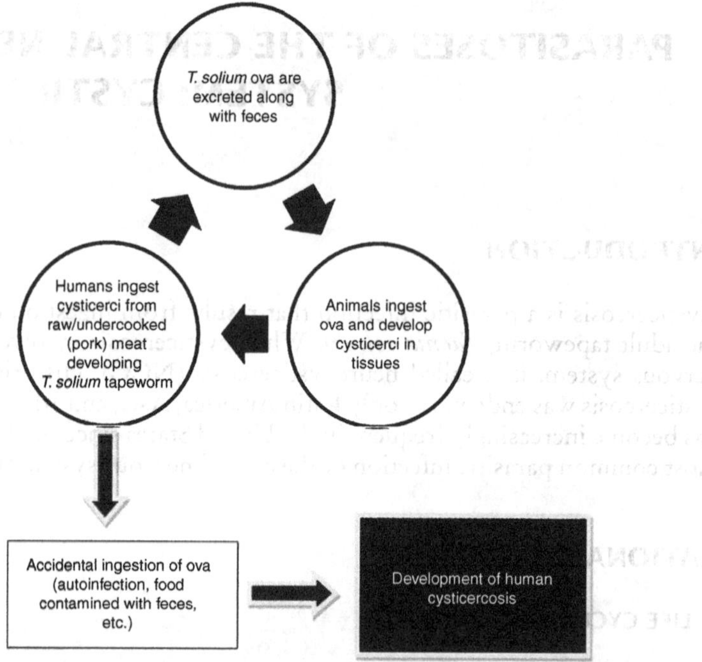

Fig. 1. Diagram of *T. solium* life cycle

rostellum armed with suckers and hooks. In the CNS, cysticerci may lodge in the brain parenchyma (most frequently), subarachnoid space, ventricular system (most commonly the 4th ventricle), or spinal cord. Once the oncosphere has passed into the parenchyma, it grows and evolves through vesicular, colloidal, nodular-granular, and calcified stages. After entering the nervous system, cysticerci elicit a scarce inflammatory reaction in the surrounding tissues. In this stage parasites have a clear vesicular fluid and a normal scolex (vesicular stage). Cysticerci may remain viable for years or, as the result of a complex immunological attack from the host, enter into a process of degeneration that ends with its death. The first stage of involution of cysticerci is the colloidal stage, in which the vesicular fluid becomes turbid and the scolex shows signs of degeneration. Colloidal cysticerci are surrounded by a thick collagen capsule, and the surrounding brain parenchyma shows astrocytic gliosis and diffuse edema. Thereafter, the wall of the cyst thickens and the scolex is transformed into coarse mineralized granules; this is called the nodular-granular stage. Finally, in the calcified stage, the parasite remnants appear as a mineralized nodule. When parasites enter into the granular and calcified stages, the edema subsides but astrocytic changes in the vicinity of the lesions become more intense than in the preceding stages.

Meningeal cysticerci elicit intense inflammation in the subarachnoid space with formation of a dense exudate composed of collagen fibers, lymphocytes, multinucleated giant cells, and hyalinized parasitic membranes, leading to abnormal leptomeningeal thickening. The optic chiasm and cranial nerves are encased in this exudate. The foramina of Luschka and Magendie may be occluded by the thickened leptomeninges with the subsequent development of hydrocephalus. Small penetrating arteries arising from the circle of Willis are also affected by this inflammatory reaction; this may cause occlusion of the lumen of the vessels and cerebral infarctions. Ventricular cysts also elicit an inflammatory reaction if they are attached to the choroid plexus or the ventricular wall. The ependymal lining is disrupted and ependymal cells are replaced by subependymal glial cells that protrude toward the ventricular cavities and block the transit of CSF, particularly when the site of protrusion is at the foramina of Monro or the cerebral aqueduct (most commonly the racemose form).

3. CLINICAL MANIFESTATIONS

Clinical manifestations of NCC depend primarily on the number and location of cysticerci and the host's immune response to infection. Involvement of brain parenchyma is common and leads to the most frequent presentation of seizures (70–90% of acutely symptomatic patients) or headache [4]. Headache usually indicates the presence of hydrocephalus, meningitis, or increased intracranial pressure. Extraparenchymal ventricular and subarachnoid cysts are also found. These carry a worse prognosis and often lead to obstructing hydrocephalus requiring surgical intervention. Fourth ventricle cysts can create a subacute hydrocephalus via a valve-and-ball mechanism. However, head movement can suddenly increase the intracranial pressure (Brun's syndrome). Cysticerci within the basilar cisterns or Sylvian fissures may enlarge to 10–15 cm in diameter. Those within the cisterns may also cause serious vasculitis and stroke. The mortality rate of patients with hydrocephalus or increased intracranial pressure is higher than the mortality rate of patients with seizures. Patients with intrasellar cysticerci present with ophthalmological and endocrinologic disturbances similar to those produced by pituitary tumors. Spinal NCC is rare. It may present with root pain or motor and sensory deficits that vary according to the level of the lesion.

4. IMAGING STUDIES

Due to the poor sensitivity of MRI for the detection of calcifications, CT remains the best screening neuroimaging procedure for patients with suspected neurocysticercosis, and MRI is the imaging modality of choice for the evaluation of patients with intraventricular cysticercosis, brainstem cysts and small cysts located over the convexity of cerebral hemispheres. MRI is also superior to CT in the follow-up of the patients after therapy.

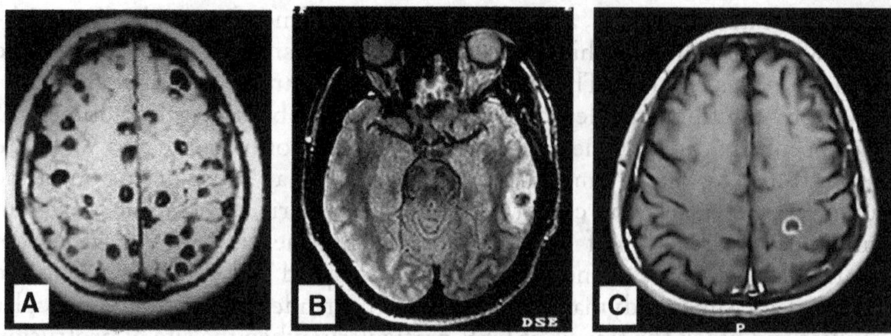

Fig. 2. Neurocysticercosis in its different stages of evolution. **A** Multiple viable cysts (vesicular stage). **B** Granular stage with abundant perilesional edema. **C** Single granular lesion with scarce edema

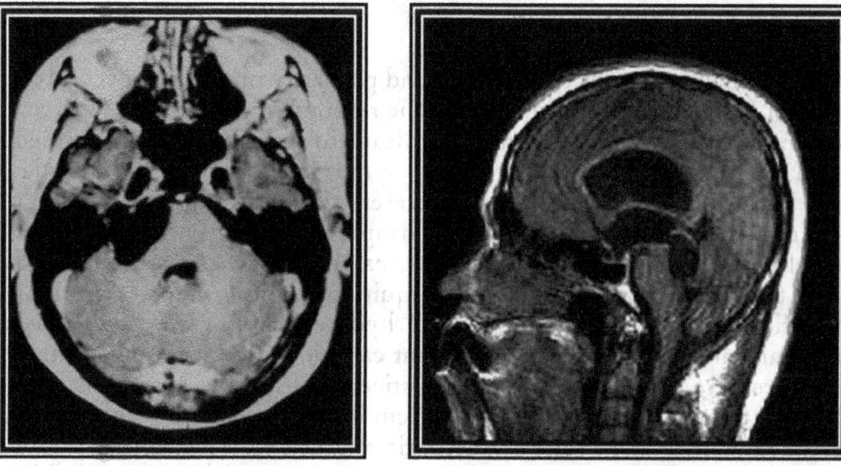

Fig. 3. *Left*: Vesicular cyst in posterior fossa. *Right*: Obstructive hydrocephalus secondary to aqueductal cysticercosis

CT and MRI findings in parenchymal neurocysticercosis depend on the stage of development of the parasites (Fig. 2). Vesicular (living) cysticerci appear on CT as small and rounded low-density areas without perilesional edema or enhancement after contrast medium administration (Fig. 3). On MRI, vesicular cysts appear with signal properties similar to those of CSF in both, T1 and T2-weighted images. The scolex is usually visualized within the cyst as a high intensity nodule giving the lesion a pathognomonic "hole-with-dot" imaging. Sometimes, these parasites are so numerous that the brain resembles a "swiss cheese". On MRI, the wall of the colloidal cysticerci becomes thick and hypointense and there is marked perilesional edema, better visualized on T2-weighted images. Granular cysticerci appear on CT as nodular hyperdense lesions surrounded by edema after contrast administration. On MRI,

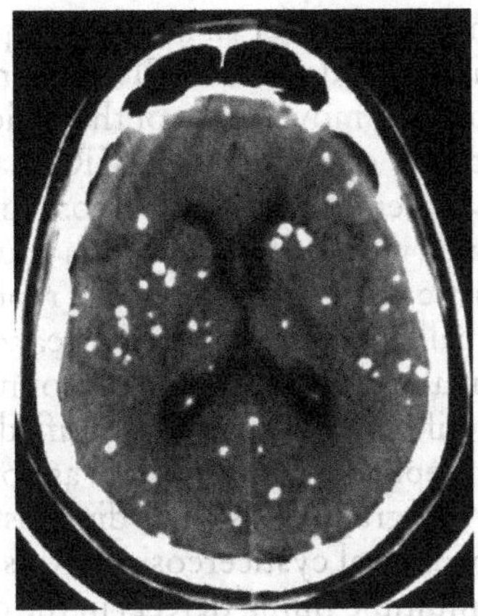

Fig. 4. Multiple calcificated cysts

granular cysticerci are visualized as areas of signal void on both T1 and T2-weighted images surrounded by edema or gliosis with hyperintense rims around the area of signal void. Calcified (dead) cysticerci normally appear on CT as small hyperdense nodules without perilesional edema or abnormal enhancement after contrast medium administration (Fig. 4).

Hydrocephalus, caused by inflammatory occlusion of the foramina of Luschka and Magendie, is the most common neuroimaging finding in patients with subarachnoid neurocysticercosis (Fig. 3). Acute hypertensive hydrocephalus is associated with periventricular lucencies representing interstitial edema due to transependymal migration of CSF. In contrast, chronic and relatively normotensive forms of hydrocephalus are not associated with this CT pattern. The fibrous arachnoiditis that is responsible for the development of hydrocephalus is seen on CT or MRI as areas of abnormal leptomeningeal enhancement at the base of the brain after contrast medium administration. Ischemic cerebrovascular complications of subarachnoid neurocysticercosis are well visualized with CT or MRI but these are nonspecific.

Ventricular cysticerci appear on CT as hypodense lesions that distort the ventricular system causing asymmetric or obstructive hydrocephalus. The administration of positive intraventricular contrast medium allows precise localization of intraventricular cysticerci by CT. The administration of contrast medium is usually performed by transcutaneous puncture of the antechamber of a ventricular shunt or through a ventriculostomy tube. Positive contrast medium may also be administered through a lumbar puncture; however, this procedure should be conducted cautiously since intracranial pressure may induce the development of brain herniation in patients with hydrocephalus or intraventricular masses. Most ventricular cysts are readily visualized on MRI. In some cases, the ventricular cyst is only visualized in the proton density sequence or with FLAIR techniques, where they appear barely hyperintense with regard to the CSF. Cyst mobility within the ventricular cavities in response to movements of the patient's head, the "ventricular migration sign", is better observed with MRI than with CT. This finding facilitates the diagnosis of ventricular cysticercosis in some patients.

On MRI, intramedullary cysticerci appear as rounded or septated lesions that may have an eccentric hyperintense nodule representing the scolex. The periphery of the cyst usually enhances due to a breakdown of the blood-spinal barrier in the parenchyma of the spinal cord surrounding the cyst. The spinal cord is seen enlarged and if the scolex is not identified it is difficult to differentiate this condition from ependymomas, cystic astrocytomas, or primary syringomyelic cavities. Myelography is still of diagnostic value in patients with suspected spinal leptomeningeal cysticercosis. In this form of the disease, myelograms usually show multiple filling defects in the column of contrast material corresponding to the cysts. Leptomeningeal cysts may be freely mobile within the spinal subarachnoid space and may change their position during the exam according to movements of the patient in the exploration table.

DECISION-MAKING

1. DIAGNOSTIC CRITERIA

Del Brutto et al. provided diagnostic criteria for neurocysticercosis based on objective clinical, imaging, immunologic, and epidemiologic data [6]. These include four categories of criteria stratified on the basis of their diagnostic strength, including the following:

1.1 Absolute

- Histologic demonstration of the parasite from biopsy of a brain or spinal cord lesion.
- Cystic lesions showing the scolex on CT or MRI.
- Direct visualization of subretinal parasites by funduscopic examination.

1.2 Major

- Lesions highly suggestive of neurocysticercosis on neuroimaging studies.
- Positive serum enzyme-linked immunoelectrodiffusion transfer blot (EITB) for the detection of anticysticercal antibodies.
- Resolution of intracranial cystic lesions after therapy with albendazole or praziquantel.
- Spontaneous resolution of small single enhancing lesions.

1.3 Minor

- Lesions compatible with neurocysticercosis on neuroimaging studies.
- Clinical manifestations suggestive of neurocysticercosis.
- Positive CSF enzyme-linked immunosorbent assay (ELISA) for detection of anticysticercal antibodies or cysticercal antigens.
- Cysticercosis outside the CNS.

1.4 Epidemiologic

- Evidence of a household contact with *Taenia solium* infection.
- Individuals coming from or living in an area where cysticercosis is endemic.
- History of frequent travel to disease-endemic areas.

Interpretation of these criteria permits two degrees of diagnostic certainty:

1.5 Definitive diagnosis

- One absolute criterion, or
- Two major plus one minor and one epidemiologic criterion.

1.6 Probable diagnosis

- One major plus two minor criteria, or
- One major plus one minor and one epidemiologic criterion, or
- Three minor plus one epidemiologic criterion.

2. IMMUNOBLOT

The Western blot for cysticercosis or the EITB, which uses lentil lectin purified glycoprotein (LLGP) antigens extracted from the metacestode of *T. solium*, has been the "gold standard" serodiagnostic assay since it was first described in 1989. It gives close to 100% specificity and a sensitivity varying from 70 to 90%. This high sensitivity decreases when the number of cysticerci is low. The EITB is more efficient using serum instead of cerebrospinal fluid (CSF).

3. ELISA

ELISA, when used in serum, has 65% of sensitivity and 63% specificity. Sensitivity is higher with CSF. In developing countries ELISA is preferred because of its better availability, simplicity and lower cost compared to EITB. When used for detecting cysticerci antigens in CSF, ELISA gives close to 85% sensitivity and 100% specificity, with the advantage of identifying the active forms of the larvae.

I personally recommend to perform stereotactic biopsies when a doubtful single lesion shows no radiographic improvement with clinical treatment, even with a positive serology, because of the high incidence of gliomas (Fig. 5).

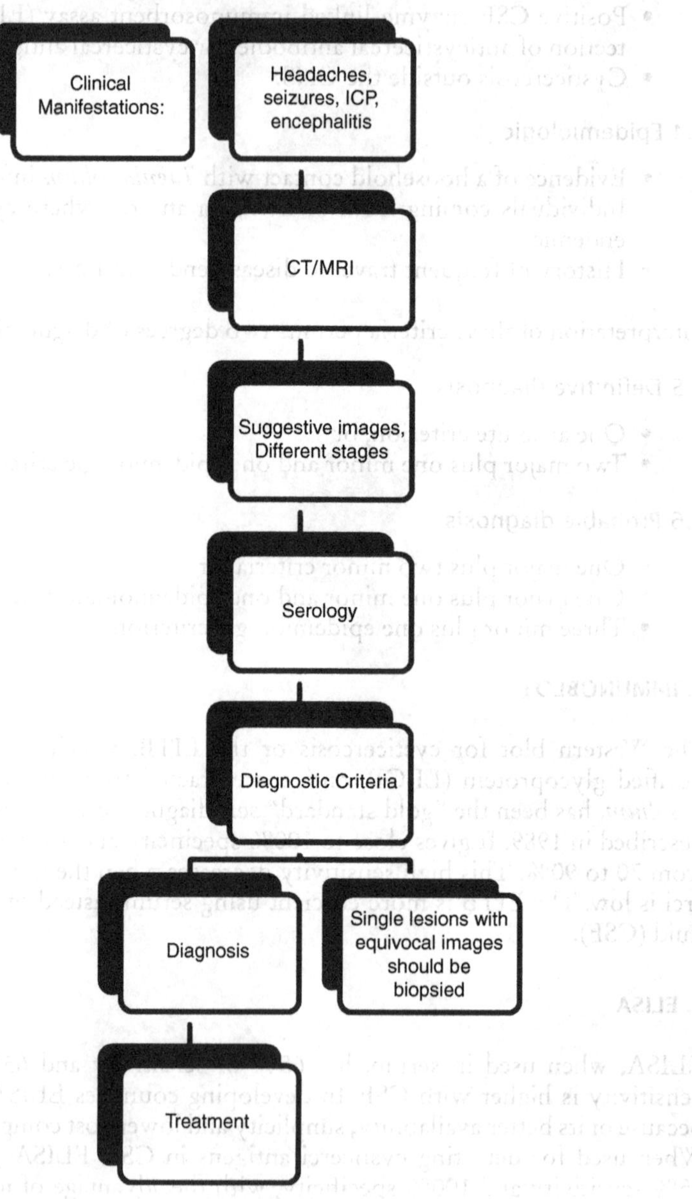

Fig. 5. Diagnostic approach to neurocysticercosis

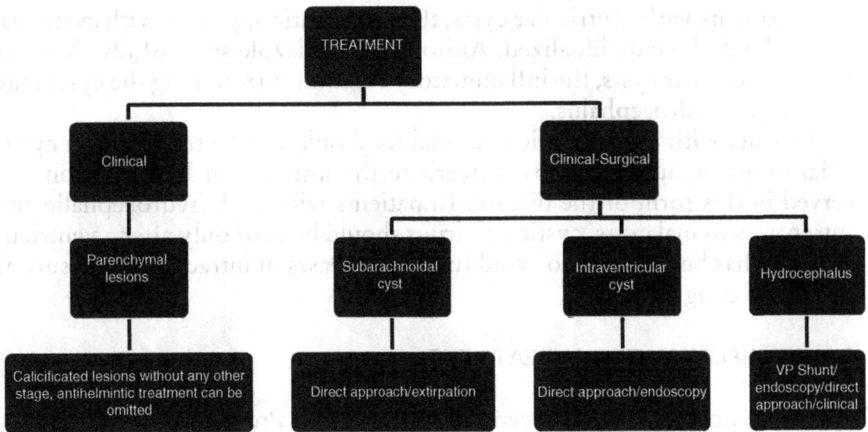

Fig. 6. Decision-making for the treatment of neurocystercosis

TREATMENT

Cysts' number, location, stage and the hosts immune response are to take into consideration for a proper and individualized treatment that usually includes a combination of symptomatic drugs, cysticidal drugs, surgical resection of lesions, and placement of ventricular shunts (Fig. 6).

1. ANTIHELMINTICS

For intraparenchymal NCC with viable cysts, albendazole (ABZ) (15 mg/kg/ day orally for seven days or longer) is associated with destruction of most cysts, and a decrease in seizures of at least 45% (higher in seizures with generalization). Praziquantel (PZQ) can be used orally in a single-day regimen of three doses of 25 mg/kg given at two-hour intervals, or the standard 15-day regimen of 50–100 mg/kg/day [3]. PZQ has a slightly lower cysticidal efficacy than ABZ. Steroids decrease serum levels of PZQ. Serum levels of phenytoin and carbamazepine may also be lowered as the result of simultaneous praziquantel administration [11].

Patients with single enhancing lesions may not need specific therapy as most of these lesions disappear spontaneously. Dead, calcified cysts do not need to be treated with anti-parasitic drugs. Steroids can shorten the duration of the edema but they might not affect the frequency of subsequent edema episodes.

For subarachnoid cysticercosis treatment with albendazole for 4 weeks is recommended, sometimes requiring more than one course. Cysticidal drugs must be used with caution in patients with giant subarachnoid cysts because the host's inflammatory reaction in response to the destruction of parasites may occlude leptomeningeal vessels surrounding the cyst.

In patients with ventricular cysts, the therapeutic approach with cysticidal drugs should be individualized. Although albendazole successfully destroys many ventricular cysts, the inflammatory reaction surrounding the cysts may cause acute hydrocephalus.

Patients with cysticercotic encephalitis should not be treated with cysticidal drugs because this may exacerbate the intracranial hypertension observed in this form of the disease. In patients with both hydrocephalic and intraparenchymal cysts, cysticidal drugs should be used only after a ventricular shunt has been placed to avoid further increases of intracranial pressure as a result of drug therapy.

2. ANTI-INFLAMMATORY TREATMENT

Dexamethasone in doses between 4.5 and 12 mg/day. Prednisone at 1 mg/kg/day may replace dexamethasone when long-term steroid therapy is required [5].

Corticosteroids are the primary form of therapy for cysticercotic encephalitis, angiitis, and arachnoiditis causing progressive entrapment of cranial nerves. In such cases, up to 32 mg per day of dexamethasone may be needed for control of symptoms. In patients with cysticercotic encephalitis, corticosteroids may be used in association with mannitol at doses of 2 mg/kg per day [2].

Simultaneous administration of corticosteroids and cysticidal drugs ameliorate the secondary effects of headache and vomiting that may occur during cysticidal drug therapy. Headache and vomiting are not due to toxic effects of the drugs but rather to the destruction of parasites within the brain and are reliable indicators of drug efficacy. In patients with giant subarachnoid cysticerci, ventricular cysts, spinal cysts, and multiple parenchymal brain cysts, corticosteroids must be administered before, during, and even some days after the course of cysticidal drugs to avoid cerebral infarction, acute hydrocephalus, spinal cord swelling, and massive brain edema, respectively.

3. SURGICAL TREATMENT

The main problem in ventricular shunt placement is the high prevalence of shunt dysfunction; indeed, it is common for patients with hydrocephalus secondary to neurocysticercosis to have two or three shunt revisions [8]. Maintenance steroid therapy and antihelmintic drugs may decrease the frequency of shunt blockages [10]. Neuroendoscopy can be used for resection of intraventricular cysts, with much less morbidity than with open surgery.

3.1 Surgical treatment basis

Surgical treatment of NCC is an option when clinical treatment is not effective. Surgery should be the first choice of treatment in the presence of increased intracranial pressure secondary to giant cysts causing mass effect and hydrocephalus due to CSF circulation blockage.

The modality of the treatment is chosen according to the localization of cysticerci. The most common procedures are ventriculo-peritoneal shunting for treating hydrocephalus and neuroendoscopy for both cyst resection and extraction and management of hydrocephalus [1]. For those cysts localized in the 3rd and 4th ventricles, surgery is targeted to resection and extraction of the lesions, and resolution of the intracranial hypertension secondary to the hydrocephalus, all at the same time (Figs. 7–9). For cysts localized in the lateral ventricles, neuroendoscopic resection can be performed simultaneously with a ventriculocysternotomy for treating hydrocephalus.

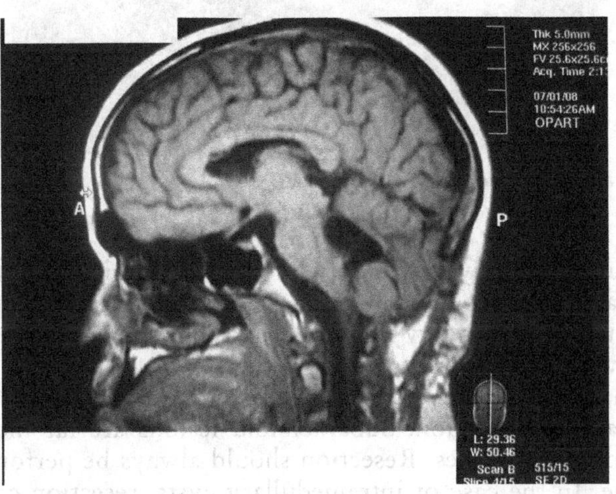

Fig. 7. Residual cysts in 4th ventricule, after surgery

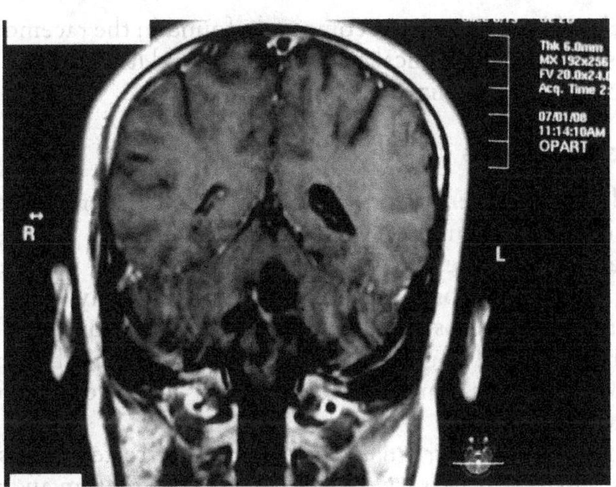

Fig. 8. Residual cysts after surgery in 4th ventricle

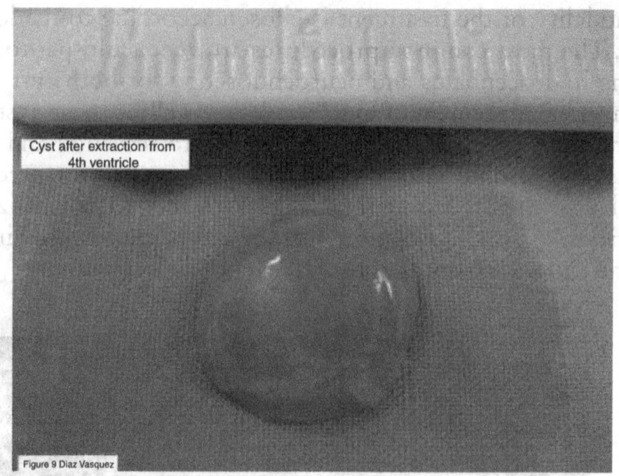

Fig. 9. Cyst after extraction from 4th ventricle

Intraparenchymal cysts will only be managed surgically, in the setting of severe intracranial hypertension.

Pseudotumors secondary to giant subarachnoid cysts, must be managed surgically whenever clinical treatment fails.

In spinal cord involvement, surgery is always mandatory in presence of medullary compression. Subarachnoid lesions are far more common than the intramedullaries. Resection should always be performed using a microscope. In the case of intramedullary cysts, resection constitutes an exceptional diagnosis without the evidence of a concomitant intracranial lesion.

Subarachnoid cysts are most commonly found in the racemous form. Surgery is considered when clinical treatment fails, and it consists in the resection under microscope of localized lesions.

3.2 Surgical techniques

The installation of a ventriculo-peritoneal shunt is performed in a classic manner, with the implantation of a mid-pressure valve, taking into consideration the side of the lesion. For the abdominal time, we prefer the transumbilical approach for aesthetic purposes, mainly in children and young women. We choose ventriculocysternostomy over shunting whenever possible. Shunt dysfunction due to obstruction of the catheter is one of the most common complications, which leads to a revision for its reinstallation.

Free-floating intraventricular cysts should be treated endoscopically. In many cases it may be necessary passing through the septum and performing a ventriculocysternostomy in the same intervention.

For cysts in the 4th ventricle, we choose a suboccipital classic approach, paying special attention to microsurgery, and a thorough irrigation with normal saline.

Lesions in the lateral ventricles are assessed through a frontal trepanus with the introduction of the neuroendoscope. The site and angle of entrance will vary depending on the number of vesicles. Sometimes it can be necessary an additional entry point in order to perform a simultaneous ventriculo-cysternoscopy. Septum pellucidum fenestration is a common procedure and carries no major consequences. The cyst may accidentally rupture without leading to complications.

In some subarachnoid cysts, stereotactic localization is needed: (1) giant cysts causing mass effect, (2) encephalitis secondary to cerebral edema (exceptionally).

CONCLUSIONS

Neurocysticercosis is a parasitic infection that has become worldwide due to its easy spread through travelers. It has multiple forms of presentation like epilepsy, syndrome of intracranial hypertension, and hydrocephaly. Intraparenchymal neurocysticercosis has a favorable course and responds well to clinical treatment. Subarachnoid and intraventricular cysts have a greater morbi-mortality, since these can grow to the development of intracraneal hypertension with mass effect. Hydrocephaly secondary to CSF obstruction and arachnoiditis require decompression surgery. A large number of patients treated with ventriculo-peritoneal shunts, need reintervention to release obstruction. The vast majority of patiens need anticonvulsive therapy. True disease control is only achieved by avoiding transmission, with proper sanitary measures.

References

[1] Bergsneider M (1999) Endoscopic removal of cysticercal cysts within the fourth ventricle. J Neurosurg 91: 340-345

[2] Carpio A, Santillan F, Leon P, Flores C, Hauser WA (1995) Is the course of neurocysticercosis modified by treatment with antihelminthic agents? Arch Intern Med 155: 1982-1988

[3] Cruz M, Cruz I, Horton J (1991) Albendazole versus praziquantel in the treatment of cerebral cysticercosis: clinical evaluation. Trans R Soc Trop Med Hyg 85: 244-247

[4] Del Brutto OH, Santibanez R, Noboa CA, Aguirre R, Diaz E, Alarcon TA (1992) Epilepsy due to neurocysticercosis: analysis of 203 patients. Neurology 42: 389-392

[5] Del Brutto OH, Sotelo J, Roman GC (1993) Therapy for neurocysticercosis: a reappraisal. Clin Infect Dis 17: 730-735

[6] Del Brutto OH, Wadia NH, Dumas M, Cruz M, Tsang VC, Schantz PM (1996) Proposal of diagnostic criteria for human cysticercosis and neurocysticercosis. J Neurol Sci 142: 1-6

[7] Garcia HH, Gonzales AE, Evans CAW, Gilman RH (2003) Taenia solium cysticercosis. Lancet 362: 547-556

[8] Madrazo I, Flisser A (1992) Cysticercosis. In: Apuzzo MLJ (ed) Brain surgery: complication avoidance and management. Churchill Livingstone, New York, pp 1419-1430

[9] Roman G, Sotelo J, Del Brutto O, Flisser A, Dumas M, Wadia N, et al. (2000) A proposal to declare neurocysticercosis an international reportable disease. Bull WHO 78: 399-406

[10] Suastegui Roman RA, Soto-Hernandez JL, Sotelo J (1996) Effects of prednisone on ventriculoperitoneal shunt function in hydrocephalus secondary to cysticercosis: a preliminary study. J Neurosurg 84: 629-633

[11] Vazquez ML, Jung H, Sotelo J (1987) Plasma levels of praziquantel decrease when dexamethasone is given simultaneously. Neurology 37: 1561-1562

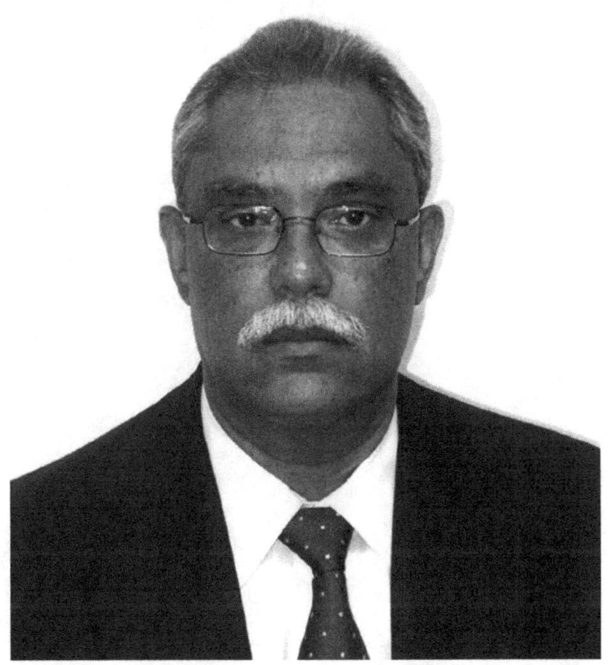

Pedro Pablo Diaz Vasquez

Pedro Pablo Diaz Vasquez is currently Professor of Neurosurgery and Neuroanatomy in the Universidad Autonoma de Santo Domingo and works as an adult and pediatric neurosurgeon in the Universidad Central del Este Medical Center, Santo Domingo.

He is president, founder and director of the French Hospital of Santo Domingo Foundation (Fundacion Hospital Frances de Santo Domingo), a non-profit, non-governmental institution dedicated specially to neurosciences. He was decorated as "Meritorious Gentleman" by the French Government.

He graduated as doctor in medicine from the Universidad Autonoma de Santo Domingo (Autonomous University of Santo Domingo). He completed his subspecialty training in neurosurgery, neuroradiology, anatomy of the central nervous system, microsurgery and fundamental and clinical neuropsychopharmacology at the University of Aix Marseille II, Marseille, France.

He was the President of the Dominican Society of Neurology and Neurosurgery and also President of the International Congress of Neurosurgery, Santo Domingo 1997 and of the 57th Congres de Neurochirurgie de Langue Francaise, Punta Cana, 2007.

Contact: Pedro Pablo Diaz Vasquez, Fundacion Hospital Frances de Santo Domingo, Calle Duarte #359, Zona Colonial, Santo Domingo
E-mail: ppdiazvasquez@hotmail.com

CONTENTS

Volume 1: Cranial Approaches, Vascular, Traumas, Cerebrospinal Fluid, Infections

Volume 3: Spine, Functional, Peripheral Nerves, Education

9783211848197